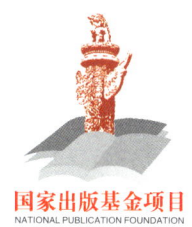

National Key Book Publishing Planning Project of the 13th Five-Year Plan

"十三五"国家重点图书出版规划项目

International Clinical Medicine Series Based on the Belt and Road Initiative

"一带一路"背景下国际化临床医学丛书

Regional Anatomy

局部解剖学

Chief Editor　Zhang Yanru

主编　张雁儒

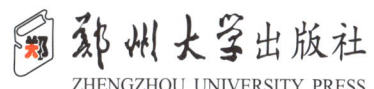

图书在版编目(CIP)数据

局部解剖学 = Regional Anatomy：英文 / 张雁儒主编. — 郑州：郑州大学出版社，2020.12

("一带一路"背景下国际化临床医学丛书)

ISBN 978-7-5645-5996-0

Ⅰ.①局… Ⅱ.①张… Ⅲ.①局部解剖学-英文 Ⅳ.①R323

中国版本图书馆 CIP 数据核字(2019)第 006066 号

局部解剖学 = Regional Anatomy：英文

项目负责人	孙保营 杨秦予	策划编辑	孙保营
责任编辑	刘 莉	装帧设计	苏永生
责任校对	陈文静	责任监制	凌 青 李瑞卿
出版发行	郑州大学出版社有限公司	地 址	郑州市大学路40号(450052)
出版人	孙保营	网 址	http://www.zzup.cn
经 销	全国新华书店	发行电话	0371-66966070
印 刷	河南文华印务有限公司		
开 本	850 mm×1 168 mm 1/16		
印 张	31.5	字 数	1 214 千字
版 次	2020 年 12 月第 1 版	印 次	2020 年 12 月第 1 次印刷
书 号	ISBN 978-7-5645-5996-0	定 价	153.00 元

本书如有印装质量问题，请与本社联系调换。

Staff of Expert Steering Committee

Chairmen

Zhong Shizhen   Li Sijin   Lü Chuanzhu

Vice Chairmen

Bai Yuting	Chen Xu	Cui Wen	Huang Gang	Huang Yuanhua
Jiang Zhisheng	Li Yumin	Liu Zhangsuo	Luo Baojun	Lü Yi
Tang Shiying				

Committee Member

An Dongping	Bai Xiaochun	Cao Shanying	Chen Jun	Chen Yijiu
Chen Zhesheng	Chen Zhihong	Chen Zhiqiao	Ding Yueming	Du Hua
Duan Zhongping	Guan Chengnong	Huang Xufeng	Jian Jie	Jiang Yaochuan
Jiao Xiaomin	Li Cairui	Li Guoxin	Li Guoming	Li Jiabin
Li Ling	Li Zhijie	Liu Hongmin	Liu Huifan	Liu Kangdong
Song Weiqun	Tang Chunzhi	Wang Huamin	Wang Huixin	Wang Jiahong
Wang Jiangang	Wang Wenjun	Wang Yuan	Wei Jia	Wen Xiaojun
Wu Jun	Wu Weidong	Wu Xuedong	Xie Xieju	Xue Qing
Yan Wenhai	Yan Xinming	Yang Donghua	Yu Feng	Yu Xiyong
Zhang Lirong	Zhang Mao	Zhang Ming	Zhang Yu'an	Zhang Junjian
Zhao Song	Zhao Yumin	Zheng Weiyang	Zhu Lin	

专家指导委员会

主任委员
  钟世镇 李思进 吕传柱

副主任委员（以姓氏汉语拼音为序）
  白育庭 陈 旭 崔文黄 黄 钢 黄元华 姜志胜
  李玉民 刘章锁 雒保军 吕 毅 唐世英

委 员（以姓氏汉语拼音为序）
  安东平 白晓春 曹山鹰 陈 君 陈忆九 陈哲生
  陈志宏 陈志桥 丁跃明 杜 华 段钟平 官成浓
  黄旭枫 简 洁 蒋尧传 焦小民 李才锐 李国新
  李果明 李家斌 李 玲 李志杰 刘宏民 刘会范
  刘康栋 宋为群 唐纯志 王华民 王慧欣 王家宏
  王建刚 王文军 王 渊 韦 嘉 温小军 吴 军
  吴卫东 吴学东 谢协驹 薛 青 鄢文海 闫新明
  杨冬华 余 峰 余细勇 张莉蓉 张 茂 张 明
  张玉安 章军建 赵 松 赵玉敏 郑维扬 朱 林

Staff of Editor Steering Committee

Chairmen

Cao Xuetao   Liang Guiyou   Wu Jiliang

Vice Chairmen

Chen Pingyan   Chen Yuguo   Huang Wenhua   Li Yaming   Wang Heng
Xu Zuojun   Yao Ke   Yao Libo   Yu Xuezhong   Zhao Xiaodong

Committee Member

Cao Hong	Chen Guangjie	Chen Kuisheng	Chen Xiaolan	Dong Hongmei
Du Jian	Du Ying	Fei Xiaowen	Gao Jianbo	Gao Yu
Guan Ying	Guo Xiuhua	Han Liping	Han Xingmin	He Fanggang
He Wei	Huang Yan	Huang Yong	Jiang Haishan	Jin Chengyun
Jin Qing	Jin Runming	Li Lin	Li Ling	Li Mincai
Li Naichang	Li Qiuming	Li Wei	Li Xiaodan	Li Youhui
Liang Li	Lin Jun	Liu Fen	Liu Hong	Liu Hui
Lu Jing	Lü Bin	Lü Quanjun	Ma Qingyong	Ma Wang
Mei Wuxuan	Nie Dongfeng	Peng Biwen	Peng Hongjuan	Qiu Xinguang
Song Chuanjun	Tan Dongfeng	Tu Jiancheng	Wang Lin	Wang Huijun
Wang Peng	Wang Rongfu	Wang Shusen	Wang Chongjian	Xia Chaoming
Xiao Zheman	Xie Xiaodong	Xu Falin	Xu Xia	Xu Jitian
Xue Fuzhong	Yang Aimin	Yang Xuesong	Yi Lan	Yin Kai
Yu Zujiang	Yu Hong	Yue Baohong	Zeng Qingbing	Zhang Hui
Zhang Lin	Zhang Lu	Zhang Yanru	Zhao Dong	Zhao Hongshan
Zhao Wen	Zheng Yanfang	Zhou Huaiyu	Zhu Changju	Zhu Lifang

编审委员会

主 任 委 员
　　曹雪涛　梁贵友　吴基良
副主任委员（以姓氏汉语拼音为序）
　　陈平雁　陈玉国　黄文华　李亚明　王　恒
　　徐作军　姚　克　药立波　于学忠　赵晓东
委　　　员（以姓氏汉语拼音为序）
　　曹　虹　陈广洁　陈奎生　陈晓岚　董红梅　都　建
　　杜　英　费晓雯　高剑波　高　宇　关　颖　郭秀花
　　韩丽萍　韩星敏　何方刚　何　巍　黄　艳　黄　泳
　　蒋海山　金成允　金　清　金润铭　李　琳　李　凌
　　李敏才　李迺昶　李秋明　李　薇　李晓丹　李幼辉
　　梁　莉　林　军　刘　芬　刘　红　刘　晖　路　静
　　吕　滨　吕全军　马清涌　马　望　梅武轩　聂东风
　　彭碧文　彭鸿娟　邱新光　宋传君　谈东风　涂建成
　　汪　琳　王慧君　王　鹏　王荣福　王树森　王重建
　　夏超明　肖哲曼　谢小冬　徐发林　徐　霞　许继田
　　薛付忠　杨爱民　杨雪松　易　岚　尹　凯　余祖江
　　喻　红　岳保红　曾庆冰　张　慧　张　琳　张　璐
　　张雁儒　赵　东　赵红珊　赵　文　郑燕芳　周怀瑜
　　朱长举　朱荔芳

Editorial Staff

Honorary Editor in Chief
    Zhong Shizhen
Reviewer
    Huang Wenhua   Southern Medical University
Chief Editor
    Zhang Yanru   Ningbo University
Editorial Board Member
    Chen Hao   Lanzhou University
    Chen Xi   University of South China
    Chen Yiyong   Ningbo University
    Cheng Jiamao   Dali University
    Cui Xiaojun   Guangdong Medical University
    Ke Lining   Fujian Medical University
    Lu Wei   Zhunyi Medical University
    Luo Gang   Hainan Medical University
    Meng Buliang   Yunnan University
    Meng Yanbin   Xiangnan University
    Sun Chenyou   Wenzhou Medical University
    Tan Jianguo   University of South China
    Wang Degui   Lanzhou University
    Wang Mingyan   Xiamen University
    Xian Dehai   Southwest Medical University
    Yang Lin   Zhunyi Medical University
    Zhang Bensi   Dali University
    Zhang Hongwu   Southern Medical University
    Zhu Jianhua   Dali University

作者名单

名誉主编
  钟世镇

主　审
  黄文华　　　　南方医科大学

主　编
  张雁儒　　　　宁波大学

编　委（以姓氏汉语拼音为序）
  陈　昊　　　　兰州大学
  陈　熙　　　　南华大学
  陈一勇　　　　宁波大学
  成家茂　　　　大理大学
  崔晓军　　　　广东医科大学
  柯荔柠　　　　福建医科大学
  卢　巍　　　　遵义医学院
  罗　刚　　　　海南医学院
  蒙艳斌　　　　湘南学院
  孟步亮　　　　云南大学
  孙臣友　　　　温州医科大学
  谭建国　　　　南华大学
  王德贵　　　　兰州大学
  王明炎　　　　厦门大学
  先德海　　　　西南医科大学
  杨　琳　　　　遵义医学院
  张本斯　　　　大理大学
  张洪武　　　　南方医科大学
  朱建华　　　　大理大学

Preface

At the Second Belt and Road Summit Forum on International Cooperation in 2019 and the Seventy-third World Health Assembly in 2020, General Secretary Xi Jinping stated the importance for promoting the construction of the "Belt and Road" and jointly build a community for human health. Countries and regions along the "Belt and Road" have a large number of overseas Chinese communities, and shared close geographic proximity, similarities in culture, disease profiles and medical habits. They also shared a profound mass base with ample space for cooperation and exchange in Clinical Medicine. The publication of the International Clinical Medicine series for clinical researchers, medical teachers and students in countries along the "Belt and Road" is a concrete measure to promote the exchange of Chinese and foreign medical science and technology with mutual appreciation and reciprocity.

Zhengzhou University Press coordinated more than 600 medical experts from over 160 renowned medical research institutes, medical schools and clinical hospitals across China. It produced this set of medical tools in English to serve the needs for the construction of the "Belt and Road". It comprehensively coversaspects in the theoretical framework and clinical practicesin Clinical Medicine, including basic science, multiple clinical specialities and social medicine. It reflects the latest academic and technological developments, and the international frontiers of academic advancements in Clinical Medicine. It shared with the world China's latest diagnosis and therapeutic approaches, clinical techniques, and experiences in prescription and medication. It has an important role in disseminating contemporary Chinese medical science and technology innovations, demonstrating the achievements of modern China's economic and social development, and promoting the unique charm of Chinese culture to the world.

The series is the first set of medical tools written in English by Chinese medical experts to serve the needs of the "Belt and Road" construction. It systematically and comprehensively reflects the Chinese characteristics in Clinical Medicine. Also, it presents a landmark achievement in the implementation of the "Belt and Road" initiative in promoting exchanges in medical science and technology. This series is theoretical in nature, with each volume built on the mainlines in traditional disciplines but at the same time introducing contemporary theories that guide clinical practices, diagnosis and treatment methods, echoing the latest research findings in Clinical Medicine.

As the disciplines in Clinical Medicine rapidly advances, different views on knowledge, inclusiveness, and medical ethics may arise. We hope this work will facilitate the exchange of ideas, build common ground while allowing differences, and contribute to the building of a community for human health in a broad spectrum of disciplines and research focuses.

Nick Lemoine

Foreign Academician of the Chinese Academy of Engineering
Dean, Academy of Medical Sciences of Zhengzhou University
Director, Barts Cancer Institute, London, UK
6th August, 2020

Foreword

With the rapid development of education in China's economic society and higher medical science, more and more foreign students come to China to study medicine in medical colleges and universities. Anatomy is one of the most important and basic courses in medicine, it is very important to combine the reading habits of foreign medical students in China with the teaching materials of medical colleges and universities in China, so we have organized a group of teachers from different medical schools with rich experience in anatomy teaching and foreign learning to compile this textbook, hoping to contribute to the improvement of the training quality of foreign medical students in China.

The biggest characteristic of this textbook is that it is suitable for China's teaching system and meets the requirements of the syllabus, This consistent exposure to students who are studying systemic anatomy for the first time and others who are reviewing anatomy during their residency training period helps to keep us informed of students needs and how certain body parts could be more completely or more clearly demonstrated in the atlas. In order to enhance students' interest in learning, the integration of basic and clinical knowledge is strengthened, so, more attention were paid to the clinical cases in the description of the anatomical structures.

We both encourage and welcome users of this edition to write to us for your kind comments and for offering suggestions of how this textbook might be improved.

Our appreciation also goes to academician of Zhong Shizhen and professor Huang Wenhua of Southern Medical University and Zhengzhou University Publishing House for their enthusiastic efforts and a lot of work in the contributiors to write and publish this edition.

It is a great challenge to compile this English book. If you find any errors or mistakes that might exist in the book, please let us know. We are always open to suggestions and comments, and strive to improve it for a better edition.

Authors

Contents

Introduction 1

Chapter 1   The Head 8
   1.1 Introduction 8
   1.2 The face 9
   1.3 The cranium 18
   1.4 Main contents of the head 23

Chapter 2   The Neck 97
   2.1 Introduction 97
   2.2 Superficial structures and cervical fascia 99
   2.3 Sternocleidomastoid and anterior region of the neck 102
   2.4 The lateral region of the neck 107
   2.5 Main contents of neck 108

Chapter 3   The Thorax 138
   3.1 Introduction 138
   3.2 Thoracic wall and cavity 140
   3.3 The pleura and pleural cavity 144
   3.4 The mediastinum 149
   3.5 The diaphragm 155
   3.6 Main contents of the thorax 156

Chapter 4   The Abdomen 207
   4.1 Introduction 207
   4.2 The anterolateral abdominal wall and the inguinal region ... 210
   4.3 The peritoneum and peritoneal cavity 221
   4.4 Organs in the supracolic compartment 229
   4.5 Organs in the infracolic compartment 239
   4.6 Retroperitoneal space 246
   4.7 Main contents of the abdomen 250

Chapter 5   The Pelvis and Perineum 278
   5.1 Introduction 278
   5.2 The pelvis 280
   5.3 Pelvic organs 284
   5.4 The perineum 294

  5.5 Main contents of the pelvis and perineum ··· 304

Chapter 6 The Upper Limb ··· 330
  6.1 Introduction ··· 330
  6.2 The pectoral region and axillary region ·· 332
  6.3 The anterior region of the arm, the elbow, the forearm, and the wrist ·· 340
  6.4 The posterior region of the arm, the elbow, the forearm, and the wrist ·· 351
  6.5 Main contents of the upper limb ·· 351

Chapter 7 The Lower Limb ··· 401
  7.1 Introduction ··· 401
  7.2 The front and medial aspects of the thigh ··· 402
  7.3 The gluteal region, the back of the thigh and the popliteal fossa ·· 413
  7.4 The anterior and lateral region of the leg ·· 422
  7.5 The region of the ankle and foot ·· 428
  7.6 Main contents of lower limb ·· 440

Chapter 8 The Back and Vertebral Region ·· 481
  8.1 Introduction ··· 481
  8.2 The layers and structures of the back ··· 482

References ·· 490

Introduction

The *Systemic Anatomy* presents the structures of the human body on the basis of the functional systems, so it helps us to understand how the human body is built for its functions. As a continuation of *Systemic Anatomy*, the *Regional Anatomy* presents the structures of the human body on the basis of defined local regions, rather than functional systems. In this course, the human body is divided into a number of regions, such as the head, the neck, the thorax, the abdomen, the pelvis, and the upper and lower limbs. And it describes what organs or structures exist in each of the regions and what are their three-dimensional relationships. For important organs in each region, it provides detailed information about their position, shape, size, blood supply, nerve control and lymphatic drainage. This knowledge helps you to understand if an organ is ill or injured, what will happen, how to examine it and how to treat it. In other words, the *Regional Anatomy* helps you to understand how clinical applications, such as physical examinations, instrumental examinations and surgical operations are designed and performed. Therefore, the *Regional Anatomy* is also called the "Clinical Anatomy".

Here, we take one example to explain why you need to study *Regional Anatomy*. You have learned an organ—the thyroid gland. It belongs to the endocrine system and is located in the anterior region of the neck. A common disease related with this gland is called the goiter. It is a noncancerous overgrowth of the gland caused by lack of iodine. For this disease, the enlarged thyroid gland must be removed partly. The operation is called the subtotal thyroidectomy. In the operation, we must make an incision on the skin, separate tissues in the front of the gland to expose it, and then cut and remove part of the gland. Now questions are raised: How to make an incision on the skin in the anterior region of the neck, transversely or longitudinally? How to separate the tissues in front of the gland to expose it? How to cut the gland without severe bleeding? And how to avoid injury of nearby structures such as some important nerves? It is clear, if you want to answer these questions, you must learn the detailed anatomy of the thyroid gland and its three-dimension relationship with other organs or structures in the anterior region of the neck.

It is no doubt that dissection is the best way to study anatomy. By dissecting the human body, you can learn the three-dimension relationships of human organs as they are in original positions; and you can touch very small structures, such as vessels and nerves, to feel their texture, rigidity and strength. This experience cannot be obtained just by reading the textbook or watching the video of anatomy on a computer. In addition, through the course of dissection, you can learn the dissecting techniques. This is also important, because these techniques are very similar to those used in surgical operations. For example, in your dissection course, you will learn how to hold a scalpel, a pair of forceps or scissors, and how to use them to cut tissues or separate fine structures. These techniques are the same when used in a surgical operation. Therefore, people usually say that anatomy is the background of surgery. Here, it refers not only to the knowledge, but also the techniques.

The cadaver that you will use for dissection was donated by a person who wished to make a contribution to your education as a physician. It is not possible to put into words the emotions experienced by that individual as he or she made the decision to become a body donor. It goes without saying that the value of the gift that the donor has made to you cannot be measured, and can only be repaid by the proper care and use of the cadaver. The cadaver must be treated with the same respect and dignity that are usually reserved for the living patient. So medical students should cherish and consciously respect the dead, love the cadaver. Respect and treasure the corpse are mainly manifested as operating carefully and getting the most out of it. At the same time, the cadaver should be carefully preserved and not dried or decomposed due to poor management. To this end, these should be done in the anatomy and custody of the body.

After disection, cover the cadaver with a damp cloth and plastic cloth. In anatomic class, open only the part that needs dissection and observation, and the rest is still covered. Spraying water and preservative solution regularly to keep the cadaver fresh and moist instructions, and blind cutting, damage to the body and anatomical instruments are not allowed.

Anatomical terms (for *Systemic Anatomy* only)

Before you begin to do dissection, you must first learn some special terms used in anatomy.

(1) Anatomical position

As you know, in a dissection laboratory the cadaver is lying on the dissecting table. However, to describe the human body more precisely, we must establish a standard and universally accepted position, the anatomical position. In this position, persons are described as if they were standing erect with the face forward and the feet together. The arms are by the side with the palms facing anteriorly.

(2) Direction terms

Based on the anatomical position, we can use five pairs of direction terms to describe the locations of any organs or structures in the human body. The first pair are the superior and inferior. Superior means closer to the head end of the body; and inferior, to an opposite direction, away from the head end. You should note that all the direction terms must be used with a reference. For example, if you want to describe the location of the nose, you must first choose at least one reference. If taking the eyes as the reference, the nose is inferior to the eyes. But if taking the mouth as the reference, the nose is superior to the mouth. That means with different reference, the same location has different descriptions.

The second pair of the direction terms are the anterior and posterior. Anterior means closer to or at the front of the human body, and posterior, closer to or at the back. Sometimes, we also use ventral or dorsal to express the corresponding meanings.

The third pair of the direction terms are the medial and lateral. These two terms are used with the median plane of the body as reference. The median plane is a vertical plane that passes through the center of the human body and divides it exactly into a right and a left halves. Medial means closer to the plane and lateral, away from it.

Superficial means closer to the surface of the human body, and deep, away from the surface.

The terms of proximal and distal are used when taking the origin of a structure, an organ or a part of the body as reference. Proximal means closer to the origin and distal, away from it. For example, the origin of the lower limb is the inferior end of the trunk. The thigh is closer to this origin than the leg. Therefore, the thigh is proximal to the leg.

(3) Plane terms

In addition to the direction terms, there are three standard plane terms: the sagittal, the coronal and the transverse planes. The sagittal plane refers to any longitudinal planes that divide the human body into a right and a left parts. The coronal plane refers to any vertical planes that divide the body into an anterior and a posterior parts; and the transverse plane refers to any horizontal planes that divide the body into an upper and a lower parts.

(4) Variation

In anatomy, variation refers to any structures found in some normal individuals which deviate from those observed in the majority of the population. Here, we emphasize that the individual who has variational structures is normal. This means the difference does not affect the physiological functions. If the difference affects the function, we call it distortion rather than variation. The variation is frequently observed when you dissect the human body. In fact, there is no one whose all structures exactly match the descriptions of the textbook. So if you find any variational structures during the dissection, do not become confused, and ask all others to have a look.

Dissecting techniques (for *Regional Anatomy* only)

(1) Dissecting instruments (Figure 0-1)

A pack of instruments has been prepared for your dissection course. In each pack, there are two pairs of forceps, one probe, two pairs of hemostatic forceps, one pair of scissors and two scalpels with detachable blades.

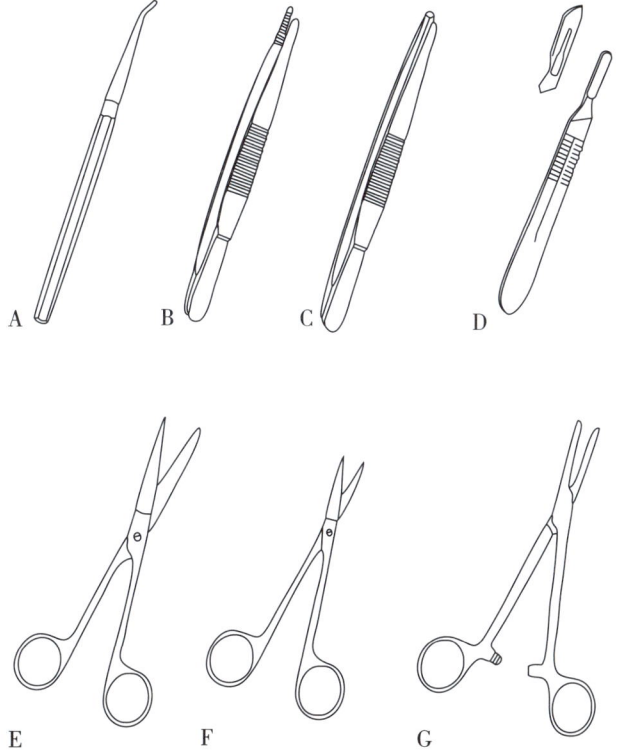

A. Probe; B. Forceps; C. Tissue (rat-toothed) forceps; D. Scalpel and removable blade; E. Large scissors; F. Small scissors; G. Hemostat.

Figure 0-1 Personal dissection instruments

Probe, the primary dissecting tool, after your fingers. A probe is designed to tear connective tissue and allow the user to feel nerves and vessels before they are damaged.

There are two kinds of forceps, one with teeth at its ends and the other without. The forceps with teeth are called toothed forceps. In surgery, the toothed forceps are used just for holding the skin. You can not use them to deal with other soft tissues, because this may cause injury of a delicate living tissue. So in dissection course, the toothed forceps are also allowed only to handle the skin.

Hemostatic forceps are used in surgery for clamping blood vessels to stop bleeding. Here, in dissection, we use them to handle structures and fix skin flaps. Please note that the hemostatic forceps should be held with your thumb and ring finger. Do not use the middle finger.

Scissors are used to cut, blunt dissection, and transection and separate soft tissue. Please note that the scissors should be also held with your thumb and ring finger. Two pairs of scissors are recommended: a large, heavy pair of dissecting scissors (about 15 cm in length) and a small pair of scissors with two sharp points for the dissection of delicate structures (Figure 0-2).

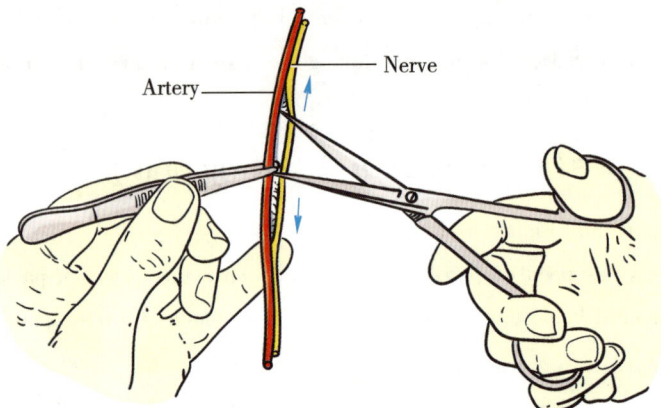

Figure 0-2 Scissors technique for separating structures
(Closed scissors are inserted between structures, then opened)

The scalpel includes a handle and a detachable blade. Before use, you must mount the blade onto the handle with hemostatic forceps. And after each round of dissection, the blade must be detached from the handle for safety reason. The scalpel is primarily used as a skinning tool. Scalpels are not recommended for general dissection, because they cut small structures without allowing you to feel them. The scalpel handle should be made of metal (not plastic). The blade should be about 3.5-4.0 cm long. The cutting edge must have some convexity near the point. A sharp blade must be used at all times, because no one can do good work with a dull scalpel. Therefore, a sufficient supply of blades will be needed.

After each anatomical operation, the disectting instruments must be scrubbed clean and kept in order to avoid loss.

(2) Dissecting terms

This dissection manual repeatedly uses a number of dissection terms. Before beginning to dissect, learn the meaning of the following.

1) Dissect—to cut apart. In the context of this dissection manual, the meaning of dissect is to tear apart. The dissection approach throughout this manual is to dissect as much as possible with the fingers, to next use a probe, and to then use scissors. A scalpel is used only as a tool of last resort for crude cuts or to dissect extremely tough connective tissues.

2) Blunt dissection—to separate structures with your fingers, a probe, or scissors by tearing (not

cutting) connective tissues.

3) Scissors technique—a method of blunt dissection in which the tips of a closed pair of scissors are inserted into connective tissue and then opened, tearing the connective tissue with the back edge of the tips. The scissors technique is an effective way to dissect vessels and nerves.

4) Sharp dissection—to dissect by use of a scalpel. Sharp dissection is discouraged and will be recommended only in rare situations.

5) Clean—to remove fat and connective tissue by means of blunt dissection (preferred) or sharp dissection.

Clean the surface of a muscle—to remove all fat and connective tissue so that the muscle fascicles become obvious and the direction of force can be understood.

Clean the border of a muscle—to define the border by using fingers or a probe to break the loose connective tissue that binds the muscle to surrounding structures.

Clean a nerve—to use a probe (or scissors technique) to tear the connective tissue around the nerve for purposes of observing its relationships and branches.

Clean a vessel—to use a probe (or scissors technique) to strip the fat and connective tissue off the surface of a vessel and its branches to illustrate its relationships.

6) Define—to use blunt dissection to enhance a structure to better illustrate its relationships. Defining a structure usually involves bluntly dissecting the loose connective tissue away from it by use of a probe.

7) Retract—to pull a structure to one side to visualize another structure that lies more deeply. Retraction is a temporary displacement and is not intended to harm the retracted structure.

8) Transect—to cut in two in the transverse plane, as in transection of a muscle belly or tendon.

9) Reflect—to fold back from a cut edge, as in folding back a transected muscle to view what is beneath it. The reflected tissue should remain attached to the specimen.

10) Strip a vein—to remove a vein and its tributaries from the dissection field so that the artery and related structures can be seen more clearly. Veins are stripped by blunt dissection using a probe.

(3) How to do your dissection efficiently?

There are two important suggestions about how to do good job in your dissection.

1) Read the related contents in your textbook before each round of practical. That means you must have got an outline of the region you want to dissect. For example, what organs and structures exist in the area, and what are their three-dimensional relationships.

2) Work step by step exactly according to the guide in the dissection and observation in your textbook.

Some other suggestions are offered.

• Prepare before the lab. Read the dissection assignment in this book and become familiar with the new vocabulary, the structures to be dissected, and the dissection approach. You must deliberately search for structures, and a small amount of advance preparation will make the exercise go more quickly.

• Use a good atlas in the dissection lab. This dissection manual provides references to five excellent atlases to help you quickly find illustrations that support the dissection.

• Palpate bony landmarks and use them in the search for soft tissue structures.

• Remove fat, connective tissue, and smaller veins to clean up the dissection.

• Review the completed dissection at the end of the dissection period and again at the start of the next dissection period. To help you do this, review exercises are included at strategic points in each chapter.

• Complete each dissection before proceeding to the next because each new dissection is an extension of the previous dissection.

▶▶ Lab safety

While in the laboratory, protect your clothing by wearing a long laboratory coat or apron. For sanitary reasons, this outer layer of clothing should not be worn outside of the dissection laboratory. Do not wear sandals or opentoed shoes in the laboratory because a dropped scalpel can seriously injure your foot. Gloves must be worn to prevent contact with human tissue and fixatives. When cutting bones, wear glasses or goggles to protect your eyes against flying chips.

(4) Commonly used techniques

There two commonly used techniques: the first is used in reflecting the skin. The skin of a dead body becomes very strong and a little hard after chemical fixation (fixation with formal dehyde). So reflecting the skin is somewhat a hard work. The most effective way to do this is stripping the skin off, rather than cutting. As shown in the figure, you can make a stab incision in the skin flap, insert a finger into it. And then pull the flap forcibly. By this way, you can see numerous white and fine collagen fibers along the interface between the skin and the underlying fatty tissues. Use the sharp edge of a blade to slightly cut the fibers while stripping the skin off.

The second technique is called blunt dissection. For separation of a nerve from a vessel, you can insert the sharp ends of scissors between the two structures, and separate them by gently spreading the scissors. You can also use a hemostatic forceps to do this, but do not use a scalpel because it may cause injury of the fine structures. We call this "insert and spread". For big organs, for example two tightly attached muscles, you can gently push and separate them with your hands. We call this second technique "push and spread". Here, it must be emphasized that, if you want to cut or remove any organ or structure, you must first separate it from the surrounding tissues by blunt dissection. This is a very important rule not only for the dissection, but also for surgical operations. Therefore, throughout the course of dissection, you must keep the rule in your mind—separate before cut.

(5) Procedure of common disection

1) Skin incision

The thickness of the skin is 1-2 mm, and the thickness of each part varies, generally the ventral side is thinner, dorsal side is thicker, in order to avoid damaging the deep structure of the skin, the palm with the knife should be in contact with the specimen when cutting, cutting the skin with a sharp point, not too deep (Figure 0-3).

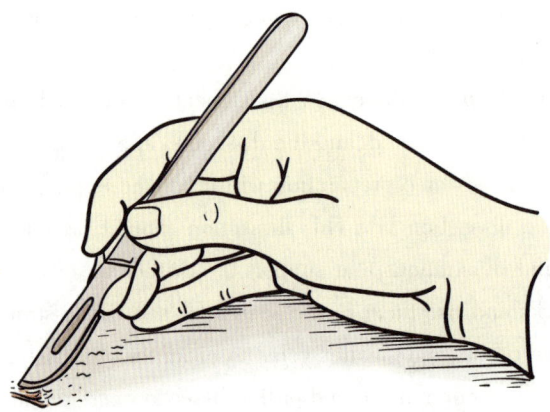

Figure 0-3　When dissecting, rest the hand to reduce unsteady movements

2) Fold the skin

With tweezers to clamp the corners of the cut flap, with a knife carefully to cut off the white fiber skin that connect the skin with the superficial fascia, so that the shallow fascia to stay in place. If you open a large piece of skin, you can first cut off a small hole in the stripped flap, insert the index finger and tighten the flap and isolate the skin and shallow fascia with scalpel. This method is more effortless than holding the flaps with tweezers.

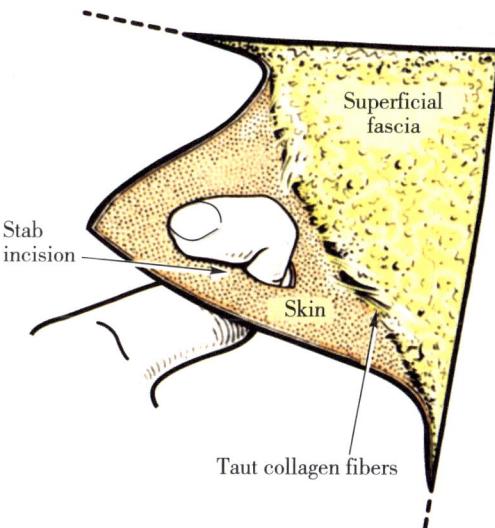

Figure 0-4 When removing skin, make a stab incision to help you apply traction

(Use the scalpel blade to cut the collagen fibers from the deep surface of the skin where the fibers are taut)

3) Stripping the superficial fascia

The superficial fascia contains fat, and its thickness varies greatly in different parts. the superficial fascia contains cutaneous nerves and blood vessels, especially many small veins. Multi-fat superficial fascia is best isolated by hand blunt, or closed blunt forceps or blunt scissors.

4) Separate and repair the muscles

Separate the loose connective tissue between the muscles with a finger or blunt probe and remove the connective tissue from the muscle surface with a knife and tweezers. Repair the edge, origin and insertion of the muscles to distinguish the direction of muscle fibers.

5) Separate and dissect vascular nerve bundles

First separate the vascular nerve bundle and the surrounding structure with the fingers or knife or blunt probe, and then use scissors to open its connective tissue sheath, with tweezers to clamp the vascular nerve bundles, with the scissors to separate the blood vessels and nerves in the bundle along the long axis of nerve tract.

Zhang Yanru

Chapter 1

The Head

1.1 Introduction

The head is the top part of the human body. Its skeleton is the skull that encloses the cranial cavity and constitutes the bony shelf of the face.

1.1.1 Boundary and division of the head

The head connects inferiorly with the neck, the boundary between them is a line linking the base of mandible, the angle of mandible, the mastoid process, and the external occipital protuberance.

The head is usually divided into two parts by a line along the upper border of the orbit, the zygomatic arch, the upper margin of the external acoustic foramen and the root of the mastoid process. The part above this line is the cranium that can be sub-divided into the calvaria, the cranial cavity and the cranial base. The boundary between the first two is a line linking with the supra-orbital margin and superior margin of external acoustic meatus. The part under the cranium is called the face.

1.1.2 Surface anatomy

In addition to a number of useful landmarks such as the upper border of the orbit, the zygomatic arch, the base and the angle of mandible, the mastoid process, and the external occipital protuberance, there are several structures that are either important clinically or the outlets for the vessels and nerves supplying the superficial structures of the head (Figure 1-1).

(1) The stylomastoid foramen is a pore on the lower surface of the cranial base, between the roots of the mastoid process and the styloid process. It is the outlet of the canal for facial nerve and from it the facial nerve emerges out.

(2) The supraorbital foramen (located on the upper margin of the orbit), the infraorbital foramen (below the lower margin of the orbit) and the mental foramen (at mid-point between the upper and lower edges of the body of the mandible) are three important outlets with the same named nerves and vessels emerging out. They are aligned along a vertical line about 2.5 cm lateral to the anterior median line.

(3) The pterion is an H-shaped suture on the lateral surface of the skull, formed by junction of the

frontal bone, the parietal bone, the temporal bone and the greater wing of sphenoid bone. It is the thinnest place of the calvaria with the anterior branch of the middle meningeal artery passing through a groove on its inner surface. Thus a blow on the lateral side of the head may cause the fracture at pterion, which may rupture the artery, leading to sever intracranial hemorrhage.

(4) The bregma (anterior fontanelle) is a diamond and membrane-sealed gap at the crossing place of the sagittal and coronal sutures in fetal skull. It is usually ossified before two years old. Therefore, a soft bregma in the children at this age is an alert for acalcerosis.

(5) The lambda is a membrane-sealed suture at the junction of the sagittal and lambdoid sutures in fetal skull.

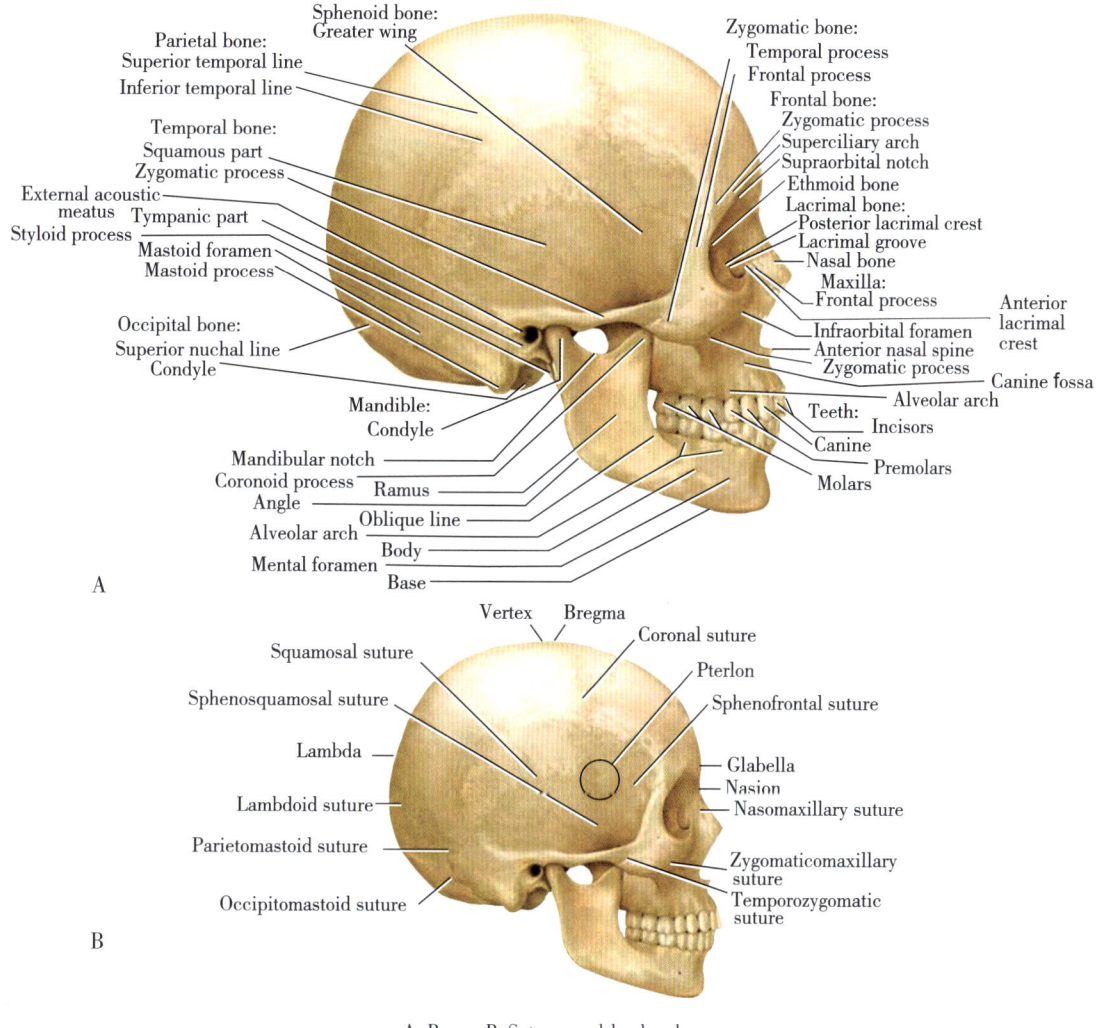

A. Bones; B. Sutures and landmarks.

Figure 1-1 Bone of the head

1.2 The face

For the descriptive purpose, the skin, the superficial fascia and the facial muscles (expression muscles) are together defined as the superficial structures of the face, and those deep to the ramus of the mandible are termed the deep structures of the face.

1.2.1 Superficial structures of the face

1.2.1.1 Skin

Compared with other parts of the body, the skin of the face is relatively thinner, softer and smoother, and its surface shows regularly arranged cleavage lines. For this reason, incisions of the operation on the face should be made along these natural lines and be sutured with fine needle and thread.

1.2.1.2 Superficial fascia

The superficial fascia of the face is composed of loose connective tissues. It contains little fat, but numerous blood and lymphatic vessels. This is why edema appears frequently in the face, especially in the upper eyelid, in patients with renal or heart diseases. In addition to the vessels, the superficial fascia also contains several groups of skeletal muscles (facial or muscles of facial expression) and both motor and sensory nerves.

(1) Facial muscles

The facial muscles are the cutaneous muscles that originate from the facial bone or the fascia and insert into the overlying skin (Figure 1-2, Figure 1-3). Functionally, these muscles allow a wide variety of facial postures to express complex emotions and help to open and close the eyes and mouth. For example, contractions of the orbicularis oculi and the orbicularis orisclose the eyes or mouth more tightly. All the facial muscles are supplied by the facial nerve.

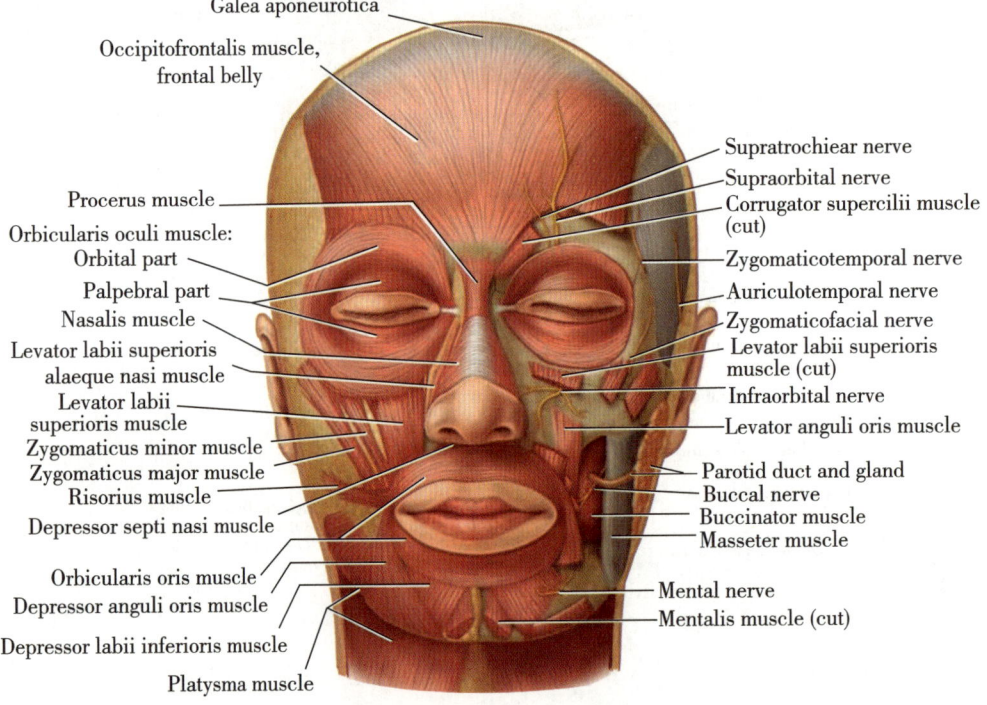

Figure 1-2 Musles of the face

(2) Nerves

1) The facial nerve

The facial nerve (the cranial nerve Ⅶ) emerges through the stylomastoid foramen and then enters the parotid gland, where it divides and anastomoses to form a plexus and finally reorganizes into five groups of terminal branches.

● The temporal branches, usually 1 to 2, emerge out from the superior edge of the parotid gland and run to the temporal and frontal areas.

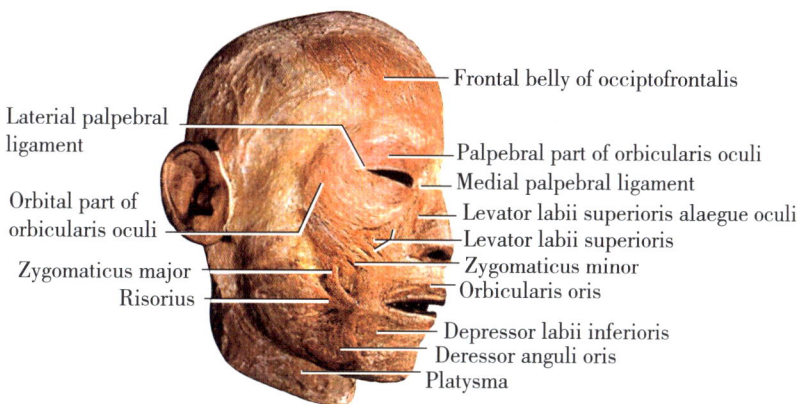

Figure 1-3　Musles of the face (right side)

- The zygomatic branches, usually 2 to 3, leave the parotid gland at its superior and anterior edges and run towards zygomatic process.
- The buccal branches, usually 3 to 5, emerge out from the anterior edge of the parotid gland and pass anteriorly on the surface of the masseter muscle.
- The mandibular branch, usually 1 or 2, emerge out from the inferior edge of the parotid gland and run anteriorly along the base of the mandible.
- The cervical branch, usually only 1, leaves the parotid gland at its inferior edge and goes inferiorly to the neck to supply the platysma muscle.

All of these terminal branches of the facial nerve supply the muscles of the facial expression (the platysma muscle is also an expression muscle, but it has degenerated in human beings) (Figure 1-4, Figure 1-5).

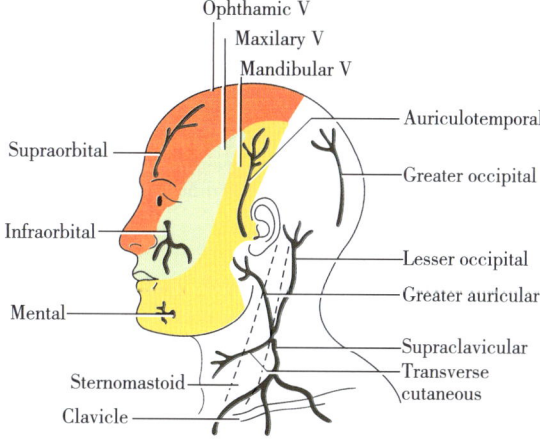

Figure 1-4　The main sensory nerves of face and neck

2) Terminal branches of the trigeminal nerve

The skin of the face is supplied mainly by the terminal branches of the three divisions of the trigeminal nerve. The major branches are follows (Figure 1-6).

- The supraorbital nerve that is a branch of the ophthalmic nerve, emerges from the supraorbital foramen and supplies the area above the eye. Accompanying along its medial side, there is another small terminal branch of the ophthalmic nerve, called the supratrochlear nerve.
- The infraorbital nerve, a branch from the maxillary nerve, which emerges from the infraorbital foramen and supplies the skin between the eye and the mouth.
- The mental nerve that is derived from the mandibular nerve, emerges from the mental foramen and supplies the area below the mouth.

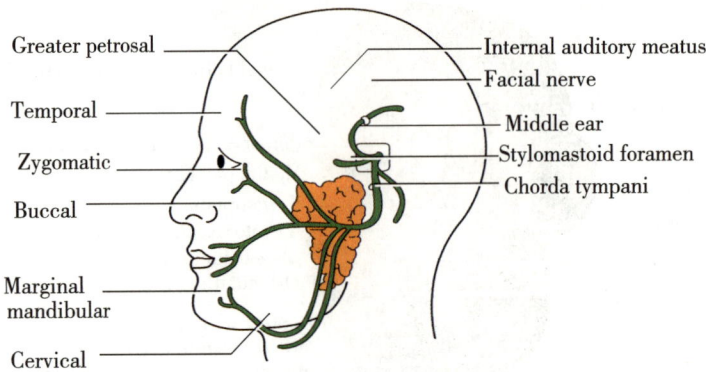

Figure 1-5 The course of the facial nerve

(The nerve passes through the middle ear and the parotid gland)

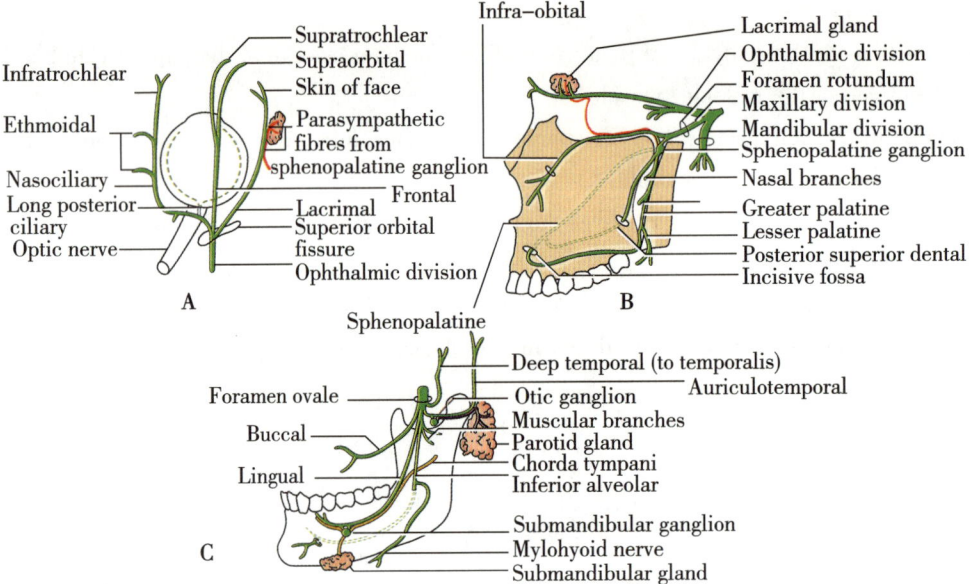

A. The course and branches of the ophthalmic division of the trigeminal nerve; B. The course and branches of the maxillary division of the trigeminal nerve. Parasympathetic fibres are shown in orange; C. The course and main branches of the mandibular division of the trigeminal nerve. The fibres of the chorda tympani are shown in yellow.

Figure 1-6 The sensory divisions of trigeminal nerve

• The auriculotemporal nerve, a branch of the mandibular nerve, which passes superiorly through the parotid gland and finally supplies the temporal and parietal areas of the head.

The trigeminal neuralgia is a disease with unknown reason. It is characterized by a very sharp pain repeatedly appearing in the area supplied by the trigeminal nerve. An emergency treatment for this disease is the block anaesthesia, in which the anaesthetic is injected into the supraorbital, infraorbital and mental foramens to release the pain.

(3) Vessels

The superficial structures of the face are supplied by the superficial temporal artery and the facial artery, both of them are derived from the external carotid artery (Figure 1-7).

1) The superficial temporal artery

The superficial temporal artery arises within the parotid gland. It runs superiorly, enters into the

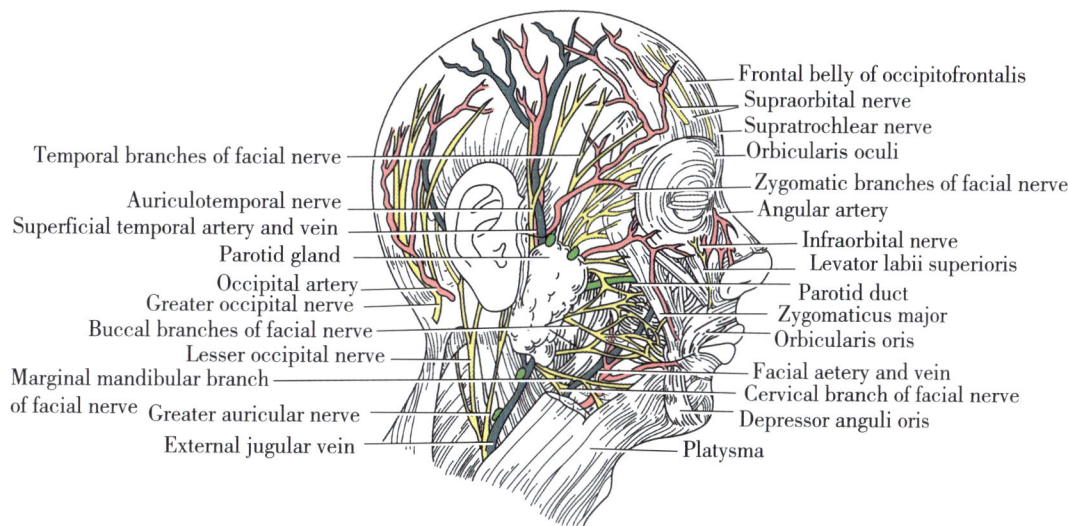

Figure 1-7   Vessels and nerves of the face (right side)

superficial fascia after emerging out from the upper edge of the gland and splits into two branches to supply the scalp. Before leaving the parotid gland, it gives off the transverse facial artery that runs anteriorly on the surface of the masseter muscle to the cheek.

2) The facial artery

The facial artery arises from the external carotid artery in the carotid triangle. It runs upwards and then anteriorly to cross the lower edge of the mandible at the anterior margin of the masseter. After entering the face, it runs superiorly and anteriorly in a tortuous way to the medial angle of the eye, where it continues into the angular artery. During its course, it gives off the inferior and superior labial arteries to the lips and the lateral nasal artery to side of the nose.

3) The facial vein

The facial vein is continued from the angular vein at the medial angle of the eye. It accompanies the facial artery (usually posterior to the artery), but takes a relatively straight and superficial way. After crossing the lower margin of the mandible, it joins the anterior branch of the retromandibular vein and is finally drained into the internal jugular vein. The facial vein drains the area where the facial artery supplies, but its angular vein communicates through the superior ophthalmic vein with an intracranial venous sinus called the cavernous sinus. In the lateral side of the face, the facial vein has a couple of deep tributaries called the deep facial veins that connect to the pterygoid venous plexus located between the muscles deep to the ramus of the mandible. This venous plexus can also communicates with the cavernous sinus through several ways, for example, the inferior ophthalmic veins. Thus the facial vein establishes an important communication approach between the intracranial and extracranial venous systems. The facial vein has no valves. For this reason, infections of the face may spread to the cavernous sinus through the counterflow in the facial vein. This condition may be initiated by squeezing the "pimples" on the face, especially on the triangular area bounded by the bilateral nasolabial grooves and oral fissure. That is why clinically, this triangular area is called the "dangerous triangle of face".

1.2.2 Parotid gland

Parotid gland is the largest among three major salivary gland and surrounded by a capsule derived from the investing layer of deep cervical fascia.

1.2.2.1 Position and division

The parotid gland is located on the lateral surface of the oral cavity, between the ramus of the mandible and the sternocleidomastoid muscle. It can be divided into three parts by the facial nerve that passes through it. The portion lateral to the nerve is its superficial part, and medial to the nerve is the deep part. The junction between the two is called the isthmus. The parotid gland is the major salivary gland of the digestive system. It secretes saliva into the oral cavity through the parotid duct that emerges from the anterior edge of the gland, runs anteriorly along the surface of the masseter muscle, about 1 cm below the zygomatic arch. At the anterior margin of the masseter muscle, it pierces the buccinator and finally opens to the oral cavity opposite to the second upper molar tooth.

1.2.2.2 Important structures through parotid gland

Several important structures pass through the parotid gland(Figure 1-8). The vessels and nerves that pass the gland longitudinally include the external carotid artery with its terminal branch, the superficial temporal artery and accompanied auriculotemporal nerve, and the retromandibular vein. Those that pass the gland transversely are the transverse facial artery and the facial nerve. Of these, the most superficial are branches of the facial nerve which run forwards to the face and pass superficial to the retromandibular vein and its tributaries. The deepest is the termination of the external carotid artery. Among these structures, the relationship of the facial nerve with the parotid gland is the most important clinically. The nerve branches in a fan-like way and these branches anastomose to form a network within the gland, called the parotid plexus. This makes the operation on the gland very difficult. In some parotid gland diseases such as the parotitis or carcinoma, the inflammation or the growing tumor may invades or compress the facial nerve and its branches, leading to the facial paralysis.

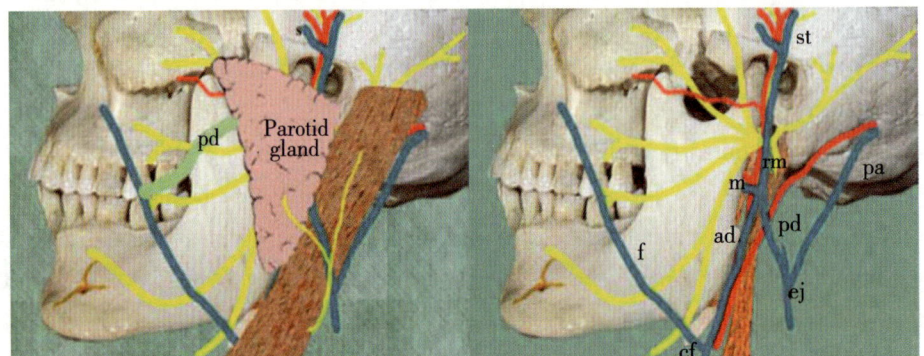

pd—posterior division; st—superficial temporal; rm—retromandibular vein; m—maxillary vein; ad—anterior division; f—facial; cf—common facial; pa—posterior auricular; ej—external jugula.

Figure 1-8　The structures pass through parotid gland

1.2.3　The deep part of lateral face (infratemporal fossa)

This fossa lies deep to the ramus of the mandible. It's boudared superior wall is infratemporal surface of sphenoid bone; ant wall is posterior surface of maxilla; internal wall is external plate of sphenoid bone; external wall is ramus of mandible.

The most prominent structures in this fossa are the two pterygoid muscles. The lateral pterygoid muscle arises fron the lateral pterygoid plate and runs posterioly inserting to the mandibular neck and articular capsule. The medial pterygoid arises from the medial surface of lateral pterygoid plate and maxilla, it runs downward and backward, finally insertis to the medial surface of the angle of mandibl.

Additionally the mandibular division of the trigeminal nerve and its branches, and the maxillary vessels and their branches also lie in this fossa. Adjacent to the fossa is the temporamandibular joint.

1.2.3.1 Maxillary artery

Maxillary artery is the large terminal branch of the external carotid artery arising within the parotid gland(Figure 1-9). It travels along the deep of the neck of mandible, the lower margin of lateral pterygoid, and the superficial surface of the lateral pterygoid, finnally enters the pterygopalatine fossa.

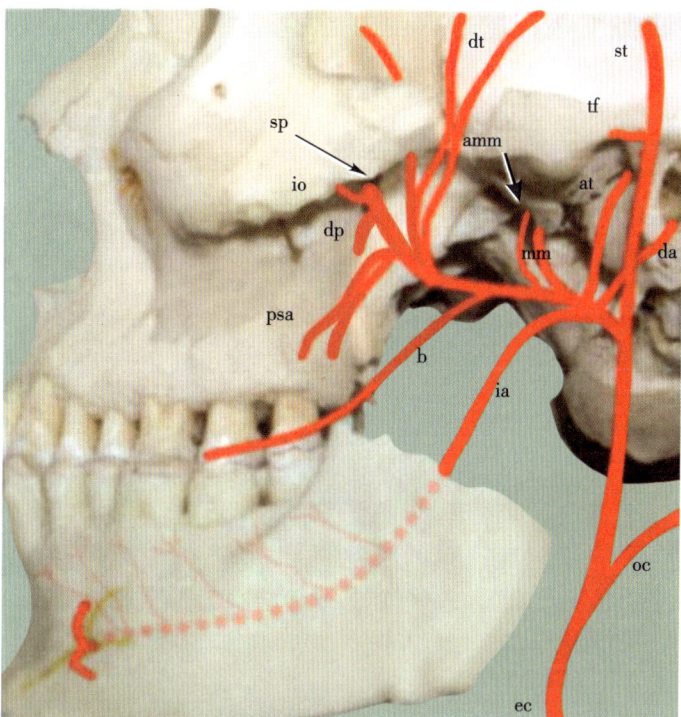

da—deep auricular; at—anterior tympanic; mm—middle meningeal; amm—accessory middle meningeal; ia—inferior alveolar; b—buccal; dt—deep temporal; psa—posterior superior alveolar; dp—descending palatine; io—infraorbital; sp—sphenopalatine; oc—occipital; tf—transverse facial; st—superficial temporal; ec—external carotid.

Figure 1-9   Maxillary artery and external carotid artery

This artery is divided into three portions: the fitst portion, from the beginning of the artery to the lower margin of lateral pterygoid, gives rise two branches, one is the inferior alveolar artery, the other is the middle meningeal artery. The inferior alveolar artery decends in companeing with its corresponding vein and nerve and then passes throug the foremen of mandible into the mandibular canal. And the middle meningeal artery that runs upward between the two roots of the auriculatemporal nerve and then passes through the spinous foremen and erters the cranial cavity.

Superficial or deep to the lateral pterygoid is the second portion of the artery. It gives off the buccal artery and some branches to masticatory muscles. Before entering the pterygopalatine fossa, the third one gives off the posterior superior alveolar and infraorbital arteries.

1.2.3.2 Pterygoid venous plexus

Pterygoid venous plexusis located between lateral and medial pterygoid and aroud maxillary artery. It converges backward to form a short trunk called the maxillary vein, the maxillary vein then joins with superf temporal vein to form the retromandibular vein in the parotid gland. The pterygoid venous plexus communicates with both introcranial and extracranial veins.

1.2.3.3 Mandibular nerve

Mandibular nerve is located in the deep of lateral pterygoid muscle and contains sensory and motor fibres(Figure 1-10). It is divided into anterior and posterior trunks. The anterior trunk is slender and mainly motor. It gives off the branches to masticatory muscles (motor) and buccal nerve to the cheek (sensory). Please note among these branches, only the buccal nerve is sensory. Posterior trunk is large and mainly sensory. It has three branches, the auriculotemporal, lingual (joined by chorda tympani) and inferior alveolar nerve(gives off mylohyoid nerve).

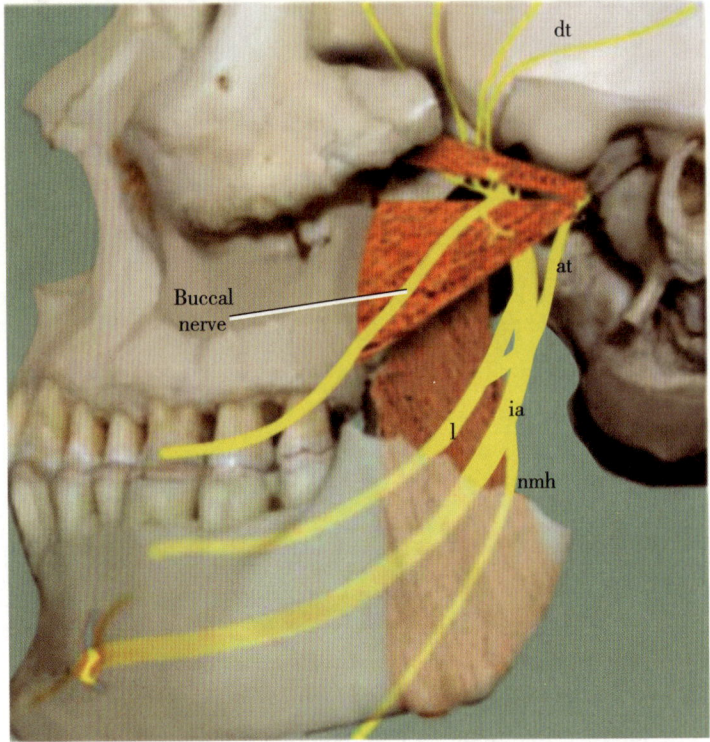

dt—deep temporal; at—auriculotemporal; ia—inferior alveolar; nmh—nerve to the mylohyoid; l—lingual; branches to lateral pterygoid (not labeled). Not shown: meningeal branch, nerve to masseter.

Figure 1-10 The branches of mandibular nerve

- The auriculotemporal nerve arises by two roots which clasp the origin of the middle meningeal artery. The nerve passes backwards behind the tempotamandibular joint and then ascends and emerges out from the upper edges of the parotid gland in company with the superfical tempora vessels.
- The lingual nerve inclines downwards and forwards between the pterygoids, in the floor of the mouth it runs forwards lateral to the hyoglossus muscle, and then turns medially to pass inferior to the submandibular duct and enters the base of the tongue. it conveys gerneral sensation from the anterior two-thirds of the tongue. Near the low border of the lateral pterygoid, the lingual nerve is joined by the chorda tympani(a branch of the facial nerve).
- The inferior alveolar nerve descends and gives rise to a motor branch to supply mylohyoid and the anterior belly of digastric. Thereafter the inferior alveolar nerve enters the mandibular foramen in the ramus of the mandible and runs forwards in the mandibular canal accompanning with the atery and supplying the lower teeth. Its mental branch emerges from the mental foramen to supply skin overlying the chin.

Infratemporal and submandibular regious are seen in Figure 1-11.

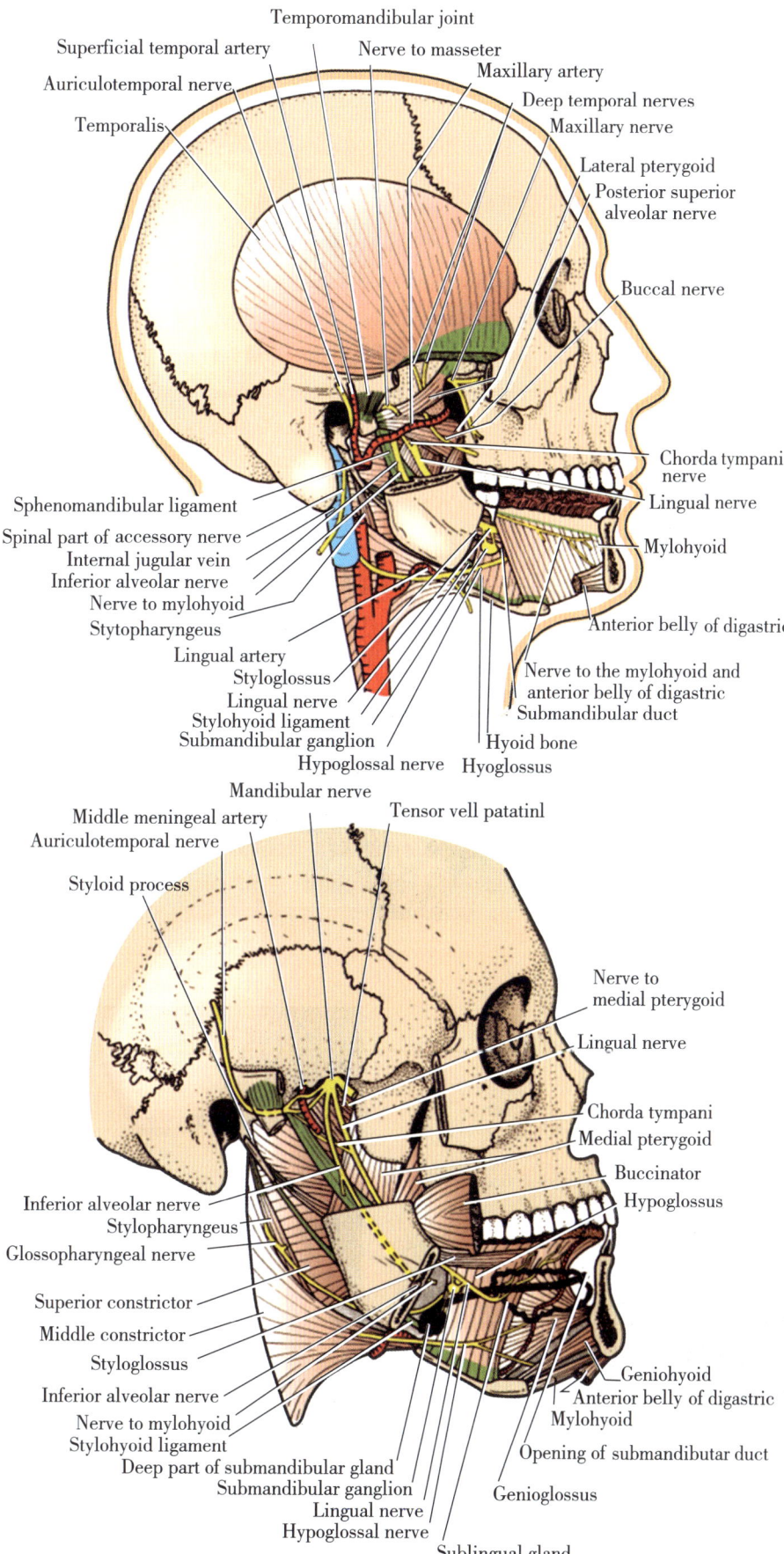

Figure 1-11 Infratemporal and submandibular regions

1.3 The cranium

1.3.1 Frontoparietooccipital region

Let's start with the scalp. The scalp is the soft tissue that covers the calvaria. It is composed of five layers with different tissue components (Figure 1-12). From out surface to deep, they are the skin, the superficial fascia, the epicranial aponeurosis, the subaponeurotic connective tissues and the pericranium among these five layers, the outer three are tightly adhered and are very difficult to be separated. So they are usually taken as one layer, called the scalp proper. The epicranial aponeurosis is the aponeurotic portion of the occipitofrontalis between its two bellies, the frontal and the occipital. The contraction of the two bellies will add strong stress on the scalp. Therefore, clinically, when sewing a wound on the scalp, the aponeurosis must be strongly sutured together with the skin even though it is not injured.

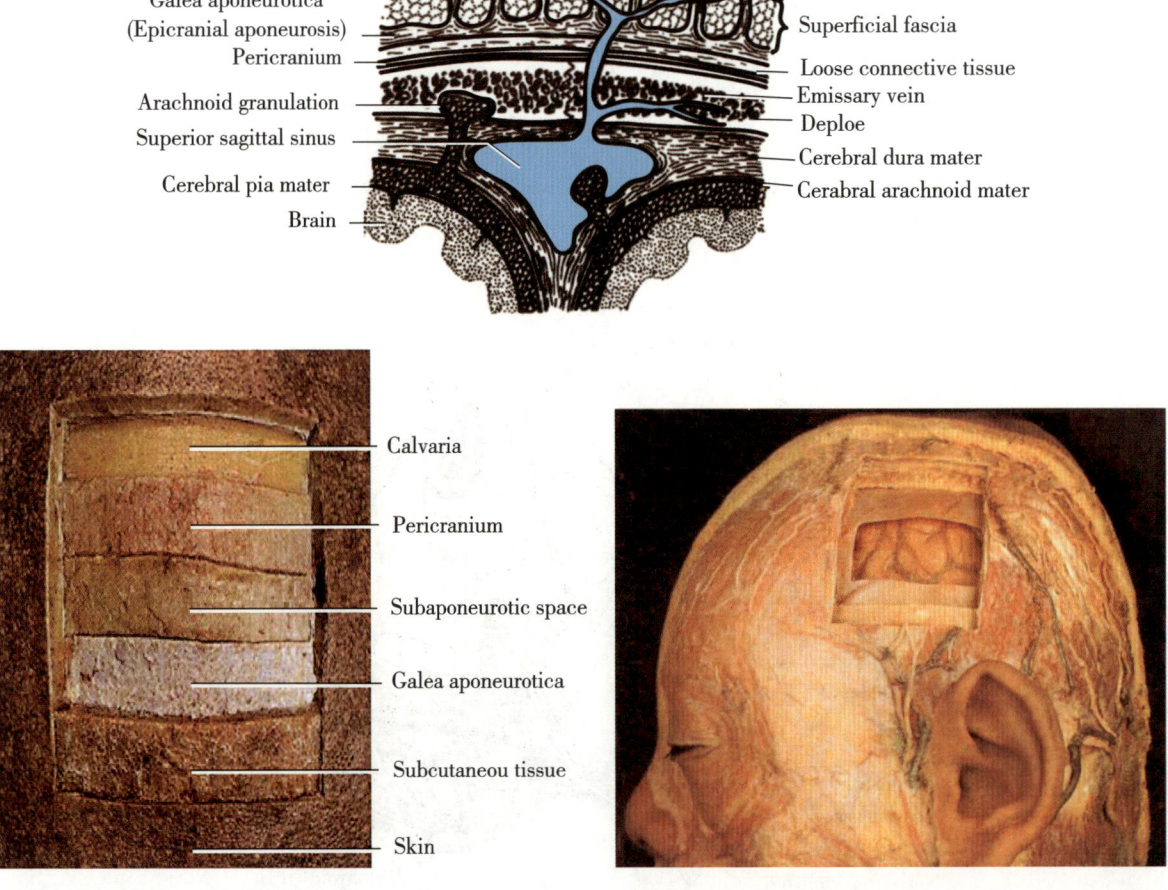

Figure 1-12 Layers of frontoparietooccipital region

The vessels and the nerves supplying the scalp are distributed in the superficial fascia. They are generally divided into three groups. The anterior group includes the supratrochlear and the supraorbital nerves with their accompanying vessels. The middle group contains mainly the auriculotemporal nerve accompanying the superficial temporal vessels anterior to the auricle, and the less occipital nerve accompanying the posterior auricular vessels behind the auricle. The posterior group includes the greater occipital nerve and the occipital vessels. All the nerves and vessels pass from the lower margin of the calvaria to the top (Figure 1-13). Thus incisions of the operation on the cranium should be made in a manner to keep lower margin of the skin flap as its root.

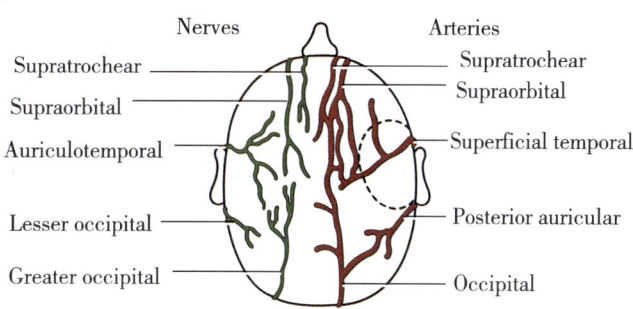

Figure 1-13 The nerves and blood vessels of the scalp (the dotted line shows a temporal "flap")

1.3.2 Temporal region

The temporal region (fossa) is one of the areas of calvaria, in order to be convenient for learning and operating, we'll deal with this region in advance.

The temporal region (ortemporal fossa) is bounded by the superior temporal line and the zygomatic arch. It is a transitional part between the scalp and the face so that its layers have the characteristics of both. Like the scalp, the outer two layers of the temporal fossa are the skin and the superficial fascia, but the epicranial aponeurosis disappears and is replaced by the temporal fascia. In the superficial fascia, the structures emerg from the upper edge of the paroitd gland and pass anterior to the auricle. From anterior to posterior, they are arranged as follows: the temporal branch of facial nerve, the superficial temporal artery, the auriculotemporal nerve and superficial temporal vein. The temporal fascia is a dense deep fascia that attaches superiorly to the superior temporal line. Below its attachment, it splits into two layers. The superficial layer extends inferiorly and attaches onto the superficial surface of the zygomatic arch. The deep layer covers the temporalis and attaches onto the deep surface of the zygomatic arch. The space between two layers is called the temporal fascial space and filled by fatty tissue. The temporalis is a fan-shaped masticatory muscle with the function similar to the masseter.

1.3.3 The cranium

The cranium is divided into the calvaria, cranial cavity and cranial base before, the calvaria is subdivide into the temporal region and the frontoparietooccipital region.

1.3.3.1 Internal surface of the cranial base

The internal surface of the cranial base is naturally divided into three regions, the anterior cranial fossa that houses the frontal lobes of the brain, the middle cranial fossa that lodges the temporal lobes and the posterior cranial fossa occupied by the brain stem and the cerebellum. The central part of the meddle cranial fossa, formed by the upper surface of the body of the sphenoid bone, is called the region of sella turcica, we can obsver several bony structures such as the tubercle of sellae, the sulcus chiasma, hypophysial fossa, dorsum sellae and the sphenoidal sinus within the body of the sphenoid bone in the region. This region holds several structures such as the hypophysis (pituitary gland) and the cavernous sinus. These structures and their relations are clinically important (Figure 1-14).

1.3.3.2 Cerebral dura mater and venous sinus

The cerebral dura mater is composed of two layers: the outer periosteal layer and the inner meningeal

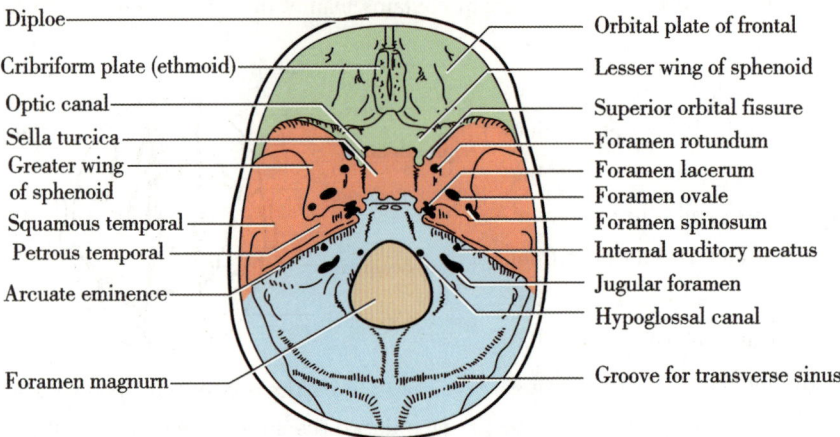

Figure 1-14 The internal surface of the cranial

layer (Figure 1-15). The meningeal layer forms distinct septa, they are the cerebral falx, the tentorium of cerebellum, the cerebellar falx, and the diaphragma sellae. In certain regions, the two layers separate to enclos the dural sinuses: the majar dural sinuses incloudes the superior sagittal sinus lying in the fixed margin of the cerebral falx, the inferior sagittal sinus lies in its free lower margin and runs posteriorly and finally ends by merging with the great cerebral vein to form the the straight sinus. the straight sinus runs inferoposteriorly to the cerebellar tentorium to join the confluence of sinuese. The confluence of sinuese is formed by the junction of the straight sinus and the superior sagittal sinus near the internal occipital protuberance. The dura space at both sides of the hypophysial fossa are the cavernous sinus.

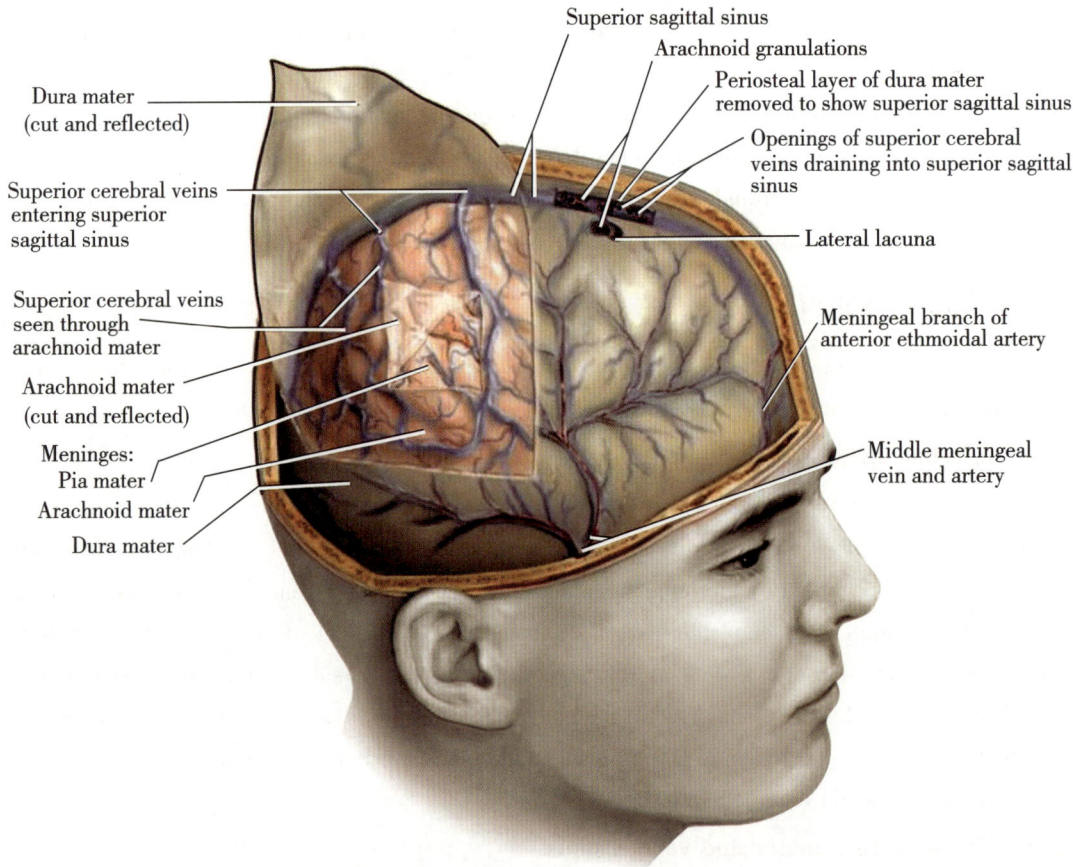

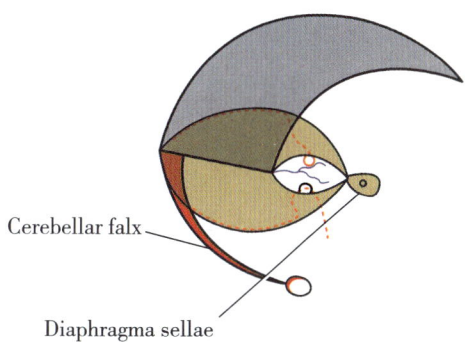

Figure 1-15　The cerebral dura mater and venous sinus

　　The cavernous sinuses are a pair of sponge-like dural venous sinuses on each side of the sella turcica. It receives blood from the bilateralsphenoparietal sinus, the superficial middle cerebral veins intacranially, and the superior and inferior ophthalmic veins extracranially. Posteriorly the cavernous sinus drains though the superior and inferior petrosal sinus into the transverse sinus and the internal jugular vein.

　　The cavernous sinus has very complex relations. From superior to downwards, the oculomotor nerve [cranial nerve(CN)], the trochlear nerve (CN Ⅳ), the ophthalmic nerve (CN V_1) and the maxillary nerve (CN V_2) pass through its lateral wall between the endothelium and the dura. The internal carotid artery with the accompanying sympathetic plexus, and the abducent nerve (CN Ⅵ) run anteriorly through it (Figure 1-16). Because of these relations, the patient with the thrombophlebitis of the cavernous sinus may have very complex syndromes such as the abnormal eye positions, pupil changes and skin sensations on the involved side of the face.

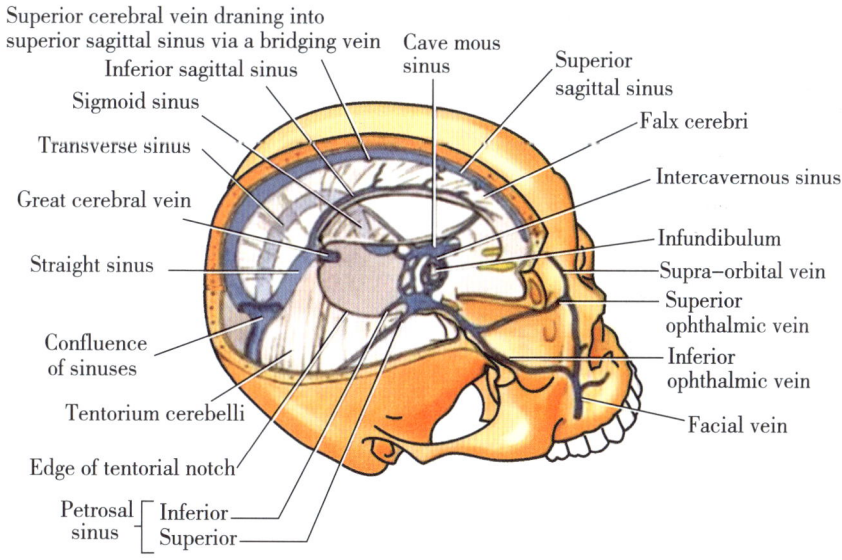

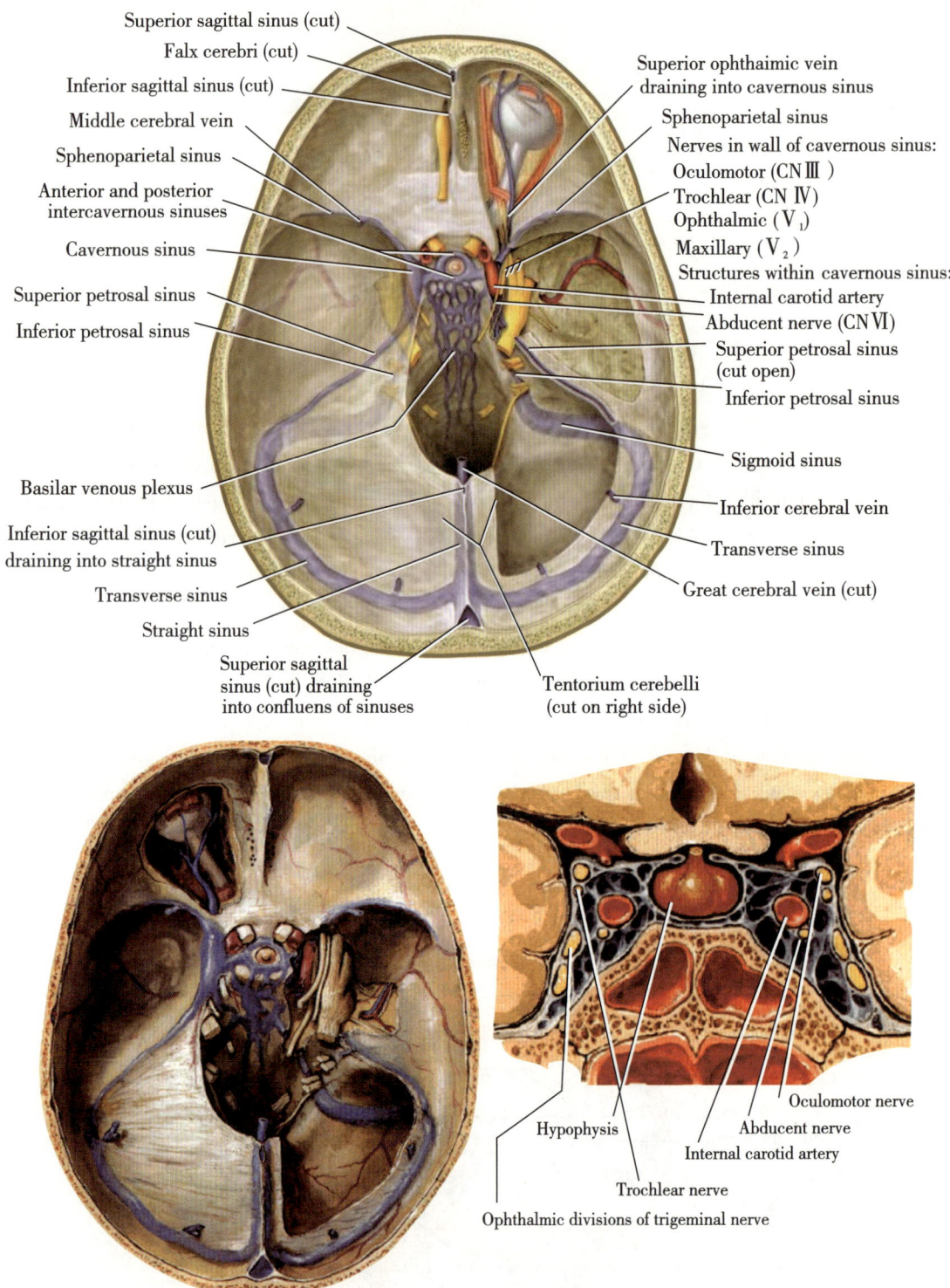

Figure 1–16 Sinuses of duramater

1.3.3.3 Hypophysis

The hypophysis is an oval-shaped endocrine organ located in the hypophysial fossa, below the diaphragma sella. The diaphragma sella is a double-layer dural septum that attaches on the dorsum and tubercle of sellae. It has a central hole from which the infundibulum passes through to connect the hypophysis to the hypothalamus.

The hypophysis is related anteriorly to the tubercle of sellae and posteriorly to the dorsum sellae. Laterally, it is flanked by the cavernous sinuses and inferiorly, it is separated from the sphenoidal sinus by a thin layer of bone. Superiorly, it is related through the diagragma sella to the optic chiasma. This is very important clinically, because a growing pituitary tumor may expand superiorly to compress the chiasma, leading to the bitemporal hemianopia.

1.4 Main contents of the head

1.4.1 Face and scalp region

Overview of skull bones
The skeletal framework for this area is comprised of cranial and facial bones
The skull contains a series of intercommunicating cavities including: ✓ Cranial cavity—this large cavity encases the brain and the beginnings and exits of the cranial nerves ✓ Nasal cavity—is concerned with respiration, olfaction, and heat exchange ✓ Oral cavity—is concerned with taste, suckling, chewing, swallowing, speech, and respiration ✓ Vestibulo-cochlear cavity—is concerned with hearing and balance and is contained in the temporal bone
Orbital cavity—is concerned with protection of sight functions since it contains the globe
Calvaria

✓ The roof of the cranial cavity protects the cerebral hemispheres
✓ In neonates, the calvaria may be considerably misshapen as moulding of these bones occurs when the baby passes through the birth canal
✓ During childhood, the calvarium expands to allow for brain expansion
✓ This bony encasement limits the swelling of the brain and its meningeal coverings in adults
✓ Individual bones included in the calvarium are as follows:
  ◊ Frontal bone
  ◊ Parietal bone
  ◊ Occipital bone

Frontal bone
✓ This bone was originally paired but the two bones become fused in most adults ✓ The original suture that connected the two frontal bones is called the metopic suture ✓ It persists in some children and adults and should not be confused with a fracture line ✓ Supraorbital foramen or notch—transmits the supraorbital nerve, artery, and vein ✓ The orbital rim is located inferiorly and contributes to extremely hard orbital encasement that protects the globe ✓ The frontal paranasal sinuses form in later childhood within this bone ✓ The frontal bone eventually forms bony sutures with the nasal, temporal, maxillary, zygomatic, temporal, sphenoid, parietal bones

Parietal bones

- ✓ Parietal bones are paired bones connected by a sagittal suture
- ✓ The anterior sutural connection with the frontal bones is known as the coronal suture
- ✓ They contain emissary foramina that connect the veins within the loose connective tissue layer of the scalp with the dural venous sinuses inside the cranium
- ✓ They protect the cerebral hemispheres

Occipital bone

- ✓ This bone has a prominent landmark—the external occipital protuberance
- ✓ This bone contains the foramen magnum
- ✓ Its inner surface cradles the cerebellar hemispheres
- ✓ It forms a bony suture lines with the temporal bone (lambdoidal suture)

Facial skeleton—provides protection for special sensory organs (eye, nose)

Nasal bones

- ✓ Nasal bones are paired bones
- ✓ They are frequently fractured and repaired/remodeled during a surgical procedures known as a rhinoplasty
- ✓ These form suture lines with the frontal and maxillary bones and articulate with the nasal cartilages

Maxilla

- ✓ Paired bones that are small in the infant but enlarge as teeth erupt. Thus the maxilla develops an alveolar portion that holds the deciduous and permanent teeth
- ✓ Maxilla contributes to the inferior orbital rim and contains a canal and infraorbital foramen
- ✓ Maxilla contains a maxillary sinus making it a hollow, lightweight bone that helps the voice resonate

Temporal bones

- ✓ Temporal bones are paired bones
- ✓ Contain a squamous portion that is the thinnest portion and is occasionally fractured with life-threatening consequences due to laceration of the underlying middle meningeal artery
- ✓ Contains a tympanic portion and external acoustic meatus (external ear canal)
- ✓ Develops a mastoid process due to the pull of the sternocleidomastoid muscle as infants develop the ability to hold their heads without support
- ✓ The inner extremely hard portion (petrous portion) contains the inner ear
- ✓ Zygomatic process is an arch that forms a suture with the zygomatic bone

Zygomatic bones

- ✓ Zygomatic bones are paired "cheek" bones
- ✓ The arch portion is frequently fractured
- ✓ Forms visible sutures with the maxilla, frontal bone and temporal bones
- ✓ Contains zygomaticofacial and zygomaticotemporal foramina

Lacrimal bones

- ✓ Lacrimal bones are paired bones within the orbit
- ✓ They form the exit funnels that direct tears downward into the nasolacrimal ducts

Mandible

✓ Paired bones that fuse
✓ Contains a mental foramen where terminal branches of the inferior alveolar nerve, artery, and vein emerge
✓ Contains an alveolar portion that is tooth bearing. In infants who have not developed their primary dentition, the mandible is small and underdeveloped
✓ In older edentulous (toothless) adults, mandibular bone is reabsorbed and the mandible is easily fractured
✓ Contains condylar processes that articulate with the skull at the temporomandibular joint
✓ Other portions consist of the ramus, a mandibular notch and coronoid process

Surface regions on the face

✓ Frontal eminence—prominence of the forehead
✓ Superciliary ridge—bony ridge above the eyebrow
✓ Glabella—flattened area between the eyebrows
✓ Orbital rim—a dense bony socket that protects the globe
✓ Lateral and medial canthi—lateral/medial angles of the eyes
✓ Palpebral—having to do with the eyelids
✓ Pinna or auricle (outer ear where sound waves are collected)
✓ Tragus—cartilaginous lump anterior to external auditory canal
✓ Nasion—depression at root of nose; location of fronto-nasal suture
✓ Nares—external nasal openings
✓ Alae—wings at the side of nose
✓ Columella—the central inferior dividing skin between the nares
✓ Philtrum—vertical groove between the columella and upper lip
✓ Labial tubercle—thickening in the upper lip below the philtrum
✓ Labial commissure—junction of the upper and lower lips
✓ Vermillion—the reddish covering of the lips
✓ Mental protuberance—anterior prominence of the chin
✓ Zygoma—lateral prominence of the upper cheek
✓ You will use this nomenclature to describe the exact location of skin lesions/lacerations that you observe during physical exams

Cutaneous innervation of face, scalp, and neck

The trigeminal nerve (CN V)

✓ The vast majority of nerve components in this nerve are sensory
✓ Pseudo-unipolar nerve cell bodies reside in a ganglion (a collection of nerve cell bodies)
✓ This extremely large 3-part ganglion is known as the trigeminal or semilunar ganglion
✓ The semilunar ganglion is equivalent to a dorsal root ganglion like you have seen near the spinal cord
✓ All ganglia (including this largest sensory example) are derived from neural crest cells

✓ Ganglia can be affected by viral infection known as herpes zoster. When a patient becomes immuno-compromised, the skin that is supplied by this nerve develops a painful skin rash known as shingles

✓ This ganglion is also affected (stimulated, irritated) by unknown causes. This condition is called trigeminal neuralgia or tic douloureux—an excruciatingly painful condition

✓ Concept: all nerves feeding into the trigeminal ganglion from the peripheral territory of CN V are a part of the dermatome pattern for this cranial nerve. Thus the head is a place where all the peripheral nerves and the dermatomes are identical. A pain sensation arriving from a peripheral nerve in the mandibular division can become magnified and impossible to localize. The brain interprets the pain throughout the entire distribution of the mandibular division. On rare occasions, the pain is experienced over all three divisions

Ophthalmic (V_1) division of the trigeminal nerve

✓ Innervates the skin of the tip and bridge of the nose

✓ Innervates the forehead up to the top of the cranial vault

✓ Innervates the upper eyelid and medial canthal region (corner of the eye)

✓ Innervates the cornea—those of you that have experienced a corneal abrasion from a foreign body in the eye or from contact lens can appreciate the extreme sensitivity of this area

✓ The sensory branches to the conjunctiva and cornea form the afferent limb of the blink reflex. Sensory loss over the cornea can lead to corneal ulceration

✓ Cutaneous branches of this division have the following names (to name a few):

  ◊ Supratrochlear nerve

  ◊ Supraorbital nerve—a main supplier of the forehead and frontal scalp. Infiltration of local anesthetic carefully placed in the vicinity of this branch can render it possible to pick out glass, dirt or place sutures in the forehead/scalp skin

  ◊ Infratrochlear nerve

  ◊ Lacrimal nerve—sends a palpebral branch to the lateral portion of the eyelid

  ◊ External nasal nerve—a branch of the anterior ethmoidal nerve and "ouch" nerve when patients have a fractured nose

Maxillary (V_2) division of the trigeminal nerve

✓ Passes forward through foramina and canals to enter the maxilla where it then emerges from various foramina

✓ Innervates skin of the upper lip, lateral nose, lower eyelid, lower conjunctival sac, cheek, temporal region of scalp, palate, upper teeth and gingiva, maxillary sinus

✓ Cutaneous branches of this division that appear on the face are as follows:

  ◊ Infraorbital nerve

  ◊ Zygomaticofacial nerve

  ◊ Zygomaticotemporal nerve—innervates the scalp over the temples

Mandibular (V_3) division of the trigeminal nerve

✓ Innervates the skin of the lower lip, the skin over lower jaw, temporal region

✓ Innervates the lower teeth and gingiva, external auditory meatus, outer eardrum

✓ Cutaneous branches of this division that appear on the face are as follows:

♢ Auriculotemporal nerve—travels with the superficial temporal artery
  ◆ This nerve has a long course superiorly to the vertex of the scalp
♢ Buccal nerve—should not be confused with the buccal branch of the facial nerve
  ◆ This nerve is sensory to the lining of the cheek
♢ Mental nerve—a terminal branch of the inferior alveolar nerve
  ◆ This is a nerve to remember if you are responsible for suturing a lower lip or chin and need to supply local anesthetic

Cutaneous branches of the cervical plexus

✓ This plexus receives contributions from the anterior rami of C_2, C_3, C_4
✓ All these cutaneous nerves emerge on the superficial regions of the neck by winding around the posterior border of the sternocleidomastoid muscle
✓ Several travel upward to the face or behind the ear
✓ Others remain in the vicinity of the neck
✓ Lesser occipital nerve (C_2, C_3)—supplies skin posterior to the ear
✓ Great auricular nerve (C_2, C_3)—supplies lower cheek and skin anterior to the ear
✓ Transverse cervical (anterior) nerve (C_2, C_3)
✓ Supraclavicular nerves (C_3, C_4)—medial, intermediate, lateral branches travel downward in the neck to provide sensation over the clavicles and onto the upper pectoral region

Cutaneous branches from the posterior (dorsal) rami

✓ Great occipital nerve (C_2)—the largest member of the dorsal group. It courses upward to supply skin over the occipital bone and upward to the vertex of the scalp
✓ 3rd occipital nerve (C_3)—courses to the upper neck skin
✓ C_3–C_6—courses to lower neck skin

Arterial supply to face/scalp

Internal carotid artery and several important branches

✓ Supratrochlear artery
  ♢ Distributed to the glabella and medial brow region
  ♢ Located near the trochlear pulley where the superior oblique muscle takes a turn
✓ Supraorbital artery
  ♢ Emerges from the supraorbital notch/foramen
  ♢ Extends upward to the vertex of the skull
✓ External nasal artery
  ♢ Distributed to the bridge of the nose

External carotid artery and several important superficial branches

✓ Infraorbital artery
  ♢ A terminal branch of the maxillary artery
  ♢ It emerges from the infraorbital foramen with the nerve and vein
  ♢ Its territory includes the lower eyelid, cheek
  ♢ It is an important artery to the mid-face

- ✓ Zygomaticofacial artery
  - ◊ Small artery emerging from a foramen in the zygomatic bone
- ✓ Zygomaticotemporal artery
  - ◊ Small artery emerging from a foramen in the zygomatic bone
- ✓ Superficial temporal artery
  - ◊ A terminal branch of the external carotid artery
  - ◊ A key artery supplying the temporal region
  - ◊ Runs anterior to the ear and extends up to the vertex of the scalp
  - ◊ A major artery where a pulse can be palpated
  - ◊ Transverse facial artery—a branch that courses near the parotid duct

Facial artery

- ✓ A direct branch of the external carotid artery
- ✓ After supplying the tonsils and submandibular gland, this artery emerges onto the face and winds upward
- ✓ It is another convenient site where a pulse can be palpated and measured
- ✓ Branches on the face include:
  - ◊ Inferior labial artery—supplies the lower lip
  - ◊ Superior labial artery—contributes to epistaxis (nosebleeds). This is the basis for applying compression to the upper lip to staunch the flow of blood from a nosebleed
  - ◊ Lateral nasal artery—supplies the skin of the ala of the nose
  - ◊ Angular artery—supplies the medial canthus (angle of the eye)
  - ◊ Posterior auricular artery—a direct branch of the external carotid artery, supplies the scalp posterior to the ear and the pinna itself
  - ◊ Occipital artery—a direct branch of the external carotid artery, supplies the posterior scalp all the way to the vertex. This is a major source of blood loss when individuals fall, hit the back of their scalp and knock themselves unconscious

Concept

- ✓ The face and scalp are exceedingly well supplied with a rich series of anastomotic channels. Lacerations or deliberate excisions by a surgeon bleed profusely and typically require suturing
- ✓ The rich supply of vessels makes it possible to swing local flaps of skin to cover tissue defects that are made when tumors are excised
- ✓ The rich supply of vessels makes infections and wound healing problems rather rare since there is usually adequate supply of oxygen, nutrients and delivery of immune cells

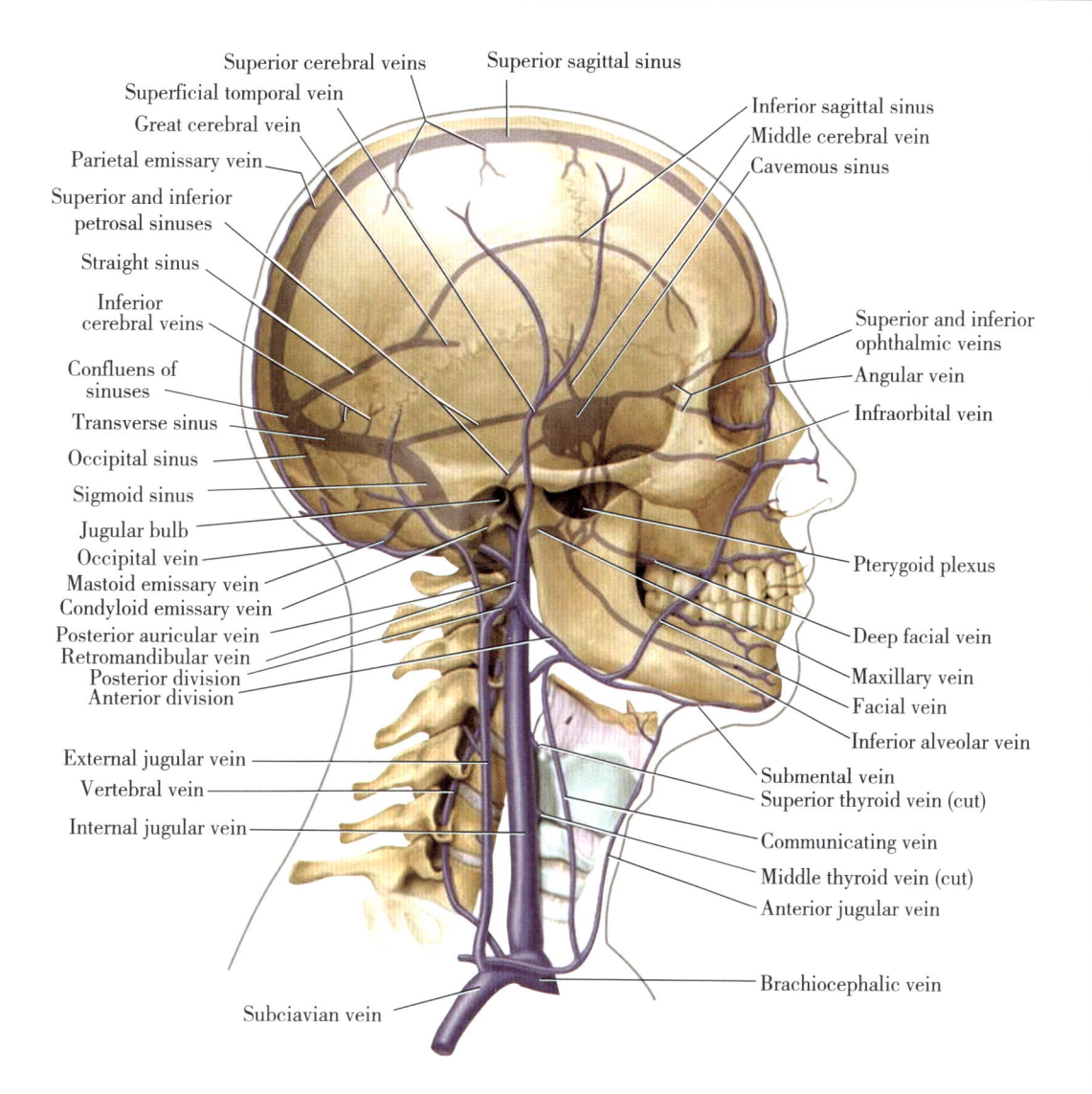

Lymphatic drainage of face/scalp

Groups of lymph nodes form a "pericervical collar" at the head/neck junction as follows:
- ✓ Occipital nodes
- ✓ Retro-auricular (mastoid) nodes
- ✓ Parotid nodes
- ✓ Submandibular nodes
- ✓ Submental nodes

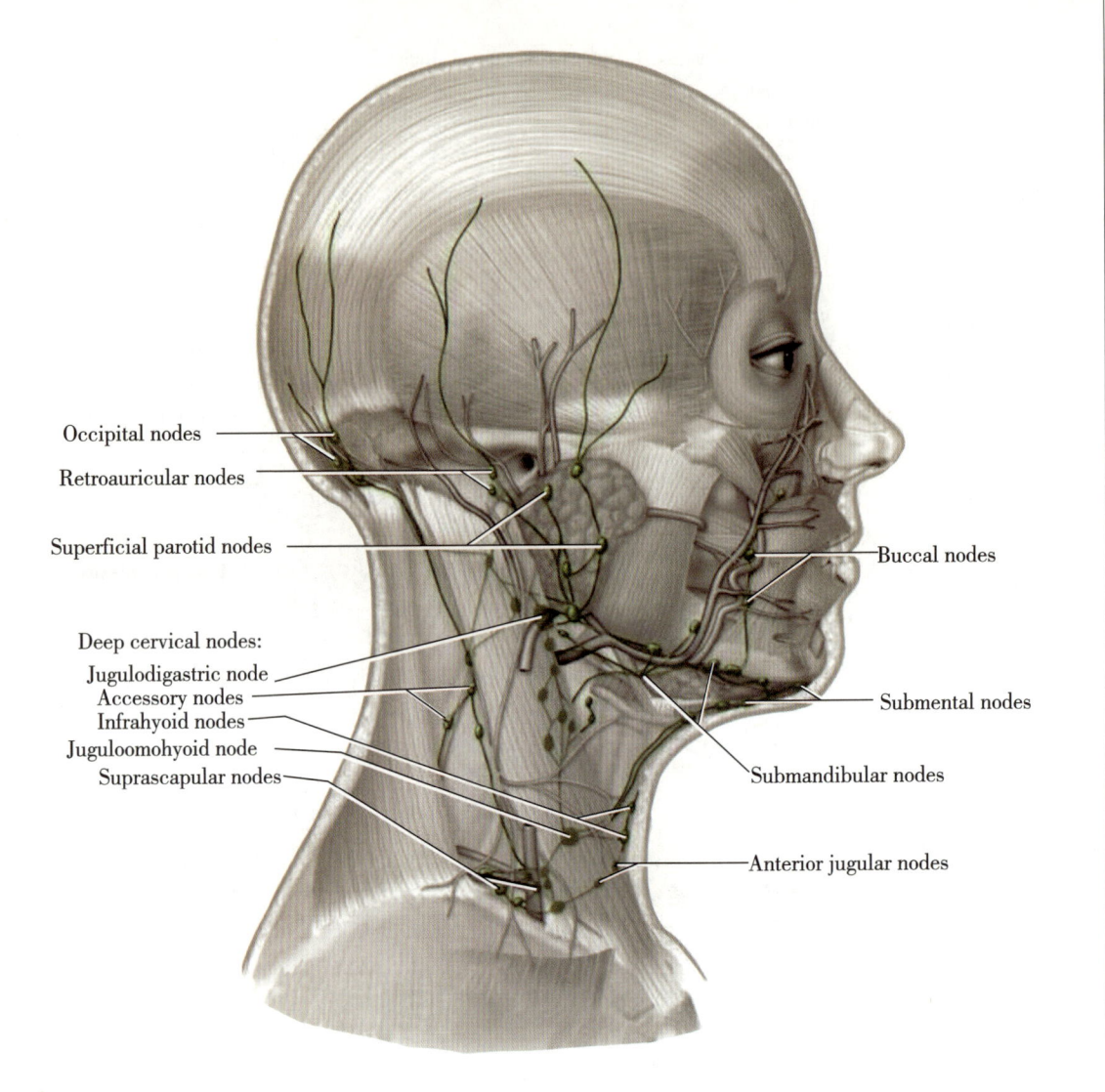

✓ Superficial lymph node chains accompany the anterior and external jugular veins
✓ Superficial lymph nodes ultimately drain into the deep cervical lymph nodes
✓ Deep cervical lymph nodes (upper and lower) parallel the internal jugular veins
✓ The deep sets empty into the systemic venous return at the jugulovenous angle (the junction of the internal jugular veins and subclavian veins
✓ Sentinel node mapping is now performed in tracing the specific drainage
✓ A radical neck dissection is an aggressive surgical removal of these cervical lymphatic nodes, their lymphatic chains, and the internal jugular vein

Concept

✓ The skin on the face/scalp is the most exposed to harmful ultraviolet rays and lesions (melanomas, squamous cell carcinomas and basal cell carcinomas) are common on ears, lips, noses and scalp. This is the rationale for being wise and wearing a hat when you are going to have prolonged exposure to the sun
✓ The oral cavity, esophagus, larynx is exposed to constant intake from food or tobacco over a lifetime. Head and neck tumors of deep origin are also common and can spread through these lymphatic channels

Muscles of facial expression

✓ These unusual muscles arise from neural crest cells that migrate and proliferate into the subcutaneous region over the 2nd branchial (pharyngeal) arch

✓ The facial nerve (CN VII) provides motor innervation to all muscular derivatives from the 2nd arch

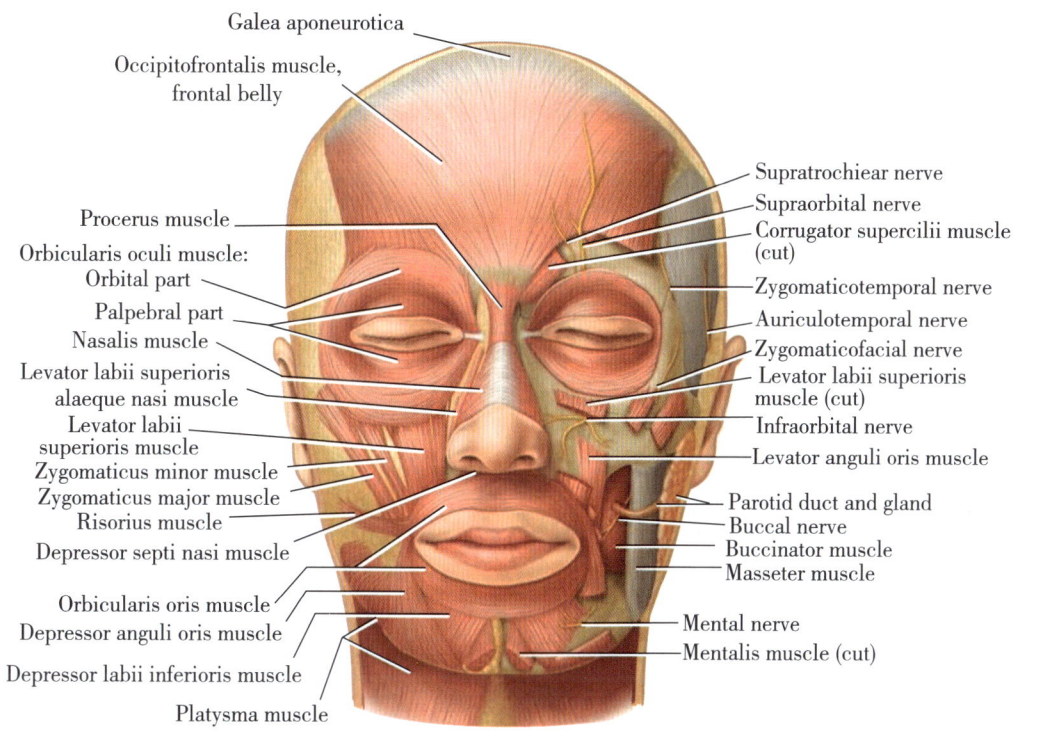

✓ Innervation reached these muscles very early during the developmental process. Later the parotid gland branched and expanded into this region. Unfortunately, the branches of the facial nerve were eventually encased by the parotid tissue. Thus you will note that CN VII must pass through the parotid gland where its branches are at risk of damage if there is a tumor, surgical resection, laceration or trauma to the face

✓ Muscles of facial expression may originate on bone, but most arise in the skin and insert into skin

✓ These muscles are responsible for the wrinkles that inevitably develop along Langer's Lines as a person ages and the skin experiences a lifetime of pull in a certain direction

✓ Surgeons deliberately orient their incisions in these lines of tension whenever possible in order to reduce the development and visibility of scars

✓ The function of these muscles is for facial expression (to convey body language)

✓ Equally important functions include work as sphincters and dilators of the openings on the face

◊ These muscles control the ability to blink or to close the lips to keep saliva from drooling. They dilate the nostrils during extreme physical exertion and they raise the brows to keep eyelid skin from obstructing the visual field, etc

Epicranial complex—important muscles of the scalp

Frontalis muscle

✓ It is located over the frontal bones

✓ This muscle raises the brow skin and keeps the skin out of the eyes

Occipitalis muscle

- ✓ It is located over the occipital bone

Galea aponeurotica

- ✓ This is the intervening facial layer that connects the two muscles
- ✓ It is located over the top of the scalp
- ✓ When this layer is transversely cut, the cut ends retract anteriorly and posteriorly causing the scalp to gap open. These injuries typically requires suturing since they expose the underlying loose connective tissue over the pericranium of the skull opening up the possibility of infection
- ✓ Auricular group
  - ◊ Useful for entertaining at anatomy parties

Orbicularis oculi muscle—the important muscle since it forms the sphincter of the orbit

- ✓ Orbital portion—eye squenching
- ✓ Palpebral portion
  - ◊ Essential for blinking/eyelid closure
  - ◊ Essential in preventing the conjunctiva from drying out
  - ◊ Helps distribute tears across the conjunctiva sac
- ✓ Lacrimal portion—pumps tears down the lacrimal apparatus into nose Plate 78

Procerus muscle, corrugator supercilii muscle

- ✓ Can be deliberately paralyzed with botulism toxin to alleviate wrinkling
- ✓ If you were obtaining patient consent for this procedure, what important complication would you need to warn about? Hint: what do you think happens if the toxin drains into nearby muscles in this vicinity?

Nasal—mostly useful if you run in the Boston Marathon or Olympics

Oral muscles—forming a sphincter and opener to the oral cavity
- ✓ Orbicularis oris—the most important sphincter of rima oris
- ✓ Levator labii superioris muscle
- ✓ Other muscles of lesser importance—levator labii superioris alaque nasi, zygomaticus major, minor, levator anguli oris, depressor anguli oris, depressor labii inferioris, mentalis
- ✓ Risorius—the grin or grimace muscle, activated when tests are returned one way or the other

Cheek

- ✓ Buccinator—functions primarily in mastication to keep food between the teeth
- ✓ Prevents patients from looking like a hamster when they chew food, useful to babies (sucking, feeding), also called the trumpeter's muscle

Neck

- ✓ Platysma—mains the tone and beauty of the neck in youth but becomes increasingly wrinkled and droopy during the later decades of life

Cranial nerve VII—innervation of the muscles of facial expression

✓ This cranial nerve emerges from the base of the cranium at the stylomastoid foramen
✓ It passes through the parotid gland—at risk here from parotid tumors
✓ It emerges on the face as five major branches: temporal, zygomatic, buccal, mandibular, cervical

Idiopathic paralysis of CN VII (Bell's palsy) can present with the following symptoms

✓ The eye cannot be tightly closed; lower lid droops; tears overflow (epiphora)
✓ The eye cannot be blinked increasing the risk of corneal drying or infectiona, i.e., the efferent limb of the blink reflex is deficient
✓ The corner (commissure) of the mouth droops, saliva drools, the patient can't whistle, has trouble producing labial sounds, has a crooked smile from contralateral muscles that do work and are not opposed by the opposite side
✓ The affected cheek accumulates food in the vestibule because the buccinator doesn't maintain tone in the cheek
✓ Re-animation of the muscles of facial expression is possible following traumatic damage to CN VII. Surgeons place myocutaneous gracilis flaps into the affected side and reanastomose the neurovascular pedicle into nearby nerves (CN VII or CN XII) and arteries into branches of the external carotid. After a period of one year or so the nerves grow back down the perineurial sheath and the facial muscles can once again work

External eye

Connective tissue—protection for the globe

✓ Superior and inferior tarsal plates—provide stiffness to eyelids
✓ Lateral and medial palpebral (canthal) ligaments hold the eyelid aligned in correct position
✓ Orbital septum separates the anterior conjunctival sac from the posterior globe and periorbital fat

Blood supply

✓ Palpebral branches supply the eyelid structures from all vessels in the vicinity
✓ These include supraorbital artery and vein, supratrochlear, infraorbital, lacrimal, angular vein
✓ When this area is traumatized (car crash, flying ball, flying fist), ecchymosis (bruising, bleeding) is quite visible through the thin, highly distensible skin
✓ Blood also follows the pull of gravity and settles downward producing a "shiner"

Lacrimation

✓ The lacrimal gland is tucked away in the lateral superior orbital region
✓ Basal levels of secretions (tears) are swept across the conjunctival surface from lateral to medial. They function to maintain moisture levels and irrigate the conjunctival sac and retard the growth of pathogens
✓ Superior and inferior iacrimal papillae are raised bumps with centrally placed lacrimal puncta where tears enter the superior and inferior lacrimal canaliculi in the canthal area
✓ Tears (secretions) accumulate in the lacrimal sac between blinks
✓ Tears are expelled from thelacrimal sac by the action of the lacrimal portion of the orbicularis oculi muscle
✓ The nasolacrimal duct conducts tears downward to the nasal cavity where they emerge inferior to the inferior nasal conchae. This is the explanation for having a "runny nose" when your eye is irritated or when you cry

✓ The lacrimal caruncle is located in the medial canthal region. It is a bulge of mucosa with a laterally placed fold known as the plica semilunaris. This is where the "Sandman" is reputed to visit

SCALP

S—skin

✓ A common site for sebaceous cysts, basal cell carcinomas, actinic keratoses (precancerous lesions), squamous cell carcinomas, malignant melanomas since the top of the head is most often exposed to harmful UV irradiation that has a cumulative outcome on cells in the epidermis

C—connective tissue

✓ Here one finds especially dense dermis, containing fat that is loculated by vertically tethered
✓ Fibrous septa
✓ This is the level where the dermal blood vessels and nerves are located
✓ In fact this is among one of the most richly supplied vascular areas of the body. This is in marked contrast with circulatory problems found in the leg/foot region
✓ Lacerations into this level bleed profusely because the cut vessels are held open by the density of the connective tissue
✓ By contrast, in other tissues the small arteries recoil and constrict, a mechanism that naturally staunches blood loss
✓ Lacerations into this connective tissue layer nearly always require suturing
✓ Lacerations can be life-threatening due to extensive hemorrhage

A—aponeurosis

✓ Over the region of the cranial vault, this layer is termed the galea aponeurotica
✓ This facial layer is continuous with the frontalis muscle and occipitalis muscles
✓ Tension from the contraction of these muscles pulling on the galea aponeurotic causes transverse cuts into this layer to gap open. Lacerations to this layer require suturing

L—loose connective tissue

✓ This loose "areolar" tissue plane is the cleavage plane where scalping injuries occur
✓ Scalping injuries typically result when a patient's hair becomes entangled in either an industrial machine or lawnmower
✓ This tissue layer is also a danger zone where scalp infections can easily spread either laterally or penetrate through emissary veins into bone (osteomyelitis) or dural sinuses (the venous outflow pathway from the brain)

P—pericranium (periosteum)

✓ This is technically the periosteal layer of the bones of the calvarium

Parotid gland

✓ This is the largest of the salivary glands
✓ This gland originates as an outgrowth from the oral cavity
✓ It is encased in an unyielding fibrous capsule that is continuous with the deep cervical fascia in the neck

Clinical notes: The gland is often infected with viral pathogens (the mumps). This is especially painful when one moves the mandible or begins to salivate, because the fascial covering is tight and unyielding when the gland swells

Parotid duct (Stensen's duct)

✓ This outflow tract for parotid secretions passes from the horizontal anterior edge of the gland to pierce the buccinator muscle
✓ The opening of the duct empties into the vestibule of the mouth near the upper 2nd maxillary molar tooth
✓ The duct can be palpated one finger breadth beneath the zygomatic arch

Clinical notes: The duct can be severed when patients have facial lacerations such as are typical following dog bites, car wrecks, knifing wounds. The duct can be blocked by calculi (stones)

Blood supply

✓ Arterial contributions arriving from the external carotid pass through this gland and provide the fluid that is used for its secretions
  ▷ Superficial temporal artery and its branch the transverse facial artery
  ▷ Maxillary artery and many of its branches
✓ Sympathetic contributions (periarterial plexi) also arrive by this route. Thus the vasoconstriction caused by sympathetic stimulation acts to "dry up" the basal levels of parotid secretions. This is one reason why speakers experience a "cotton mouth" and why a pitcher of water is usually located near the speaker podium
✓ Venous drainage is by the retromandibular vein

Clinical notes: Tumors of the parotid gland are common, thus lymphatic drainage is important for providing patients with prognostic information. Superficial and deep parotid nodes drain into both the superficial and deep cervical nodes. These lymphatic channels accompany the internal jugular vein

Nerve supply

The parasympathetic contributions

✓ Parasympathetic neurons residing in the brainstem send presynaptic axons forward. These fibers exit the cranium through the foramen ovale and synapse on post-synaptic neurons of the otic ganglion
✓ These post-synaptic parasympathetic neurons reach the parotid gland by hitchhiking a ride along the auriculotemporal nerve (a branch of CN V_3)
✓ Parasympathetic stimulation along this pathway triggers a thin watery serous type of saliva

The sympathetic contributions

✓ Presynaptic neurons originate in the IML at the upper thoracic levels
✓ Axons from these presynaptic neurons exit the spinal cord through ventral roots and these white rami arrive in the sympathetic chain and travel upward to synapse on post-synaptic neurons in the middle cervical ganglion
✓ Axons from these post-synaptic neurons exit the ganglia as grey rami, jump ship and become periarterial plexi traveling along the external carotid branches
✓ Arteries supplying the parotid gland bring in these nerves that act to constrict blood flow and change the secretions into a more viscous, mucous-like saliva

Structures within the parotid gland

- ✓ The facial nerve passes onto the face and then fans out as a pes anserinus formation
- ✓ External carotid artery—divides into superficial temporal and maxillary arteries
- ✓ Retromandibular vein
  - ◊ Formed from the union of the superficial temporal and maxillary veins
  - ◊ Joins the post auricular vein to form the external jugular vein
  - ◊ Is superficial to the branches of the external carotid artery

1.4.2 Nasal cavities and paranasal sinuses

The nose

- ✓ The nose is the part of the respiratory tract that contains the peripheral organ of smell. It is divided into right and left nasal cavities by the nasal septum
- ✓ The nose and each nasal cavity perform the following functions:
  - ◊ Olfaction (smelling)—superior 1/3 of nasal mucosa is the olfactory area
  - ◊ Respiration (breathing)—inferior 2/3 of nasal mucosa is the respiratory area
  - ◊ Filtration of dust
  - ◊ Humidification of inspired air (accomplished by rich plexus of nasal veins)
  - ◊ Reception of secretions from the paranasal sinuses and nasolacrimal ducts

External nose

- ✓ A mainly cartilaginous projection from the face; the cartilage is covered by skin that contains many sebaceous glands
  - ◊ Root—superior angle of dorsum of nose; located between the eyes
  - ◊ Apex—"tip of nose"; farthest anterior projection of the external nose
- ✓ Nares (nostrils, anterior nasal aperture)—two piriform openings on the inferior surface of nose
- ✓ Alae ("wings of nose")—lateral boundaries of the nares
- ✓ Nasal septum—midline structure that separates nares externally and nasal cavities internally
- ✓ Vestibule—dilated area inside nares where stiff hairs (vibrissae) are located; lined by skin; extends to limen, the junction between the skin and the mucous-membrane (no vibrissae)
- ✓ Skeleton of external nose—the supporting skeleton of the nose is composed of bone and cartilage

Bony part of the external nose

- ✓ Nasal bones
- ✓ Frontal processes of maxillae
- ✓ Nasal part of the frontal bone and its nasal spine

Cartilaginous part of nose consists of five main cartilages

- ✓ Two lateral cartilages
- ✓ Two alar cartilages—U-shaped nasal cartilages that move with constriction and dilation of nares
- ✓ One septal cartilage

Nasal septum—bony and cartilaginous nasal septum that divides the chamber of the nose into two nasal cavities, composed of:

✓ Perpendicular plate of ethmoid—superior part of the nasal septum that descends from the cribiform plate and is continued superiorly as the crista galli
✓ Vomer—a thin, flat bone that forms the posteroinferior part of the nasal septum with some contributions from the nasal crests of the maxillary and palatine bones
✓ Septal cartilage—articulates with the edges of the bony septum

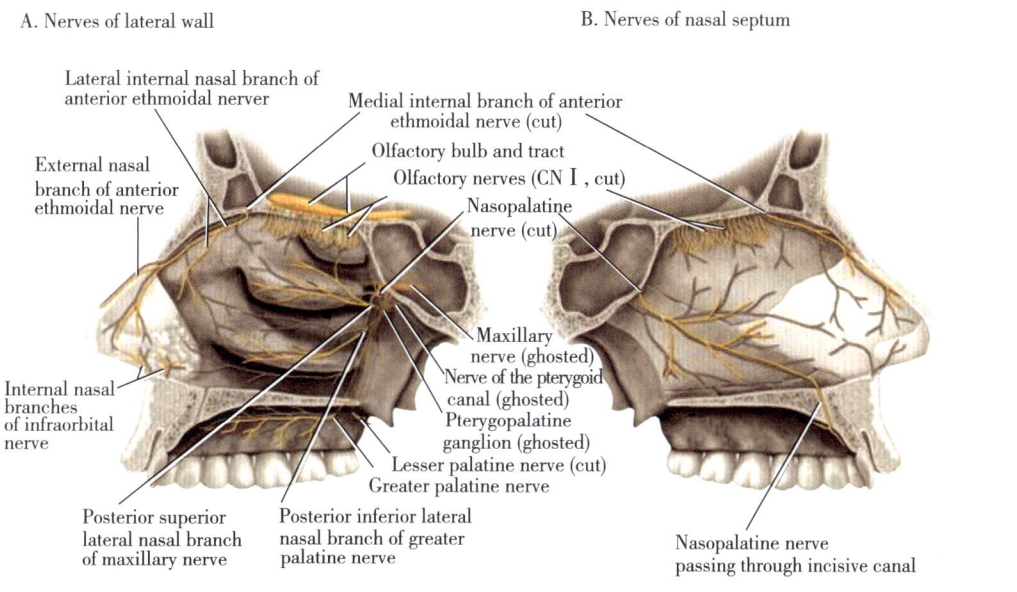

The nasal cavity

✓ It entered anteriorly through the nares and opens posteriorly into the nasopharynx through the choanae. It is lined by mucosa (except for the vestibule), which is firmly bound to the periosteum and perichondrium of the supporting bones and cartilage of the nose. The mucosa is highly vascular for heat exchange, humidification, and regulation of airflow. The inferior 2/3 of the nasal mucosa is the respiratory area and the superior 1/3 is the olfactory area, which contains the peripheral organ of smell; sniffing draws air to the area. The central processes of olfactory cells in the olfactory epithelium unite to form nerve bundles that pass through the cribiform plate and enter the olfactory bulb of the brain

Bony boundaries of the nasal cavity

✓ Roof—curved and narrow, except at its posterior end; has three components
  ◊ Frontonasal—formed by nasal spine of frontal bone and nasal bone
  ◊ Ethmoidal—formed by perpendicular cribiform plates of ethmoid bone
  ◊ Sphenoidal nasal—formed by crest of the sphenoid
✓ Floor—wider than the roof; has two components
  ◊ Palatine process of the maxilla
  ◊ Horizontal plate of the palatine bone
✓ Medial wall—nasal septum composed of perpendicular plate of ethmoid, vomer, and septal cartilage (discussed previously)
✓ Lateral wall—irregular because of three scroll-shaped elevations, the nasal conchae, that project from the lateral wall. The conchae curve inferomedially and form a roof for a groove or meatus—a passage in the nasal cavity

✓ Nasal conchae—superior, middle, and inferior conchae divide the nasal cavity into four nasal passages: the sphenoethmoidal recess, superior meatus, middle meatus, and inferior meatus
  ◊ Superior and middle nasal conchae—part of the ethmoid bone
  ◊ Inferior nasal conchae—separate bones
  ◊ Nasal meatuses—the spaces beneath the conchae; named according to the conchae lying superior to it with the exception being the sphenoethmoidal recess

Paranasal sinuses

✓ They are four air-filled extensions of the respiratory part of the nasal cavity; named according to the bones in which they reside; functions include acting as resonating chambers for the voice, warming and humidifying air, decreasing the weight of the skull, and adding contours to the face

Sphenoid sinus

✓ They located in body of sphenoid bone and may extend into the wings of this bone
✓ Vital anatomical structures in proximity—the optic nerves, the optic chiasm, the pituitary gland, the internal carotid arteries, and the cavernous sinuses
✓ Drainage—into sphenoethmoidal recess above superior nasal conchaeinnervation—posterior ethmoidal nerve (CN V_1)
✓ Arterial supply—posterior ethmoidal artery

Frontal sinus

✓ Located between outer and inner tables of the frontal bone; posterior to the superciliary arches and the root of the nose; these sinuses vary greatly in size
✓ Vital anatomical structures in proximity—depending on its size, its roof may form the floor of the orbit and its roof may form the floor of the anterior cranial fossa
✓ Drainage—via frontonasal duct into ethmoidal infundibulum, which opens into the semilunar hiatus of the middle meatus
✓ Innervation—branches of the supraorbital nerves (CN V_1)
✓ Arterial supply—supraorbital artery off ophthalmic artery

Maxillary sinus

✓ They are the largest of the paranasal sinuses; pyramid-shaped cavities occupy the body of the maxillae and its apex can extend into zygomatic bone, the base forms the inferior part of the nasal cavity, the roof is formed by the floor of the orbit, and the floor is formed by the alveolar part of the maxilla
✓ Vital anatomical structures in proximity—infraorbital nerve (CN V_2) and vessels, roots of maxillary molar teeth, and superior alveolar nerves

Clinical notes: ①Unfortunate placement of maxillary ostium (located high on the superomedial walls) leads to poor drainage. ②When maxillary molar teeth are removed, a communication between the sinus and the oral cavity may result and an infection can occur. ③The maxillary teeth and the mucosa of the maxillary sinus have the same innervation (superior alveolar nerve), so inflation of the sinus mucosa can lead to sensation of a toothache in the molar teeth
✓ Drainage—via maxillary ostium into semilunar hiatus of the middle meatus
✓ Innervation—anterior, middle, and posterior superior alveolar nerves—branches of the maxillary nerve (CN V_2)

√ Arterial supply—mainly from superior alveolar branches of the maxillary artery; branches of the greater palatine artery supply the floor of the sinus

Ethmoidal sinuses

√ They comprise several cavities; located in lateral mass of ethmoid bone between the nasal cavity and orbit. Innervated by the anterior and posterior ethmoidal branches of the nasociliary nerves.
√ Anterior ethmoidal cells—drain directly or indirectly through the ethmoidal infundibulum into the semilunar hiatus of the middle meatus
√ Middle ethmoidal cells—open directly into the middle meatus and are sometimes called "bullar cells", because they form the ethmoidal bulla, a swelling on the superior border of the semilunar hiatus
√ Posterior ethmoidal cells—open directly into the superior meatus

Sphenoethmoidal recess

√ They receives the opening of the sphenoid sinus; lying superoposterior to the superior concha

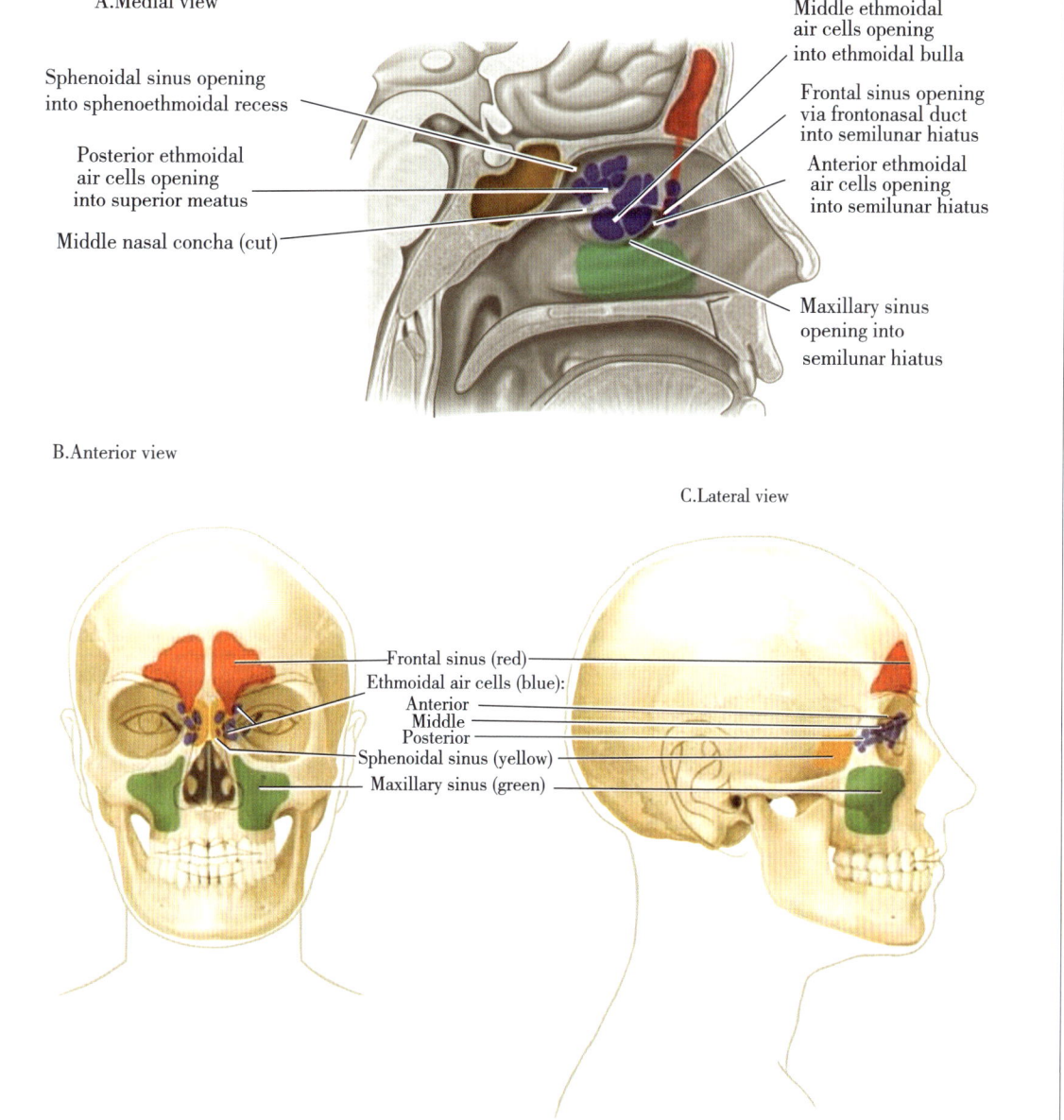

Superior meatus—receives posterior ethmoidal sinuses by one or more orifices
Middle meatus—receives the drainage from the frontal sinus (via frontonasal duct which empties into the ethmoidal infundibulum and eventually the semilunar hiatus), the anterior ethmoidal cells (via semilunar hiatus), middle ethmoidal cells (drain directly into meatus around the ethmoidal bulla), and the maxillary sinus (drains into posterior end of semilunar hiatus)
Inferior meatus—receives the nasolacrimal duct (not associated with the paranasal sinuses), which drains tears (lacrimal fluid) from the lacrimal lake, a triangular space at the medial aspect of the eye where tears collect, into the anterior part of this inferior nasal meatus. The nasolacrimal duct has a dilated superior component called the lacrimal sac. Tears enter the lacrimal sac (via the lacrimal canaliculi) and then travel to the nasal cavity, where they flow posteriorly into the nasopharynx and are swallowed
Nerves of the nasal cavity—primarily involved in general sensory information but sympathetic and parasympathetic nerves can ride on these nerves
Olfactory nerves (CN I)—concerned only with smell
✓ Arise from cells in the olfactory epithelium on superior part of the lateral and septal walls of the nasal cavity ✓ Primary bipolar neurons whose central processes pass through the cribiform plate to synapse on neurons in the olfactory bulbs (in the forebrain)
Anterior and posterior ethmoidal nerves

✓ Arise from the ophthalmic division (CN V_1) of the trigeminal nerve (CN V)
✓ Supply the anterosuperior aspect of the nasal cavity
✓ Maxillary division (CN V_2) of the trigeminal nerve (CN V)—returns from the nasal cavity by passing through the pterygopalatine fossa and entering the cranial cavity via the foramen rotundum; branches of the maxillary nerve innervate the majority of the posteroinferior aspect of the nasal cavity
   ◊ Nasopalatine nerve—supplies posteroinferior part (1/2 to 2/3) of the nasal septum before leaving nasal cavity through the sphenopalatine foramen; also passes through the incisive foramen of palate to supply mucosa of the hard palate and gingiva proper (fibrous tissue covered with mucosa located within the oral cavity)
   ◊ Greater palatine nerve—supplies posteroinferior part (1/2 to 2/3) of the lateral nasal wall via its posterolateral nasal branches (superior and inferior); also passes through the greater palatine foramen to give innervation to the hard palate

Maxillary division (CN V_2) of trigeminal nerve (CN V)—also supplies the paranasal sinuses
✓ Anterior superior alveolar nerve—a branch off the infraorbital nerve (which passes through the roof of the maxillary sinus), innervates mucosa of maxillary sinus, anterior part of inferior conchae, upper incisor teeth, and labial gingiva; runs anterolateral to the maxillary sinus ✓ Middle superior alveolar nerve—another branch off the infraorbital nerve; passes through lateral wall of maxillary sinus to provide innervation to the upper canines and premolars; innervates the maxillary sinus as well ✓ Posterior superior alveolar nerve—may be considered its own branch off the maxillary division or as a branch off the infraorbital nerve; enters the alveolar bone of the maxilla and supplies the posterior molars

✓ Greater and lesser palatine nerves—supply hard and soft palate, respectively; run in the palatine canals; lesser palatine nerve also supplies the palatine tonsil (painful during a tonsillectomy)
✓ Pharyngeal nerve—supplies nasopharynx and opening of pharyngotympanic tube

Parasympathetic and sympathetic supply of the mucosa of the nasal cavity

Parasympathetic innervation—greater petrosal nerve off the facial nerve (CN VII)

✓ Greater petrosal nerve—arises from facial nerve at the geniculate ganglion and emerges from the superior part of the petrous portion of the temporal bone to enter the middle cranial fossa→joins its travel partner the deep petrosal nerve (at the foramen lacerum)→together they travel through the pterygoid canal (forming the nerve of the pterygoid canal) and enter the pterygopalatine fossa to synapse on the pterygopalatine ganglion → postsynaptic axons (secretomotor functions) travel on branches of the maxillary division of the trigeminal nerve ($CN\ V_2$) to the nasal mucosa, sinus mucosa, and also along zygomatic branches to the lacrimal nerve of ophthalmic nerve ($CN\ V_1$) to the lacrimal gland

Sympathetic innervation—follows the deep petrosal nerve (from the internal carotid periarterial plexus)

✓ Deep petrosal nerve—postsynaptic sympathetic fibers from the superior cervical ganglion that travel along with the internal carotid artery and coalesce to form this nerve→joins its travel partner the greater petrosal nerve (at the foramen lacerum)→together they travel through the pterygoid canal (forming the nerve of the pterygoid canal) and enter the pterygopalatine fossa → distributed with the arteries that supply the nasal cavity and paranasal sinuses

Blood supply to the nasal cavity

✓ Five arteries supply nasal cavity on each side; there is a prominent anastomoses on the anterior part of the nasal septum (kiesselbach's area)

Clinical notes: All five arteries supplying the nasal mucosa contribute to epistaxis (nosebleeds); the cavernous type of nasal mucosa can result in severe bleeding in patients with coagulation anomalies or severe hypertension. The "take home message" is don't palpate your nasal cavity

✓ Sphenopalatine artery (from maxillary artery)—supplies the largest amount of blood to the nasal cavity
　◊ Posterior lateral nasal artery
　◊ Posterior septal branches—travels toward the incisive canal and anastomoses with the greater palatine artery
✓ Posterior ethmoidal artery (off the ophthalmic artery)—with septal and lateral nasal branches
✓ Anterior ethmoidal arteries (off the ophthalmic artery)
　◊ Anterior septal branches
　◊ Anterior lateral nasal artery
　◊ External nasal nasal branch—travels anteriorly on external nose; in between the nasal bone and lateral process of septal nasal cartilage
✓ Greater palatine artery—anastomoses with the posterior septal branch of sphenopalatine artery in proximity to the incisive canal

Branches of the facial artery

✓ Lateral nasal artery—alar branches
✓ Superior labial artery—nasal septal branches

The pterygopalatine fossa—a small space with the shape of an inverted pyramid that resides inferior to the apex of the orbit

Boundaries

- ✓ Anterior—posterior border of maxilla
- ✓ Lateral (no distinct wall)—pterygomaxillary fissure
- ✓ Posterior—pterygoid process of the sphenoid bone
- ✓ Medial (incomplete)—vertical plate of the palatine bone and sphenopalatine foramen
- ✓ Roof (incomplete)—greater wing of the sphenoid bone and inferior orbital fissure
- ✓ Floor—pyramidal process of the palatine bone

Contents

- ✓ Terminal portion (the 3rd part or pterygopalatine part) of the maxillary artery
- ✓ Nerve of the pterygoid canal
- ✓ Maxillary nerve (CN V_2 and its branches)
- ✓ Pterygopalatine ganglion

Communications—the pterygopalatine fossa communicates:

- ✓ Laterally—with the infratemporal fossa through the pterygomaxillary fissure
- ✓ Medially—with the nasal cavity through the sphenopalatine foramen
- ✓ Anterosuperiorly—with the orbit through the inferior orbital fissure
- ✓ Posterosuperiorly—with the middle cranial fossa through the foramen rotundum and pterygoid canal

Pterygopalatine (or 3rd) part of maxillary artery

- ✓ Passes through the pterygomaxillary fissure and enters the pterygopalatine fossa. This artery lies anterior to the pterygopalatine ganglion. This artery gives off several branches that follow the nerves in the region (with the same name)
- ✓ Posterior superior alveolar artery
- ✓ Descending palatine artery, which divides into the greater and lesser palatine arteries
- ✓ Artery of the pterygoid canal
- ✓ Sphenopalatine artery (from maxillary artery)—supplies the largest amount of blood to the nasal cavity (as discussed earlier)

Posterior lateral nasal artery

- ✓ Posterior septal branches—travels toward the incisive canal and anastomoses with the greater palatine artery
- ✓ Infraorbital artery—gives rise to the anterior superior alveolar artery and terminates as branches to the lower eyelid, upper lip, and nose. Note: as the maxillary nerve leaves the pterygopalatine fossa through the inferior orbital fissure, its name changes to the infraorbital nerve

Clinical note 1: Rhinitis—inflammation and swelling of the nasal mucosa during upper respiratory infections and allergic reactions due to increased vascularity; clinically significant as infections may spread to the anterior cranial fossa (via the cribiform plate), nasopharynx and retropharyngeal soft tissues, the middle ear (via the pharyngotympanic tube), paranasal sinuses (discussed previously), and lacrimal apparatus and conjunctiva

Clinical note 2: Sinusitis—inflammation and swelling of the mucosa of the paranasal sinuses often due to infection reaching the sinuses via the nasal cavity; sinusitis may block one or more opening of the sinuses causing improper drainage; this condition is particularly clinically significant in the ethmoidal sinuses where infections may break through the fragile medial wall of the orbit leading to blindness; the posterior ethmoidal cells lie in close proximity to the optic canal which houses the optic nerve and ophthalmic artery. Infection from these cells could also affect the dural nerve sheath of the optic nerve, a condition known as optic neuritis

Clinical note 3: Cerebrospinal fluid (CSF) rhinorrhea—a clear nasal discharge after a head injury. CSF rhinorrhea results from a fracture of the cribiform plate, tearing of the cranial meninges, and leakage of CSF from the nose

1.4.3 Mouth, palate and tongue

The lips

- ✓ Covered externally by skin and internally by a mucous membrane.
- ✓ Between these 2 layers are:
  - ◊ A circular sphincter muscle—the orbicularis oris muscle
  - ◊ Labial arteries
  - ◊ Labial salivary glands
  - ◊ Labial frenulum
  - ◊ Nasolabial sulcus
  - ◊ Mentolabial sulcus
  - ◊ Philtrum (love charm)

Sensory nerves of the lips

- ✓ To the upper lip—infraorbital nerve (CN V_2)
- ✓ To the lower lip—mental nerve (CN V_3)

Lymph vessels from the lips drain into the submandibular lymph nodes then onward into the deep cervical chain of lymph nodes

- ✓ Pustules in the vicinity of the upper lip are potentially dangerous (in the danger area of the face), because the infection may extend intracranially by draining through the superior labial vein, angular vein, superior ophthalmic vein to enter the cavernous sinus
- ✓ Carcinoma of the lip accounts for about 15% of all head and neck malignancies
- ✓ This is mainly due to its vulnerability for exposure to ultraviolet radiation
- ✓ The lips are important for maintaining an anterior seal during swallowing
- ✓ The lips are also important for producing certain sounds made during speech

The mouth

- ✓ An organ of digestion, speech, respiration, expression and sensation
- ✓ Rima oris is surrounded by the orbicularis oris muscle, the most superior sphincter of the gastrointestinal tract

Regional Anatomy

✓ The mouth consists of two parts separated by the teeth and alveolar processes of the mandible and maxilla

✓ With the mouth closed, the two parts communicate with each other on each side

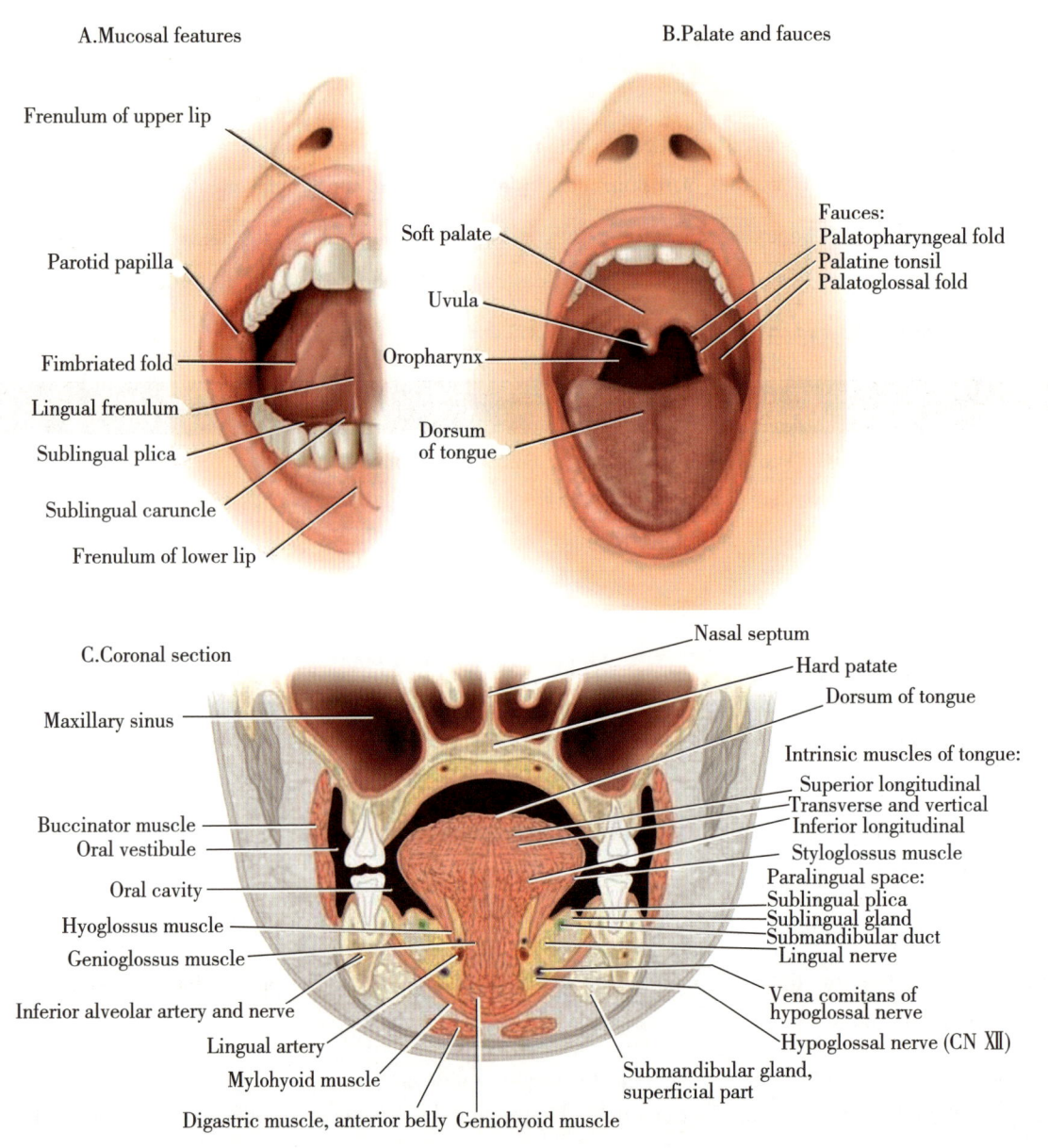

Vestibule

✓ Slit-like space between the lips and cheeks and the teeth and gingivae

✓ Features
  ◊ Superior and inferior labial frenula (can cause problems with dentures)
  ◊ Duct of parotid gland opens here (opposite the 2nd upper molar)

Oral cavity proper

Boundaries of this cavity are as follows:

✓ It is limited antero-laterally by the teeth and gums

- ✓ The roof is formed by the hard and soft palate
- ✓ The tongue rises from its floor
- ✓ The oral cavity communicates with the oropharynx posteriorly via the isthmus of the fauces

The gingivae

- ✓ Are composed of fibrous tissue that are covered with mucous membrane
- ✓ Are firmly attached to the margins of the alveolar processes (tooth sockets) of the mandible and maxilla and to the teeth
- ✓ Nerve supply
  - ◊ Alveolar nerves give branches that run up through the roots of each tooth and these also supply the gingivae in the vicinity
  - ◊ These sensory nerves include the buccal nerve, superior anterior, middle and posterior alveolar nerves, the greater palatine nerve, nasopalatine nerve, mental nerve
- ✓ Gingivitis—inflammation of the gums
- ✓ Periodontitis—inflammation and destruction of alveolar bone and periodontal ligament, often leads to tooth loss

The dentition

- ✓ Ten deciduous teeth (primary or milk teeth buds) begin to develop in the mandible before birth
- ✓ The first tooth usually erupts at 6-8 months after birth and the last deciduous tooth by 20-24 months of age. This teething stage is accompanied by inflammation, fever, fussiness
- ✓ The deciduous teeth are usually shed between 6 and 12 years of age and are replaced by permanent teeth
- ✓ Eruption of the permanent teeth (normally 16 in each jaw) is usually complete by 18, except for the third molars ("wisdom teeth")
- ✓ If teeth are malpositioned and/or impacted, they may not erupt
- ✓ Each tooth
  - ◊ Consists of 3 parts: crown, neck, root
  - ◊ Is fixed in the alveolus (tooth socket) by a fibrous periodontal ligament
  - ◊ The root number varies among the different types of teeth
  - ◊ Incisors, canines have a single root
  - ◊ Maxillary molars have 3 roots—one might suppose that they resist gravity better
  - ◊ Mandibular molars have 2 roots
- ✓ Types of teeth
  - ◊ Incisors or "cutters"—4
  - ◊ Canines or "piercers—2
  - ◊ Premolars—4
  - ◊ Molars or "grinders"—6
- ✓ Structure of a tooth
  - ◊ Composed of dentin
  - ◊ Covered by enamel over the crown and cementum over the root
  - ◊ A pulp cavity contains connective tissue, blood vessels, nerves. It is continuous with periodontal tissue through the root canal at the apical foramen

◊ Root canals transmit the nerves and vessels to and from the pulp cavity
✓ Surfaces of the teeth
　◊ Incisor and canine teeth have lingual and labial surfaces
　◊ Premolar and molar teeth have buccal, lingual and occlusal surfaces
✓ Vessels that nourish the teeth
　◊ Maxillary artery (anterior, middle, posterior superior alveolar branches)
　◊ Inferior alveolar artery
　◊ Veins accompany the arteries and drain into the pterygoid venous plexus
　◊ Lymph vessels pass mainly to the submandibular lymph nodes
✓ Innervation to the teeth
　◊ Maxillary division of CN V_2 supplies the maxillary dentition
　◊ Inferior alveolar nerve (from the CN V_3 supplies the dentition on the mandible
✓ Clinical conditions
　◊ Cavities (caries)
　　◆ If untreated, invasion of the pulp of the tooth eventually results in infection and irritation of the pulp cavity leading to a toothache—swollen pulp tissue
　　◆ If untreated, small vessels in the root canal may die owing to pressure and the infected material may pass through the apical foramen into the periodontal tissues resulting in an abscess necessitating tooth extraction
　　◆ A root canal or endodontic procedure is the ablation of the nerve to the tooth

The palate

✓ Forms the arched roof of the mouth and the floor of the nasal cavities
✓ It functions to separate the oral cavity from the nasal cavities and the nasopharynx

Hard palate

✓ Formed by the palatine processes of the maxillae and horizontal plates of palatine bones
✓ Bounded by the alveolar processes and the gingivae
✓ Posteriorly it is continuous with the soft palate
✓ The incisive foramen is the opening of the incisive canal which transmits
✓ The nasopalatine nerve
✓ The terminal branch of the sphenopalatine artery
✓ Greater palatine foramen is one opening of the palatine canal which transmits
✓ The greater palatine vessels and nerve from CN V_2 that contains components for general sensation, parasympathetics, sympathetics
✓ Lesser palatine foramen is another opening of the palatine canal which transmits
✓ The lesser palatine vessels and nerves to the soft palate containing components from CN V_2 for general sensation, parasympathetics, sympthetics
✓ The hard palate is covered by a mucous membrane that is intimately connected to the periosteum—a mucoperiostium
　◊ Deep to the membrane are mucus-secreting palatine glands
　◊ The anterior mucous membrane has 3-4 transverse palatine folds

Soft palate

- ✓ Has no bony framework but contains a membranous aponeurosis
- ✓ This palatine aponeurosis is formed by the expanded tendon of the tensor veli palatini muscle
- ✓ At rest:
  - ◊ The soft tissues hang from the posterior aspect of the palate into the cavity of the pharynx
  - ◊ This entity separates the nasopharynx superiorly from more inferior oropharynx
- ✓ During swallowing, the soft palate moves posteriorly against the wall of the pharynx, thereby preventing regurgitation of the food into the nasal cavities
- ✓ This is the posterior velopharnygeal seal
- ✓ Laterally it is continuous with the wall of the pharynx and is joined to the tongue and pharynx by the palatoglossal and palatopharyngeal arches
- ✓ If this seal is incompetent, food and liquids will pass into the nasopharynx during swallowing
- ✓ If this seal is incompetent or the muscles are spastic or the child is mentally deficient, unusual speech patterns will develop when the child tries to make certain sounds
- ✓ Palatine tonsil this 2nd arch pouch becomes invaded by lymphocytes
- ✓ It is located between the anterior and posterior pillars of the fauces
- ✓ Deep to the palatal mucosa are mucous glands

Five pairs of muscles control palatal and tongue movements

Levator veli palatini muscles

- ✓ Originate from the cartilage of the auditory tube and petrous part of temporal bone
- ✓ They insert into the palatine aponeurosis and decussate to the opposite side
- ✓ The are innervated by CN X via the pharyngeal plexus
- ✓ These muscles elevate the soft palate drawing it superiorly and posteriorly during swallowing and yawning
- ✓ They also manipulate the cartilaginous portions of the auditory tube to assist the tensor veli palatini muscles in equalizing air pressure in the middle ear and pharynx

Tensor veli palatini muscles

- ✓ Originates from the scaphoid fossa of the medial pterygoid plate, the sphenoid spine and auditory tube
- ✓ As it passes inferiorly, the tendon of this muscle hooks around the hamulus of the medial pterygoid plate before inserting into the palatine aponeurosis
- ✓ Its innervation as a 1st arch muscle is the mandibular division of CN V_3
- ✓ It tenses the soft palate by using the hamulus as a pulley, and it also pulls the membraneous portion of the auditory tube open to equalize air pressure by allowing air to pass from the nasopharynx backward into the middle ear cavity

Palatoglossus muscles

- ✓ Originates from the palatine aponeurosis
- ✓ Inserts into the lateral portion of the tongue musculature
- ✓ Forms the anterior pillar of the tonsilar fossa
- ✓ Is innervated by cranial part of CN XI through the pharyngeal branch of CN X
- ✓ Elevates the posterior part of tongue and draws the soft palate closer to the tongue and closes off the oral cavity from the oropharynx

Palatopharyngeus muscles

✓ Originates from hard palate and palatine aponeurosis
✓ Inserts into lateral wall of pharynx
✓ Forms the posterior pillar of the tonsillar fossa
✓ Innervated by cranial part of CN XI through the pharyngeal branch of CN X
✓ Tenses the soft palate and pulls the pharynx walls superiorly, anteriorly and medially during swallowing

Musculus uvulae muscles

✓ Originates from the posterior nasal spine and the palatine aponeurosis
✓ Inserts into the mucosa of the uvula
✓ Innervated by the cranial part of CN XI through the pharyngeal branch of CN X
✓ Shortens the uvula and elevates it thus assisting in closing the nasopharynx during swallowing and during phonation

Nerves of the palate

✓ Greater palatine nerve
✓ Lesser palatine nerve
✓ Nasopalatine nerve

Vessels of the palate

✓ Maxillary artery
✓ Greater palatine artery
✓ Lesser palatine artery

The tongue—is the only organ supplied by 5 cranial nerves

Features

✓ Radix (root) and corpus (body)
✓ Its mobility is enhanced by its suspension from 3 bilateral attachments: the mandible, styloid processes and hyoid bone
✓ It is a muscular organ
✓ It functions in mastication, speech, swallowing, and tasting
✓ It has a complex embryological origin thus its innervation is complex

Gross features

✓ Sulcus terminalis
✓ Foramen cecum
✓ Circumvallate papillae
✓ Oral part of tongue
  ◊ Is freely movable
  ◊ Is loosely attached to the floor of the mouth by the lingual frenulum
  ◊ On each side of the frenulum one can observe a visible blue line—deep lingual veins
  ◊ These are particularly useful for rapid absorption of certain cardiac medications
  ◊ Lingual papillae and taste buds are located on the superior surface

✓ Pharyngeal part
  ◊ Lies posterior to the sulcus terminalis and palatoglossal arches
  ◊ Has no papillae
  ◊ Has underlying lymphoid tissue (lingual tonsils that help to complete the circular ring of lymphoid tissue known as waldeyer's ring)

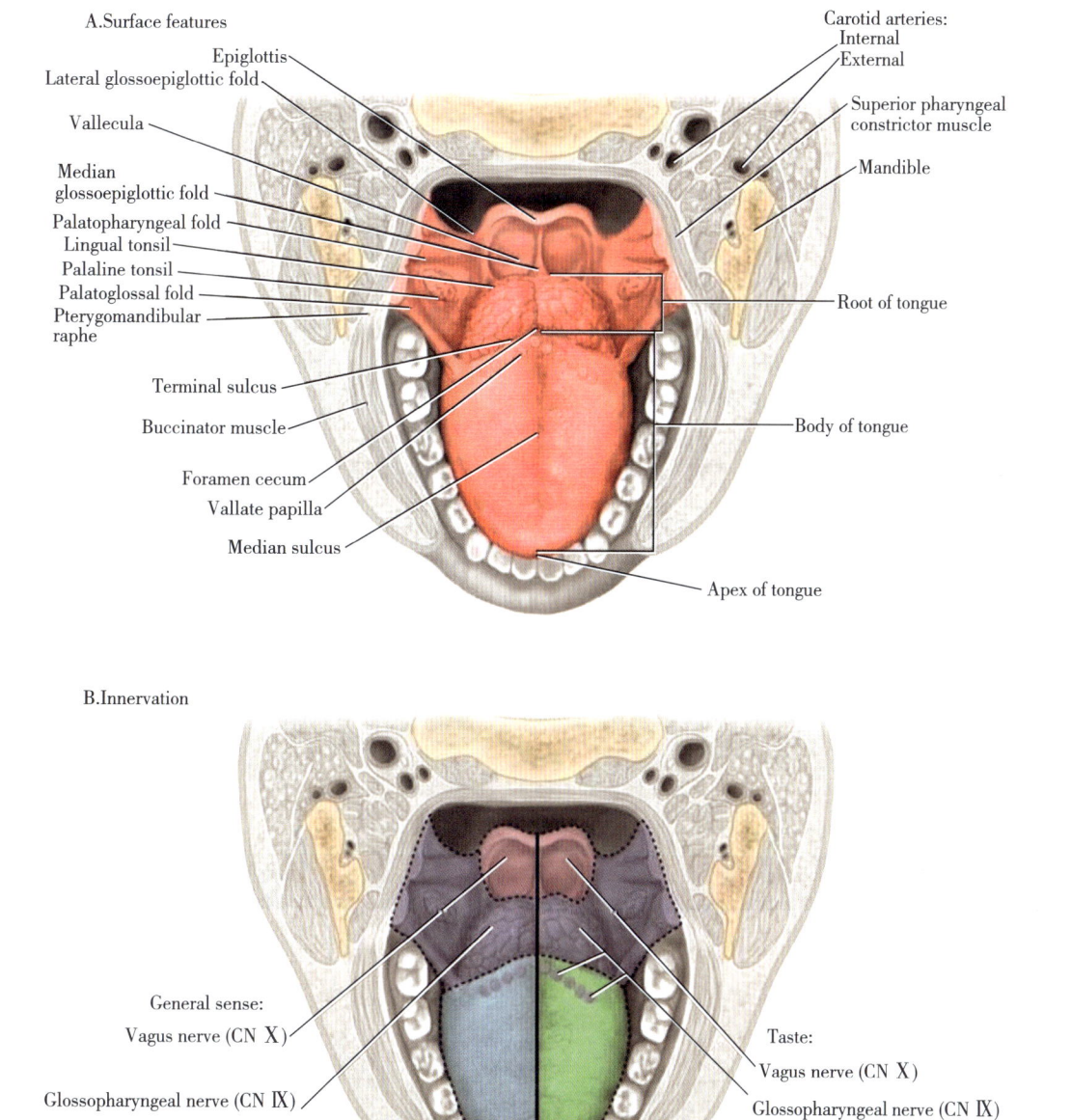

Clinical conditions

✓ The oral part of the tongue may be touched without discomfort but when the pharyngeal part is touched, the patient may gags and experience nausea
✓ Ankyloglossia (tongue-tie) occurs when the frenulum of infants extends almost to the tip of the tongue interfering with protrusion
✓ Macroglossia or microglossia are other conditions associated with breathing or speech problems

Tongue musculature

✓ All of the lingual muscles are innervated by CN XII except the palatoglossus (CN X)
✓ The tongue contains no rigid skeletal parts but is suspended in position by four pairs of muscles

Extrinsic muscles

✓ Originate outside the tongue and attach (suspend) this organ
✓ They mainly act to move the tongue, but they can alter the shape as well
✓ Below the tongue is a mobile diaphragm formed by the mylohyoid muscles
✓ Genioglossus muscles
  ◊ Originate on the superior mental spine of the mandible
  ◊ They fans out as they enters the tongue inferiorly with the most inferior fibers inserting into the body of the hyoid bone
  ◊ They depress the tongue and the posterior part functions to protrude the tongue
✓ Hyoglossus muscles
  ◊ Arise from the body and greater horn of hyoid bone
  ◊ Insert into the side and inferior aspect of the tongue
  ◊ They depress the tongue, pulling its sides inferiorly and they also aid in retrusion
✓ Styloglossus muscles
  ◊ Arise from the anterior border of the styloid process and from stylohyoid ligament
  ◊ They pass inferoanteriorly to insert into the side and inferior aspect of the tongue
  ◊ They retrude the tongue and curl its sides to create a trough during swallowing
✓ Palatoglossus muscles

Intrinsic muscles

✓ Superior and inferior longitudinal muscles—involved in shortening and thickening the tongue
✓ Transverse muscle group—narrows and increases the height of the tongue
✓ Vertical muscle group—flattens and broadens the tongue

Tongue innervation

Hypoglossal nerve

✓ Is the motor nerve of the tongue to all "glossus" muscles except palatoglossus muscle
✓ Sectioning of this nerve as typically occurs during traumatic injuries, results in paralysis and atrophy of one side of the tongue
✓ The tongue will then deviates to the side of the lesion during protrusion because of the action of the unopposed genioglossus muscle of the other side (so asking patients to stick out their tongue is a motor test for CN XII)
  ◊ Vagus nerve supplies the palatoglossus muscle
  ◊ Lingual nerve
✓ Conducts general sensations from the anterior 2/3 of the tongue
✓ Carries taste fibers supplied through the chorda tympani (from CN VII)
✓ Carries parasympathetic secretomotor fibers to the major and minor salivary glands (exception: the parotid gland receives its fibers from CN IX)

Glossopharyngeal nerve
✓ Conducts general sensations from the posterior 1/3 of the tongue ✓ Conducts special (taste) sensations from the posterior 1/3 of the tongue ✓ Supplies innervation to the stylopharngeus muscle on its course toward the tongue
Arterial supply to the tongue
✓ Lingual artery branch from the external carotid artery
Venous drainage of the tongue
✓ Two lingual veins accompany the artery ✓ Deep lingual veins ✓ Vena comitans nervi hypoglossi ✓ When quick absorption of a drug is desired, place it under the tongue where it dissolves and enters the deep lingual veins in less than a minute
Lymphatic drainage of the tongue (takes one of four possible routes)
✓ Tip of tongue—submental nodes ✓ Lateral aspects of the anterior 2/3—submandibular nodes to the deep cervical nodes ✓ Medial part of the anterior 2/3—inferior deep cervical nodes ✓ Posterior 1/3—superior deep cervical nodes on both sides ✓ Malignant tumors in the posterior 1/3 metastasize to the superior deep cervical lymph nodes whereas tumors in the anterior 2/3 metastasiz

1.4.4 Larynx

Larynx

✓ The viscera of the respiratory layer, the larynx and trachea, contribute to the respiratory function of the body
✓ The larynx is the complex organ of voice production composed of nine cartilages connected by membranes and ligaments and containing the vocal folds
✓ The main functions of the respiratory layer
    ◊ Routing air and food into the respiratory tract and esophagus respectively
    ◊ Providing a patent airway, and a means for sealing it off temporarily
    ◊ Producing voice
✓ Trachea—extends from the larynx (C_7) into the thorax and divides into the right and left main bronchi. It transports air to and from the lungs, and its epithelium propels debris-laden mucus toward the pharynx for expulsion from the mouth
✓ Larynx—located in the anterior neck at the level of the bodies of the C_3–C_6 vertebra. The larynx is the phonating mechanism designed for voice production (vocalization) and connects the inferior part of the oropharynx with the trachea. It also guards the air passages, especially during swallowing and maintains a patent airway

Laryngeal skeleton

✓ The laryngeal skeleton consists of nine cartilages joined by ligaments and membranes. Three cartilages are single—thyroid, cricoid and epiglottic and three are paired—arytenoids, corniculate and cuneiform
✓ Hyaline cartilage—thyroid, cricoid and arytenoids (bodies)
✓ Elastic cartilage—epiglottic, arytenoids (tips), corniculate and cuneiform
✓ Clinical—laryngeal fractures (contact sports, boxing, basketball, hockey)

Thyroid cartilage

✓ Largest of the cartilages
✓ Inferior 2/3 of its two platelike lamina fuse anteriorly in the median plane to form the laryngeal prominence ("Adams apple")
  ◊ 90 angle in males
  ◊ 120 angle in females
✓ Superior to this promience, the lamina diverge to form a V-shaped superior thyroid notch
✓ The posterior border of each lamina projects superiorly as the superior horn and inferiorly as the inferior horn
✓ 4th pharyngeal arch derivative
✓ Thyrohyoid membrane—superior border and superior horns attach to the hyoid bone
  ◊ Median thyrohyoid ligament—thick, median part
  ◊ Lateral thyrohyoid ligament
  ◊ Cricothyroid joints—the inferior horns articulate with the lateral surfaces of the cricoid cartilage at the cricothyroid joints (main movements are rotation and gliding of the thyroid cartilage which results in changes is the length of the vocal folds)
  ◊ Oblique line—attachments of sternothyroid and thyrohoid muscles

Cricoid cartilage

✓ Is shaped like a signet ring with its band facing anteriorly—the ringlike opening fits an average finger
✓ The posterior (signet) part of the cricoid is the lamina
✓ The anterior band is the arch
✓ Thicker and stronger than the thyroid cartilage—only complete ring of cartilage to encircle any part of the airway
✓ Attaches to the inferior thyroid cartilage by the median cricothyroid ligament
✓ Attaches to the 1st tracheal ring by the cricotracheal ligament
✓ 6th laryngeal arch derivative

Arytenoid cartilage

✓ Pairs of three-sided pyramids that articulate with the lateral parts of the superior border of the cricoid cartilage lamina
✓ Apex—superiorly
✓ Vocal process anteriorly—provides the posterior attachment to the vocal ligament
✓ Large muscular process—projects laterally from its base—serves as a lever to which the posterior and lateral cricoarytenoid muscles are attached

- ✓ The apex bears the corniculate cartilage
- ✓ 6th laryngeal arch derivative

Corniculate cartilage

- ✓ Located on the apex of the arytenoid cartilage
- ✓ Small nodules in the posterior part of the aryepiglottic fold
- ✓ 6th pharyngeal arch derivative

Cuneiform cartilage

- ✓ 6th laryngeal arch derivative
- ✓ Small nodules in the posterior part of the aryepiglottic folds
- ✓ Do not directly attach to other cartilages

Epiglottic cartilage

- ✓ Elastic cartilage—gives flexibility to the epiglottis, heart-shaped covered with mucous membrane
- ✓ Located posterior to the root of the tongue and the hyoid bone
- ✓ Located anterior to the laryngeal inlet
- ✓ Forms the superior part of the anterior wall and the superior margin of the laryngeal inlet
- ✓ Broad superior end is free
- ✓ Tapered inferior end (stalk) is attached to the angle formed by the thyroid laminae—thyroepiglottic ligament
- ✓ Hyoepiglottic ligament—attaches the anterior surface of the epiglottis to the hyoid bone
- ✓ Quadrangular ligament—thin, submucosal sheet of CT that extends between the lateral aspects of the arytenoid and epiglottic cartilages
    - ◊ Its free margin constitutes the vestibular ligament which is covered loosely by the vestibular fold
    - ◊ This fold lies superior to the vocal fold and extends from the thyroid cartilage to the arytenoid cartilage
    - ◊ The free superior margin of the quadrangular membrane forms the aryepiglottic ligament which is covered with mucosa to form the aryepiglottic fold

Cricoarytenoid joints, vocal folds and conus elasticus

Cricoarytenoid joints

- ✓ Between the bases of the arytenoids cartilages and the superolateral surfaces of the lamina of the cricoid cartilage
- ✓ Permits the arytenoids cartilages to slide toward or away from one another, to tilt anteriorly and posteriorly and to rotate
- ✓ These movements are important in approximating, tensing and relaxing the vocal folds

Vocal folds

- ✓ Extends from the junction of the lamina of the thyroid cartilage anteriorly to the vocal process of the arytenoid cartilage posteriorly
- ✓ Vocal ligament forms the skeleton of the vocal fold
- ✓ It is the thickened, free superior border of the lateral cricothyroid ligament (part of the conus elasticus)
- ✓ It blends anteriorly with the median cricothyroid ligament

Conus elasticus (conus elastus)

- ✓ Lower attachment—arch of the cricoid ligament from one arytenoid articular facet to the other
- ✓ Median part—median cricothyroid ligament
- ✓ Paired lateral parts—elastic vocal ligaments—supporting ligaments of vocal folds (free superior border of the lateral cricothyroid ligament)

Interior of the larynx

- ✓ The laryngeal cavity extends from the laryngeal inlet, through which it communicates with the laryngopharynx, to the level of the inferior border of the cricoid cartilage where it is continuous with the cavity of the trachea
- ✓ The laryngeal cavity is divided into three parts:
  - ◊ Vestibule of the larynx—superior to the vestibular folds (false vocal folds)
  - ◊ Ventricle of the larynx (laryngeal sinus)—between the vestibular folds and superior to the vocal folds
  - ◊ Infraglottic cavity—the inferior cavity of the larynx extending from the vocal folds to the inferior border of the cricoid cartilage

Vocal folds (true vocal folds)—control sound production

- ✓ The apex of each wedge-shaped fold projects medially into the laryngeal cavity
- ✓ Each vocal fold has:
  - ◊ Vocal ligament—thickened elastic tissue is the medial free edge of the lateral cricothyroid ligament
  - ◊ Vocalis (vocal) muscle—exceptionally fine muscle fibers that form the most medial part of the thyroarytenoid muscle
- ✓ The vocal folds are the source of the sounds that come from the larynx; produce audible vibrations when their free margins are closely—but not tightly—opposed during phonation and air is forcibly expired intermittently
- ✓ The vocal folds also serve as the main inspiratory sphincter of the larynx when they are tightly closed—complete adduction of the folds forms an effective sphincter that prevents entry of air

Glottis—vocal apparatus of the larynx

- ✓ Vocal folds
- ✓ Vocal processes
- ✓ Rima glottis—aperture between the vocal folds
- ✓ Shape of the rima
  - ◊ Ordinary breathing—narrow and wedge-shaped
  - ◊ Forced respiration—wide and kite-shaped
  - ◊ During phonation—rima is slit-like when the vocal folds are approximated
- ✓ Variation in the tension and length of the vocal folds, in the width of the rima glottis and in the intensity of the expiratory effort produces changes in the pitch of the voice
- ✓ The lower pitch of the voice of postpubertal males results from the greater length of the vocal folds

Vestibular folds (false vocal folds)

- ✓ Extend between the thyroid and arytenoids cartilages
- ✓ Play little or no part in voice production

- ✓ They are protective in function
- ✓ Consist of two thick folds of mucous membrane enclosing the vestibular ligaments
- ✓ The space between these ligaments is the rima vestibuli
- ✓ The lateral indentations between the vocal and vestibular folds is the ventricle of the larynx

Laryngeal muscles

- ✓ Extrinsic laryngeal muscles
  - ◊ Infrahyoid muscles—depress hyoid bone and larynx
  - ◊ Suprahyoid and stylopharyngeus muscles—elevators of the hyoid bone and larynx
- ✓ Intrinsic laryngeal muscles—move the laryngeal parts—alter the length and tension of the vocal folds and the size/shape of the rima glottis
  - ◊ All but one (cricothyroid muscle) of the intrinsic laryngeal muscles are innervated by the recurrent laryngeal nerve (CN X)
  - ◊ The cricothyroid muscle is innervated by the external laryngeal nerve (superior laryngeal nerve)
  - ◊ The actions of the intrinsic laryngeal muscles are easiest to understand when they are considered as functional groups: sphincters, adductors and abductors, and tensors and relaxers

Adductors and abductors—muscles move the vocal folds to open and close the rima glottides

Adductors

- ✓ The principal adductors are the lateral cricoarytenoid muscles which pull the muscular processes anteriorly, rotating the arytenoids so that their vocal processes swing medially
- ✓ When this action is combined with that of the transverse arytenoid muscles, they pull the arytenoids cartilages together, air pushed through the rima glottidis causes vibrations of the vocal ligaments (phonation)
- ✓ When the vocal ligaments are adducted but the transverse arytenoids do not act, allowing the arytenoids cartilages to remain apart, air may bypass the ligaments—position of whispering, when the breath is modified into voice in the absence of tone

Lateral cricoarytenoid

- ✓ Origin—arch of cricoid cartilage
- ✓ Insertion—muscular process of arytenoid cartilage

Transverse arytenoid

- ✓ Origin—one arytenoid cartilage
- ✓ Insertion—opposite arytenoid cartilage

Abductors—sole abductors are the posterior cricoarytenoid muscles

- ✓ Pull the muscular processes posteriorly, rotating the vocal processes laterally, thus widening the rima glottides

Posterior cricoarytenoid

- ✓ Origin—posterior surface of the lamina of the cricoid cartilage
- ✓ Insertion—muscular process of arytenoid cartilage

Sphincters

- ✓ The combined actions of most of the muscles of the laryngeal inlet result in sphincteric action that closes the inlet as a protective mechanism during swallowing
- ✓ Contraction of the lateral cricoarytenoids, transverse and oblique arytenoids and aryepiglottic muscles brings the aryepiglottic folds together and pulls the arytenoids cartilages toward the epiglottis
- ✓ Oblique arytenoids
  - ◊ Origin—vocal process of arytenoid cartilage
  - ◊ Insertion—opposite arytenoid cartilage

Tensors—the principal tensors are the cricthyroid muscles which tilt or pull the prominence or angle of the thyroid cartilage anteriorly and inferiorly toward the arch of the cricoid cartilage

- ✓ Increasing the distance between the thyroid prominence and arytenoid cartilages
- ✓ Because the anterior ends of the vocal ligaments attach to the posterior aspect of the prominence, the vocal ligaments elongate and tighten, raising the pitch of the voice
- ✓ Cricothyroid muscle
  - ◊ Origin—anterolateral part of the cricoid cartilage
  - ◊ Insertion—inferior margin and inferior horm of thyoid cartilage
  - ◊ Innervation—external laryngeal nerve

Relaxers—principal relaxers are the thyroarytenoid muscles which pull the arytenoid cartilages anteriorly, toward the thyroid prominence, thereby relaxing the vocal ligaments

- ✓ Thyroarytenoid muscle
  - ◊ Origin—posterior surface of thyroid cartilage
  - ◊ Insertion—muscular process of arytenoid cartilage
- ✓ Vocalis muscles—produce minute adjustments of the vocal ligaments, selectively tensing and relaxing parts of the vocal folds during animated speech and singing
  - ◊ Origin—vocal process of arytenoid cartilage
  - ◊ Insertion—vocal ligaments
- ✓ Aryepiglottic muscles—transverse and oblique arytenoids

Arteries of the larynx

Superior laryngeal artery

- ✓ Branch of the superior thyroid artery (ECA)
- ✓ Accompanies the superior laryngeal nerve through the thyrohyoid membrane
- ✓ Supplies the internal surface of the larynx

Inferior laryngeal artery

- ✓ Branch of the inferior thyroid artery (thyrocervical trunk)
- ✓ Accompanies the inferior laryngeal nerve
- ✓ Supplies the mucous membrane and muscles in the inferior part of the larynx

Nerves (CN X)

Superior laryngeal nerve

- ✓ Arises from the inferior vagal ganglion at the superior end of the carotid triangle

- ✓ Divides into two terminal branches within the carotid sheath:
  - ⬦ Internal branch—sensory and autonomic
  - ⬦ External branch—motor to cricothyroid
    - ◆ Supplies inferior constrictor muscle of the pharynx
    - ◆ Cricothyroid muscle

Inferior laryngeal nerve—continuation of the recurrent laryngeal nerve

- ✓ Enters the larynx by passing deep to the inferior border of the inferior constrictor of the pharynx
- ✓ Divides into anterior and posterior branches that accompany the inferior laryngeal artery into the larynx
  - ⬦ Anterior branch
    - ◆ Lateral cricothyroid
    - ◆ Thyroarytenoid
    - ◆ Vocalis
    - ◆ Aryepiglottic muscles
    - ◆ Thyroepiglottic muscles
  - ⬦ Posterior branch
    - ◆ Posterior cricoarytenoid
    - ◆ Transverse and oblique arytenoids muscles

1.4.5 Pharynx

Overview

✓ This musculomembranous tube is shared by the nasal and oral cavities superiorly and the respiratory and digestive channels inferiorly. Curiously, the respiratory and digestive pathways actually cross each other within the pharynx

✓ The pharynx extends superiorly from the base of the skull to the lower border of the cricoid cartilage at the level of the lower margin of the 6th cervical vertebra—level to remember for future recall

✓ Anteriorly, the pharynx is largely deficient; it lacks an anterior wall owing to the fact that the right and left nasal cavities open into it as does the oral cavity. It is deficient inferiorly since there are major openings into the respiratory and digestive systems

✓ On the basis of these openings, the pharynx is topographically and rather arbitrarily divided into the nasal pharynx (epipharynx/nasopharynx), the oral pharynx (oropharynx), the laryngeal pharynx (hypopharynx/laryngopharynx)

The nasal pharynx

✓ Normally this upper portion has a predominantly respiratory function

✓ It also serves as a conduit for air passing to the eustachian tubes to equalize air pressure within the middle ear cavity

✓ In patients with allergic rhinitis, it serves as a conduit for excessive secretions (post-nasal drip)

✓ In patients experiencing nausea, it may inadvertently serve as a conduit for gastric contents if the level of the patient's head is not optimally positioned

- ✓ This tube remains patent (it's non-collapsable) due to its bony framework
- ✓ Anterior boundary—the choanae (posterior nares) with the posterior border of the nasal septum interposed between them
- ✓ Lateral walls include the orifices of the pharyngotympanic (auditory or eustachian) tubes

The pharyngotympanic tubes

- ✓ Allow communication between the nasopharynx (external environment) and the right and left tympanic cavities
- ✓ Are inclined obliquely. This makes it possible to insert either a blunt probe or flexible tube into the lumen. To locate a tube, enter the nares, pass straight posteriorly beneath the inferior nasal conchae then turn laterally. This anatomical information is clinically useful if a physician needs to open and introduce air into a blocked eustachian tube
- ✓ The levator veli palatini muscles produce a bulge or cushion in the lower circumference of the orifice
- ✓ Expansion of this muscle belly during its contraction phase pushes the long crus of the cartilaginous tube while the tensor veli palatini muscle pulls on the short crus of tube. This dilates the lumen of the tube. This is the natural physiologic mechanism for ventilating the middle ear (important in equalizing air pressure differences between external environment and middle ear)
- ✓ Normally several deliberate swallows move these muscles of the posterior wall and "milk" air into the tube

Clinical notes: ①Special nipples must be used in feeding infants with a cleft lip and palate since milk from the oral cavity can easily enter the nasopharynx and flow into the middle ear cavity. ②Bacterial/viral pathogens from the nasopharynx/oropharynx frequently travel down this route to enter the middle ear cavity resulting in otitis media

Salpingopharyngeus muscle

- ✓ Extends from the orifice of the pharyngotympanic tubes downward where it inserts into the laryngopharynx
- ✓ It produces a ridge of mucosa known as the salpingopharyngeal fold

Tubal tonsils

- ✓ There is an extensive collection of lymphatic tissue in the mucous membrane guarding the orifice of the tube. This raises a mound of tissue known as the torus tubarius
- ✓ This tonsillar material and all others sites within Waldeyer's ring reach their peak size at a mean age of approximately 6 years old. Subsequently they undergo a steady reduction in size that continues into young adulthood
- ✓ An inflammation (swelling) in this material hinders ventilation of the middle ear. This is a condition that makes it extremely painful to fly especially during rapid descent when air pressures change rapidly. Wise parents feed their young children during this period since the sucking movement will stimulate muscles in the nasopharynx and equalize air pressure

Posterior wall/roof

- ✓ The mucous membrane in the midline at the posterior of the nasopharynx is thrown into many variable folds. This focal region of mucosa shows an accumulation of nodular and diffuse lymphoid tissue that is known as the pharyngeal tonsil ("adenoids")

✓ This lymphatic tissue also atrophies and shrinks with age

Clinical notes: ①Pharyngeal tonsils are accessible to view by gazing upward from the oral cavity. ②Enlargement of the pharyngeal tonsil impedes the flow of air and is a leading contributor to snoring in the young child. ③Removal of the pharyngeal tonsil (adenoidectomy) along with placement of tubes in the tympanic membrane (myringotomy) is a common surgical procedure that is indicated when a child is experiencing repeated and/or continuous episodes of otitis media

Pharyngeal recesses

✓ These spaces are located posterio-lateral to the orifices of the auditory tubes
✓ The pharyngeal walls here are membranous only. This area is located superior to the superior constrictor muscle; thus there is no muscular component to reinforce this site in the nasopharynx. One finds apharyngobasilar fascia that is lined internally with pharyngeal mucosa

Floor of the nasopharyngeal chamber

✓ The floor or lower portion of this chamber is largely open to allow for the passage of air
✓ An incomplete partition is formed by the posterosuperior surface of the soft palate. This flap delineates the level and opening between the nasal and the oral pharynx. The opening between the soft palate and posterior wall of the pharynx is called thepharyngeal isthmus
✓ The "Ridge of Passavant" is a physiologic "sphincter" of sorts. It is produced by the contraction of the superior constrictor muscle where it meets the uvula during deglutition. Thus every time a normal patient swallows, the palatal muscles tense and lift up the soft palate. This contracting mechanism closes the pharyngeal isthmus. If there is a paralysis of the soft palatal muscles or spasticity, this closure is deficient and food particles can enter the nasal cavity. The patient is said to have velopalatal incompetence (VPI). Normal people can mimic this spasticity when they laugh and swallow at the same time

Clinical notes: ①VPI can develop in adult patients. Examples include patients with progressive neuromuscular degeneration or a rapid onset in patients who have experienced a stroke. ②When the VPI problem is detected in small children you may suspect a mental deficiency or a child deprived of the opportunity to learn proper speech patterns. Cerebral palsy is another cause of VPI. ③In children, surgical corrections are possible and frequent visits to a speech pathologist can work to correct these problems

The oral pharynx

✓ Extends from the pharyngeal isthmus to the level of the pharyngoepiglottic folds
✓ Air and food pathways cross here
✓ Communicates with the oral cavity via the isthmus of the fauces
✓ The isthmus of the fauces is formed between the palatoglossal and palatopharyngeal arches of each side of the oral cavity
✓ A tonsillar fossa which houses the palatine tonsils fills the concavity between the arches
✓ These are landmarks used in physical diagnosis. The mucosal folds are also referred to as the anterior and posterior pillars. If select a pediatric practice, the structures between these landmarks may serve as the financial "pillars" of your early clinical practice

✓ This fossa is the former location of the 2nd pharyngeal pouch. These embryonic structures (one on each side) were lined with endoderm and were small outpockets from the lateral walls of the foregut tube that were secondarily invaded with lymphocytic tissue
✓ A capsule separates the tonsil from the underlying wall of the pharynx

Clinical notes: In the pre-antibiotic era and for several more decades, these were almost routinely removed during childhood; hence, they're often missing in cadavers. This tissue is another part of Waldeyer's Ring of Tonsillar Tissue that guards the opening of the body from foreign invaders. The tonsillar tissue itself can swell to considerable size (tonsillitis) or the pharyngeal tissue beneath it (a peritonsillar abscess). The end result is fever, malaise and tonsillar tissue that can nearly obstruct the oral cavity

Blood supply of the palatine tonsil

Arterial

✓ The tonsillar artery, a direct branch of the facial artery. This is the main artery to the tonsil
✓ The tonsillar branch of the ascending pharyngeal artery (branch of external carotid)
✓ The tonsillar branch of the ascending palatine artery (branch of facial artery)
✓ The tonsillar branch of the descending palatine artery (branch of the maxillary artery)
✓ The tonsillar branch of the dorsal lingual artery (branch of the lingual artery)

Clinical notes: Although the arterial supply is abundant, the extensive hemorrhage that occasionally occurs following tonsillectomy usually results from damage to the paratonsillar vein (external palatine vein)—a sometimes sizable tributary of the facial vein

The laryngeal pharynx (the laryngopharynx)

✓ The laryngeal pharynx imperceptibly begins at the lower end of the oropharynx
▷ Anteriorly—an epiglottis that is connected to the root of the tongue via lateral epiglottic (glossoepiglottic) folds and the median epiglottic fold, between which lie small indentations (valleculae). Saliva collects in the valleculae between swallows
✓ Food particles do usually not slip over the epiglottis and gain entrance to the larynx, nor does the epiglottis completely "close" over the laryngeal aperture like a trap door. Instead, the flow of food and liquids is deflected to either side of the epiglottis. During swallowing, the epiglottis is elevated along with the rest of the visceral feeding tube (the tongue, hyoid bone, thyroid cartilage and associated musculature). This does lower the epiglottis over the opening to the larynx. The bolus of food/liquid slides around the aperture laterally through the piriform recesses and onward and downward into the esophagus. The epiglottis mostly acts like a rock in the middle of the rapids. It deflects the flow

Clinical notes: Piriform recesses are lateral pockets where pills, fish bones, and improperly chewed food can become caught. Patients may present to the emergency room for an extraction procedure

✓ Mucosal folds in the piriform recesses are formed by the internal laryngeal nerve which passes underneath this area
✓ Posterio—laterally, the laryngeal pharynx is enclosed by the inferior constrictor musculature. Laterally there is a gap in the muscle that is filled with the thyrohyoid membrane. This membrane is pierced by the internal laryngeal nerve accompanied by the internal laryngeal artery

✓ The mucous membrane in the laryngeal pharynx contains plexiform venous networks (the pharyngeal venous plexus), which are especially dense at the entrance of the esophagus

✓ Congestive swelling due to an acute inflammatory response inglottis edema brings the danger of acute asphyxiation

✓ The loose texture of the submucosa in this area contributes considerably to the ease with which the edema tends to spread. As you can imagine, if you procrastinate before you intubate a patient who is developing this problem, the anatomic blockage can make it impossible to pass the tube through this area

✓ These veins drain directly into the internal jugular vein. Malignant cells in this area spread quickly into deep cervical lymphatic chains

Pharyngeal musculature

✓ The spatial arrangement is unique in this area compared to the rest of the digestive tube

✓ Muscles are composed of the striated skeletal variety

✓ In contrast to the intestine, the longitudinal muscles (e.g., salpingopharyngeus, glossopharyngeus, thyroepiglottic) lie internally and the circular muscles (constrictors) lie externally

✓ This necessitates a structural rearrangement of the muscle layers at the transition to the esophagus. The oblique fibers of the inferior constrictor regroup to form the outer longitudinal muscle of the esophagus

✓ A triangular area (Laimer's triangle) at the beginning of the esophagus often remains free of or thinly covered by muscular tissue and favors the formation of diverticula. This is yet another recess where pills can accumulate with life-threatening consequences

✓ The three pharyngeal constrictors originate from anterio-laterally placed structures

Superior constrictor

✓ Origins: pterygomandibular raphe, pterygoid hamulus, buccinator ridge of the mandible

✓ Insertion: the right and left muscles sweep posteriorly and superiorly. In the midline the superior attachment is to the pharyngeal tubercle on the base of the skull and the remaining muscle meets its companion muscle from the opposite side to form a mid-line pharyngeal raphe

Middle constrictor

✓ Origins: from the hyoid bone, stylohyoid ligament

✓ Insertion: meets its partner to contribute to the pharyngeal raphe

✓ The pharyngeal raphe will be apparent on those cadavers where the prevertebral cut has been performed and the pharynx is viewed from behind

Inferior constrictor

✓ Origins: from the oblique line on the cricoid and thyroid cartilages often described as having two components—thryopharyngeus and cricopharyngeus

 ↳ Diverticula may develop in the relatively weak area ("Killian's dehiscence") between the two components

- ✓ Insertion: meets its partner to contribute to the mid-line posterior raphe muscle fibers of the lower cricopharyngeus—which are horizontal—pass as an uninterrupted muscular band completely around laryngopharynx serve as the major component of the upper esophageal ("pharyngoesophageal") sphincter which keeps the esophagus closed between swallows
- ✓ Because pharyngeal constrictors blend together posteriorly to form a continuous circular (oblique) muscle, it is difficult to distinguish them from this approach. They are most readily distinguished by following them to their origins, or on the basis of structures which pass over or between their borders
- ✓ As mentioned above, the lateral portions of each constrictor muscle is discontinuous. This leaves gaps between the musculature. These areas serve to permit passages for structures that enter and leave the pharynx

Gap 1—Structures passing over the superior border of the superior pharyngeal constrictor

- ✓ Cartilaginous portion of the pharyngotympanic tube
- ✓ The levator veli palatini muscles
- ✓ The ascending palatine arteries
- ✓ The pharyngeal branch of the ascending pharyngeal arteries

Gap 2—Structures passing in the lateral gap between the origins of the superior and middle pharyngeal constrictors

- ✓ Stylopharyngeus muscle
  - ▷ This muscle is derived from the material that moves the 3rd pharyngeal arch cartilages. It runs between the styloid process superiorly and inserts onto the thyroid cartilage
- ✓ Glossopharyngeal nerve (CN IX)
  - ▷ This nerve wraps around the stylopharyngeus muscle (innervates it) and moves forward toward the oropharynx and tongue
- ✓ Stylohyoid ligament
  - ▷ This is a remnant of the 2nd pharyngeal arch cartilage. It runs between the styloid process and the superior horn of the hyoid bone

Gap 3—Structures passing between the middle and inferior pharyngeal constrictors

- ✓ This gap is spanned by the thyrohyoid membrane
- ✓ It is pierced by the internal laryngeal branch of superior laryngeal nerve
- ✓ Superior laryngeal branch of superior thyroid artery and vein

Gap 4—Structures passing under (deep to) the inferior border of the inferior pharyngeal constrictor

- ✓ Recurrent (inferior) laryngeal nerve (CN X)
- ✓ Branches of the inferior thyroid artery

Retropharyngeal space

- ✓ Infections from the tonsillar materials, abscessed teeth if untreated can eventually penetrate posterior to the constrictor muscles and gain access to the region posterior to the pharyngeal tube. This area is known as the retropharyngeal space. It is lined on its pharyngeal surface with retropharyngeal or visceral fascia that is continuous with the pretracheal fascia. This layer completely encompasses the central visceral tube. Posterior to the retropharyngeal space are the cervical neck muscles and nerves of the cervical plexuses that are encased in a prevertebral fascial sheath

> ✓ Infections that gain access to the retropharyngeal space are limited in their upward spread by the base of the skull. Infections spread downward due to gravity. They can move downward through the thoracic outlet and into the posterior mediastinal area

Vessels and nerves of the pharynx

Arteries

✓ Ascending pharyngeal artery (external carotid artery)
✓ Ascending palatine artery (facial artery, supplies mainly upper portions of pharynx as well as auditory tube, tonsils, etc.)

Veins

✓ Accompanying the above listed arteries and their branches, plus: the pterygoid venous plexus and the external palatine vein (paratonsillar vein)

Lymph vessels

✓ Drainage mainly into upper deep cervical nodes
✓ Nasal cavity, nasopharynx—retropharyngeal node (part of upper deep cervical group)

Nerves

✓ Sensory
　↳ Upper portions: glossopharyngeal nerve (CN Ⅸ)
　↳ Lower portions: vagus nerve [internal laryngeal branch of superior laryngeal nerve (CN Ⅸ)]
✓ Motor
　↳ Pharyngeal plexus: it is most probable that the motor fibers come from the cranial portion of the accessory nerve (CN Ⅺ), which are carried to the pharyngeal plexus via the vagus nerve (CN Ⅹ)
　↳ Exception: stylopharyngeus—supplied by glossopharyngeal nerve (CN Ⅸ)

1.4.6　Orbit and eyeball

The circulation of the orbit and globe

Extraocular circulation

Arteries

✓ Two sources
　↳ Internal carotid artery—ophthalmic artery. The ophthalmic artery supplies most of the extraocular structures.
　↳ External carotid artery—infraorbital artery. The infraorbital artery supplies the lower portion (floor) of the orbit. E.g., inferior rectus and oblique muscles

Veins

✓ Superior ophthalmic vein
　↳ Drains area supplied by the ophthalmic artery

- ▷ Empties posteriorly into the cavernous sinus
- ▷ Nasal branch anastomoses with angular (facial) vein anteriorly
- ✓ Inferior ophthalmic vein
  - ▷ Drains area supplied by the infraorbital artery
  - ▷ Drains to superior ophthalmic vein (cavernous sinus) and pterygoid venous plexus (infratemporal fossa)

Intraocular circulation

Arteries (all are derivatives of the ophthalmic artery)

- ✓ Retinal system
  - ▷ Central retinal artery. Central retinal artery (and vein) serves all portions of the retina except the layer of rods and cone cells (which are supplied by the choroidal vessels)
- ✓ Ciliary system
  - ▷ Anterior ciliary arteries
    - ◆ From arteries of the four rectus muscles
    - ◆ Join posterior system at the greater arterial circle within the ciliary body
  - ▷ Posterior ciliary arteries
    - ◆ 2 long posterior ciliary arteries
    - ◆ 20 short posterior ciliary arteries
    - ◆ The choroid, ciliary body, iris, cornea and structures near the limbus are supplied by the anterior and posterior ciliary arteries

Clinical notes: The cornea does not contain blood vessels, but receives its supply from capillaries at the limbus which are derived from the anterior ciliary arteries

Veins

Vortex (vorticose) veins (4):
- ✓ Primary system of drainage from the uveal tract
- ✓ Drain into superior and inferior ophthalmic veins

Innervation of the intrinsic eye muscles

- ✓ Innervation of intrinsic muscles mainly parasympathetic
- ✓ Sympathetic nerves go only to blood vessels and radial muscles of iris

Sympathetic innervation

- ✓ Presynaptic cell bodies: IML cell column of grey matter, T_1-T_3
- ✓ Presynaptic fibers follow usual course (ventral root, mixed spinal nerve, ventral ramus, white ramus communicans to sympathetic trunk)
- ✓ Presynaptic fibers ascend through cervical portions of sympathetic trunks without synapsing until reaching superior cervical ganglion
- ✓ Postsynaptic cell bodies. Postsynaptic fibers leave sympathetic trunks via cephalic arterial rami to form periarterial plexuses around the internal carotid artery. Vasomotor fibers serving vessels of the orbit then continue along vessels to their terminations. The motor fibers to nonvascular smooth muscle leave the carotid plexus as it passes near the trigeminal ganglion or its ophthalmic ($CN\ V_1$) branch

✓ Fibers joining the ophthalmic nerve (CN V₁) enter its nasociliary branch, from which:

  ⟡ Some fibers pass directly to bulb via its long ciliary branch

  ⟡ Other fibers run to the ciliary ganglion via its long root. These fibers pass through the ganglion without synapsing (they are already post-synaptic) and pass to the bulb via the short ciliary nerves

  ⟡ Still other fibers continue on in the nasociliary nerve and are distributed to the extraocular smooth muscle of the orbit

✓ Fibers following route (a) mostly continue to the dilator pupillae muscle. Fibers following route (b) mostly serve the blood vessels of the bulb

Parasympathetic innervation

✓ Presynaptic cell bodies in Edinger-Westphal nucleus (incorporated in nucleus of III)

✓ Presynaptic axons enter oculomotor nerve (CN III), passing into the short root of the ciliary ganglion

✓ Postsynaptic cell bodies in ciliary ganglion. Postsynaptic axons pass to the bulb via the short ciliary nerve, and continue to the smooth muscle of the ciliary body or to the circular muscle of the iris

Clinical notes: ① Some presynaptic parasympathetic fibers traverse the ciliary ganglion without synapsing, continuing into the ciliary nerves to synapse within microscopic episcleral ganglia (much like the enteric ganglia of the gut). ② Contraction of the ciliary muscle causes the circular ciliary body to decrease in diameter, like a sphincter; the lens, suspended in the center of the circle, thus relaxes, rounding up or thickening (near vision). Relaxation of the ciliary body increases its diameter; thus the lens suspended in its center is stretched and become thinner (far vision). ③ The movement of the iris is paradoxical compared with movements produced by the autonomic nervous system elsewhere: dilator pupillae muscle constriction (sympathetical innervated) is slow, sphincter pupillae muscle constriction (parasympathetical innervated) is fast

A lesion of III results in:

✓ Ptosis

✓ Depression and lateral rotation of bulb (superior oblique and lateral rectus unopposed—pupil is "down and out")

✓ No accommodation (lens does not thicken due to loss of parasymp. fibers)

✓ Dilation of pupil

✓ Horner's syndrome (loss of sympathetic innervation)

  ⟡ Slight ptosis (due to paralysis of smooth muscle fibers interdigitated with striated muscles of the levator palpebrae superioris muscle = superior tarsal muscles)

  ⟡ Constriction of pupil (unopposed sphincter pupillae muscle)

The globe

Location and general information about the globe

✓ Globe contains the optical apparatus of the visual system

✓ Globe occupies the anterior most portion of the bony orbit

✓ Extraocular muscles, considerable orbital fat, and vessels fill the remainder

✓ All structures in the globe are circular or spherical in shape

Layers (coats or tunics) of the globe

- ✓ Outer fibrous layer: sclera and cornea
- ✓ Middle vascular layer ("uveal tract"): choroid, ciliary body, and iris
- ✓ Inner nervous layer: includes optic and non-optic portions

Outer fibrous layer

Sclera

- ✓ Relatively avascular, white, opaque layer covering posterior 5/6 of globe
- ✓ Consists of a thick, elastic connective tissue containing irregularly arranged collagen fibers and is relatively well-hydrated
- ✓ Surrounded by the bulbar fascia that forms the true "eye socket" in which the globe is suspended in the orbit and in which it rotates
- ✓ Strongest immediately anterior to the insertion of the 4 rectus muscles
- ✓ Weakest immediately posterior to these muscular insertions
- ✓ Also weakest at the posterior portion known as the lamina cribrosa—where the optic nerve pierces the sclera

Structures piercing the sclera on their way to supply/drain underlying structures

- ✓ Anterior ciliary arteries
- ✓ Optic nerve pierces posteriorly
- ✓ Long and short ciliary arteries—branches of the ophthalmic artery
- ✓ Ciliary nerves
- ✓ Vorticose (vortex) veins

Limbus

- ✓ Angle formed by intersecting curvatures of sclera and cornea at corneoscleral junction
- ✓ 1 mm wide gray semi-transparent circle
- ✓ Numerous capillary loops here supply an avascular cornea

Cornea

- ✓ Transparent layer covering anterior 1/6 of the globe
- ✓ Major refractive medium of eye
- ✓ Avascular, receiving nourishment from periphery (capillaries of limbus, aqueous (deep surface), lacrimal fluid (external surface)
- ✓ Contains a highly regular arrangement of collagen fibers and is more dehydrated than sclera

A. Surface anatomy of the eye

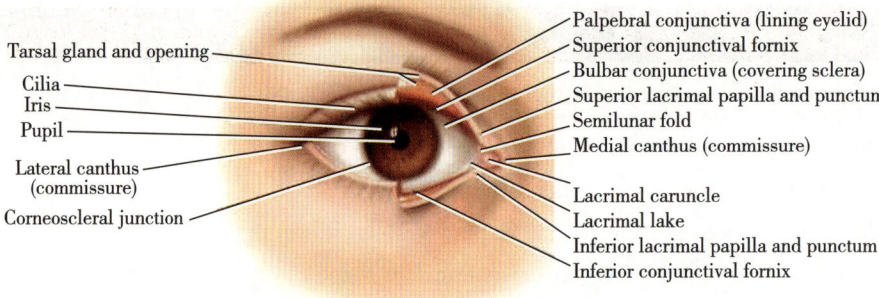

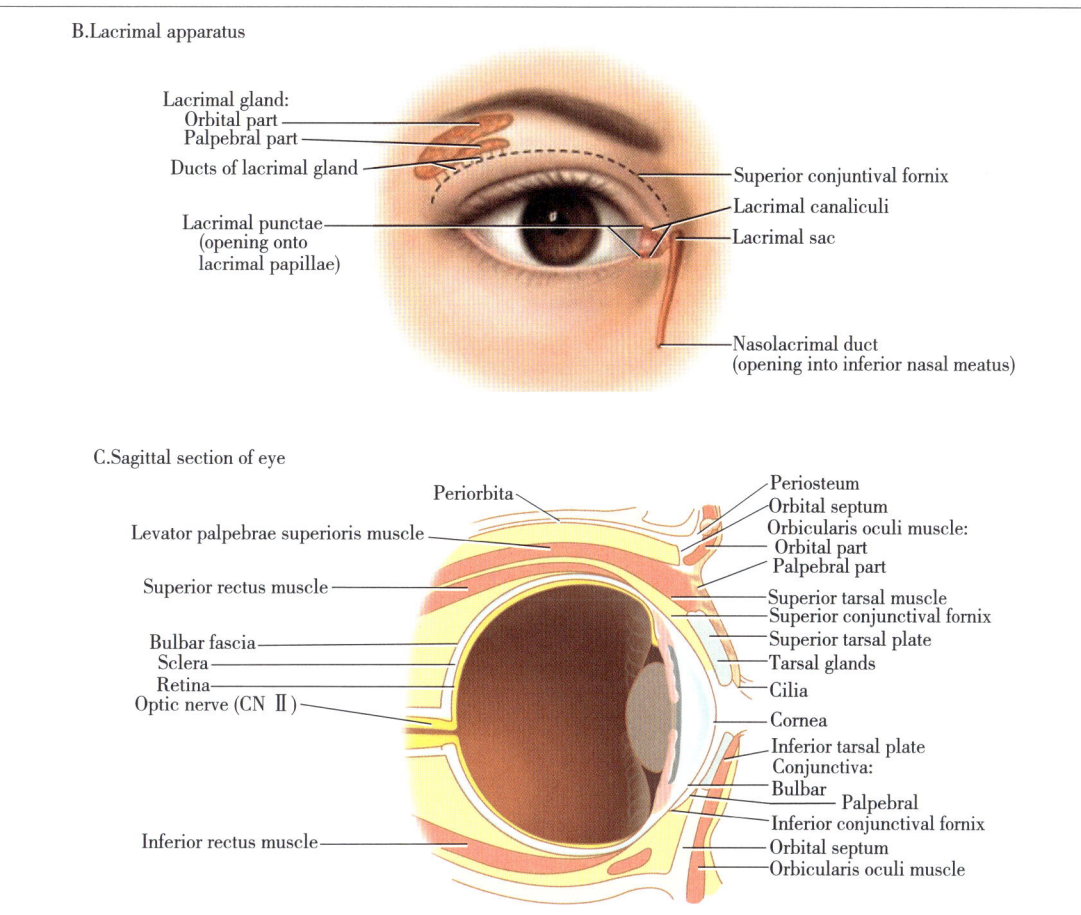

B. Lacrimal apparatus

C. Sagittal section of eye

Middle vascular layer ("uveal tract")

✓ Contains a great deal of pigment
✓ Choroid
✓ Contains a matrix of blood vessels
✓ Become progressively finer from external to internal aspect of choiroid
✓ Choriocapillaris: deepest layer, in direct contact with the retina
✓ Nourish outermost (cones and rods) layer of retina
✓ All arteries feeding choroid are branches of ophthalmic artery
✓ Veins—collect returning blood into 4 large vortex veins
✓ These veins drain into the superior and inferior ophthalmic veins

Ciliary body

✓ Comprised of blood vessels and muscle tissue
✓ Pars plana—a smooth posterior portion
✓ Corona radiata—more anterior portion
✓ Most vulnerable structure in the eye
✓ Ciliary processes
✓ 70-80 radiate outward
✓ Are attached to a circular scleral spur on the inner scleral aspect
✓ Zonular fibers attach to tips, extend to periphery of lens
✓ Secrete acqueous into posterior chamber of anterior segment

Iris
✓ Arises from the ciliary body
✓ Its free anterior margin rests on the anterior surface of the lens
✓ Composed of muscle and blood vessels
✓ Is easily injured, injuries remain unhealed for life
✓ Contains two involuntary muscles that regulate the size of the pupil

Sphincter pupillae muscle
✓ Constriction decreases the pupil size
✓ Muscle fibers circularly arranged
✓ Is under parasympathetic control

Dilator pupillae muscle
✓ Increases size of pupillary opening
✓ Muscle fibers are radially-arranged
✓ Dilation is a weaker and slower action than sphincter action

Inner nervous layer = retina

Optic (nervous) part
✓ The light sensitive portion
✓ Consists mostly of nerve cells (neural layer) and a finer pigmented layer
✓ Posterior to ora serrata
✓ Posterior border of pars plana of ciliary body
✓ Named for its scalloped appearance
✓ Lies anterior to equator of globe
✓ Cones and rods are in outermost region of optic part
✓ Is a thin transparent membrane
✓ Specialized areas of fundus (posterior interior eyeball)
◊ Optic disc
◆ "blind spot" where nerves enter eyeball and retina
◆ Elevated (papilledema) when intracranial (CSF) pressure is high since extension of subarachnoid space that surrounds optic nerve ends immediately beneath it
◊ Macula
◆ Lateral to optic disc
◆ Area of retina with cones only
◊ Fovea centralis
◆ 1.5 mm central pit
◆ Area of greatest visual acuity
◆ Visible branches of central retinal artery remain outside this area

Non-visual part
✓ Anterior to ora serrata—on ciliary body (ciliary part) and posterior aspect of iris (iridial part)

Segments of globe/refractive media
Posterior segment
✓ Posterior to lens ✓ Filled with vitreous
Vitreous
✓ Gelatinous substance that fills the interior of the globe ✓ Makes up 2/3 of the weight and volume of the globe ✓ Functions are not thoroughly understood ✓ Normally keeps retina applied against choriocapillaris by maintaining intraocular pressure (retina otherwise unattached to it) ✓ Prevents collapse of the eye ✓ Is adherent to the retina at the optic disk and ora serrata ✓ Has an anterior condensation known as the vitreous face, hyaloid membrane or anterior hyaloid ✓ Is attached to the ciliary epithelium at the pars plana ✓ In young patients—is attached to the posterior lens surface ✓ Contains an empty canal (hyaloid canal Cloquet) ✓ Remnant of a fetal vessel—hyaloid artery ✓ Extends from the optic disc to the lens
Lens

✓ Divides the globe into:
  ▷ Posterior segment—space filled with vitreous
  ▷ Anterior segment—space filled with aqueous
✓ Is held upright behind the iris by stiff, inextensibleciliary zonules
✓ Suspended from ciliary processes attached to the equator of the lens
✓ Transparent, crystalline, biconvex
✓ Surrounded by a highly elastic lens capsule
✓ Purpose—fine focus of rays of light onto the retina

Accommodation
✓ When the ciliary muscle contracts, the ciliary body moves forward and inward. This decreases the diameter of the ciliary body. Zonule fibers slacken. The lens bulges forward near objects are brought into focus ✓ As the ciliary muscle relaxes, ciliary body recedes, tightening the zonule, returning the lens to a less convex shape for distant vision
Anterior segment

✓ Filled with aqueous—a transparent, colorless fluid
  ▷ Posterior chamber—small area enclosed by the posterior surface of the iris, ciliary body and zonules and anterior lens capsule
  ▷ Anterior chamber—the much larger space between the iris and cornea
✓ Circulatory pattern for aqueous

- ✓ Ciliary processes secrete aqueous into the posterior chamber
- ✓ Flows through pupil into anterior chamber
- ✓ Absorbed at narrow periphery of the anterior chamber—the anterior chamber angle or filtration angle
- ✓ Fine strands of connective tissue form a trabecular network that filters the aqueous
- ✓ Enters venous blood stream at thesinus venosus sclerae (canal of Schlemm)
- ✓ Flows into veins of the limbal plexus
- ✓ Maintaining normal intraocular pressure requires a balance between production and outflow of aqueous
- ✓ Disturbances in this balance result inglaucoma

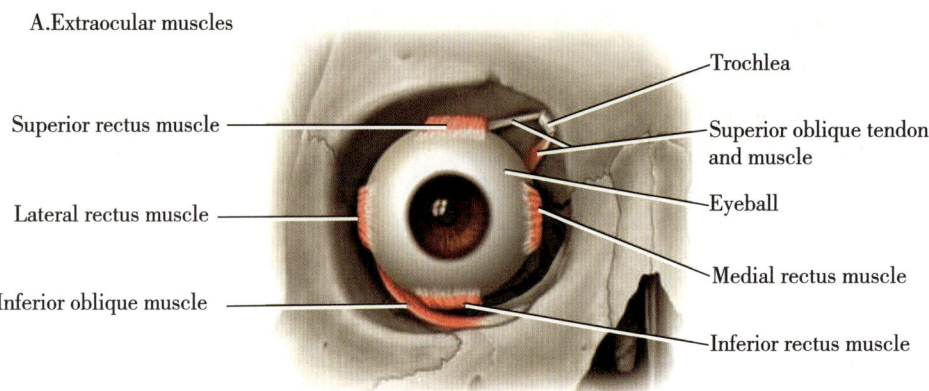

A. Extraocular muscles

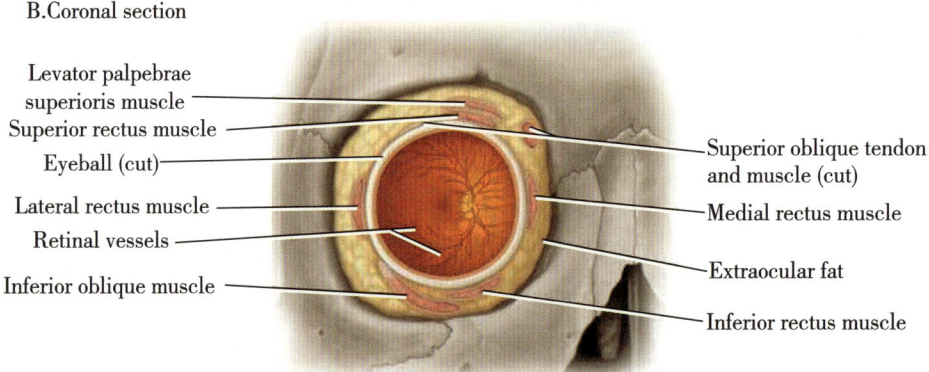

B. Coronal section

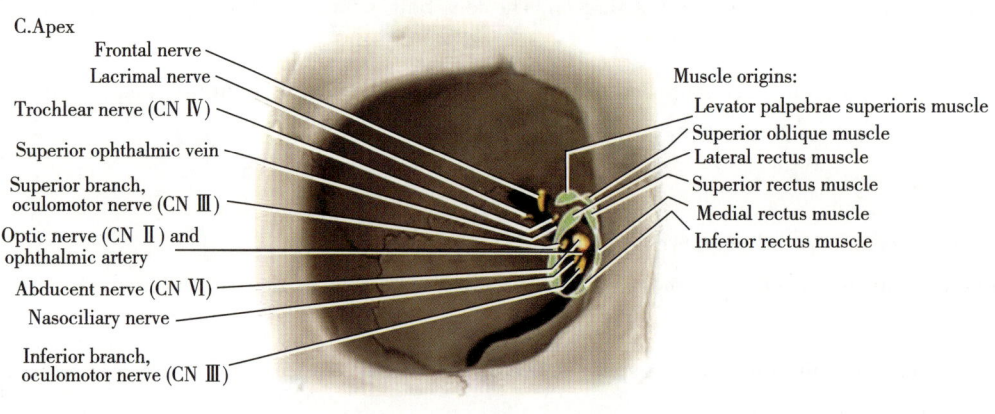

C. Apex

Cornea
✓ Antereior boundary of anterior chamber of anterior segment ✓ Major refractive ("light bending") medium of eye ✓ Lens further refracts for far and near vision ✓ Very sensitive to touch, innervated by ophthalmic nerve (CN V_1) ✓ Corneal reflex tests functional status of CN V_1 ✓ Touching cornea with wisp of cotton evokes blink

1.4.7 The ear

Overview
The ear can be divided into three parts
External ear
✓ Consisting of: 　▷ Auricle (pinna) 　▷ External auditory meatus 　▷ Tympanic membrane (ear drum)
Middle ear
✓ Tympanic cavity containing: 　▷ Ossicles 　▷ Openings of the pharyngotympanic (auditory) tube and entrance (aditus) to the mastoid air cells, which form a continuous, diagonal pathway (airway) from the mastoid bone to the nasopharynx; this continuous airway intersects the transverse line defined by the discontinuous external and internal auditory meatuses ✓ Function of the external and middle ear is to collect and conduct sound
Internal ear
✓ Consisting of: 　▷ Semicircular canals/ducts 　　◆ Sensory organs for maintenance of equilibrium (working together with visual and proprioceptive sensations) 　▷ Cochlea/cochlear duct 　　◆ Sensory organ for the perception of sound 　▷ Vestibule 　　◆ Containing the utricle, saccule and associated ducts and connecting the cochlea and semicircular canals
External ear
Auricle or pinna
✓ Designed to "catch" sound waves—works mostly in animals capable of "cocking" the ears (directing auricles toward a sound, as dogs do)

✓ In man, as ornamental as it is useful, being a poor collector of sound waves (but does hold your hat above your eyes, perhaps—and provides a purchase for earrings, etc.)
✓ Terms and components

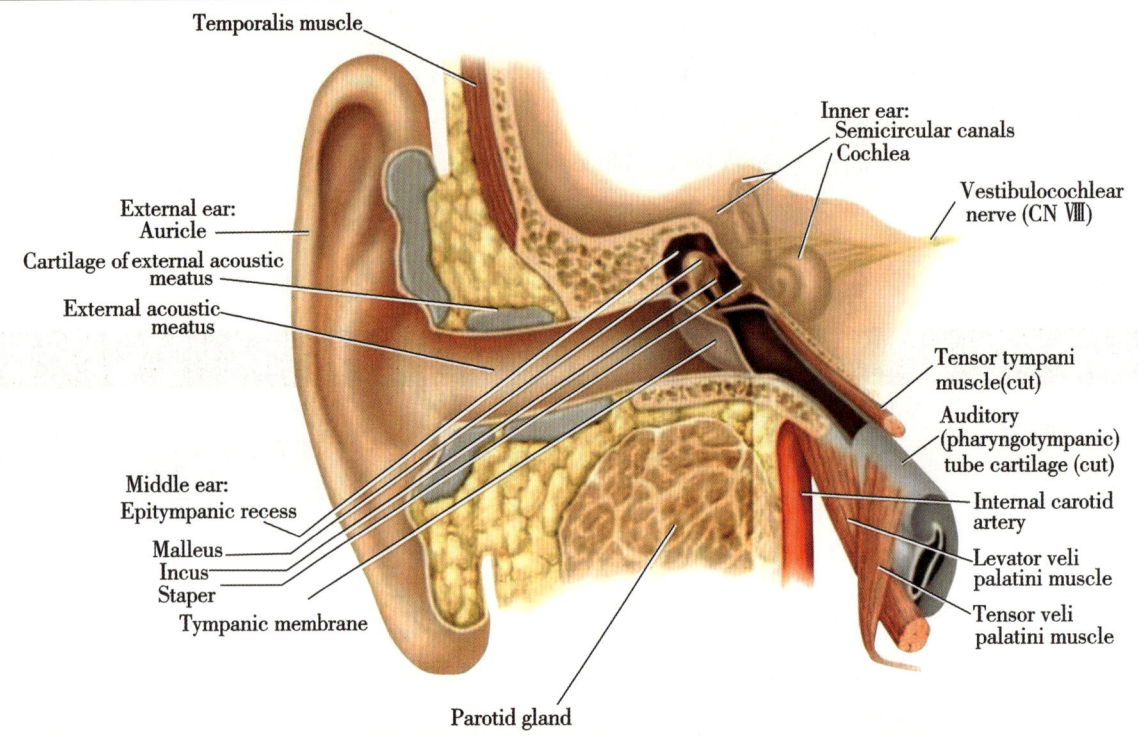

External acoustic meatus

✓ Shelters eardrum, maintaining relatively constant temperature and humidity
✓ Acts as a tubular resonator
✓ Provides a site for the accumulation of "ear wax" (not a wax at all)

Parts (in adults)

Cartilaginous (external or lateral) portion

✓ Continuous with cartilage of auricle
✓ Directed superiorly and posteriorly as it runs medially

Osseous (internal or median) portion

✓ Formed by tympanic portion of temporal bone
✓ Directly inferiorly and anteriorly as it runs medially
✓ Therefore, in inspecting the drum, one must line up the cartilaginous (moveable) half with the osseous (immovable) half by drawing the auricle superiorly and posteriorly; this facilitates the introduction of the otic speculum/otoscope and inspection of most of the drum
✓ Tube is more elliptical than round in cross-section
✓ External two-thirds becomes increasingly narrow it proceeds medially (narrowest part = the isthmus), a problem when foreign bodies lodge medial to this portion. It then widens again in its osseous part
✓ An elevation on the floor (anterior inferior surface) just lateral to the drum prevents complete drum inspection in this area

Parts (in infants)

✓ In infants (at term), there is no bony portion of the external auditory meatus (infants are not small adults); the drum lies in the same plane as the outer surface of the skull. The canal is considerably more horizontal than in the adult; therefore, the roof of the meatus and the drum are nearly on the same plane. It is also compressed so that he roof and floor frequently touch. Therefore, in examining the infant's drum, the ear lobe must be retracted inferiorly to open the canal. By age 2, the canal has relatively wide lumen

Innervation of external auditory meatus

✓ Superior aspect = trigeminal nerve (CN V) (auriculotemporal nerve from CN V_3)
✓ Inferior aspect = vagus nerve (CN X)

Tympanic membrane

Orientation, attachments

✓ Obliquely placed (45°), so its lateral surface is directly inferiorly and anteriorly
✓ It is pulled inward as a slight cone by the attachment of the manubrium (handle) of the malleus at the umbo
✓ Attached at its periphery via a fibrocartilagenous ring (yet another anulus tendineus)
✓ Kept tense (mostly) by the pull of tensor tympani (which actually attaches to the malleus which is attached in turn to the membrane

Layers of tympanic membrane (trilaminar construction)

✓ Outer layer—a continuation of skin of external auditory meatus
  ◊ It is innervated by CN V superiorly and CN X inferiorly
✓ Middle connective tissue core
  ◊ Elastic fibers arranged in a double layer, in a concentric circular arrangement crossed by radial fibers from a central hub, much in the form of a orb spider's web
✓ Inner layer—a continuation of mucous membrane of middle ear
  ◊ It is innervated by CN IX
  ◊ 1 cm in diameter, 0.1 mm thick
  ◊ Vibrations incredibly minute

Blood supply of the eardrum

External surface

✓ Most arterial twigs to the external surface are from the deep auricular branch of 1st part of the maxillary artery; the largest of these is the manubrial artery which descends from above, running along the malleolar stria (the "stripe" of the attachment of the manubrium of the malleus to the drum), while the smaller twigs radiate inward from the sides. Hence, the favorable site for piercing (lancing) the drum in middle ear infections is in its posteroinferior quadrant (certain prominent middle ear structures lies behind each quadrant. The jugular bulb of the internal. Jugular vein lies behind this quadrant, but the danger of wounding it is slight for the most part. The carotid canal is much more vulnerable in the anteroinferior quadrant—the area of the "cone of light". In the upper quadrants, the opening of the auditory tube is anterior; the long process of the incus, the stapes and the oval window of the vestibule of the inner ear lies posteriorly)

Regional Anatomy

Internal surface
✓ Anterior tympanic branch of 1ˢᵗ part of maxillary aretery
✓ Stylomastoid branch of the posterior auricular aretery

Other features of the eardrum
✓ Pars tensa
✓ Pars flaccida
✓ Posterior and anterior malleolar folds

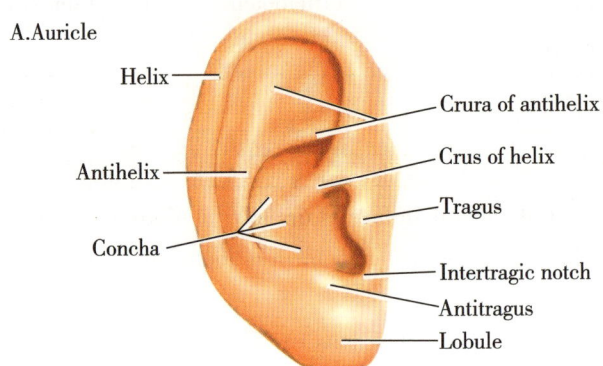

A. Auricle

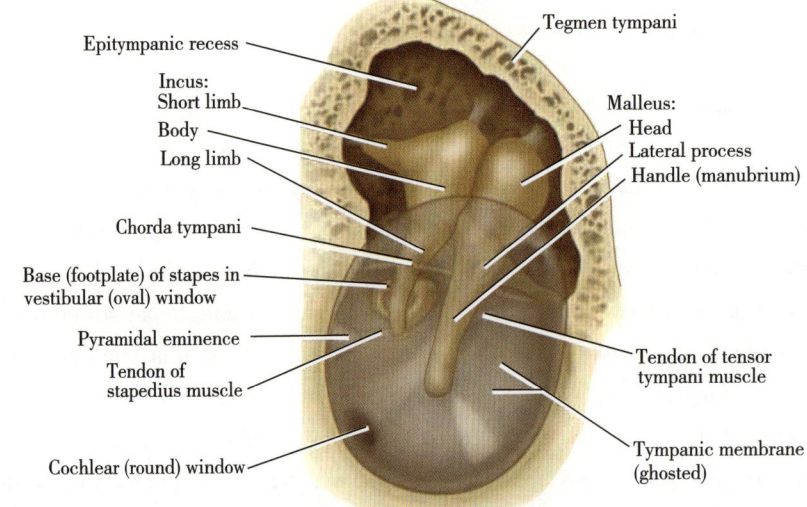

B. Tympanic membrane, lateral view

C. Ossicles of ear seen through tympanic membrane

Middle ear (tympanic cavity and contents)

Description of the tympanic cavity

✓ The tympanic cavity is biconcave (narrow from side to side in its middle portion, but wider peripherally—shaped like a lozenge or red-blood cell standing on edge). The umbo of the tympanic membrane bulges medially into the cavity from the lateral wall, and the promontory of the basal turn of the cochlea bulges laterally into the cavity from the medial side

✓ The tympanic membrane is stretched across a large round opening which occupies most of the lateral wall. The roof slants and is made of thin bone, the tegmen tympani. The roof extends higher than the superior border of the ear drum, so a space—the epitympanic recess—is formed which will house the head of the malleus and the body of the incus, two of the ear ossicles. A narrow channel is directed posteriorly from the epitympanic recess is the aditus. It leads to a common room within the mastoid process of the temporal bone, the antrum into which the many mastoid air cells open. The epitympanic recess communicates anteriorly and medially with the nasopharynx via the pharyngotympanic (formerly auditory or eustachian) tube. The floor is slightly elevated by the underlying jugular bulb (beginning of the internal jugular vein). Its anterior wall is a common one shared with the carotid canal. In its posterior wall, the facial nerve (CN VII) descends toward the stylomastoid foramen. Running through a bony wedge between the carotid artery and jugular vein is the tiny tympanic canaliculus by which the tympanic branch of CN IX enters the tympanic cavity. It will form the tympanic nerve plexus on the convex medial wall of the cavity (the promontory of the basal turn of the cochlea)

Contents of the tympanic cavity

Ossicles ("tiny bones") of the ear—lack periosteum; covered only with mucosa

✓ Malleus
  ◊ Head, neck, lateral and anterior processes
✓ Incus
  ◊ Body, short and long limbs, lenticular process
✓ Stapes
  ◊ Head, anterior and posterior limbs, base (footplate)

Joints—synovial, with all features of synovial joints

✓ Incudomallear
✓ Incudostapedial

Muscles

✓ Tensor tympani
  ◊ Arises and lies in a bony canal which parallels the pharyngotympanic tube
  ◊ Tendon turns 90° to insert into manubrium of malleus
  ◊ Innervated by branch of CN V_3 (arises from otic ganglion)
✓ Stapedius
  ◊ Smallest muscle of body
  ◊ Lies within cavity of pyramidal eminence on posterior wall of tympanic cavity
  ◊ Innervated by branch of facial nerve (CN VII)

◊ These muscles may act together as synergists in a reflex response to sounds of high intensity, protectively dampening the vibrations of the eardrum and ossicles; they also act independently as antagonists to adjust the sensitivity to sounds of different frequencies: the tensor makes the eardrum more taut and pushes the stapes more tightly into the oval window—actions which increase sensitivity to sounds of higher frequency. When acting independently, the stapes opposes the effect of the tensor on the stapes

Nerve

✓ Chorda tympani (CN VII)—"just passing through"

Internal ear

Comprised of two major components: the osseous labyrinth and the membranous labyrinth—the latter housed inside the former

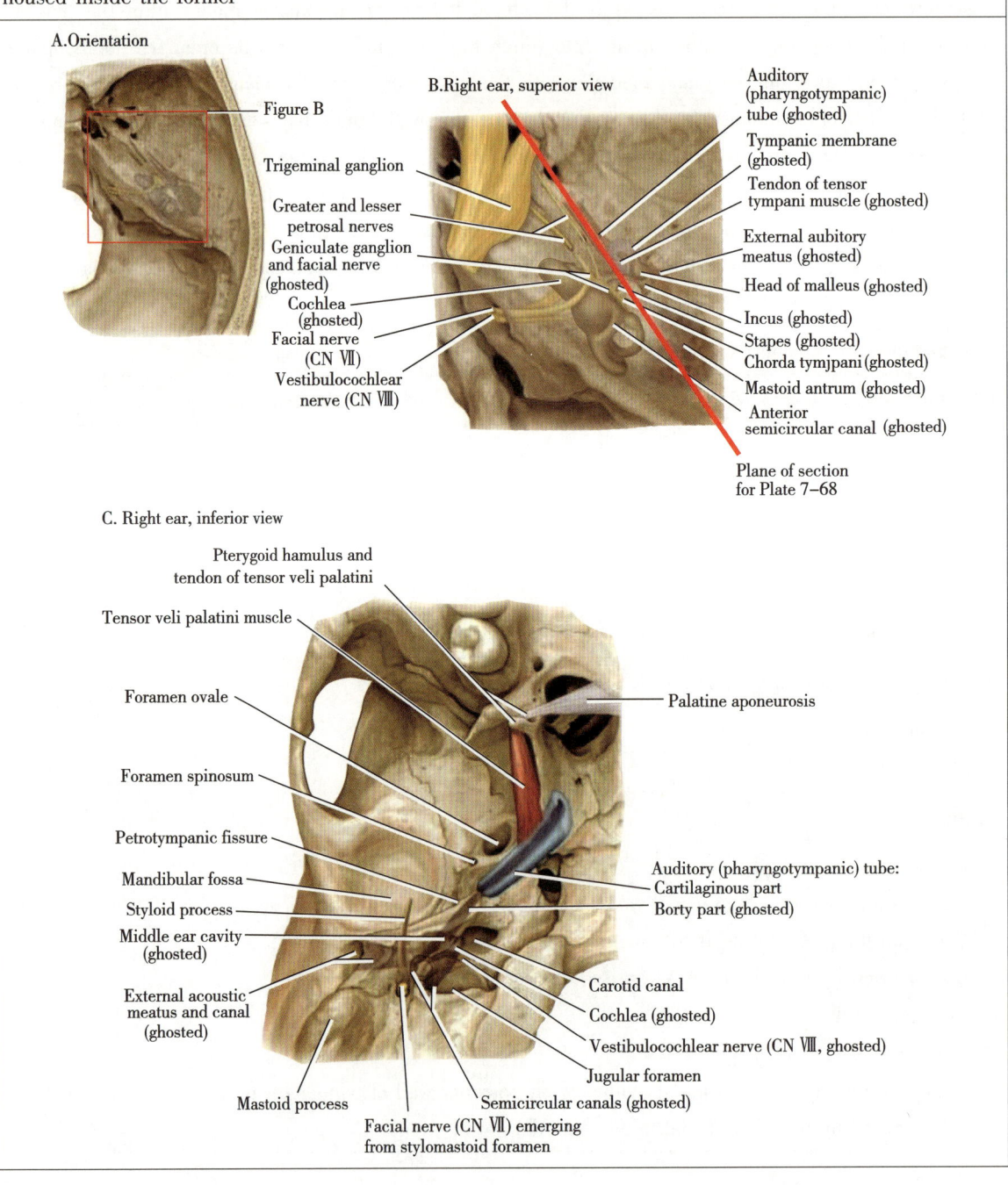

The osseous labyrinth

✓ A complex cave in solid bone
✓ The bone which forms the immediate walls of the cave (the otic capsule) is the hardest bone in the body. Hence, the experienced dissector can isolate the walls of the osseous labyrinth by removing the softer bone which surrounds it. This may be done with a dental drill

Components of the osseous labyrinth

✓ A vestibule, or large "central room" or compartment into which the other components open.
✓ Three semicircular canals (anterior or superior, posterior and lateral)
✓ The cochlea or cochlear canal

Openings (communications) into the vestibule

✓ The oval window (fenestra ovale or vestibulum)
✓ The round window (fenestra rotundum or tympanicum)
✓ The six ends of the three semicircular canals by means of five openings (superior and posterior canals have a "common crus", merging to enter together at the non-ampullary end
✓ The cochlear canal
✓ The vestibular aqueduct giving passage to endolymphatic duct
✓ The cochlear canaliculus giving passage to perilymphatic duct

  ◊ Since the osseous labyrinth is actually a space inside of the bone, it is perhaps more realistically demonstrated by means of a cast of that space
  ◊ The osseous labyrinth is filled with a fluid, the perilymph, in which the membranous labyrinth is suspended. Perilymph resembles extracellular fluid in composition (sodium salts are the predominate positive electrolyte)

The membranous labyrinth

✓ Extends into all parts of the osseous labyrinth, but occupies only a fraction of the volume of the osseous labyrinth (approx $1/16^{th}$)
✓ Walls formed by a delicate membrane
✓ Filled with endolymph. Endolymph resembles intracellular fluid (potassium is the main positively-charged ion)
The osseous labyrinth with its contained membranous labyrinth may be subdivided into the cochlea (hearing) and the vestibular apparatus (for balance and sense of orientation)

Cochlea

✓ The cochlear canal (bony labyrinth) is partially divided by a bony shelf (thespiral lamina) which winds around a hollow central bony core (the modiolus). The cochlear duct (membranous labyrinth) is attached to the "free" edge of the spiral lamina and extends to the opposite wall of the canal, creating separate tube-like compartments above (the scala vestibul) and below (the scala tympani). These two tubes, and the cochlear duct between them, spiral about the modiolus for 3/4 turns. The two scalae communicate at the apex by means of the helicotrema. The cochlear duct, being part of the membranous labyrinth, is filled with endolymph while the scalae, surrounding it, are filled with perilymph

✓ The vibrations of the footplate of the stapes are converted to variations in fluid pressure at the oval window of the vestibule of the bony labyrinth. Waves of the varying pressures are conducted up the scala vestibuli to the helicotrema and then down the scala tympani to the secondary tympanic membrane of the round window where they are "lost" to the airspace of the middle ear. The ascending and descending waves of fluid pressure distort the intervening cochlear duct, which contains the sensory organ of Corti that converts the mechanical forces to nervous action potentials

Vestibular apparatus

✓ Consists of the membranous labyrinth minus the cochlear duct
✓ Components of the membranous labyrinth include:
  ◊ Saccule
  ◊ Utricle
  ◊ Three semicircular ducts
  ◊ Tubes that connect them together (utriculosaccular duct)
✓ The saccule and the utricle have maculae—areas of specialized receptor cells with microscopic hairs. Chalky particles (otoliths) are overlying these hairs making nerve endings in the hairs sensitive to changes in gravity and acceleration
✓ The anterior, posterior and lateral semicircular ducts are arranged at right angles to each other. Each has a dilated end or ampulla in which is found the sensory area, the crista. Hair cells of the cristae act as barriers to the contained endolymph, and are deflected when changes in angular acceleration occur

Clinical correlations: Unique susceptibility of ear to trauma/disease due to structure and function
✓ Acoustic trauma → high intensity explosions
✓ Otic barotrauma → flyers and divers
✓ Menier's disease → increased amount of endolymph; can cause vertigo and tinnitus → can cause degeneration of hair cells

1.4.8 Temporal and Infratemporal fossae, Temporomandibular joint

Overview

The temporal region includes the temporal and infratemporal fossae
✓ Temporal fossa
✓ Parotid region
✓ Temporomandibular joint (TMJ)
✓ Infratemporal fossa
✓ Maxillary artery
✓ Pterygoid venous plexus
✓ Mandibular nerve (CN V_3)

Temporal fossa—"temple"

Boundries

✓ Posteriorly and superiorly—temporal lines

- ▷ Superior temporal line
- ▷ Inferior temporal line
- ✓ Anteriorly—frontal and zygomatic bones
- ✓ Laterally—zygomatic arch
- ✓ Inferiorly—infratemporal crest of the sphenoid bone
- ✓ Floor—frontal, parietal, temporal and greater wing of the sphenoid
- ✓ Roof—temporalis muscle and fascia

Sutures

- ✓ Coronal (frontoparietal)
- ✓ Squamosal (parietal-temporal)
- ✓ Frontozygomatic
- ✓ Temporozygomatic

Pterion—point marked by the earlier position of the anterolateral fontanelle; junction of the great wing of the sphenoid bone with the frontal, parietal and temporal bones; 3 cm behind and slightly above the zygomatic process of the frontal bone

Temporal fascia

- ✓ Stretches over the temporal fossa and temporalis muscle
- ✓ Inferiorly splits into two layers
    - ▷ Superficial layer—attaches to the superior margin of the zygomatic arch
    - ▷ Deep layer—passes medial to the zygomatic arch to become continuous with the fascia to the masseter muscle

Parotid region—between the mastoid process of the temporal bone (posterior) and the neck and ramus of the mandible (anterior)

Contents

- ✓ Parotid gland
- ✓ Structures within the parotid gland
    - ▷ Facial nerve (CN VII)
    - ▷ Retromandibular vein
    - ▷ External carotid artery
    - ▷ Superficial and deep parotid lymph nodes

Facial nerve (CN VII)—most superficial

- ✓ Emerges from the stylomastoid foramen
- ✓ Enters the posterior part of the parotid gland
- ✓ Divides into a superior and inferior division
    - ▷ Superior division
        - ◆ Temporal branch
        - ◆ Zygomatic branch
        - ◆ Buccal branch
    - ▷ Inferior division

◆ Mandibular branch
◆ Cervical branch
✓ Branches emerge on the anterior aspect of the parotid gland and lie on the masseter muscle
✓ Innervates the muscles of facial expression

Retromandibular vein

✓ Formed by the union of the superficial temporal and maxillary veins
✓ Descends in the parotid gland deep to the facial nerve but superficial to the external carotid artery
✓ Joins the posterior auricular vein to form the external jugular vein
✓ Forms common trunk with facial and lingual veins

External carotid artery

✓ Enters the deep surface of the parotid gland
✓ Divides into the superficial temporal and maxillary arteries

Temporomandibular joint (TMJ)

✓ The TMJ is a modified hinge type of synovial joint
✓ Articular surfaces
  ▷ Condyle of the mandible (inferior)
  ▷ Articular tubercle of the temporal bone
  ▷ Mandibular fossa of the temporal bone (squamous part)

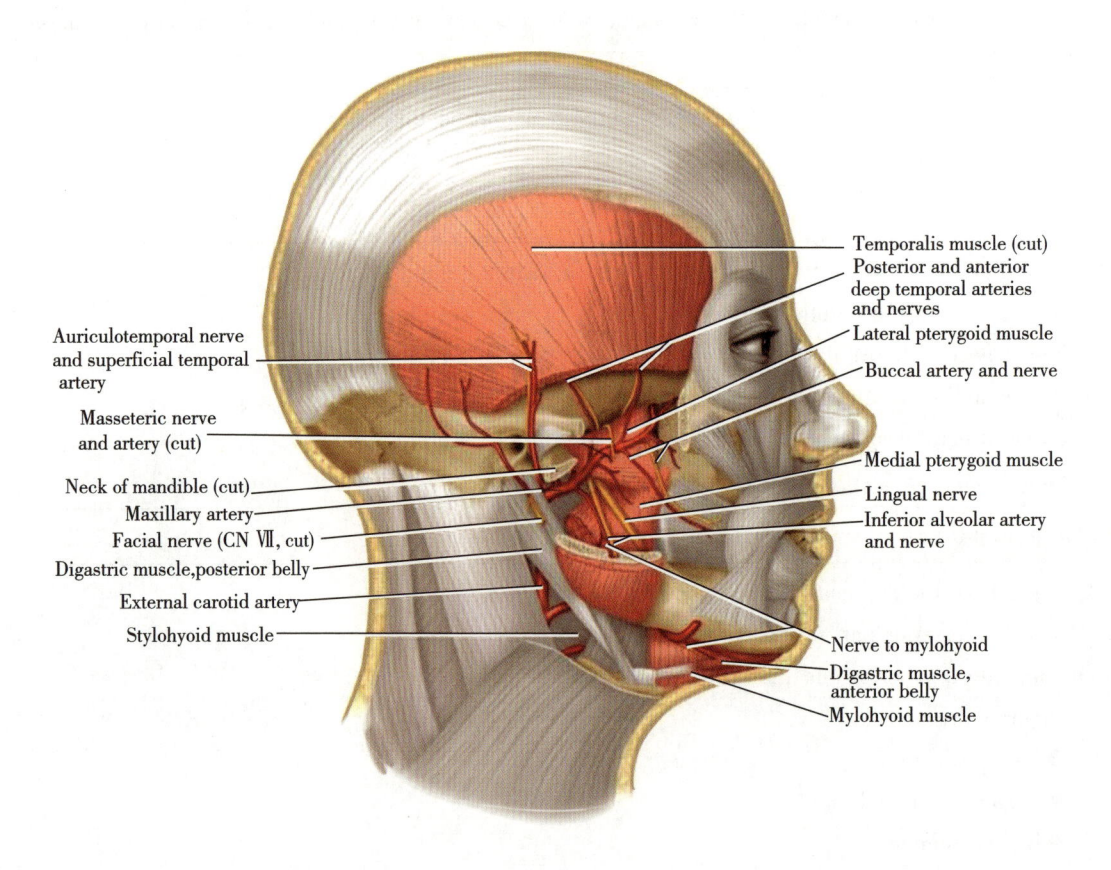

Articular capsule
The loose, fibrous capsule attaches to the margins of the articular area on the temporal bone and around the neck of the mandible ✓ Superior synovial membrane—lines the fibrous capsule superior to the articular disc ✓ Inferior synovial membrane—lines the capsule inferior to the disc
The joint is divided into two compartments by an articular disc—oval, fibrocartilage ✓ Superior compartment—gliding movements of protrusion and retrusion (translation) ✓ Inferior compartment—hinge movements of depression and elevation ✓ The disc is fused with the articular capsule which binds it superiorly to the limits of the temporal articular surface and inferiorly to the neck of the mandible. It is attached more firmly to the mandible than the temporal bone ✓ When the mouth is opened, the disc slides anteriorly on the articular surface against the posterior surface of the articular tubercle

Intrinsic ligament
The thick part of the articular capsule forms the intrinsic lateral ligament (TMJ ligament) which strengthens the TMJ laterally, prevents posterior dislocation of the TMJ

Extrinsic ligaments
✓ Stylomandibular ligament 　◊ Thickening of the fibrous capsule of the parotid gland 　◊ Extends from the styloid process of the temporal bone to the angle of the mandible 　◊ Does not contribute significantly to the strength of the joint ✓ Sphenomandibular ligament 　◊ Runs from the spine of the sphenoid to the lingua of the mandible 　◊ Primary passive support of the mandible, although the tonus of the muscles of mastication usually bears the mandible's weight 　◊ Serves as a "swinging hinge" for the mandible serving as both as fulcrum and as a check ligament for the movements of the mandible at the TMJ

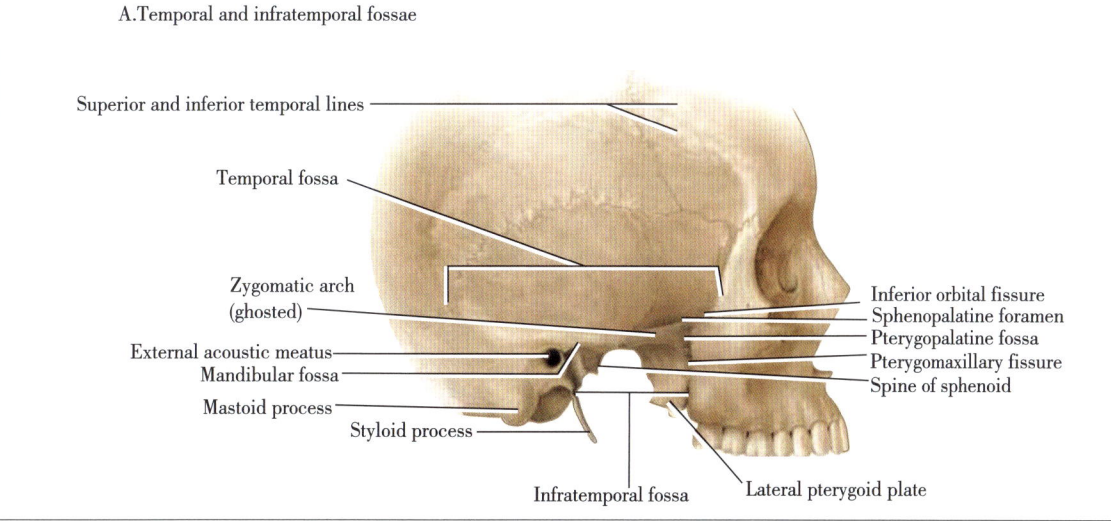

A. Temporal and infratemporal fossae

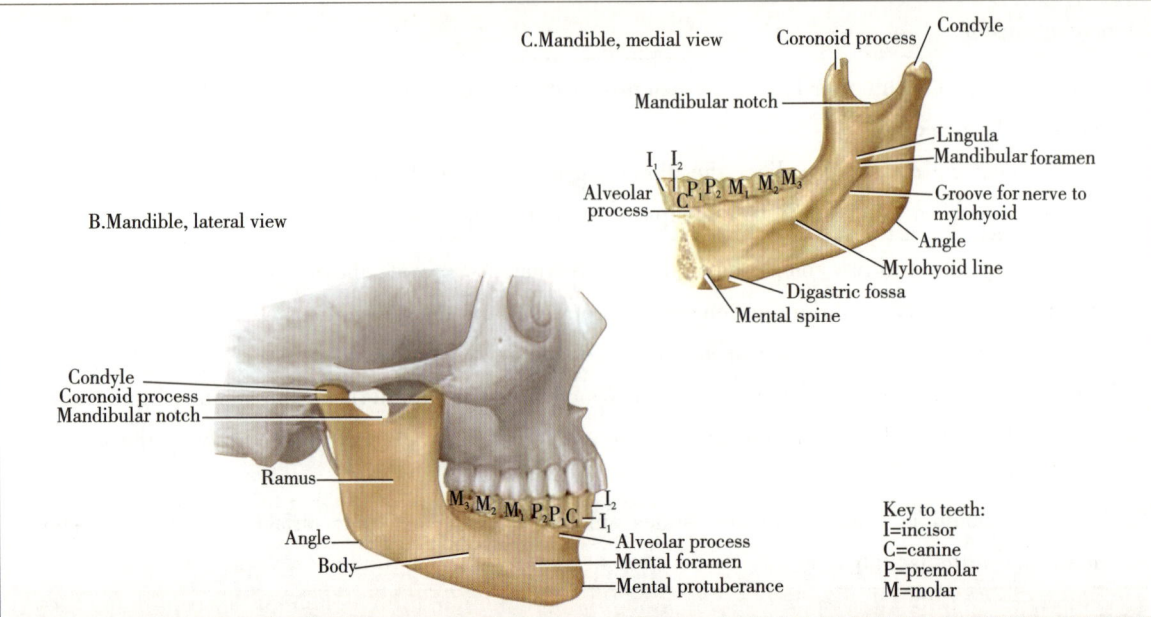

Muscles of mastication—produce movements of the mandible at the TMJ

Temporalis muscle

- ✓ Origin—floor of temporal fossa and deep surface of the temporal fascia
- ✓ Insertion—tip and medial surface of coronoid process and anterior border of ramus of mandible
- ✓ Innervation—mandibular nerve ($CN\ V_3$)
- ✓ Action
  - ◊ Elevates the mandible (closing the jaw)
  - ◊ Middle, oblique and posterior fibers retrude the mandible

Masseter muscle

- ✓ Origin—inferior border and medial surface of zygomatic arch
- ✓ Insertion—lateral surface of ramus of mandible and coronoid process
- ✓ Innervation—mandibular nerve ($CN\ V_3$)
- ✓ Action
  - ◊ Elevates and protudes the madible (closing jaws)
  - ◊ Deep fibers retrude the chin
  - ◊ Occlude teeth for biting and chewing

Lateral pterygoid

- ✓ Origin
  - ◊ Superior head—infratemporal surface and crest of greater wing of sphenoid bone
  - ◊ Inferior head—lateral surface of lateral pterygoid plate
- ✓ Insertion—neck of mandible, articular disc and capsule of TMJ
- ✓ Innervation—mandibular nerve ($CN\ V_3$)
- ✓ Action
  - ◊ Lateral pterygoids acting together—protrude the mandible
  - ◊ Acting alone and alternately—produce side to side movements

Medial pterygoid

- ✓ Origin
  - ◊ Deep head—medial surface of lateral pterygoid plate and palatine bone
  - ◊ Superficial head—tuberosity of maxilla
- ✓ Insertion—medial surface of the ramus of the mandible
- ✓ Innervation—mandibular nerve (CN V_3)
- ✓ Action
  - ◊ Acting together—elevate the mandible (closing jaw)
  - ◊ Acting together—protude the mandible
  - ◊ Acting alternatively—grinding motion

Movements of the TMJ

- ✓ Depression—open mouth
  - ◊ Gravity—prime mover
  - ◊ Suprahyoid and infrahyoid muscles mainly active against resistance
  - ◊ Note: protrusion must occur for all but minimal depression
  - ◊ Lateral pterygoid
- ✓ Elevation—close mouth
  - ◊ Temporalis
  - ◊ Masseter
  - ◊ Medial pterygoid
- ✓ Protrusion—protraction of the chin
  - ◊ Lateral pterygoid—prime mover
  - ◊ Masseter (oblique superficial fibers only)—secondary synergist
  - ◊ Medial pterygoid—secondary synergist
- ✓ Retrusion—retraction of the chin
  - ◊ Temporalis—middle oblique and posterior fibers—prime mover
  - ◊ Masseter—vertical (deep) fibers only—secondary synergist
- ✓ Lateral movement—side-to-side grinding and chewing
  - ◊ Retractors of same side (temporalis, masseter)
  - ◊ Protruders of opposite side (pterygoids)

TMJ movements

- ✓ The gliding movements of retrusion and protrusion occur in the superior compartment of the TMJ
- ✓ The hinge movements of elevation and depression occur in the inferior compartment of the TMJ
- ✓ The mandible is depressed during opening of the mouth
- ✓ The head of the mandible and articular disc move anteriorly on the articular surface until the head lies on the articular tubercle. This movement is called "translation" by dentists. If the anterior gliding occurs unilaterally, the head of the contralateral mandible rotates (pivots) on the inferior surface of the articular disc, permitting simple side-to-side chewing and grinding movements over a small range
- ✓ During protrusion and retrusion, the head and articular disc slide anteriorly and posteriorly on the articular surface of the temporal bone with both sides moving together

Nerve and vascular supply of the TMJ

- ✓ Arterial supply—branches from the maxillary artery (1st and 2nd parts)
- ✓ Nerve supply—auriculotemporal nerve

Infratemporal fossa

- ✓ The infratemporal fossa is an irregularly shaped space deep and inferior to the zygomatic arch, deep the ramus of the mandible, and posterior to the maxilla
- ✓ It communicates with the temporal fossa through the interval between (deep to) the zygomatic arch and (superficial to) the cranial bones

Boundries

- ✓ Lateral—ramus of the mandible
- ✓ Medial—lateral pterygoid plate
- ✓ Anterior—posterior aspect of the maxilla
- ✓ Posterior—tympanic plate, mastoid and styloid processes of the temporal bone
- ✓ Superior—inferior (infratemporal) surface of the greater wing of the sphenoid
- ✓ Inferior—where the medial pterygoid muscle attaches to the mandible near its angle

Contents

- ✓ Inferior part of the temporalis muscle
- ✓ Lateral and medial pterygoid muscles
- ✓ Maxillary artery
- ✓ Pterygoid venous plexus
- ✓ Nerves
  - ◊ Mandibular nerve (CN V$_3$)
  - ◊ Inferior alveolar
  - ◊ Lingual
  - ◊ Buccal
  - ◊ Chorda tympani
- ✓ Otic ganglion

External carotid artery branches

- ✓ Superior thyroid artery
- ✓ Ascending pharyngeal artery
- ✓ Lingual artery
- ✓ Occipital artery
- ✓ Facial artery
- ✓ Posterior auricular artery
- ✓ Maxillary artery
- ✓ Superficial temporal artery

Maxillary artery

✓ Arises posterior to the neck of the mandible
✓ Passes anteriorly, deep to the neck of the mandibular condyle (1st part or mandibular part)
✓ Passes superficial or deep to the lateral pterygoid muscle (2nd part or pterygoid part)
✓ Disappears through the pterygomaxillary fissure to enter the pterygopalatine fossa (3rd part or pterygopalatine part)
✓ The maxillary artery is thus divided into three parts by the lateral pterygoid muscle

Mandibular or 1st part of the maxillary artery

✓ Deep auricular artery—external acoustic meatus
✓ Anterior tympanic artery—tympanic membrane
✓ Middle meningeal artery—dura mater and calvaria (via foramen spinosum)
✓ Accessory meningeal artery—cranial cavity (via foramen ovale)
✓ Inferior alveolar artery—mandible, gingivae, teeth (via mandibular canal)

Pterygoid or 2nd part of the maxillary artery

✓ Deep temporal artery—temporal muscle
  ▷ Anterior branch
  ▷ Posterior branch
✓ Pterygoid artery—pterygoid muscles
✓ Masseteric artery—masseter muscle (deep surface)
✓ Buccal artery—buccinator muscle

Pterygopalatine or 3rd part of the maxillary artery

✓ Posterior superior alveolar (dental) artery—supplies the maxillary molar and premolar teeth, the lining of the maxillary sinus and the gingival
✓ Infraorbital artery—supplies the inferior eyelid, lacrimal sac, side of the nose and the superior lip
✓ Descending palatine artery—supplies the maxillary gingival, palatine glands, and the mucous membrane of the roof of the mouth
✓ Artery of the pterygoid canal—supplies the superior part of the pharynx, the pharyngotympanic tube, and the tympanic cavity
✓ Pharyngeal artery—supplies the roof of the pharynx, the sphenoidal sinus, and the inferior part of the pharyngotympanic tube
✓ Sphenopalatine artery—the termination of the maxillary artery; supplies the lateral nasal wall, the nasal septum and the adjacent paranasal sinuses

Pterygoid venous plexus

✓ Located between the temporal and pterygoid muscles
✓ Communicates with the cavernous sinus by emissary veins of vesalius (sphenoid emissary foramen—inconstant)
✓ Drains into the deep facial vein (common trunk with retromandibular and lingual veins)

Mandibular nerve

- ✓ Descends through the foramen ovale to enter the infratemporal fossa
- ✓ Divides into sensory and motor branches

Motor branches—muscles of mastication

- ✓ Anterior and deep temporal branch
- ✓ Masseteric branch
- ✓ Lateral and medial pterygoid branch
- ✓ Nerve to myelohyoid (anterior digastric)
- ✓ Tensor tympani and tensor veli palatini

Sensory branches

- ✓ Auriculotemporal nerve
- ✓ Inferior alveolar nerve
- ✓ Lingual nerve
- ✓ Buccal nerve

Otic ganglion

- ✓ Parasympathetic—located in the infratemporal fossa
- ✓ Inferior to the foramen ovale, medial to the mandibular nerve and posterior to the medial pterygoid muscle
- ✓ Receives presynaptic parasympathetic fibers derived mainly from the glossopharyngeal nerve (CN IX) that synapse in the otic ganglion
- ✓ Postsynaptic fibers which are secretory to the parotid gland, pass from the otic ganglion to the parotid through the auriculotemporal nerve—inferior salivatory nucleus, tympanic nerve and plexus, lesser petrosal nerve, otic ganglion, auriculotemporal nerve→parotid gland

Auriculotemporal nerve

- ✓ Encircles the middle meningeal artery
- ✓ Divides into numerous branches, the largest which passes posteriorly medial to the neck of the mandible
- ✓ Supplies sensory fibers to the auricle and temporal region
- ✓ Articular fibers to the TMJ
- ✓ Parasympathetic secretomotor fibers to the parotid gland

Inferior alveolar nerve

- ✓ Enters the mandibular foramen and passes through the mandibular canal forming the inferior dental plexus
- ✓ Sends branches to all mandibular teeth on its side
- ✓ Another branch—mental nerve, passes through the mental foramen and supplies the skin and mucous membrane of the lower lip, skin of the chin, and the vestibular gingiva of the mandibular incisor teeth
- ✓ Nerve to myelohyoid and anterior digastric muscles runs with the inferior alveolar nerve in the mandibular canal

Lingual nerve

- ✓ Lies anterior to the inferior alveolar nerve
- ✓ Enters the mouth between the medial pterygoid and ramus of the mandible

✓ Passes anteriorly under the cover of the oral mucosa just inferior to the 3rd molar tooth
✓ Sensory to the anterior 2/3 of the tongue, the floor of the mouth and the lingual gingival

Buccal nerve

✓ Emerges from deep to the ramus of the mandible and runs anteriorly on the buccinator muscle, piercing but not supplying this muscle
✓ Sends branches to thumb-sized area of skin over the cheek, and supplies the mucous membrane lining the cheek and the posterior part of the buccal surface of the gingiva

Chorda tympani nerve

✓ Branch of the facial nerve (CN Ⅶ)
✓ Joins the lingual nerve in the infratemporal fossa
✓ Carries taste fibers from the anterior two-thirds of the tongue
✓ Carries secretomotor fibers for the submandibular and sublingual salivary glands
✓ Submandibular and sublingual glands—superior salivatory nucleus, intermediate nerve, chorda tympani, lingual nerve, submandibular ganglion, submandibular and sublingual glands
✓ Taste—anterior 2/3 of the tongue, chorda tympani nerve (via lingual nerve), geniculate ganglion, intermediate nerve, tractus solitarius

1.4.9 Meninges and cranial cavity

Overview

Neurocranium = cranial vault or brain case

Calvaria = "skull cap" or top of neurocranium

Usually composed of four bones:
✓ A frontal bone (unpaired) anteriorly
✓ Two parietal bones forming the lateral walls
✓ An occipital bone (unpaired) posteriorly

Clinical notes: ①Sutural (Wormian) bones may also be present. ②Bones have not fused in children allowing molding to occur during birth

✓ Bones are separated by sutures where bones fuse
　◊ Coronal = between frontal and parietal bones
　◊ Sagittal = between two parietal bones
　◊ Lambdoid (look like a "λ") = between parietal bones and occipital bone
✓ Other important landmarks
　◊ Bregma = intersection of sagittal and coronal sutures
　◊ Pterion = intersection of the frontal, parietal, sphenoid, and temporal bones

Inferior surface of calvaria

Landmarks

✓ Sagittal groove-attachment of the superior sagittal sinus; widens posteriorly

- ✓ Foveolae granulares—pits or depressions in the calvaria
  - ◊ More numerous and evident in old age
  - ◊ Formed by arachnoid granulations, where cerebrospinal fluid (CSF) is returned to the dural venous sinuses
  - ◊ Occur mostly along the superior sagittal sinus
- ✓ Grooves for branches of middle meningeal vessels (located in parietal bones)

Cut surface of calvaria allows visualization of three layers of the cranial walls

- ✓ Most flat bones of the skull have two lamina (or tables) of compact bone
- ✓ Inner layer is distinctly thinner and thus more prone to injury. In fact, the inner layer can fracture with outer table still intact
- ✓ Two lamina are separated by the diploë—a layer of cancellous (spongy) bone
  - ◊ Diploë contains bone marrow and canals which transmit diploic veins—vein that drain either into the veins of the scalp or dural venous sinuses. Veins pass through all three layers of the skull and connect the dural venous sinuses with veins outside the skull are called emissary veins. These veins are highly variable in number and location
- ✓ Thickness of cranium varies among regions, which is best visualized when holding the skull up to the light. Usually most thin in regions covered by muscles

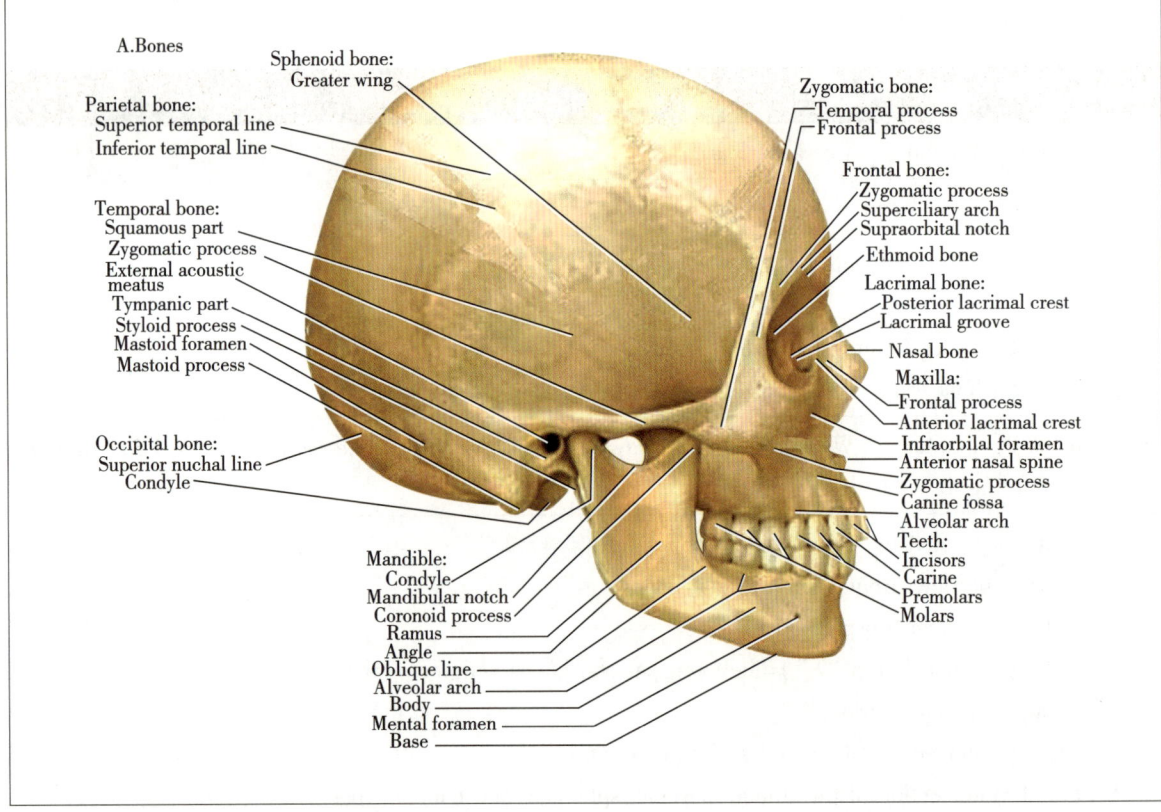

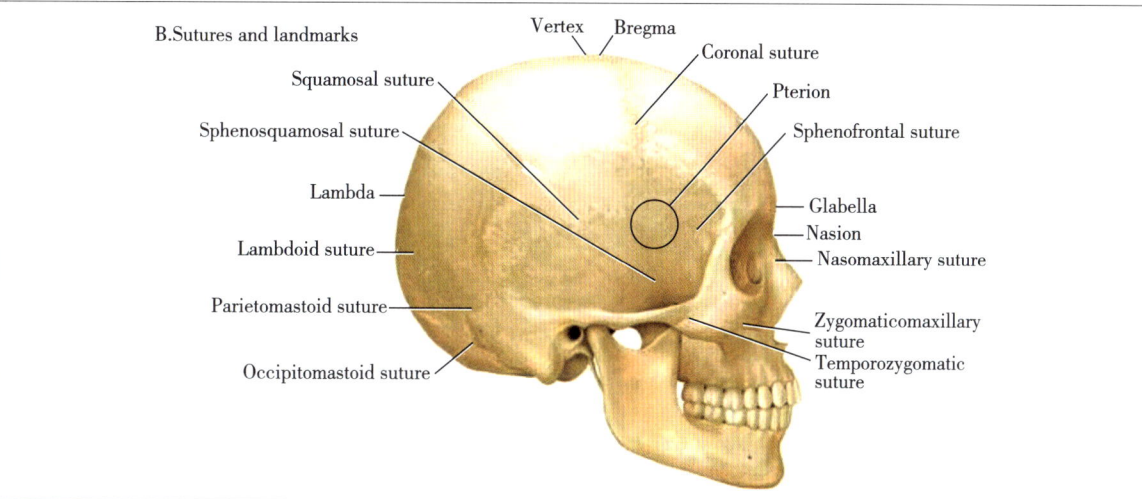

B. Sutures and landmarks

Cranial meninges

Functions

- ✓ Protect the brain
- ✓ Serve as supporting framework for arteries, veins, and dural venous sinuses
- ✓ Enclose the subarachnoid (leptomeningeal) space, where blood vessels and CSF reside

Contains same three layers previously studied: dura mater, arachnoid mater, and pia mater

Dura mater

Composed of two layers that are (usually) fused

- ✓ Endosteal (outer) layer of dura = internal periosteum of the skull
  - ◊ Continuous with external periosteal layer through the various foramina
  - ◊ Not continuous with the dura mater of the spinal cord
  - ◊ Can also be called the endocranium
- ✓ Meningeal (inner) layer of dura = equivalent of spinal dura mater
  - ◊ Continuous with the dura mater of the spinal cord at foramen magnum
  - ◊ Not continuous with the spinal epidural space

Clinical notes: Epidural anesthesia can not ascend to enter the skull

- ✓ Layers of the dura mater form two very important structures: septa and dural venous sinuses
- ✓ Septa—reflections of the meningeal layer of the dura that partially separate parts of the brain
- ✓ Falx cerebri—largest dura reflection located in the median sagittal plane separates left and right cerebral hemispheres and forms a vertical partition
- ✓ Attaches to the frontal crest and cristi galli anteriorly and to the internal occipital protuberance as well as the cerebellar tentorium posteriorly
- ✓ Becomes continuous with the cerebellar tentorium, forming the walls of the straight dural venous sinus

Cerebellar tentorium

- ✓ The tent of the cerebellum; 2nd largest dural fold
- ✓ Separates cerebellum from occipital lobe of the brain

✓ Attaches to the clinoid processes of the sphenoid bone anteriorly, to the petrous portion of the temporal bone laterally, and the internal surfaces of the occipital and parietal bones. This septum must be cut to remove the brain from the skull
✓ Divides the cranial cavity into supratentorial and infratentorial compartments
✓ The anterior portion of the cerebellar tentorium has an opening called the tentorial incisure or tentorial notch through which the midbrain will pass

Clinical notes: In general, space-occupying lesions (tumor, arterial bleeding, or blockage of cerebrospinal fluid are examples) occur below the cerebellum tentorium (i.e., located infratentorially) in children. In adults, most space-occupying lesions occur above the cerebellar tentorium (i.e., located supratentorially). Supratentorial lesions can cause increased intracranial pressure (ICP) and lead to herniation of the uncus (the most medial part of the temporal lobe of the brain) inferiorly through the tentorial notch (incisure). This clinical condition is called uncal herniation

✓ A patient with uncal herniation has three cardinal symptoms
✓ Decreased level of consciousness (due to compression of the reticular formation in the midbrain), so patient acts lethargic
✓ Ipsilateral (same-side as lesion) dilation of the pupil (due to compression of the parasympathetic division of the oculomotor nerve, CN III, which controls the pupillary sphincter). The oculomotor nerve exits anterior to the tentorial incisure from the midbrain, which is why it is compromised
✓ If the ICP is not relieved, the patient can die due to tonsillar herniation, where lowest part of cerebellum (tonsil) is pushed inferiorly into the foramen magnum; this results in a compressed medulla and its structures of the brain that are important for vital functions (including consciousness, breathing, heart rate, etc.)

Falx cerebelli

✓ Sickle-shaped vertical septa between cerebellar hemispheres
  ◊ Lies inferior and attaches to the tentorium cerebelli
  ◊ Occipital venous sinus is located in its base

Diaphragma sellae

✓ Small, circular, and horizontal sheet of dura
✓ Covers hypophyseal fossa in the sella turcica ("Turkish saddle"). Infundibulum of the pituitary gland penetrates this septum; causing infundibular stalk to break when brain is removed in lab. Therefore, the pituitary gland will remain inside the hypophyseal fossa of the sella turcica

Clinical notes: ① Pituitary tumors will cause this septum to be displaced superiorly. ② Can lead to endocrine symptoms (obesity, genital shrinking, etc.), due to the involvement of the pituitary and hypothalamus superiorly. ③ Can also compress the optic chiasm—leading to bitemporal hemianopsia (or blindness in temporal halves of the visual field, "tunnel vision")

Dural venous sinuses—venous channels formed between the meningeal and endosteal layers of the dura (equivalent to internal vertebral venous plexus of the spinal cord, which is located between the periosteum and dura of vertebral canal); drain all blood from the brain via the jugular foramen; continuous with cerebral veins; have no valves; lined with endothelium; no muscles in their walls; equivalent to internal vertebral venous plexus in the spinal cord as the venous sinuses (usually) lie between periosteal and endosteal layers of the cranial dura

Superior sagittal sinus
✓ Lies in the median plane in superior border of the falx cerebri
✓ 60% of cases ends in right transverse sinus
✓ Receives superior cerebral veins. These veins are clinically important as they can be torn following a blow to the "front" of the head. This results in a subdural hemorrhage—bleeding into the potential space between the arachnoid and dura
✓ Contains protrusions from subarachnoid space called arachnoid villi, which return CSF into venous system

Inferior sagittal sinus
✓ Occupies posterior 2/3 of the free inferior edge of the falx cerebri
✓ Ends in the straight sinus

Straight sinus
✓ Formed by the inferior sagittal sinus and great cerebral vein of Galen
✓ Runs inferoposteriorly along falx cerebri to tentorium cerebelli
✓ Empties into a transverse sinus (usually the left)
✓ Helps form confluence of sinuses—dilation of the venous channels posteriorly; where the superior sagittal, straight, occipital, and transverse sinuses meet

Transverse sinuses
✓ Paired sinuses (left and right)
✓ Pass lateral from the confluence of sinuses
✓ Form deep grooves in the occipital (and part of the parietal) bones
✓ Become the sigmoid sinus at the posterior aspect of the petrous temporal bone as they leave the tentorium cerebelli

Sigmoid sinuses
✓ Paired sinuses with a S-shaped course in the posterior cranial fossa
✓ They receive the inferior petrosal sinuses directly

Occipital sinus
✓ Found posterior to foramen magnum
✓ Lies in attached border of falx cerebelli
✓ Communicates inferiorly with internal vertebral plexus
✓ Drains superiorly in the confluence of sinuses

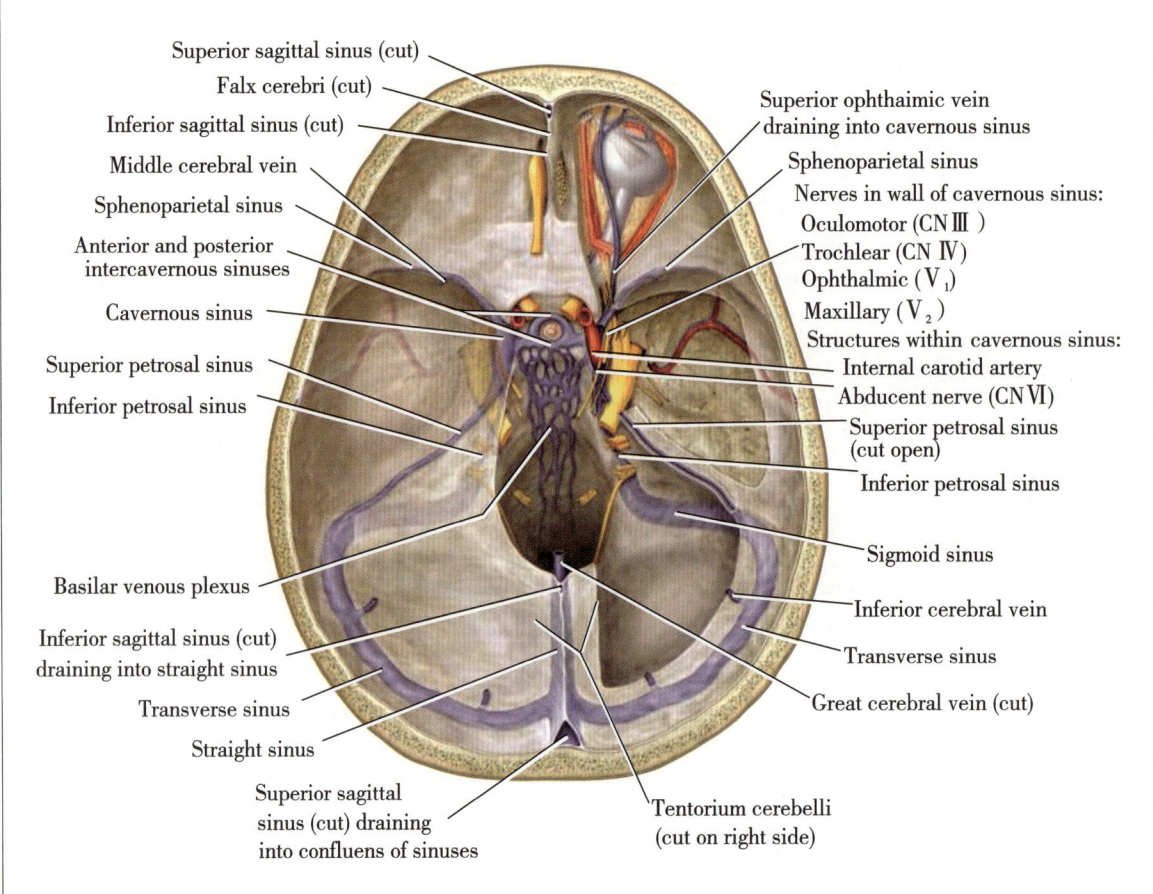

Cavernous sinuses

✓ Rather large, paired sinuses (2 cm long, 1 cm wide)
✓ Extend from superior orbital fissure to petrous part of the temporal bone
✓ Differ from the other sinuses as they are transversed by numerous trabeculae, which give them a spongy appearance
✓ Drain through the superior and inferior petrosal sinuses
✓ Receives drainage of the sphenoparietal sinus (along the crest of the lesser wing of the sphenoid), middle cerebral veins, and ophthalmic veins
  ▷ Ophthalmic veins communicate with the angular veins of the facial vein
    ◆ Infection from the forehead, eyes, nose, and lips may spread to the cavernous sinus
✓ Many structures transverse the cavernous sinuses
  ▷ The internal carotid artery and its periarterial nervous plexus (sympathetics)
  ▷ The abducens nerve (CN VI)
  ▷ The oculomotor nerve (CN III)
  ▷ The trochlear nerve (CN IV)
  ▷ The ophthalmic (CN V_1) and maxillary (CN V_2) divisions of the trigeminal nerve
  ▷ CN III, CN IV, and the divisions of CN V lie laterally in the cavenous sinus

Superior petrosal sinuses

✓ Paired sinuses that lie superior to the petrous ridge of the temporal bone

- ✓ Drain the cavernous sinuses and empty into transverse sinuses
- ✓ Lie in attached margin of tentorium cerebelli

Inferior petrosal sinuses

- ✓ Paired sinuses that drain directly into the internal jugular vein on either side; also drain the cavernous sinuses

Emissary veins

- ✓ Clinically important because infections within the scalping plane can spread to the bone via these veins or the foramina through which they pass
- ✓ Usually carry blood away from the brain; however, they contain no valves. Therefore, blood can potentially flow in both directions
- ✓ Size and number vary

Frontal emissary vein

- ✓ Passes through foramen cecum, connects superior sagittal sinus with veins of the frontal sinuses and nasal cavities
- ✓ Parietal emissary vein (parietal foramen)
- ✓ Mastoid emissary vein—passes through mastoid canal
  - ◊ Connects sigmoid sinus with occipital or posterior auricular vein
- ✓ Posterior condylar emissary vein—passes through condylar canal
  - ◊ Connects sigmoid sinus through condylar canal

Vasculature and innervation of the dura mater

Blood supply to the dura

- ✓ Is rather scant since the dura is relatively inactive metabolically; therefore, most of the blood in the "meningeal" arteries is distributed to the bones of the skull
- ✓ The middle meningeal artery is the largest and most important
  - ◊ Supplies most of the supratentorial dura except the floor of the anterior cranial fossa (which is supplied by branches of the anterior and posterior ethmoidal arteries from the ophthalmic artery)
    - ◊ Branch of the maxillary artery (from external carotid)
    - ◊ Enters middle cranial fossa via foramen spinosum
    - ◊ Forms deep grooves in the inner lamina of bone; thus, subject to injury

Nervous innervation of the dura

- ✓ In general terms, the dura is supplied by the trigeminal nerve (CN V) supratentorially and the 2nd and 3rd cervical nerve (infratentorially)
- ✓ Anterior cranial fossa—innervated by anterior meningeal branches of the ethmoidal nerve (CN V_1) in the anteriomedially and the meningeal branches of the maxillary nerve (CN V_2) posteriolaterally. The meningeal branches of the mandibular nerve (CN V_3) supply the lateral walls of the cranial vault and small part of the anterior cranial fossa laterally

- ✓ Middle cranial fossa—innervated by meningeal branches of the mandibular nerve (CN V_3) primarily, which also supply the lateral walls of the cranial vault. The meningeal branches of the maxillary nerve (CN V_2) supply a small part of this fossa anteriorly.
- ✓ Posterior cranial fossa—innervated by sensory branches from dorsal roots of the 2nd and 3rd cervical nerves (C_2 and C_3) infratentorially. However, the dura of the roof of the posterior cranial fossa (or tentorium cerebelli) is innervated by the tentorial branches of the ophthalmic nerve of CN V_1

Leptomeninges

- ✓ Consists of arachnoid (spider-like; a thin delicate membrane) and pia mater (adherent to brain tissue), connected with each other by the arachnoid trabeculae, but otherwise separated by the subarachnoid space, which collapses after death

Subarachnoid space consists of

- ✓ Arachnoid trabeculae, a network of connective tissue
- ✓ Cerebrospinal fluid (CSF) which bathes the brain tissue and helps distribute and equalize pressure within the skull. Remember your physics: fluid is incompressible
- ✓ Blood vessels—all major vessels of the brain lie in the subarachnoid space before entering the parenchyma

Cisterns

- ✓ Dilations or enlargements of the subarachnoid space where CSF pools. Remember, the pia is attached to the surface of the brain, while the arachnoid follows closely the shape of the dura. Cisterns include:
  - ◊ Cerebellomedullary cistern (or cisterna magna)—spans between the posterioinferior surface of the cerebellum and posterior part of the medulla. This is the largest cistern
  - ◊ Pontine cistern—lies over the pons of the hindbrain
  - ◊ Interpeduncular cistern—lies over the ventral surface of the brain in the area of the midbrain
  - ◊ Lumbar cistern—extends inferiorly from approximately the level of L_2 to the level of S_2 where the dural sac ends. It is in direct communication with the CSF of the brain

Subarachnoid hemorrhage

- ✓ Rupture of a blood vessel within the subarachnoid space (where the CSF travels)
- ✓ Usually due to rupture of an aneurysm (dilation of an artery)
- ✓ An aneurysm located within the Circle of Willis (the arterial vessels that form a concentric ring around the sella turcica) is the most common locatation for this type of hemorrhage. This condition is called a Berry aneurysm
- ✓ Rupture of a vessel in the subarachnoid space will turn the CSF red or pink. Remember, never take a spinal tap, obtaining CSF from the lumbar cistern with a syringe, when a mass occupying lesion is expected. The increased ICP will cause the brain to herniate through the tentorial notch
- ✓ Patient will present with the three cardinal symptoms: ①a sudden onset of the "worst headache of their life", ②nuchal ridgity (stiff neck), and ③loss (or decreased level) of consciousness
- ✓ Unlike subdural (a blow to the front of the head) and epidural (a blow to the side of the head) hemorrhages, a subarachnoid hemorrhage usually does not occur following head trauma

Cerebrospinal fluid (CSF)

✓ Filtrate of the blood that helps protect the brain and may provide nutrients to the structures it bathes. CSF is secreted by the choroid plexus within the ventricles, which are located inside the brain, and it is found in the ventricles, the subarachnoid space, and the cisterns, which are all continuous with one another. The CSF is returned into the superior sagittal venous sinus by arachnoid villi, which are essentially a one-way valve for the CSF to re-enter the bloodstream

Arterial supply to the brain—from vertebral arteries and the internal carotid arteries

Internal carotid arteries

✓ Formed following bifurcation of common carotid (level C_4)

✓ Enters the carotid canal, runs toward and superior to the foramen lacerum, travels anteriorly through the cavernous sinus toward the optic canal, give off the ophthalmic artery, turns posteriorly 180° to travel over the carotid sinus, and ends as it branches into the middle and anterior cerebral arteries

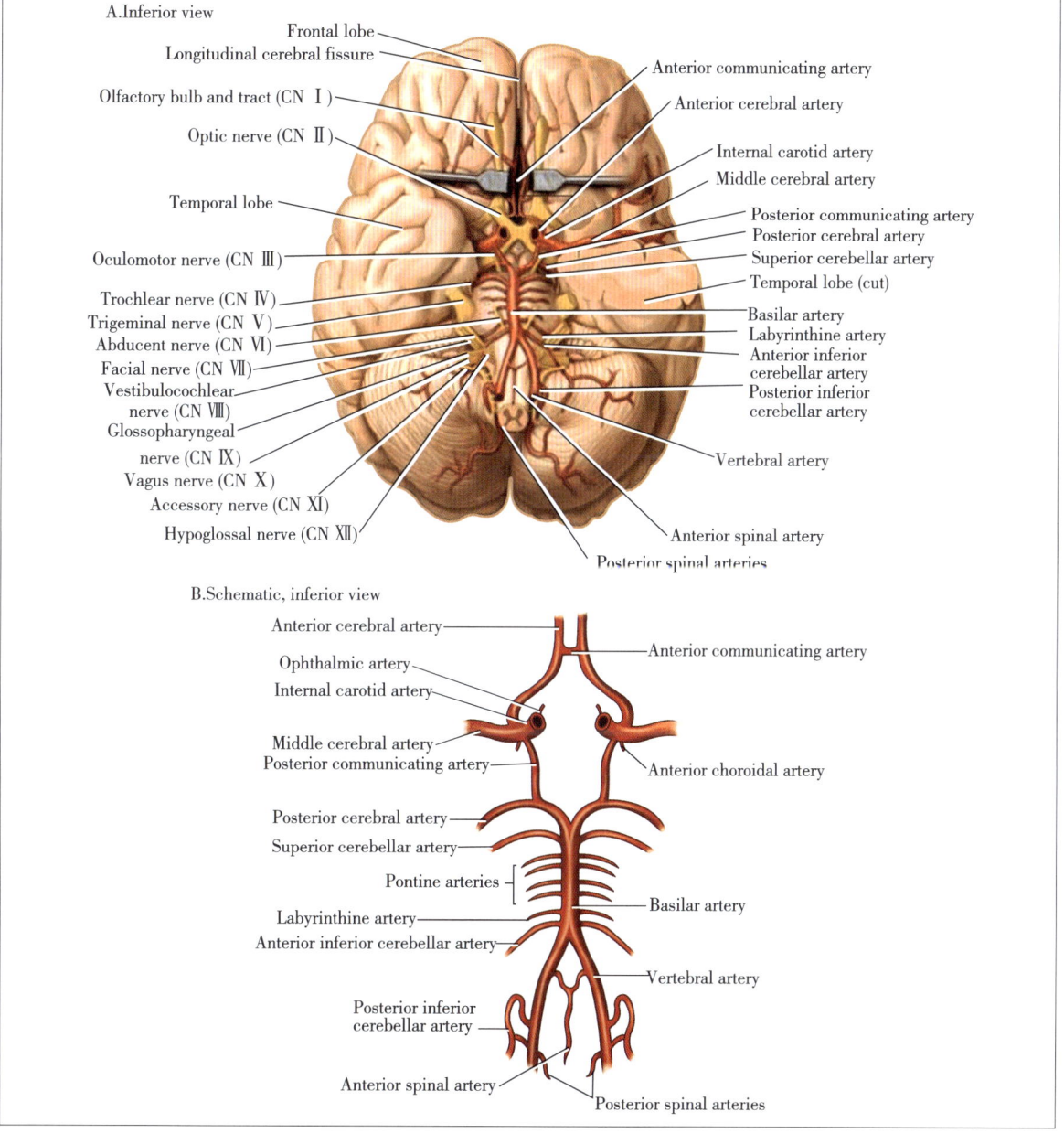

A. Inferior view

B. Schematic, inferior view

Vertebral arteries
1st branch of each subclavian artery
✓ Enter transverse foramina of C_6 and ascend superiorly through C_1, travel posteromedially along vertebral groove in posterior arch of the atlas, pierce the atlantooccipital membrane, enter the cranial via the foramen magnum, then run along the anterolateral surface of the medulla, and join other vertebral artery at caudal portion of the pons to form the basilar artery, which eventually gives off the posterior cerebral arteries on either side

Wang Degui, Lu Wei, Yang Lin, Zhang Yanru

Chapter 2

The Neck

2.1 Introduction

The neck is the major conduit between the head and trunk, and upper limbs. The neck contains bones, vessels, nerves and other structures connecting these areas. It also contains important endocrine glands such as the thyroid gland. The skeleton of th neck is formed by the seven cervical vertebrae, hyroid bone, manubrium of the sternum, and clavicles. The neck is enclosed by investing and superficial fasciae and skin.

2.1.1 Boundary of the neck

The neck is bounded superioly by a line linking the base of mandible, the angle of mandible, the mastoid process, and the external occipital protuberance, and inferiorly by the upper border of sternum, the clavicle, the acromion and the spine of the 7th cervical verbra (Figure 2-1).

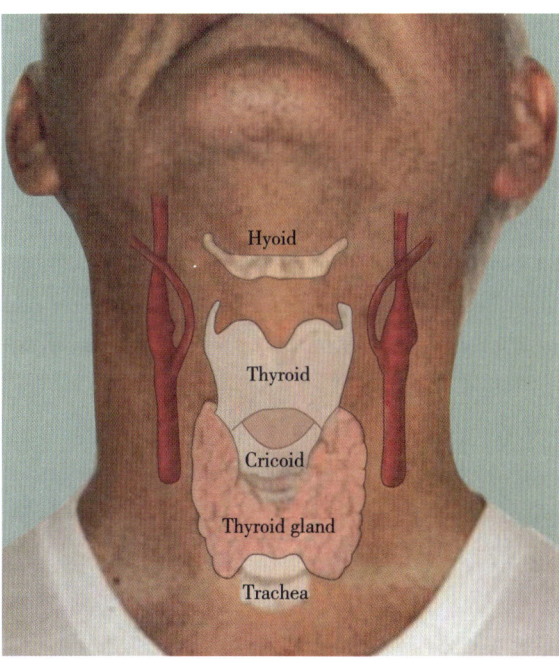

Figure 2-1　Boundary of the neck

2.1.2 Division of the neck

The neck is divided into two portions: the anterolateral and posterior by the anterior margin of the trapezius (Figure 2-2). The former is also called the side of the neck and the posterior is also termed the nucha. To facilitate description of cervical anatomy, each side of the neck is divided into anterior, lateral and sternocleidomastoid regions by the anterior and posterior edges of the sternocleidomastoid. The anteiror region of the neck is further divided into superahyoid and inferahyoid regions by the hyoid bone. The superahyoid region consists of the submental triangle and the both side of the submandibular triangles. While the inferahyoid region is composed of the carotid and muscluar triangles.

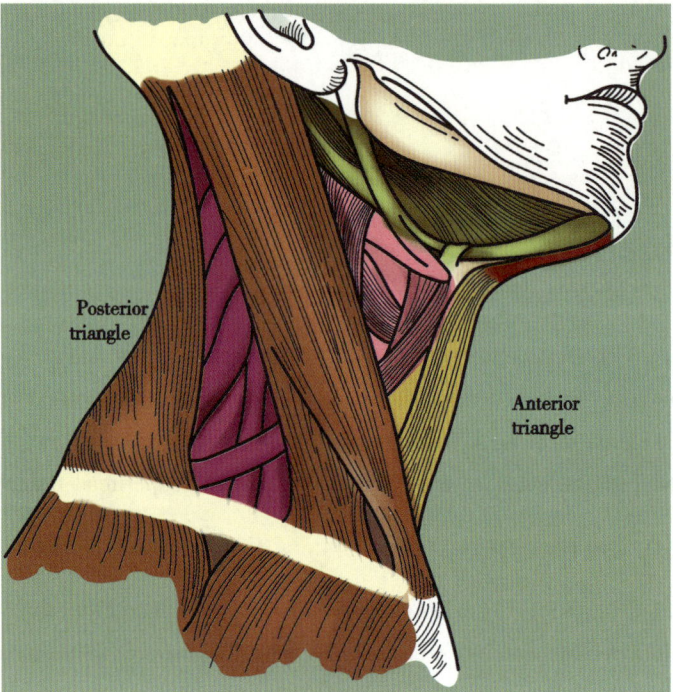

Figure 2-2 Divisions of the neck

2.1.3 Surface landmarks

Before you begin, examine the surface landmarks of the anterior and lateral neck in the cadaver. You can palpate the following structures.

(1) The hyoid bone, an U-shaped bone, can be felt at the level with the body of C_3 in the median plane inferior to the chin. When the neck is relaxed, the tips of the greater horns can be palpated.

(2) The thyroid cartilage is located inferior to the hyoid bone at the level of C_4-C_5.

(3) The cricoid cartilage lies at the level of C_6 vertebra inferior to the thyroid cartilage, where the pharynx joins the oesophagus and the larynx and trachea join each other.

(4) The suprasternal fossa is a large, visible depression at the superior border of the manubrium of the sternum and between the clavicular notches, in which the trachea can easily be palpated.

(5) Sternocleidomastoid. It can be palpated throughout its length and is clearly visible when the head is turned to the opposite side.

(6) The greater supraclavicular fossa is a large depression superior to the middle one third of the clavicle. The pulsation of the subclavian artery can be felt on the floor of the fossa.

2.2 Superficial structures and cervical fascia

2.2.1 Superficial structures

2.2.1.1 Skin

The skin of the neck is thin and very movable. Its cleavage lines are constant and run almost horizontally around the neck. Thus, incisions of the operation on the neck should be made along these natural lines.

2.2.1.2 Superficial fascia

Beneath the skin is the superficial fascia that contains cutaneous nerves, blood and lymphatic vessels, and variable amount of fat; anterioly it also contains the platysme (Figure 2-3).

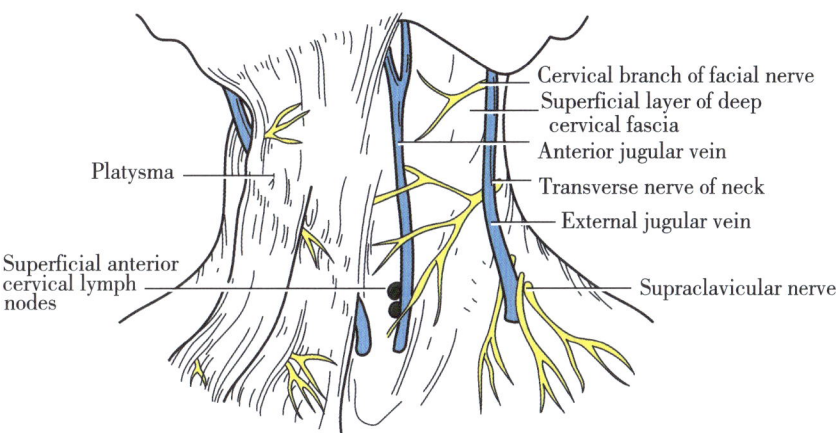

Figure 2-3 Superficial structures of the neck (anterior view)

(1) Platysma

The platysma is a thin layer of muscle arising from the fascia of pectoralis major and inserting mainly into mandible.

(2) Superficial veins

The anterior jugular vein descends anterioly on each side of the midline from the chin to the jugular notch. Each vein pierces the deep fascia above the jugular notch and passes latterally to join the external jugular vien. The external jugular vein, superiorly formed by the union of the posterior branch of the retromandibular vein and the posterior auricular vein, runs downwards and backwards from the anterior to the posterior of the sternocleidomastoid, and then pierces the deep fascia (at the posterior border of the sternocleidomastoid muscle) above the clavicle and receives the anterior jugular vein before joining the subclavian vein.

(3) Cutaneous nerves

In the superfical fascia, the cutaneous nerves run to the skin. The lesser occipital and great auricular nerves run upwards behind the ear, they supply, respectively, the skin behind the ear, and the skin below and before the ear. The transverse cervical nerve runs anteriorly across the neck and innervates most part of the anterior neck, while the supraclavicular nerve decends over the clavicle and innervates the area over the clavicle and shoulder. All the nerves appear from beneath the sternocleidomastoid muscle at the middle of the its posterior border. The point that the nerves all seem to emerging is called the nerve point. It is the site for the cervical plexus block. Additionally, the cervical branch of the facial nerve also lies in this layer and supplies the platysma(Figure 2-4).

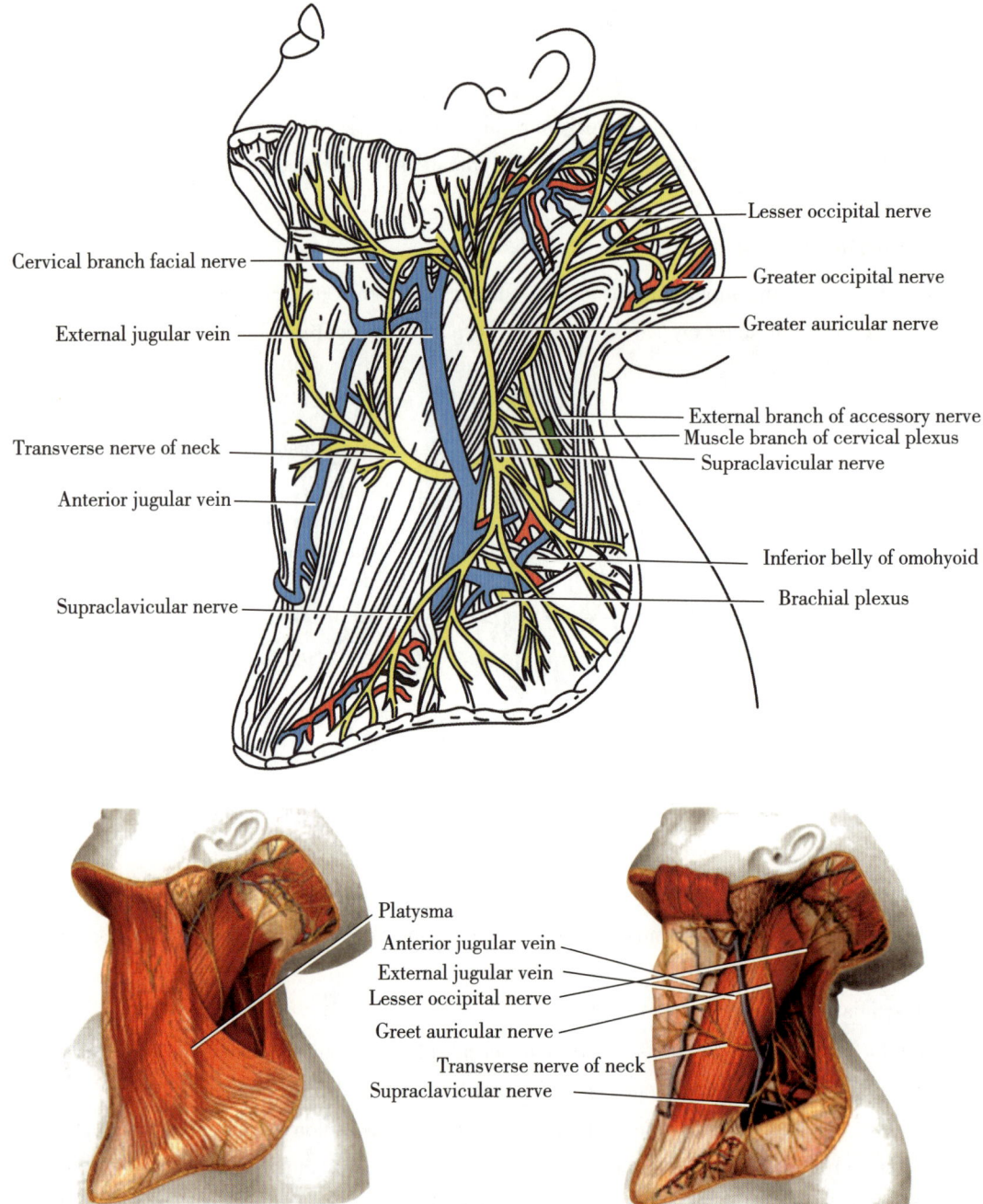

Figure 2-4 Superficial structures of the neck

2.2.2 Cervical fascia and fascial spaces

The cervical fascia lies deep to the superficial fascia and platysma and is composed of three facia layers: superficial, middle(pretracheal), and deep(prevertebral)(Figure 2-5).

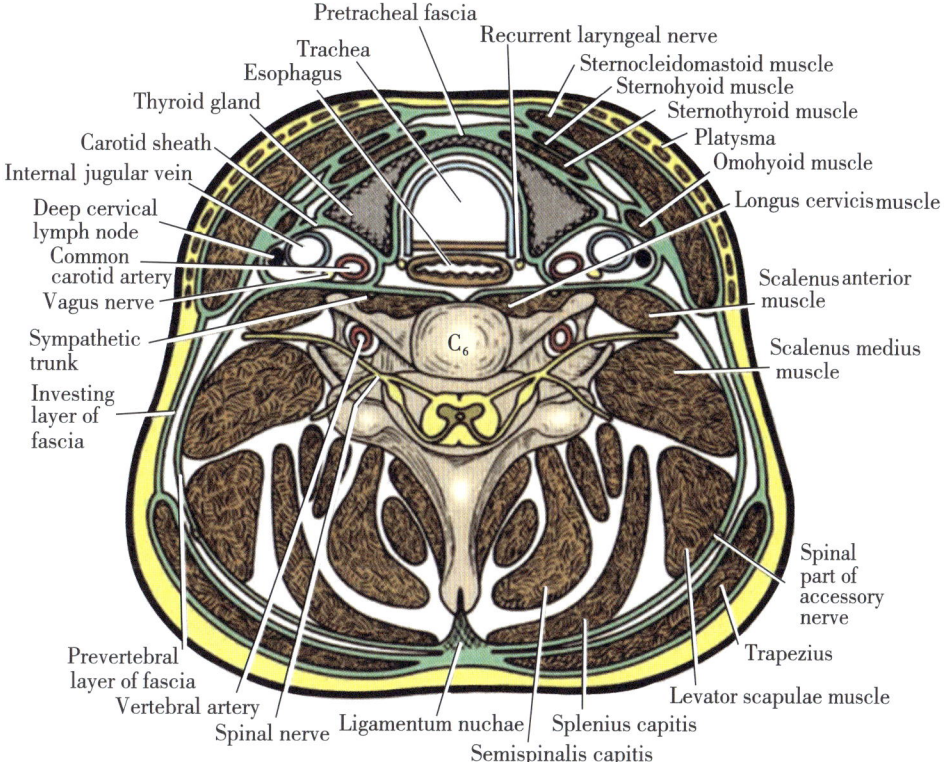

Figure 2-5 Deep cervical fascia (transvers section of neck at the level of sixth cervical vertebra) (superior view)

2.2.2.1 Superficial layer

The superficial layer of the cervical fascia is also termed investing or enveloping fascia. It's tube-shaped and surrounds the major structures of neck. It attaches superiorly to the superir nuchal line of the occipital bone, the mastoid processes of the temporal bones, the zygmatic arches, the inferior border of the mandible, the hyoid bone and the pinous processes of the 7th cervical vertebra, inferiorly to the manubrium of the sternum, the clavicles, the acromions and the spines of the scapula. At the four places of the neck, the superficial layer splits into superificial and deep layers of fascia to enclose the sternocleidomastoid, the trepezius, and the submandibular and parotid glands. Just superorly to the manubriumm of the sternum, the investing layer of fascia is divided into the two layers with outer layer attaching to the anteior and the inner to the posteriot surface of the manubrium. Thus the interval between the two layers is called the superasternal space which encloses the jugular venous arch, fat, and a few deep lymph nodes.

2.2.2.2 Middle layer

The middle layer is also termed visceral or pretracheal layer. It is a thin layer and limited to the anterior aspect of the neck. It extends inferiorly from the hyoid bone into the thorax where it fuese with the fibrous pericardium. The middle layer surrounds infrahyoid muscles (i.e., sternohyoid, sternothyroid, thyrohyoid, omohyoid) and splits to enclose the thyroid gland, trachea, eaophagus and other viscera. It is continuous posteriorly and superiorly with the buccopharyngeal fascia. The pretracheal layer of deep cervical facia blends laterally with the carotid sheaths.

2.2.2.3 Deep layer

The deep layer (prevertebral fascia) of deep cervical fascia forms a tubular sheath for the vertebral column and muscles associated with it and extends from the base of the skull to the 3rd thoracic vertebra, where it fuses with the anterior longitudinal ligament. It extenedes laterally to cover the scalenus anterior and medius, the levator scapulae, and forms the axillary sheath which surround the axillary vessels and brachial plexus. It also forms the floor of the posterior region of the neck and continues with the deep fascia of the muscles of the nape (Figure 2-6).

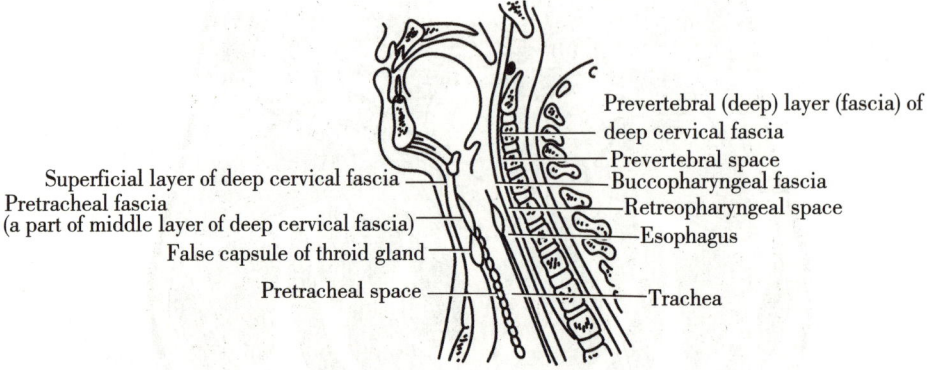

Figure 2-6 Deep cervical fascia (median sagittal section of the neck) (right side)

2.2.2.4 Carotid sheath

Carotid sheath is a tubular, dense fibrous investment that extends from the base of the skull to the root of the neck. It encloses the common and internal carotid ateries, the internal jugular vein and the vagus nerve. This facial sheath blends anteriorly with the investing and pretrachel layers of fascia and posteriorly with the prebertebral layer of deep cervical fascia.

2.2.2.5 Fascial spaces

There are several fascial spaces between or within the fascial layers, which include: the pretracheal space between the posterior surface of the pretracheal fascia and the cervical part of the trachea. The pretracheal lymph nodes, inferior thyroid vein, unpaired thyroid venous plexus, brachiocephalic trunk and left brachiocephalic vein are in this space, the upper part of the thymus is also in the space in children. The retropharyngeal space is a potential space between the pretracheal fascia and prevertebral fascia, so the infection in this region can spread downwards into the mediastinum through the ways from behind the esophagus as well as from in front of the trachea.

2.3 Sternocleidomastoid and anterior region of the neck

2.3.1 Sternocleidomastoid region

Sternocleidomastoid region refers to the area overly by sternocleidomastoid muscle. As the structures superficial to it have already been deal with, we'll focues on the structures deep to it. After cut and reastoid, the large vessls and nerves which run through the neck can be seen.

(1) Ansa cervicalis

Ansa cervicalis is a loop of nerve formed by the union of two roots derived from the anterior branches of the first three cervical spinal nerves. The fibres from the first cervical nerve (C_1 spinal nerves) run together the hypoglossal nerve for a short distance, and leaving it as the upper root of theansa cervicalis, thereafter this root decends along the medial side of internal jugular vein. The fibres from the anterior branches of the C_2 and C_3 form the inferior root of the ansa cervicalis. Most commonly, the roots merge and form the ansa cervicalis on the carotid sheath and then innervate the infrahyoid muscles execpt the thyrohyoid muscle. The sternohyoid and the sternothyroid innervated inferiorly by the branches from ansa cervicalis must be trandected at the middle of their bellies in the thyroidectomy, so it is important to advoide injured these branches clincly.

(2) Carotid sheath and its contents

The carotid sheath is a tube-like fascial structure containing the common carotid and internal carotid arteries, internal jugular vein and vagus nerve. From lateral to medial, on the leteral side is the inernal jugular vein, and medial to it is the commom artery, while the vagus nerve lies posterior and between the vein and atery. There are several important structures or orangs adjecnt to the carotid sheath. Anterior to it are the sternocleidomastoid, sternohyoid, sternothyoid and omohyoid muscles, and the ansa cervicalis. Posterior to it are the sympathetic trunk and the inferior thyroid artery, while medial to it are the pharynx, esophagus, larynx, trachea, the recurrent laryngeal nerve and the lateral lobe of thyroid gland.

Addtionaly, the cervical plexus, the cervical portion of sympathetic trunk and the external branch of accessory nerve also lie deep to the sternocleidomastoid. They are separeted from the carotid vessles and vagus nerve by the prevertebral layer of the cervical fascia.

2.3.2　Anterior region of the neck

The anterior region of the neck is formed anteriorly by the median line of the neck, superiorly by the inferior border of the mandible, and posteriorly by the anerior border of the sternocleidomastoid(Figure 2-7). The anterior region of the neck is subdivided in to suprahyoid and infrahyoid regions by the hyoid bone. The superahyoid region is consists of the submental triangle and the both side of the submandibular triangles. While the inferahyoid region is composed of the carotid and muscluar triangles.

2.3.2.1　Carotid triangle

The carotid triangle is bounded posteriorly by the anterior border of the sternocleidomastoid, superiorly by the posterior belly of the digastric and inferiorly by the superor belly of the omohyoid. On the medial side of the internal jugular vein is the common carotid artery. The common carotid artery ends by dividing into the internal and external carotid arteries at the upper border of the thyroid cartilage. There is a slight dilation at the beginning of the inernal carotid artery or at the upper end of the common carotid atery. This dilation is termed the carotid sinus with the pressure receportor in the wall of it. In the bifurcation, closely adherent to the internal carotid artery is the carotid body. It is an ovoid mass of tissue with the chemical receptor in it, the carotid body monitors blood oxygen and carbon dioxide levels (O_2 and CO_2). The external carotid artery runs upward to the neck of the mandible where it divieds into its two terminal branches, the maxillary and the superficial arteries. Acending for a short distance the external carotid artery gives off most of its branches in carotid triangle. On the medial aspect of the external carotid artery are the superior thyroid artery, lingual artery, facial artery, on the lateral aspect of it are the occipital artery and posterior auricular artery, on the posteior aspect is the ascending pharyngeal artery, these arteries supply their corresponding regions that we have dealed with in the course of the systemic antomy.

The superior thyroid artery inclines downwards and forwards from the anterior surface of the external carotid to supply the thyroid gland and the larynx. The lingual artery passes forwards from the anterior surface of the external carotid artery into the base of the tongue. The facial artery, another anterior branch,

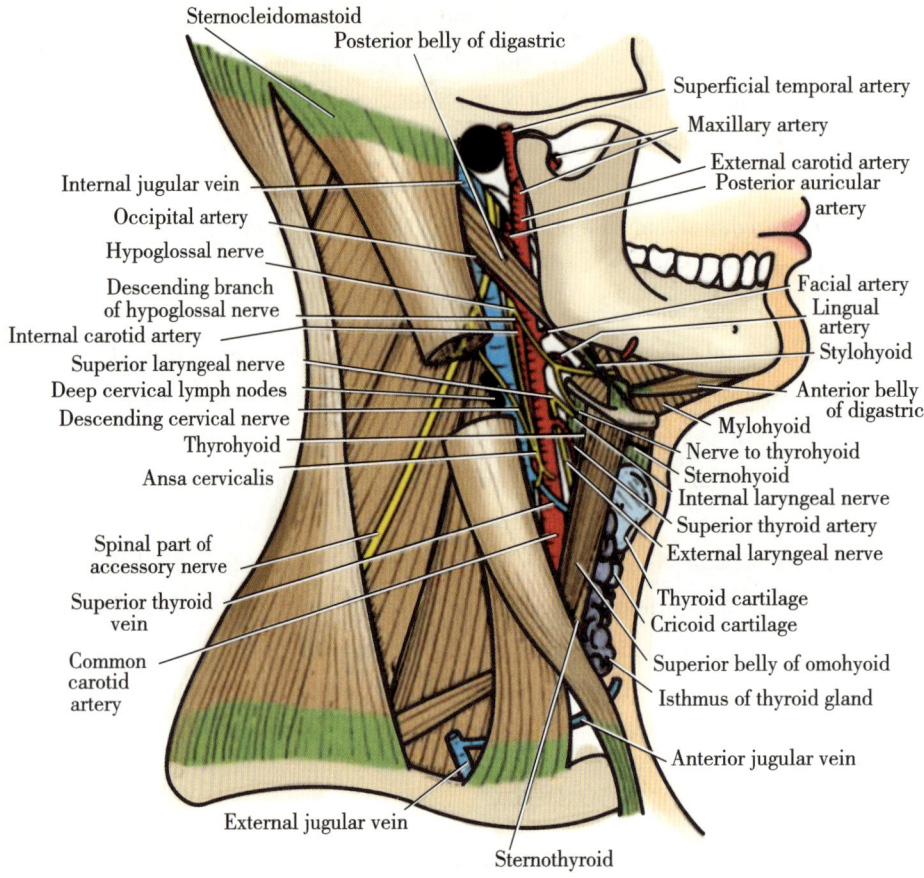

Figure 2-7 Anterior triangle of the neck

supplies the face. Arising from the posterior surface of the external carotid artery, the occipital artery passes upwards and backwards deep to sternomastoid to supply the posterior part of the scalp. The posterior auricular artery arises just above the posterior belly of the digastric muscle. It passes upwards and backwards to supply the scalp posterior to the auricle and the auricle itself.

(1) Internal jugular vein

The internal jugular vein begins in the base of the skull as the continuation of the sigmoid sinus and decends vertically lateral to the common carorid artery. It receives tributaries corresponding to most branches of the external carotid artery.

(2) Hypoglossal nerve

The hypoglossal nerve is the motor nerve of the tongue. It enters the upper angle of the carotid triangle deep to the posterior belly of the digastric, and curves forward, crosses the internal and external carotid arteries, thereafter it continuous upwards and enters the submandibular triangle. It gives off a descending branccch and a hyoid branch in the triangle. The descending branch passes more or less vertically downwards in front or within the carotid sheath to join the inferior root of the ansa cervicalis to form the a loop known as the ansa cervicalis, fibers from the ansa cervicalis supply the sternothyroid, sternohyoid and the omohyoid.

(3) Vagus nerve

The vagus nerve is a mixed neve, it leaves the skull throught the jugular foramen. The main trunk of it decends vertically downward in the neck, lying posteriorly in the carotid sheath between the internal jugular vein and the internal or comon carotid atery, to pass into the thorax. The superior laryngeal nerve arise from the vagus at the superior angle of the carotid triangle. It runs behind the carotid atery and divides into internal and external laryngeal nerves in company with the superior larygeal and the superior thyroid arteries. The internal and external laryngeal branches supply, respectively, sensation to larynx above the vocal folds, and motor fibres to cricothyroid. The small cardiac branches of the vegus originate in the neck as well as in the thorax and pass downwards along the suface of the common carotid artery into the thorax to join the cardiac plexus.

2.3.2.2 Muscular triangle

The muscular triangle is bounded by the superior belly of the omohyoid muscle, the anterior border of the sternocleidomastoid, and medially by the midline. Its name refers to the infrahyoid muscles which it contains, the sternohyoid, superior belly of omohyoid muscle, sternothyroid and thyrohyoid.

(1) Thyroid gland

The important structure in this triangle, deep to the muscles, is the thyroid gland. It is an H-shap endcrion organ (from the level of C_5 to T_1 vertebrae). It consists of right and left lobes and joined by isthmus that extends anterior to the 2nd and 3rd tracheal cartilages (Figure 2-8). A pyramidal lobe is present in about 50% of people, which ascends from the isthmus of the thyroid gland, toward the hyoid bone. In front of the gland, there are the skin, the superficial fascia, the enveloping fascia, the inferahyoid muscles and the pretracheal fascia, from outside to inwards. The posteromedial aspect of each lobe contacts with the larynx and trachea, the pharynx. In the interval between the esophagus and trachea, the recurrent laryngeal nerve curse upward towrd the larynx. Lateral to the lateral lobes are the carotid sheathh and the sympathetic trunk.

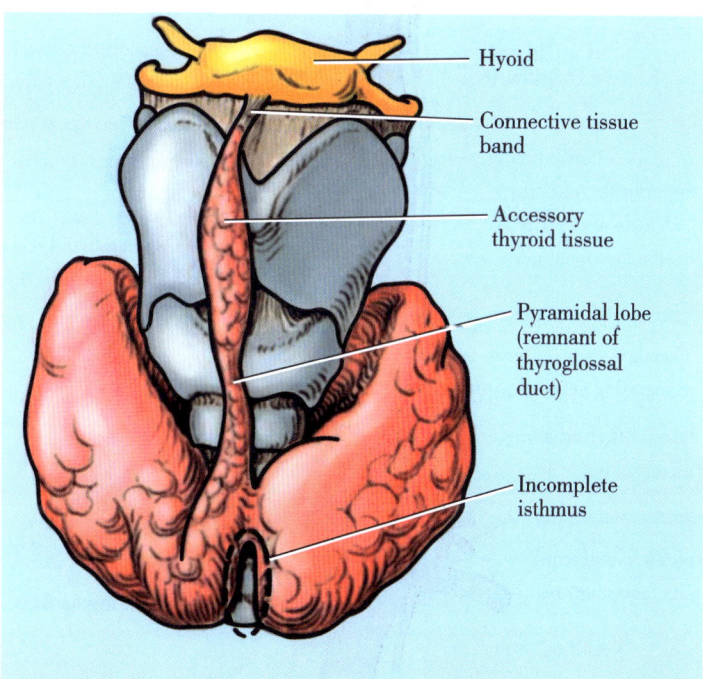

Figure 2-8   Thyroid gland(anterior view)

(2) Vessels of the thyroid gland

The arteries supplying the gland are the superior thyroid from the external carotid, the inferior thyroid from the thyrocervical trunk, a branch of the subclavian artery and occasionally the lowest thyroid artery from the brachiocephalic trunk or aortic arch. The veins draining the gland are the superior and middle thyroid veins which pass laterally and join the internal jugular vein, and the inferir thyroid veins, one on each side, pass downwards and join the (left) brachiocephalic vein.

(3) The superior thyroid artery and the superior laryngeal nerve

The superior laryngeal nerve is one of the branches of the vagus nerve. At the thyroid cartilage, it divides, forming a motor external laryngeal branch and a sensory internal laryngeal branch. The external laryngeal nerve supplies the cricothyroid muscle, and the internal laryngeal nerve supplies the mucous membrane of the larynx above the vocal cords. Usually the arteries supply to the thyroid gland comes from the superior and inferior thyroid arteries. The superior thyroid atery descends and accompanies with the superior laryngeal nerve and its external laryngeal nerve, and then leaves the nerve to the upper pole of the gland. It also gives off the superior laryngeal artery which company with the internal laryngeal nerve into the larynx. The extenal laryngeal nerve deviates from the artery about 1 cm distant to the upper pole of lateral lobe to innervare the cricothyroid muscle.

(4) The inferior thyroid artery and the recurrent laryngeal nerve

The inferior thyroid artery ascends along the medial border of the scalenus anterior, and then turns medially at the level of the cricoid cartilage, thereafter it passes across the vertebral artery behind the vagus nerve and the common caroid artery to reach the posteroraspect of the thyroid gland and giving off branches to supply the lower pole and posterior part of the gland, the trachea and esophagus (Figure 2-9).

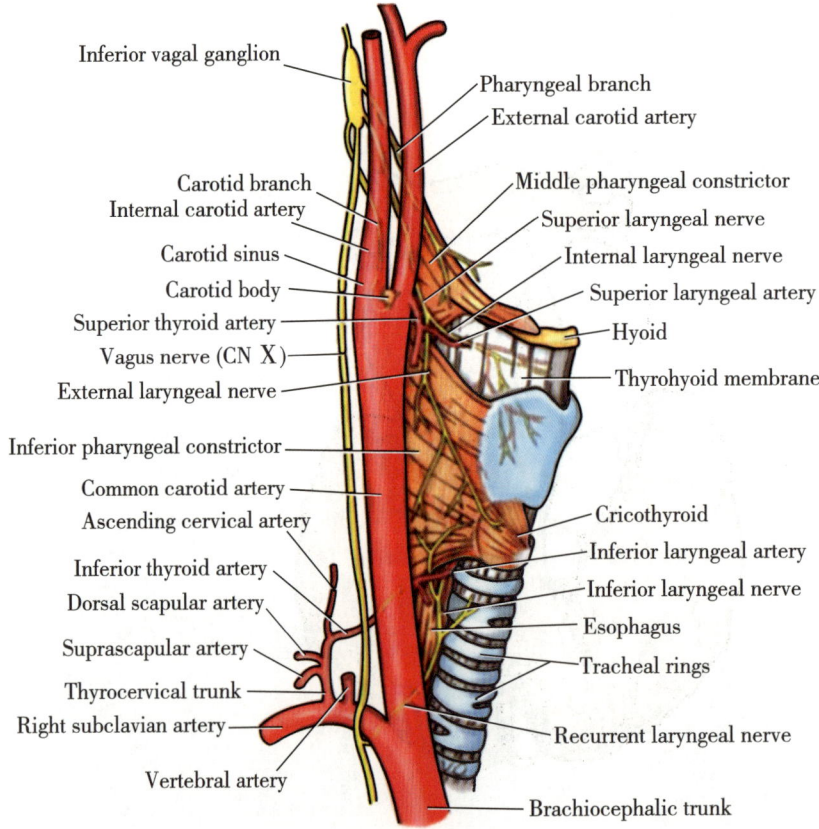

Figure 2-9　The inferior thyroid artery and the recurrent nerve (lateral view)

The recurrent nerve is another branch of the vagus nerve. On the left side, the right recurrent nerve hooks around the arch of the aorta, on the right hooks around the subclavian atery. After hooking, both recurrent laryngeal nerve ascends from the root of the neck in the groove between the trachea and oesophagus. Near the gland, the right recurrent nerve crosses in front or behind the inferior thyroid artery, while the left one crosses behind the inferior thyroid artery. The terminal branches of the recurrent laryngeal nerve supply all the laryngeal muscles except the cricothyroid and the mucosa below the vocal cords.

(5) Clinical notes about the thyroid vessels and the laryngeal nerves

1) The superior thyroid artery is ligated near the upper pole of the gland because the external laryngeal nerve deviates the artery about 1 cm above superior pole of the gland.

2) The inferior thyroid artery is ligated in some distance lateral to the gland because the recurrent laryngeal nerve especially the right one, is closely related to the artery

3) Hypoparathyroidism following thyroidectomy may caused by the injury to the parathyroid or to the gland's blood supply, or actual removal of the gland.

2.4 The lateral region of the neck

Posterior triangle of the neck is in the lateral region of the neck (Figure 2-10).

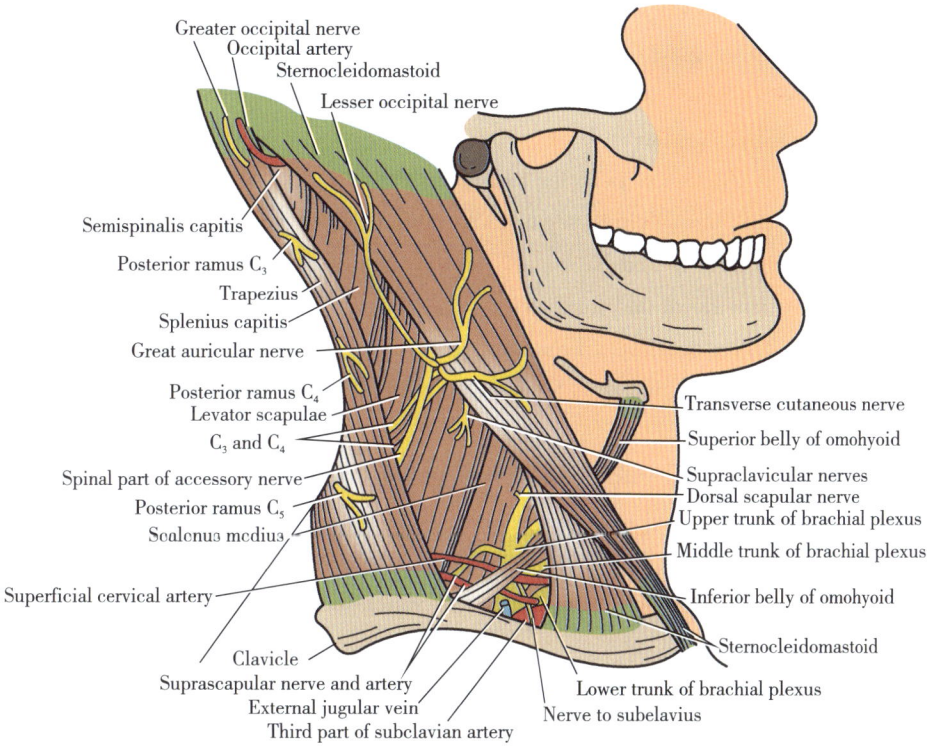

Figure 2-10 Posterior triangle of the neck

2.5 Main contents of neck

2.5.1 Root of neck

Cervical vertebrae
Typical cervical vertebra (3rd–6th)
Bony features
✓ Body elongated transversely   ✓ Upper surface like a seat (sides raised)   ✓ Lower surface is the counterpart   ✓ Lateral edges of C_3–C_6 vertebrae often come in contact, forming pseudo-synovial uncovertebral joints   ✓ Located at posterolateral margins of IV discs   ✓ Articular surfaces develop cartilage, joint space contains fluid   ✓ Frequent sites of spur (osteophyte) formation   ✓ Pedicles arise from side of body and project lateral and posterior   ✓ The vertebral foramen is triangular   ✓ Articular processes—at junction of pedicles and laminae   ✓ Form a bony column cut obliquely into segments to permit flexion and extension   ✓ Superior concave facets face up and back   ✓ Inferior convex facets face down and forward   ✓ The nearly horizontal facets describe a broad arc   ✓ Allows flexion, extension, some rotation (torsion) and lateral flexion (sideways bending)   ✓ Spinous processes—bifid, short   ✓ Transverse processes—two roots and two tubercles (costal and transverse), and a perforation (foramen transversarium)   ✓ Foramen transmits vertebral artery and vein (except C_7—vein only)   ✓ Closed by costotransverse bar which forms a gutter in which the ventral ramus of the spinal nerve runs
Vascular relationships
✓ Vertebral artery supplies bodies, discs and prevertebral musculature   ✓ Deep cervical artery supplies neural arches, deep (posterior) cervical musculature
Nervous relationships
✓ Between all vertebrae from C_3 down, a typical intervertebral foramen is formed to transmit the spinal nerves   ✓ Nerve C_1 exits above atlas and below occipital bone thus not truly "intervertebral"   ✓ Nerve C_2 exits between atlas and axis   ✓ Ventral rami of both nerves pass posterior and lateral to superior articular processes of their respective vertebrae

Atypical cervical vertebrae

Atlas (1st cervical vertebra)

✓ Loses its body, acquires an anterior arch
✓ The lost body becomes the dens of the axis, so the atlas rotates around its own body
✓ Anterior arch—anterior to dens and has a facet on its posterior aspect for the dens
✓ Posterior arch—grooved for vertebral artery; encircles large vertebral foramen
✓ Lateral mass
✓ Each has an upper and lower weight-bearing facet
✓ Upper facet fits occipital condyle and so is oval and concave
✓ A tubercle for the transverse ligament of the atlas, which retains the dens in position, projects medially (into the vertebral foramen) from each mass. Actually, the ligament itself will form the anterior border of the true spinal canal
✓ The transverse processes are long levers that help to rotate the atlas on the axis; only the lumbar transverse processes are longer

Axis (2nd cervical vertebra)

✓ Typical inferiorly but atypical superiorly due to the presence of the dens
✓ The dens is constricted at its root where the transverse ligament grips it, and it has a facet anteriorly where it contacts the atlas
✓ The superior articular facet, being weight-bearing, is large and lies entirely anterior to the plane of the inferior articular process
✓ The bifid spine and laminae are massive

7th cervical vertebra

✓ Has a long, non-bifid spine (vertebra prominens in 70% of the population—it is C_6 in 20% and T_1 in 10%)
✓ Transverse foramen transmits small veins (but not the vertebral artery)

Anomalies

✓ Fusion of occipital bone and atlas (occasional)
✓ Fusion of axis and C_3 (common)
✓ Vertebra C_7 may carry cervical ribs

Craniovertebral joints

✓ Synovial joints (no IV discs) between skull (occipital bone), atlas, and axis
✓ A greater range of movement is possible between these adjacent bones than is possible between adjacent vertebrae of rest of vertebral column
✓ Additionally, the associated ligaments are loose through most of the range of movement, becoming taut only at the extremes, checking further movement

Synovial joints involved

✓ Paired joints (two)
  ◊ Atlantooccipital (AO) joints—condyloid joints between superior facets of atlas and occipital condyles

◊ Lateral atlantoaxial joints—zygapophyseal (gliding) joints between articular processes of atlas (C_1) and axis (C_2)

Median; unpaired joint

✓ Median atlantoaxial joint—between dens and anterior arch of the atlas

Movements

✓ We flex and extend the neck, rotate and laterally flex (as in looking up sideways)
✓ At the atlantooccipital joints, we nod our heads "yes" and rock slightly
✓ Of the 130° of flexion and extension (40° of flexion; 90° of extension) possible in the neck, most (110°) occurs via the aggregated movements of the lower cervical (C_2-C_7) vertebrae (25° of flexion; 85° of extension) and 20° (5° of flexion; 15° of extension) occurs in the suboccipital region (craniovertebral joints)
✓ At the atlantoaxial joints, we shake our heads "no"
✓ Head and C_1 rotate as a unit on C_2
✓ Of the 65° of unilateral rotation possible for neck, 15° occurs here
✓ Total rotation of head from left to right = 130°, of which 100° occurs in the lower cervical region and 30° occurs in the suboccipital region
✓ About 40° of unilateral lateral flexion occurs in the lower cervical region (C_2-C_7), with an addition of up to 8° occurring at the craniovertebral joints
✓ Movement is freer in the cervical region than in rest of vertebral column because IV disks are relatively thick compared to size of vertebral bodies
✓ Articular surfaces of zygapophyseal joints are large, the joint planes are almost horizontal, and joint capsules are loose
✓ Neck is slender

Special ligaments

Transverse ligament of the atlas

✓ Extends between tubercles on the medial aspects of the lateral masses of the atlas
✓ Passes posterior to the root of the dens, forming posterior wall of the "socket" which receives and pivots about the ends
✓ A synovial joint occurs between the front of the dens and the anterior arch of the atlas and another between the back of the dens and the transverse ligament
✓ The head of the dens cannot easily be withdrawn from this ring
✓ Weak superior and inferior bands pass from transverse ligament to the occipital above and to the body of the axis below, giving the whole the appearance of a cross. Hence, cruciform ligament

Alar ligaments (bilateral)

✓ Short, very stout cords
✓ Pass from the side of the apex of the dens laterally and slightly upward to the tubercle on the occipital condyle
✓ Together, the two alar ligaments hold the skull tightly applied to the atlas and axis, while limiting the rotation of the skull and atlas on the axis

General ligaments and their derivatives
Anterior longitudinal ligament
✓ Becomes a cord at the axis and ascends to the anterior tubercle of the atlas and onto the basi-occipit ✓ Above the axis, its side parts are membranous—anterior atlantoaxial membrane which continues superior to the atlas as the anterior atlantooccipital membrane
Posterior longitudinal ligament
✓ Passes from the post surface of the body of the axis to the inner surface of the occipital, spanning atlas and transverse ligament, as the tectorial membrane
The ligamentum flavum
✓ Becomes the relatively weak posterior atlantoaxial and posterior atlantooccipital membranes seen during the dissection of the suboccipital region

Clinical correlations: Reading X-rays (lateral)—relationship between occiput (foramen magnum) and C_1 (odontoid)
✓ McGregor's line—posterior nasal spine to lowest part of occipital bone
✓ McRae's line—plane of foramen magnum
✓ Wackenheim's line—slope of clivus
✓ Power's ratio—most reliable indicator of OA instability
✓ Instability at C_1-C_2
✓ Atlanto-dens interval (ADI)
    ◊ <4 mm in children < 8 years old
    ◊ <3 mm in older children or adults
    ◊ >10 mm = all ligaments have failed
✓ Space available for cord (SAC)
    ◊ "Rule of thirds" or "Steele's rule"
    ◊ At the level of the dens—1/3 area in C_1 occupied by odontoid; 1/3 by spinal cord, remaining by empty space
✓ Normal relationships in lateral C-spine

Anatomic differences between children (< 8 years old) and adults—fulcrum of movement

✓ Fulcrum higher in children due to large head size
✓ Progresses caudad as spine matures
    ◊ Children<8 years old = maximal mobility = C_1-C_3
    ◊ 8-12 years old = C_3-C_5
    ◊ 12 years old = C_5-C_6 (adult pattern)
✓ Thus, flexion-extension injuries, as in MVA tend to result in high C-spine injury in children—in fact most common level of injury in a small child involves occiput-C_1-C_2 complex

Vertebral ligaments in neonates
✓ Newborn spine—ligamentous structures stretch 5.08 cm, cord only 0.64 cm

- ✓ Increased elasticity of pediatric spine allows injury to the cord without bony disruption
- ✓ 27% of children have delayed onset of neurologic signs (30 minutes to 4 days, mean 1.4 days)

Review of cervical fascia, compartments and spaces

Superficial cervical fascia

Investing layer of deep cervical fascia

Splits to invest

- ✓ Muscles of "4 corners" of neck (trapezius, sternocleidomastoid)
- ✓ Submandibular and parotid glands (superiorly)
  - ▷ Stylomandibular ligament is a thickened portion of this fascia
- ✓ Suprasternal space (inferiorly)

Pretracheal layer of deep cervical fascia

Muscular portion—encloses infrahyoid muscles

- ✓ Thickenings form "trochleae" for intermediate tendons of digastric and omohyoid muscles
- ✓ That for digastric tendon suspends hyoid bone in neck

Visceral portion—encloses cervical viscera

- ✓ Enclosed space is continuous inferiorly with mediastinum
- ✓ Goiter can spread into mediastinum

Prevertebral layer of deep cervical fascia

- ✓ Surrounds vertebral column and associated intrinsic muscles
- ✓ Extends laterally as axillary sheath
- ✓ Blends inferiorly with anterior longitudinal ligament

Cervical musculature

Functional groups of "somatic" neck musculature

Superficial layer

- ✓ Sternocleidomastoid
- ✓ Trapezius

Intrinsic muscles (within prevertebral fascia)

Anterior group (prevertebral muscles)

- ✓ Muscles lying medial to cervical/brachial plexus
- ✓ Clothe anterior aspect of cervical vertebrae forming a relatively flat prevertebral surface
- ✓ Important mostly because they form the posterior relationship of the carotid arteries, internal jugular veins, pharynx and esophagus, and are also intimately related to the cervical nerves (plexus), sympathetic trunks and CN IX, X, XI and XII
- ✓ Produce flexion of cervical vertebra column, and of head on column
  - ▷ Rectus capitis anterior
  - ▷ Longus capitis

- ◊ Longus cervicis (colli)
- ◊ Scalenus anterior

Lateral group

Lateral to the plexuses:
- ✓ Rectus capitis lateralis
- ✓ Scalenus medius and posterior
- ✓ Levator scapulae

Clinical notes: The scalene muscles (and sternocleidomastoid) play a role in labored respiration by elevating the first and second ribs. Use of these during labored breathing muscles is evidence of extreme respiratory distress, as in an asthma attack

Posterior group

Extend neck, innervated by dorsal rami
- ✓ Spinotransverse group—splenius muscles
    - ◊ External layer of intrinsic muscles of upper back/neck
    - ◊ Acting together, extend neck; acting alone, rotate toward ipsilateral shoulder
- ✓ Sacrospinal group—longissimus muscles (intermediate layer)
- ✓ Transversospinal group—semispinalis muscles (deep layer)
- ✓ Suboccipital group
    - ◊ Deepest posterior group of intrinsic muscles
    - ◊ Act and/or detect movement (proprioception) at atlanto-occipital and atlanto-axial joints

Structures in root of neck

- ✓ Extend up to level of upper border of T_1 vertebra (head of 1st rib), and can be inadvertently punctured during central line placement, etc.
    - ◊ Cervical pleura is reinforced by suprapleural membrane (Sibson fascia)
- ✓ Thoracic duct
    - ◊ Emerges from behind carotid sheath
    - ◊ Ascends to C_7 level, then descends, arching anteriorly over subclavian artery
    - ◊ Passes anterior to insertion of left anterior scalene, phrenic nerve and thyrocervical trunk to enter venous angle

Nerve structures in root of neck

Phrenic nerves

- ✓ Forms anterior to anterior scalene, descends on muscles anterior surface, then passes posterior to subclavian veins to enter mediastinum

Vagus nerves

- ✓ Descend through neck in carotid sheaths, pass anterior to subclavian arteries, posterior to brachiocephalic veins to enter mediastinum

Sympathetic trunks

- ✓ Embedded in prevertebral fascia

Subclavian artery
✓ Arch superior, posterior, and then lateral, grooving pleura of lung ✓ At apex, pass posterior to anterior scalene muscle ✓ As descend, pass posterior to midpoint of clavicle ✓ Anterior scalene divides each subclavian into three parts
Medial to muscle
✓ Vertebral artery—ascends between scalene and longus muscles; (vertebral triangle) ascends through foramina of C_6 through C_1; suboccipital part of the vertebral artery courses in a groove on the posterior arch of the atlas, before enters cranial cavity ✓ Internal thoracic artery ✓ Thyrocervical trunk—which gives off suprascapular, transverse cervical, and inferior thyroid, and ascending cervical arteries
Posterior to muscle
✓ Costocervical trunk—branches into superior intercostal (1st two intercostal spaces) and deep cervical arteries (deep cervical muscles)
Lateral to muscle
✓ Dorsal scapular artery
Vein
Subclavian vein
✓ Passes over first rib, anterior to scalene tubercle, anterior to anterior scalene, and then under clavicle. Attachment to these bony structures make collapse impossible; thus it is an ideal target for puncture (central line placement) ✓ Joins the IJV posterior to medial clavicle—venous angle ◊ Right—site of right lymphatic trunk drainage ◊ Left—site of thoracic duct drainage

2.5.2 Autonomic innervations of neck

Generalities concerning the ANS as a whole also apply for head/neck innervation
Type of innervation
✓ The ANS is an entirely motor nervous system (the visceral subdivision of the motor portion of the nervous system)
Structures innervated
✓ The ANS innervates involuntary muscle (smooth and cardiac) and glands
Smooth muscle
✓ Blood vessels

✓ Erector pilorum muscles
✓ Smooth muscle of globe and orbit
◊ Dilator pupillae
◊ Orbital smooth muscle (e.g., tarsal muscles)
◊ Constant pupillae
◊ Ciliary body

Glands
✓ Sweat glands
✓ Lacrimal glands
✓ Mucous glands of nose and palate
✓ Salivary glands
◊ Parotid
◊ Submandibular
◊ Sublingual
◊ Minor salivary glands
◊ Buccal, labial, lingual

Neurons involved, location of nerve cell bodies
✓ Autonomic innervation always involves two neurons, a pre- and a post-synaptic neuron, always in tandem

Thoracolumbar (sympathetic) nervous system
✓ Presynaptic neurons
◊ Intermediolateral cell column (IML), T_1–T_6 (CNS)
✓ Post-synaptic neurons
◊ Cervical portion of paravertebral chain ganglia (sympathetic trunks)
(for all of the head and much of the neck, the superior cervical ganglion is the most important of the three cervical ganglia)
◊ Post-synaptic fibers leave the cervical ganglia via:
◆ Gray rami communicans → cervical spinal nerves (parietal neck)
◆ Arterial rami → carotid periarterial plexuses (visceral neck and all of head)
◆ Cervical (cardiopulmonary) splanchnics → thoracic viscera [i.e., these arise in the neck but distribute to thorax (outside of head and neck)]

Craniosacral (parasympathetic) nervous system
✓ Presynaptic neurons
◊ Cell bodies located in CNS (motor nuclei of brain)
◊ Presynaptic fibers emerge from CNS only via certain cranial nerves: oculomotor (CN Ⅲ), facial (CN Ⅶ), glossopharyngeal (CN Ⅸ) and vagus (CN Ⅹ) (these are the "parent nerves" of the presynaptic fibers)
◊ The presynaptic fibers soon leave their parent nerve, run independently for some distance, and finally join a branch or branches of the trigeminal nerve (CN V)

✓ Post-synaptic neurons
   Generally, the cell bodies are located in 1 of 4 discrete cranial parasympathetic ganglia, all associated with branches of trigeminal nerve
   ◊ Ciliary ganglion—associated with nasociliary nerve (CN V_1)
   ◊ Pterygopalatine ganglion—associated with maxillary nerve (CN V_2)
   ◊ Otic ganglion—associated with the trunk of the mandibular nerve (CN V_3)
   ◊ Submandibular ganglion—associated with the lingual nerve (CN V_3)
   ◊ The post-synaptic fibers continue along branches of the trigeminal nerve to reach their end organ

Clinical notes: Intrinsic ganglia do exist in the head; that is, post-synaptic parasympathetic cell bodies which are not located in any of the four cranial parasympathetic ganglia but rather are found in or on the structure being innervated. For purposes of this course, however, we will generalize and consider them all to occur in the four head ganglia

Cranial nerves

✓ Are bundles of nerve fibers exiting the cranial cavity
✓ Are covered initially by sheaths derived from the cranial meninges
✓ Are 12 (pairs) in number
✓ Are identified by a name and/or a number in Roman Numerals

Cranial nerves convey one or more (up to five) of the following six components

Somatic motor (GSE)

✓ Innervate striated muscles-not derived from embryonic pharyngeal (branchial) arches
✓ Includes extraocular muscles of orbit and tongue muscles

Branchial motor (SVE)

✓ Innervate striated muscles—derived from pharyngeal (branchial) arches
✓ Includes muscles of mastication, facial expression, pharyngeal and laryngeal muscles

Visceral motor (GVE)

✓ Parasympathetic fibers innervating smooth muscle and glands
✓ E.g., sphincter pupillae and lacrimal gland

Visceral sensory/visceral afferent (GVA)

✓ Convey unconscious (reflex) information from visceral structures
✓ E.g., parotid gland, carotid body and sinus, middle ear, pharynx, larynx, thoracic viscera and abdominal viscera (GI tract) to left colic flexure

General sensory (GSA)

✓ General sensation from skin and mucous membranes which may or may not be experienced consciously
✓ Travel mainly via CN V, but also through CN VII, IX and X

Special sensory

✓ SVA: taste and small
✓ SSA: vision, hearing and balance
✓ Some cranial nerves are wholly sensory; others are wholly motor, and several are mixed

✓ Four cranial nerves (CN Ⅲ, Ⅶ, Ⅸ, and Ⅹ) convey presynaptic parasymathetic (GVE) fibers from the brainstem (collectively constituting the "cranial outflow" of the craniosacral nervous system)
✓ Within the CNS, afferent fibers terminate in relation to aggregates of neurons forming sensory nuclei; efferent fibers arise in motor nuclei

Olfactory nerve

✓ Special sensory (SVA) only—sense of smell
✓ Olfactory (neurosensory) cells
  ◊ Are biploar neurons
  ◊ Have their cell bodies located in the olfactory epithelium in the superior nasal cavity
  ◊ Have central processes which form about 20 bundles (olfactory nerves or fila) that collectively constitute CN Ⅰ
✓ Olfactory nerves traverse foramina of the cribriform plate of the ethmoid bone, the arachnoid and dura to enter the olfactory bulbs
✓ Are lost at an as average rate of 1%/year(i.e., 50% by age 50)

Optic nerve

✓ Special sensory (SSA) only—sense of vision
✓ 3 sets of neurons occur within the retina
  ◊ 1st set = rods and cones (optic neurosensory cells)
  ◊ 2nd set = retinal bipolar cells
  ◊ 3rd set = retinal ganglion cells
✓ Axons of retinal ganglion cells
  ◊ Form CN Ⅱ, which begins as the axons pierce the sclera (opaque part of fibrous outer coat of eyeball)
  ◊ From the nasal (medial) half of the retina decussate in the optic chiasm and join uncrossed fibers from the temporal (lateral) half of the opposite eye to form the optic tract
  ◊ Terminate in the lateral geniculate bodies of the thalamus
✓ The optic nerve (CN Ⅱ)
  ◊ Leaves the orbit through the optic canal to enter the middle cranial fossa
  ◊ Is actually a tract of the CNS which was "extruded" from the diencephalon during the development of the eye
  ◊ Is surrounded by subarachnoid space and extensions of the cranial meninges (the optic sheath)

Oculomotor nerve

✓ Somatic motor (GSE) and visceral motor (GVE)
✓ The oculomotor nerve (CN Ⅲ)
  ◊ Conveys somatic motor fibers to the levator of the upper eyelid and to 4 of 6 extraocular muscles
    ◆ Superior rectus
    ◆ Medial rectus
    ◆ Inferior rectus
    ◆ Inferior oblique
  ◊ Conveys presynaptic parasympathetic (GVE) fibers to the ciliary ganglion

- ▷ Postsynaptic fibers go to the sphincter of the pupil (protects retina from excessive light) and the ciliary muscle (allows lens to thicken for near vision)
- ✓ Characteristic signs of a complete lesion of CN III
  - ▷ Ptosis (drooping of upper eyelid)
  - ▷ Pupil depressed and abducted ("down and out") due to unopposed superior oblique and lateral rectus
  - ▷ Pupil dilated (dilator unopposed) and no pupillary (light) reflex
  - ▷ No accommodation of lens

Trochlear and abducent nerves

- ✓ Somatic motor (GSE) to one ocular muscle
  - ▷ Trochlear (CN IV) to superior oblique
  - ▷ Abducent (CN VI) to lateral rectus
- ✓ Have different courses within the cranial cavity
  - ▷ CN IV is the only nerve to arise from the dorsal aspect of the brainstem
  - ▷ Although both nerves run long intradural courses, CN VI has the longest intradural course of all cranial nerves, entering the dura of the clivus
  - ▷ Although both nerves are closely related to the cavernous sinus, CN IV runs in the dura of the lateral wall; CN VI runs in the sinus itself
- ✓ Both traverse the supraorbital fissure to reach the orbit

Lesions

- ✓ Trochlear nerve—impaired ability to direct gaze inferomedially
- ✓ Abducent nerve—eye assumes fully adducted ("crossed") position; unable to abduct
- ✓ Both nerve injuries cause diplopia (double vision)

Trigeminal nerve

Components

Proximally (before and after cranium is traversed)

- ✓ General sensory (GSA) from skin of (and mucous membranes deep to) face, external ear and palate
  - ▷ Unipolar cell bodies located in trigeminal ganglion
  - ▷ Central processes form sensory root of trigeminal nerve
  - ▷ Peripheral processes are distributed by all 3 divisions
    - ◆ Ophthalmic nerve (CN V_1)—via superior orbital fissure
    - ◆ Maxillary nerve (CN V_2)—via foramen rotundum
    - ◆ Mandibular nerve (CN V_3)—via foramen ovale
- ✓ Branchial motor (SVE) to the derivatives of the 1st (mandibular) arch
  - ▷ Muscles of mastication, mylohyoid, anterior belly of digastric, and tensors palati and tympani
  - ▷ Distributed only via mandibular nerve (CN V_3)

Distally (after emerging from cranium)

The following fibers join the branches of the trigeminal nerve extracranially

Special sensory fibers

✓ From facial nerve (CN Ⅶ) to lingual nerve (CN V_3) via chorda tympani

✓ Distributed to anterior 2/3 of tongue

Visceral motor (parasympathetic—GVE) fibers

✓ Although CN V is not part of the cranial outflow of the PNS (i.e., it conducts no presynaptic parasympathetic fibers out of the CNS or cranium), each of the four parasympathetic ganglia of the head are associated with a specific division of the trigeminal nerve, and its distal branches convey the postsynaptic fibers to their destinations

◊ Intraocular muscles (sphincter pupillae and ciliary body)
◊ Lacrimal gland
◊ Nasal glands
◊ Palatine and pharyngeal glands
◊ Sublingual and submandibular salivary glands
◊ Parotid gland

Facial nerve

✓ Exits cranial cavity via internal acoustic meatus

✓ Intermediate nerve arises separately from brain, but becomes part of (merges with) facial nerve within the internal acoustic meatus

Components

Branchial motor (SVE)

✓ Innervate the derivatives of the 2nd (hyoid) arch

✓ Within facial canal: stapedius

✓ After emerging from facial camal via stylomastoid foramen: muscles of facial expression (cutaneous muscles of face, neck, scalp and auricle), plus stylohyoid and posterior belly of digastric

Visceral motor (GVE—presynaptic parasympathetic)

✓ Originally part of intermediate nerve

✓ Facial nerve is parent nerve for fibers (delivers them out of CNS/cranium), but is not involved in the distribution of the postsynpatic fibers

✓ Exit facial nerve via two nerves

◊ Via greater petrosal nerve
  ◆ Conveys presynaptic fibers to pterygopalatine ganglion
  ◆ Postsynaptic fibers distributed (via CN V) to lacrimal gland, nasal glands, palatine and pharyngeal glands

◊ Via chorda tympani
  ◆ Conveys presynaptic fibers to submandibular ganglion
  ◆ Postsynaptic fibers distributed (via CN V) to sublingual and submandibular salivary glands

Special sensory (SVA)

✓ Unipolar neurons with cell bodies in the geniculate ganglion (sensory ganglion of facial nerve)

- ✓ The great majority of peripheral processes conduct taste from anterior 2/3 of tongue (via lingual nerve of CN V_3 and chorda tympani)
- ✓ A few peripheral processes travel with the visceral motor branches to the pterygopalatine ganglion, from which they continue on (without synapse) to sparse taste buds of the nasopharynx and soft palate
- ✓ Central processes traverse internal acoustic meatus, becoming part of intermediate nerve

Visceral sensory (GVA)

- ✓ Relatively insignificant
- ✓ Unipolar neurons with cell bodies in the geniculate ganglion (sensory ganglion of facial nerve)
- ✓ The few peripheral processes travel with the visceral motor branches to the pterygopalatine ganglion, from which they continue on (without synapse) to supply general semsibility to a small part of the naso-palatal-pharyngeal area
- ✓ Central processes traverse internal acoustic meatus, becoming part of the intermediate nerve

Somatic sensory (GSA)

- ✓ Also quite insignificant
- ✓ Unipolar neurons with cell bodies in the geniculate ganglion (sensory ganglion of facial nerve)
- ✓ Peripheral processes exit skull via stylomastoid foramen, become part of the posterior auricular branch of CN VII, which distributes them to a small area of skin on the posterior aspect of the auricle
- ✓ Central processes traverse internal acoustic meatus, becoming part of the main stem of the facial nerve

Vestibulocochlear nerve

Actually consists of two nerves, both composed entirely of special sensory (SSA) fibers

Vestibular nerve

- ✓ Cell bodies of bipolar neurons located in vestibular ganglion (at the depth of the internal acoustic meatus)
- ✓ Peripheral processes extend to the hair cells of the cristae of the three otic ampullae and those of the utricular and saccular maculae
- ✓ Sensory for the function of equilibriation
- ✓ Stimulated either by changes in position, changes in rate of movement, or both
- ✓ Central processes traverse internal acoustic meatus, becoming part of vestibulocochlear nerve (CN VIII)

Cochlear nerve

- ✓ Cell bodies of bipolar neurons located in the spiral ganglion in the modiolus of the cochlea
- ✓ Short peripheral processes extend to the hair cells of the organ of Corti, the major receptor for auditory stimuli
- ✓ Central processes traverse internal acoustic meatus, becoming part of vestibulocochlear nerve (CN VIII)

Glossopharyngeal nerve

- ✓ Includes 5 of the 6 types of nerve fibers (all except special sensory)
- ✓ Central processes of all sensory components traverse jugular foramen as part of main stem of nerve

Visceral sensory (GVA)

- ✓ Unipolar cell bodies located in the inferior (petrosal) ganglion of CN IX

✓ Lower and larger of two sensory ganglia located in jugular foramen
✓ Peripheral processes travel via main trunk of CN IX to pharyngeal plexus, providing general sensibility to the mucous membrane of the pharynx and the posterior third of the tongue
✓ A small bundle exits the main trunk as it passes near the bifurcation of the common carotid as the carotid branch (carotid sinus nerve), conveying:
  ◊ Pressoreceptor sensation from the carotid sinus
  ◊ Chemoreceptor sensation from the carotid body
✓ An additional small branch, the tympanic nerve, recurs through the tympanic canaliculus, forming the tympanic plexus of the middle ear
✓ Provides sensation to the mucous membrane of the tympanic cavity, mastoid antrum and pharyngotympanic (auditory) tube

Visceral motor (GVE, presynaptic parasympathetic)

✓ Traverse tympanic nerve and tympanic plexus with visceral sensory fibers
✓ Tympanic plexus sends a branch—the lesser petrosal nerve—through roof of tympanic membrane (tegmen tympani) into middle cranial fossa
✓ Passes through foramen ovale to reach otic ganglion, associated with mandibular nerve (CN V_3)
✓ Postsynaptic fibers conveyed by auricultemporal nerve to parotid gland
✓ Branchial motor (SVE)
✓ Supplies one striated muscle derived from the 3rd arch: stylolpharyngeus

Special sensory (SVA)

✓ Cell bodies in inferior (petrosal) ganglion
✓ Travel with visceral sensory (GVA) fibers to pharyngeal plexus
✓ Innervate taste buds of posterior 1/3 of tongue and adjacent pharyngeal wall

General sensory

✓ Cell bodies in superior (jugular) ganglion of CN IX
✓ Peripheral processes join auricular branch of vagus (CN X) to small areas of skin of auricle and external auditory meatus

Vagus nerve

✓ Also includes 5 of the 6 types of nerve fibers (all except special sensory)
✓ Central processes of all sensory components traverse jugular foramen as part of main stem of nerve

Visceral motor (GVE, presynaptic parasympathetic)

✓ Fibers enter main trunk of vagus, traverse neck in carotid sheath and enter thorax
✓ Supply parasympathetic innervation (synapse on postsynpatic cell bodies comprising intrinsic ganglia) of the thoracic viscera and abdominal viscera to the left colic flexure

Visceral afferent (GVA)

✓ Cells bodies lie in the inferior (nodose) ganglion of CN X (lower and larger of two sensory ganglia related to the jugular foramen)
✓ Peripheral processes, which pass to:
  ◊ The pharyngeal plexus to supplement visceral afferents from CN IX

◊ The laryngeal mucosa (afferent limb of cough reflex) via the internal laryngeal branch of the superior laryngeal nerve

◊ Esophageal and tracheal mucosa via the recurrent laryngeal nerve

◊ Viscera of thoracic and abdominal cavity (viscera above the pelvis)

✓ Includes all reflex afferents (unconscious sensation)

✓ Includes pain fibers from viscera above thoracic pain line, i.e., from:

◊ Larynx and tracheobronchial tree

◊ Pharynx and esophagus

Branchial motor (SVE)

✓ Fibers emerge from brainstem as cranial root of accessory nerve (CN IX)

✓ Merge with vagus while traversing jugular foramen

✓ Pass via the pharyngeal branch of CN X to the pharyngeal plexus

✓ Supply muscles derived from the 4th and 6th arches

◊ Most of the pharyngeal muscles (superior, middle and upper part of inferior pharyngeal constrictors, salpingo- and palato-pharyngeus muscles, but not stylopharyngeus)

◊ Palatine muscles (levator palati, palatoglossus and uvular, but not tensor veli palati)

◊ Pass via external laryngeal branch of superior laryngeal nerve to the cricothyroid muscle (4th arch)

◊ Pass via the recurrent laryngeal nerve to the muscles derived from the 6th arch

◆ Lower part of inferior pharyngeal constrictor (cricopharyngeus)

◆ Striated muscle of upper esophagus

◊ Enter larynx via inferior laryngeal nerve to innervate all intrinsic muscles of larynx (except cricothyroid)

Special sensory (SVA)

✓ Cell bodies in inferior (nodose) ganglion of vagus

✓ Pass via pharyngeal branches and plexus to a few epiglottic taste buds

General sensory (GSA)

✓ Cell bodies in superior (jugular) ganglion of vagus

✓ Peripheral processes pass to

◊ Recurrent meningeal branch of vagus

◊ Innervated subtentorial dura of posterior cranial fossa

◊ Auricular branch of vagus

◊ Small area of skin on posterior auricle, external auditory meatus (floor) and (lower half of) tympanic membrane

Accessory nerve

✓ Cranial root—discussed under "C" for vagus nerve (CN X) above

✓ Spinal root

◊ Arises from cervical portion of spinal cord, ascends between dorsal and ventral roots to enter cranial cavity via foramen magnum, exits via jugular foramen

◊ Only branchial motor (SVE) fibers are conducted as nerve exits cranium

◊ Pain and proprioceptice fibers join CN XI in posterior triangle

◊ Supplies innervation to sternocleidomastoid and trapezius muscles

Hypoglossal nerve

✓ Somatic motor fibers (GSE) only
✓ Exits cranial cavity via hypoglossal foramen/canal
✓ Supplies all intrinsic and extrinsic ("-glossal") muscles (except palatoglossus, which is actually a palatine muscle), which arise from occipital myotomes
✓ The hypoglossal nerve also conveys
  ◊ Somatic motor fibers from the C_1-C_2 loop of the cervical plexus to the superior root of the ansa cervicalis for innervation of infrahyoid muscles
  ◊ General sensory fibers from C_2 (retrograde through hypoglossal canal) to dura of posterior cranial fossa
  ◊ Both of these components join the hypoglossal nerve extracranially
  ◊ Neither are considered as components of the hypoglossal nerve

2.5.3 Superficial neck and posterior triangle

Overview

The neck is the major conduit between the head, trunk and limbs. Many important structures are crowded together in the neck, such as muscles, glands, arteries, veins, nerves, lymphatics, trachea, esophagus and vertebra
✓ Bony landmarks
✓ Fascial layers and compartments
✓ Superficial structures of the neck
✓ Posterior triangle of the neck
✓ Cervical plexus
✓ Laboratory exercise

Bony landmarks of the posterior triangle of the neck

Temporal bone

✓ Mastoid process
✓ Styloid process
✓ External acoustic meatus

Occipital bone—superior nuchal line

Mandible ("jaw bone")

✓ Ramus
✓ Angle
✓ Body

Hyoid bone (C_3)

✓ Lies in the anterior part of the neck at the level of the C_3 vertebra in the angle between the mandible and the thyroid cartilage. The hyoid bone is suspended by muscles that connect it to the manidble, styloid process, thyroid cartilage, manubrium and scapula. Functionally, the hyoid serves as an attachment for anterior neck muscles and as a prop to keep the airway open

- ✓ Body
- ✓ Lesser horn
- ✓ Greater horn

Laryngeal cartilages

- ✓ Epiglottis
- ✓ Thyroid cartilage (C_4–C_5)
- ✓ Cricoid cartilage (C_6)
- ✓ Trachea (C_7)

Cervical vertebra

Fascial layers and compartments of the neck

Cervical fascia

- ✓ Superficial cervical fascia
- ✓ Deep cervical fascia
    - ◊ Investing layer of deep cervical fascia
    - ◊ Pretracheal layer of deep cervical fascia
        - ◆ Muscular portion—fascia of infrahyoid muscles
        - ◆ Visceral portion—thyroid gland, larynx/trachea, pharynx/esophagus
        - ◆ Buccopharyngeal fascia of the pharynx (posteriorly)
        - ◆ Carotid sheath (laterally)
    - ◊ Prevertebral layer of deep cervical fascia

Compartments

- ✓ Retropharyngeal
- ✓ Lateral pharyngeal space

Superficial cervical fascia

Thin layer of subcutaneous tissue lying between the dermis of the skin and the investing layer of the deep cervical fascia

- ✓ Platysma
- ✓ Superficial veins
- ✓ Cutaneous nerves
- ✓ Lymphatics

Deep cervical fascia—investing layer of deep cervical fascia

- ✓ Encloses and covers the structures of the neck
- ✓ Surrounds all deeper structures of the neck
- ✓ Splits around the sternocleidomastoid (SCM) and trapezius
- ✓ Single sheet of fascia around the anterior and posterior triangles
- ✓ Suprasternal space of burns—anterior and posterior attachments of investing fascia to the sternum, anterior jugular vein traverses through this space

Pretracheal layer of deep cervical fascia—limited to the anterior part of the neck; extends inferiorly from the hyoid bone (C_3) into the thorax where it blends with the fibrous pericardium covering the heart

Muscular portion—thin layer of muscular fascia covering the infrahyoid muscles

✓ Superficial infrahyoid muscles
    ◊ Sternohyoid
    ◊ Omohyoid
✓ Deep infrahyoid muscles
    ◊ Sternothyroid
    ◊ Thyrohyoid

Visceral portion—encloses the thyroid gland, larynx/trachea, and esophagus
✓ Continues posteriorly and superiorly with the buccopharyngeal fascia of the pharynx ✓ Blends laterally with the carotid sheaths

Central visceral tube
✓ Trachea ✓ Esophagus ✓ Recurrent laryngeal nerve

Prevertebral layer of deep cervical fascia—forms a tubular sheath for the vertebral column and the muscles associated with the vertebral column; extends from the base of the skull to the T_3 vertebra where it fuses with the anterior longitudinal ligament; extends laterally as the axillary sheath which surrounds the axillary vessels and brachial plexus
    ✓ Anteriorly—longus colli and capitis
    ✓ Laterally—scalenes
    ✓ Posteriorly—deep cervical muscles
    ✓ Spinal nerves of the brachial plexus (C_5–T_1)
    ✓ Sympathetic trunk embedded in this layer of fascia

Carotid sheath—tubular, fascial investment that extends from the base of the skull to the root of the neck; blends anteriorly with the investing and pretracheal layers of fascia and posteriorly with the prevertebral layer of deep cervical fascia
    ✓ Common and internal carotid arteries (anterior medial)
    ✓ Internal jugular vein (anterior lateral)
    ✓ Vagus nerve (CN X)
    ✓ Deep cervical lymph nodes
    ✓ Carotid sinus nerve
    ✓ Carotid periarterial plexuses (sympathetic nerve fibers)

The carotid sheath and pretracheal fascia communicate freely with the mediastinum of the thorax inferiorly and the cranial cavity superiorly. These communications represent potential pathways for the spread of infection and extravasated blood

Compartments

Retropharyngeal space—largest and most important interfascial space in the neck
✓ Potential space consisting of loose CT between the prevertebral layer of deep cervical fascia and the buccopharyngeal fascia surrounding the pharynx superficially ✓ The alar fascia forms a further subdivision of the retropharyngeal space

◊ Extends from the skull to the C_7 vertebra

◊ Extends laterally and terminates in the carotid sheath

✓ The retropharyngeal space permits movement of the pharynx, esophagus, larynx, and trachea relative to the vertebral column during swallowing

◊ This space is closed superiorly by the base of the skull and on each side by the carotid sheath and opens inferiorly into the superior mediastinum

Lateral pharyngeal space—potential space between the pharynx, pterygoid muscles, parotid gland and carotid sheath

✓ Stylopharyngeus and styloglossus muscles reside

Superficial structures of the neck—superficial cervical fascia

Platysma muscle

✓ Origin—skin, subcutaneous tissue overlying the pectoralis major and deltoid

✓ Insertion—skin over the mandible, mandible

✓ Action—muscle of facial expression, draws mouth down

✓ Innervation—facial nerve (CN VII), cervical branch

✓ 2nd pharyngeal arch derivative

Superficial veins

External jugular vein (EJV)—drains most of the scalp and side of the face

✓ Arises from the posterior auriculuar and retromandibular veins at the angle of the mandible

✓ Superficial to the SCM, deep to the platysma

✓ Moves into the posterior triangle of the neck

✓ Pierces the investing layer of the deep cervical fascia approximately 2 cm above the clavicle

✓ Empties into the subclavian vein at the venous angle

✓ Has 2 pairs of valves—located 4 cm above the clavicle

◊ Nonfunctional valves

◊ Venous jugular distention—increase pressure in the right side of the heart (atrium/ventricle), causes backflow of blood into these veins

◊ EJV serves as an internal barometer of increased venous pressure, e. g., heart failure

Veins emptying into the EJV

✓ Suprascapular vein—skin and muscle of the supra/infraspinatus

✓ Transverse cervical vein—skin and muscle of the rhomboid area and neck

✓ Anterior jugular vein

Anterior jugular vein

✓ Begins near the hyoid bone

✓ Confluence of the submental and submandibular veins

✓ Lies in the suprasternal space of Burns—communicates with opposite side

✓ Empties into the EJV

✓ No valves

Communicating vein—vein sometimes occurring between the facial vein and the anterior jugular vein

Superficial cutaneous nerves—supplies sensation to the skin over the lateral and anterior neck (superficial to deep)

- ✓ Ascending
  - ◊ Lesser occipital nerve (C_2–C_3)
  - ◊ Greater auricular nerve (C_2–C_3)
- ✓ Transverse cervical nerve (C_2–C_3)
- ✓ Descending—supraclavicular nerve (C_3–C_4)
  - ◊ Medial, intermediate, lateral branches
  - ◊ Provide articular sensation for the SC and AC joints

Lymphatics

Head

- ✓ Occipital nodes—occipital region of skull
- ✓ Retroauricular nodes (mastoid)—behind ear
- ✓ Preauricular nodes—in front of ear
- ✓ Superficial parotid nodes—lateral face and cheek
- ✓ Facial nodes
  - ◊ Infraorbital nodes—below orbit
  - ◊ Buccal nodes—angle of the mouth
  - ◊ Mandibular nodes—mandible
- ✓ Neck submental nodes—chin, lower lip, cheek
- ✓ Submandibular nodes—submandibular gland, tongue
- ✓ Anterior jugular nodes—anterior jugular vein
- ✓ External jugular nodes—external jugular vein

Deep cervical

- ✓ Superior deep cervical nodes
  - ◊ Retropharyngeal nodes—nose and nasal sinus
  - ◊ Deep parotid nodes—middle ear, external acoustic meatus
  - ◊ Jugulodigastric nodes—tongue and palatine tonsil
  - ◊ Juguloomohyoid nodes—submental and tongue
- ✓ Inferior deep cervical nodes
  - ◊ Supraclavicular nodes
  - ◊ Jugular trunk—confluence of IJV and EJV

Lymphatics empty into the left thoracic duct (left subclavian vein) or right lymphatic duct (right subclavian vein)

Triangles of the neck

- ✓ Posterior triangle of the neck
  - ◊ Occipital
  - ◊ Supraclavicular (omoclavicular, subclavian)

- ✓ Anterior triangle of the neck
  - ◊ Submental
  - ◊ Submandibular
  - ◊ Muscular
  - ◊ Carotid

Boundaries/borders of the posterior triangle of the neck

- ✓ Anterior—SCM muscle
- ✓ Posterior—trapezius muscle
- ✓ Inferior/base—clavicle
- ✓ Apex superiorly—SCM and trapezius
- ✓ Roof—investing layer of the deep cervical fascia and skin
- ✓ Floor—prevertebral fascia overlying scalenes, levator scapula and splenius

2.5.4 Axilla and brachial plexus

Axilla

- ✓ The axilla is the name given to an area that lies underneath the glenohumeral joint, at the junction of the upper limb and the thorax
- ✓ This region is a passage by which structures such as vessels and nerves can enter and leave the upper limb

Borders of axilla

- ✓ The overall 3D shape of the axilla looks slightly like a pyramid. The borders consist of four sides and a base with an opening at the apex
  - ◊ Apex—also known as the axillary inlet, this is formed by lateral border of the first rib, superior border of scapula, and the posterior border of the clavicle
  - ◊ Lateral wall—formed by intertubecular groove of the humerus containing the portions of coracobrachialis and biceps brachii
  - ◊ Medial wall—consists of the serratus anterior and the thoracic wall (ribs and intercostal muscles)
  - ◊ Anterior wall—contains the pectoralis major and the underlying pectoralis minor and the subclavius muscles, clavipectoral fascia and suspensory ligaments of axilla
  - ◊ Posterior wall—formed by the subscapularis, teres major and latissimus dorsi
- ✓ The size and shape of the axilla regionvaries with arm abduction. It decreases in size most markedly when the arm is fully abducted. At this point, the contents of the axilla are at most risk of injury

Contents of axilla

- ✓ Axillary fat
- ✓ Axillary lymph nodes
  - ◊ The axillary lymph nodes filter lymph that has drained from the upper limb and pectoral region. In women, axillary lymph node enlargement is an non-specific indicator of breast cancer
    - ◆ Anterior (pectoral) set—along the lateral thoracic vein

◆ Posterior (subscapular) set—subscap vein
◆ Lateral (humeral) set—brachial vein
◆ Central set—axillary vein
◆ Apical set—upper axillary/subclavian vein

✓ Axillary artery
  ♢ It is the main artery supplying the upper limb
  ♢ It is commonly refered as having three parts, one medial to the pectoralis minor, one posterior to pectoralis minor, and one lateral to pectoralis minor
  ♢ The medial and posterior parts travel in the axilla
    ◆ 1st part: supreme thoracic artery
    ◆ 2nd part: thoracoacromial artery (trunk), lateral thoracic artery
    ◆ 3rd part: subscapular artery, anterior circumflex humeral artery, posterior circumflex humeral artery

✓ Axillary vein
  ♢ The main vein draining the upper limb, its two largest tributaries are the cephalic and basilic veins

✓ Brachial plexus
  ♢ A collection of spinal nerves that form the peripheral nerves of the upper limb
  ♢ Note: axillary artery through brachial plexus are enveloped by axillary sheath

Spaces associated with axilla

✓ Quadrangular space
  ♢ Borders—teres major, teres minor, long head of the triceps brachii muscles, and the surgical neck of the
  ♢ Contents—axillary nerve and posterior circumflex humeral artery

✓ Triangular interval
  ♢ Borders—long and lateral heads of the triceps brachii (or humeral shaft) and the teres major muscles
  ♢ Contents—radial nerve and deep brachial artery

✓ Triangular space
  ♢ Borders—teres major, teres minor, and the long head of the triceps brachii muscles
  ♢ Contents—circumflex scapular artery

Brachial plexus

✓ Roots—(C_5–T_1) pass between the anterior and middle scalenes with the subclavian artery (subclavian vein courses anterior to the anterior scalene muscle)
✓ Dorsal scapular nerve—(C_5) pierces the middle scalene, descends deep to the levator scapulae, rhomboideus muscles
✓ Along with the deep branch of the transverse cervical artery supplying both rhomboideus muscles

Levator scapulae

✓ Long thoracic nerve—(C_5–C_7) descends posterior to the roots of the plexus and the axillary artery, descends along
✓ The lateral surface of the serratus anterior muscle with the lateral thoracic artery while supplying the muscle

- ✓ Trunks (superior, middle, inferior) — emerge between anterior and middle scalenes and descend towards the clavicle
- ✓ Suprascapular nerve — (C_5, C_6) branches off the upper trunk, courses across the posterior triangle of neck
- ✓ Through the suprascapular foramen, inferior to the transverse scapular ligament (suprascapular artery and vein pass superior
- ✓ To the transverse scapular ligament to supply the supraspinatus muscles; continues through the greater scapular

Notch to supply the infraspinatus muscles

- ✓ Nerve to the subclavius — (C_5, C_6) branches off the upper trunk to the subclavius muscles

2.5.5 Carotid, submandibular and submental triangles of the neck

Overview of the major triangles of the anterior neck

- ✓ The anterior cervical triangle is formed by the three boundaries listed below, and is a space that is further subdivided into three paired triangles and one unpaired triangle for descriptive purposes. The triangles provide a framework from which the muscles and geographically related structures can be readily located and identified
- ✓ Boundaries (provided below): the triangle that is created has its inferior border or apex at the jugular notch, a floor that is composed of the pharynx, larynx, thyroid gland, and the prevertebral fascia, and a roof that consists of the investing layer of deep cervical fascia that arches from one sternocleidomastoid muscle to the other
    - ▷ Mandible
    - ▷ Anterior border of the sternocleidomastoid muscle
    - ▷ Median line of the neck (anterior midline of the neck)

Triangles located within the "anterior cervical triangle"

- ✓ Submandibular triangle (paired): boundaries of this triangle are the inferior border of the mandible, the anterior surface of the posterior digastric, and the posterior surface of the anterior digastric. This is a glandular area that is on occasion referred to as the "digastric triangle" (the submandibular gland nearly fills the triangle)
- ✓ Carotid triangle (paired): boundaries are the superior belly of the omohyoid, the posterior belly of the digastric muscle, and the anterior border of the sternocleidomastoid muscle. This is a vascular area, where the common carotid artery ascends and the pulse can be palpated
- ✓ Muscular triangle (paired): boundaries are the superior belly of the omohyoid muscle, the anterior border of the sternocleidomastoid muscle, and the median plane of the neck. This triangle contains the infrahyoid muscles and viscera of the neck (thyroid and parathyroid glands)
- ✓ Submental triangle (unpaired): boundaries are the hyoid bone inferiorly, and the right and left bellies of the anterior digastrics laterally

Osteology with important cartilage structures

✓ Mandible (landmarks include: body, angle, ramus, digastric fossa, mylohyoid groove, and the mental spine)

✓ Hyoid bone (located at approximately the C_3 level, and includes the following landmarks: body, greater horn and lesser horn)

✓ Styloid process

✓ Thyroid cartilage [(located at approximately the C_{4-5} level, and is responsible for producing the laryngeal prominence (Adam's apple)]

✓ Cricoid cartilage (found at approximately the C_6 level)

✓ Others involved with this region include the scapula and the sternum (i.e., for origin of the omohyoid muscle)

Muscles associated with the anterior triangle of the neck

✓ Hyoid muscles: there are eight of these, four infrahyoids that function to depress the hyoid bone, and four suprahyoids that function to elevate the hyoid bone. As a group, they function to steady or move the hyoid bone and the larynx. The hyoid bone provides attachments for the suprahyoid muscles superior to it and the infrahyoids inferior to it

✓ Infrahyoids: collectively, there are four infrahyoid muscles found inferior to the hyoid bone

✓ Sternohyoid (superficial plane): the muscle runs parallel and adjacent to the anterior median line

   ◊ Arises from the manubrium of the sternum and the medial end of the clavicle

   ◊ Inserts into the body the hyoid bone

   ◊ Functions to depress the hyoid bone after it has been elevated (as would be the case with swallowing, etc.)

   ◊ Innervated by the C_1–C_3 roots, a branch of the ansa cervicalis

Omohyoid (superficial plane): located laterally to the sternohyoid muscles

✓ Arises from the superior border of the scapula near the suprascapular notch

✓ Inserts into the inferior border of the hyoid bone

✓ The muscle consists of two muscle bellies united by an intermediate tendon, which are indirectly connected to the clavicle via a fascial sling

✓ Functions to depress, retract, and steady the hyoid bone

✓ Innervated by the C_1–C_3 roots, a branch of the ansa cervicalis

Sternothyroid (found at a slightly deeper level and the muscle is wider than the sternohyoid muscle)

✓ Arises from the posterior surface of the manubrium of the sternum

✓ Inserts on the oblique line of the thyroid cartilage

✓ Functions to depress the hyoid and larynx, also covers the lateral lobe of the thyroid gland

✓ Innervated by the C_2–C_3 roots, a branch of the ansa cervicalis

Clinical notes: The location of this muscle limits the upward expansion of the thyroid gland. This is noteworthy clinically with the development of goiter, where the expansion is forced inferiorly and anteriorly into the mediastinum

Thyrohyoid (found at a slightly deeper level than the sternohyoid)
✓ Arises from the oblique line of the thyroid cartilage ✓ Inserts into the inferior border of the body and greater horn of the hyoid bone ✓ Functions to depress the hyoid bone and elevate the larynx ✓ Innervated by the C_1 root, via the hypoglossal nerve
Clinical notes: Collectively the four infrahyoid muscles are considered to be "strap muscles", that cover the front and much of the sides of the larynx, trachea, and thyroid gland
Suprahyoid muscles
✓ Collectively there are four suprahyoid muscles, if the anterior and posterior bellies of the digastrics are viewed as one functional muscle. As a group, these are superior to the hyoid and connect it to the skull. Digastrics (there are two of these, the anterior and posterior digastric)—the two digastrics are interconnected by an intermediate tendon that is attached to the hyoid bone. While these two muscles share this common point of insertion, they are innervated by two different cranial nerves (CN V and CN VII). The intermediate tendon is attached to the body and greater horn of the hyoid by a fibrous sling that slides anteriorly and posteriorly

✓ Anterior digastric
    ◊ Arises from the digastric fossa of the mandible
    ◊ Inserts onto the intermediate tendon
    ◊ Innervated by the mylohyoid nerve, a branch of the inferior alveolar nerve (stemming from the V_3 branch of CN V (trigeminal), with an embryologic origin from the 1st pharyngeal arch)
✓ Posterior digastric
    ◊ Arises from the mastoid notch of the temporal bone
    ◊ Inserts into the intermediate tendon to the hyoid bone (body and greater horn)
    ◊ Innervated by the facial nerve (CN VII)
✓ Function: the two digastrics collectively function to depress the mandible and raise and steady the hyoid bone during swallowing and speaking

Clinical notes: Noteworthy points associated with digastrics are that the two bellies are developmentally separate, since they are supplied by two different cranial nerves (CN V and CN VII), and there is a fibrous sling (the intermediate tendon) that interconnects the two muscles
Stylohoid muscle
✓ Arises from the styloid process of the temporal bone ✓ Inserts onto the body of the hyoid bone (and is found nearly parallel to the belly of the posterior digastric muscle) ✓ Functions to elevate and retract the hyoid bone, thereby elongating the floor of the mouth ✓ Innervated by the cervical branch of the facial nerve
Clinical notes: The distal portion of the stylohyoid muscle that inserts into the hyoid bone is pierced (or split), by the intermediate tendon of the digastrics

Geniohyoid muscle—superior to the mylohyoid and the two geniohyoid muscles help reinforce the floor of the mouth
✓ Arises from the inferior mental spine of the mandible ✓ Inserts onto the body of the hyoid bone ✓ Functions to pull the hyoid anterosuperiorly, shortens the floor of the mouth, and widens the pharynx ✓ Innervated by the C_1 nerve root, via the hypoglossal nerve
Mylohyoid muscle—forms the floor of the mouth
✓ Arises from the mylohyoid line of the mandible ✓ Inserts onto the raphe and body of the hyoid bone ✓ Functions to elevate the hyoid bone, floor of the mouth, and tongue, during swallowing and speaking ✓ Innervated by the mylohyoid nerve, a branch of the inferior alveolar nerve (V_3 branch of CN V, the trigeminal)
Sternocleidomastoid muscle—the anterior border of the SCM muscle serves as the posterior boundary for larger "anterior triangle" of the neck, and more specifically for the carotid and muscular triangles

✓ Arises from the lateral surface of the mastoid process of the temporal bone, and the lateral half of the superior nuchal line
✓ Inserts distally via two heads:
  ◊ Sternal head: inserts into the anterior surface of the manubrium of the sternum
  ◊ Clavicular head: inserts into the superior surface of the medial third of the clavicle

Functions to laterally side bend and rotate the head to the opposite side
Innervated by the spinal root of the accessory nerve (spinal accessory nerve, or CN XI)
Clinical correlation: tracheotomy

✓ The easiest and most rapid approaches to opening an airway into the trachea
  ◊ Cricothyrotomy—incision is made between the thyroid and cricoid cartilages. The location of this type of incision is above the isthmus of the thyroid gland, to avoid damaging this important gland
  ◊ An alternate approach is an inferior (low) tracheotomy that is done inferior the level of the isthmus of the thyroid gland
✓ Membranes involved with a tracheotomy
  ◊ Thyrohyoid membrane
  ◊ Cricothyroid membrane (median cricothyroid ligament)
  ◊ These two membranes are under the cover of the infrahyoid muscles

Carotid artery, sheath, and related structures
Carotid artery and sheath—a tubular fascial condensation that begins at the root of the neck and ends at the base of the skull; formed by three layers of deep cervical fascia that fuse together
Contents of the inferior portion of the carotid sheath
✓ Internal jugular vein—located laterally in the sheath ✓ Common caroid artery—located medially in the sheath (superiorly in the sheath, the common carotid artery is replaced by the internal carotid artery)

✓ Vagus nerve (CN X)—posteriorly located in the sheath
✓ Ansa cervicalis—usually is embedded in the anterolateral aspect of the sheath
✓ Deep cervical lymph nodes—numerous nodes lie along the sheath and the IJV

Clinical notes: The cervical sympathetic trunk lies posterior to the carotid sheath. Thus, while closely related, the sympathetic trunk remains outside the sheath in the prevertebral fascia

Carotid arteries—begins as the common carotid artery and bifurcates into the internal and external carotids at the level of the superior border of the thyroid cartilage (approximately at the C_4 level)

The carotid arteries run upward on each side of the trachea, arising from

✓ On the right—from the bifurcation of the brachiocephalic trunk
✓ On the left—common carotid arises directly from the arch of the aorta
✓ Internal carotid artery (ICA)
✓ No branches in the neck—used as a means of clearly identifying the ICA
✓ Supplies the structures within the cranial and orbital cavities—enters the skull through the carotid canals

Clinical correlate: Carotid endarterectomy—a procedure done to remove athlerosclerotic plaques that have developed within the intima of the artery to increase blood flow. While a necessary procedure when occlusion of the artery reaches a critical level (often identified by doppler studies or clinically from transient ischemic attacks), two real risks associated with a carotid endarterectomy are cerebral vascular accidents (from any remnants of the plaque that flows into a smaller cerebral artery), and injury of one or more of the following nerves [CN IX, X (including the superior laryngeal nerve, a branch of X), CN XI, and XII]

External carotid artery (ECA)

✓ Lies anterior to the ICA
✓ Supplies almost all structures of the head and neck, outside of the cranial cavity (exception is the middle meningeal artery)
✓ There are eight direct branches from the ECA
  ◊ Superior thyroid artery—supplies the thyroid gland, and the larynx (from a branch, the superior laryngeal artery). This is the most inferior branch of the three anterior branches of the ECA
  ◊ Lingual artery—passes deep to the hypoglossal nerve, stylohyoid and posterior belly of the digastric
  ◊ Ascending pharyngeal artery—typically the first or second branch off of the ECA (sends branches to the pharynx, prevertebral muscles, middle ear and the cranial meninges)
  ◊ Occipital artery

Facial artery—often arises in common with the lingual artery, or immediately superior to it. Hooks around middle of the mandible and enters the face. This is a site where pulsations can be felt

Clinical notes: 20% of the time, the facial and lingual arteries arise from a common branch
✓ Posterior auricular artery
✓ Maxillary artery—an important branch off of the maxillary artery is the middle meningeal artery (that passes through the foramen spinosum and supplies the dura mater and calvaria)
✓ Superficial temporal artery

Structures associated with the carotid artery

✓ Carotid sinus of the internal carotid artery (slight dilation of the proximal part of the ICA)
  ◊ At this location, the walls of the carotid artery are thinner, less muscular, and consequently more elastic—the dilation may also involve the common carotid artery
  ◊ Pressoreceptors (associated with CN IX and X)—an increase in blood pressure results in a decrease in heart rate
  ◊ Pressure placed on the carotid sinus can depress the heart rate and result in fainting
✓ Carotid body
  ◊ Small mass of dark tissue in the region of the carotid bifurcation, lying on the medial (deep) side
  ◊ Chemoreceptors (associated with CN IX and X)
    ◆ Responds to either an increase in CO_2, a decrease in the O_2 level or the pH level. Stimulation of this reflex results in increased rate and depth of respiration, cardiac rate, and blood pressure

The internal jugular vein

✓ Largest vein of the head and neck—begins at the jugular foramen as a continuation of the sigmoid sinus
✓ Collects blood from the brain, superficial face, and from the neck
✓ Lies lateral to the carotid artery in the carotid sheath
✓ Near its termination, the vein has a single bicuspid valve to prevent an upward flow of blood (i.e., when an individual is upside down, such as standing on their head). This dilation is known as the inferior bulb of the IJV

Tributaries

✓ Sigmoid sinus
✓ Inferior petrosal sinus—leaves the skull through the jugular foramen
✓ Lingual veins—facial and lingual are often associated by a common trunk
✓ Pharyngeal veins
✓ Facial veins (no valves—thus, the spread of infection via this vein is an issue)
✓ Thyroid veins—superior and middle thyroid veins

The IVC unites with the subclavian vein to form the brachiocephalic vein

Thoracic duct on the left and lymphatic duct on the right, are found at the junction of the IJV and the subclavian veins (left and right venous angles)

Parasympathetic nerve supply, glands and lymphatics

Vagus nerve

✓ Lies behind and between the common carotid artery and the internal jugular vein
✓ Branches include pharyngeal and laryngeal
  ◊ Superior—further divides into the internal (sensory) and external laryngeal (motor to the cricothyroid muscle), and innervates the larynx
  ◊ Inferior laryngeals—a continuation of the recurrent laryngeal nerve (branch of the vagus). The motor nerve of the larynx, supplying all of the muscles of the larynx except the cricothyroid muscle (see superior laryngeal nerve above)

◊ Cardiac nerves—superior and inferior branches

Lymphatics

Deep cervical chain

✓ Largest group of nodes in the neck, lying lateral and posterior to the IJV
✓ Two groups of cervical lymphatics: superior deep cervical and inferior deep cervical

Clinical notes: resection of these nodes may occur in a radical neck dissection, sometimes used to stop the spread of cancer in this region

The four triangles of the neck (subcomponents of the larger anterior triangle of the neck)

Submandibular triangle (digastric)

✓ Boundaries
  ◊ One boundary is the inferior border of the mandible
  ◊ The two bellies of the digastrics (anterior and posterior) constitute the other two borders
  ◊ Floor—created by the mylohyoid, hyoglossus, and middle constrictor of the pharynx
✓ Contents
  ◊ Submandibular gland—nearly fills this triangle
  ◊ Submandibular lymph nodes—lie on each side of the submandibular gland
  ◊ Submandibular duct—approximately 5 cm in length, runs parallel to the tongue and opens into the oral cavity (the openings are the sublingual papilla)
  ◊ Hypoglossal nerve (CN XII)—motor to the intrinsics and extrinsics of the tongue
  ◊ Nerve to the mylohyoid—supplies the anterior belly of the digastric muscle
  ◊ Parts of the facial artery and vein (including the submental artery)

Carotid triangle

✓ Boundaries
  ◊ One boundary is the superior belly of the omohyoid
  ◊ Second boundary is the posterior belly of the digastric
  ◊ Third boundary is the anterior border of the SCM
✓ Contents
  ◊ Common carotid artery (with ECA and ICA)
  ◊ Carotid sheath [contains the carotid artery (sinus and body), IJV, and vagus nerve]
  ◊ Superior root of the ansa cervicalis
  ◊ Deep cervical lymph nodes
  ◊ Thyroid, larynx and pharynx
  ◊ CN XI and XII
  ◊ Superior and inferior laryngeal nerves (branch of CN X)

Muscular triangle

✓ Boundaries
  ◊ One boundary is the superior belly of the omohyoid muscle
  ◊ Second boundary is the anterior border of the SCM
  ◊ Third boundary that splits the triangle into two pieces is the median plane of the neck

✓ Contents
  ◊ Infrahyoid muscles
  ◊ Viscera of the neck (includes the thyroid gland and the parathyroid gland)

Submental triangle (an unpaired triangle)

✓ Boundaries
  ◊ One boundary is the hyoid bone (inferiorly)
  ◊ Laterally, the other two boundaries are the right and left anterior belly of the digastrics
  ◊ Floor consists of the two mylohyoid muscles—these two muscles meet in a median fibrous raphe

✓ Contents
  ◊ Submental lymph nodes—these nodes receive lymph from ①the tip of the tongue, ②the floor of the mouth, ③mandibular incisor teeth and gums, ④central part of the lower lip, and ⑤skin of the chin
  ◊ Small veins—these unite to form the anterior jugular vein

The ansa cervicalis

✓ Loop formed from superior root (C_1) and a nerve formed from branches of C_2 and C_3 (inferior root), hook-up with the hypoglossal nerve (CN XII)

✓ Branches from this supply the sternohyoid, sternothyroid and omohyoid muscles

✓ Nerves to the sternohyoid and sternothyroid enter at their posterolateral borders

✓ Nerve to the superior belly of the omohyoid enters at its lateral border

Ke Lining, Chen Hao

Chapter 3

The Thorax

3.1 Introduction

3.1.1 Boundaries and divisions

3.1.1.1 Boundaries

The thorax lies at the upper part of the trunk between the neck and the abdomen. Below it is separated from the abdomen by the diaphragm, above it is continuous with the neck, laterally it is separated from the upper limb by the anterior and posterior margins of the deltoid.

Its upper boundary is formed by a line drawing from thejugular notch or suprasternal notch, along the superior margins of the clavicles to the acromions, and then to the spinous process of the 7th cervical vertebra.

The lower boundary is formed by thexiphoid process in front, the costal arch nd the free border of 11th and 12th ribs on both sides, and the spinous process of the 12th thoracic vertebra posteriorly.

The lateral boundaries of the thorax separating from the upper limb are the anterior and posterior margins of the deltoid.

The apex of the lung and the cupula of pleura project into the neck through the superior aperture of the thorax. Some organs of the abdomen are covered by the thoracic cage, and are separated from the viscera of the thorax by the diaphragm.

3.1.1.2 Divisions

Maybe everyone knows that a bottle consists of two parts: the wall and the cavity of the bottle. The thorax is similar to the bottle, it consists of the wall and the cavity. The wall includes the thoracic wall and the diaphragm.

(1) The thoracic wall can be divided into two regions: The anterolateral thoracic region is located between the anterior median line and posterior axillary line, and the thoracodorsal region between the posterior axillary line and the posterior median line.

(2) The diaphragm.

(3) The thoracic cavity is occupied by the mediastinum, the lungs and pleural sacs. The mediastinum is in the middle, the lungs and pleural sacs are in both sides.

3.1.2　Surface anatomy

3.1.2.1　The surface landmarks

(1) The jugular notch or suprasternal notch

It is a shallow notch on the superior margin of the manubrium.

(2) The clavicle

It is subcutaneous and easily palpable.

(3) The xiphoid process.

(4) The costal arch (costal margin)

It is formed by the 7th to 10th costal cartilages.

(5) The infrasternal angle

It lies between the two costal arches.

(6) The nipple

In the male, the nipple usually lies in the 4th intercostal space about 10 cm from the midline. In the female, its position is not constant.

(7) The sternal angle (angle of louis)

It is an important surface landmark. It is the transverse ridge on the anterior surface of sternum between the manubrium and the body of the sternum, and is easily palpable. It forms a landmark for counting the second rib. If we make a level by the angle, the level is called the level of the sternal angle. Posteriorly the level is opposite to the lower margin of the 4th thoracic vertebra. There are some important structures on the level. The angle and the level mark the following structures: ①counting the ribs; ②bifurcation of trachea; ③the origin and the terminal of the aortic arch; ④the second constriction of the esophagus; ⑤arch of azygos vein; ⑥the interface of mediastinum, the level is the boundary line between the superior and inferior mediadtina; ⑦the lower border of the 4th thoracic vertebra.

3.1.2.2　The orientational lines on the thoracic wall (Figure 3-1)

(1) The anterior median line

It is the anterior median line over the sternum.

(2) The sternal line

It runs vertically just lateral to the widest part of the sternum.

(3) The midclavicular line

It runs vertically through the midpoint the clavicle.

(4) The parasternal line

It runs vertically midway between the sternal and the midclavicular lines.

(5) The anterior axillary line

It runs vertically through the anterior axillary fold.

(6) The midaxillary line

It runs vertically through the middle of the axilla.

(7) The posterior axillary line

It runs vertically through the posterior axillary fold.

(8) The paravertebral line

It runs vertically just lateral to the transverse processes of the vertebrae.

(9) The scapular line

It runs vertically through the inferior angle of the scapula.

(10) The posterior median line

It runs vertically through the tips of the spinous processes of the vertebrae.

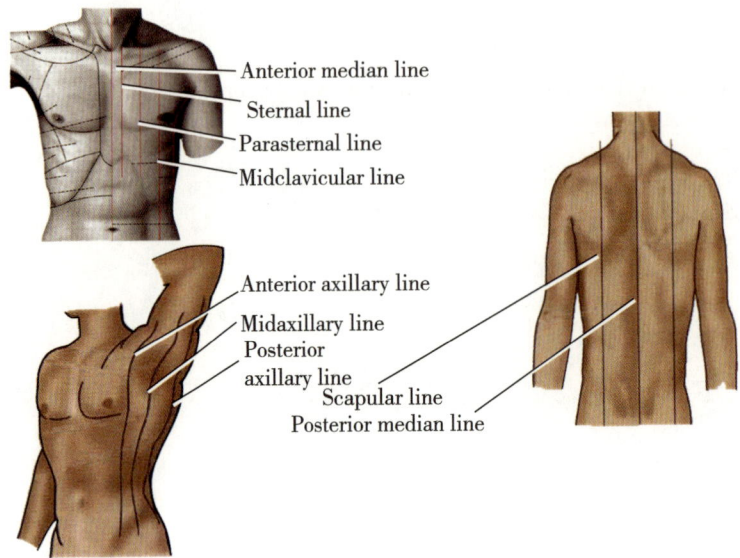

Figure 3-1 Reference lines of thorax

3.2 Thoracic wall and cavity

The layers of the thoracic wall are as follows.

3.2.1 The skin

It varies in texture, tending to be thin in front and thick behind. The skin can slide easily except the anterior region of the sternumuscle.

3.2.2 The superficial fascia

It contains the adipose tissue, the superficial blood vessels, lymphatic vessels, the cutaneous nerves and the breast.

(1) The cutaneous nerves

The skin of the anterior thoracic wall above the second rib is supplied by the supraclavicular nerves. The segmentary distribution of the thoracic nerves is important. The 2nd intercostal nerve is at the level of the sternal angle. The 4th intercostal nerve is at the level of nipple in male. The 6th intercostal nerve is at the level of xiphisternal synchondrosis.

(2) The superficial blood vessels

The anterior perforating branches of the internal thoracic artery supply the superficial fascia and skin of the anterior thoracic wall. The lateral and posterior cutaneous branches of the posterior intercostal artery supply the superficial fascia and skin of the lateral and posterior thoracic walls.

The superficial veins anastomose with each other to form the venous network in the superficial fascia and contribute to the thoracoepigastric vein which run downwards to connect with the venous network around the umbilicus and upwards to drain into the axillary vein by way of the lateral thoracic vein.

(3) The breast(mamma) (Figure 3-2)

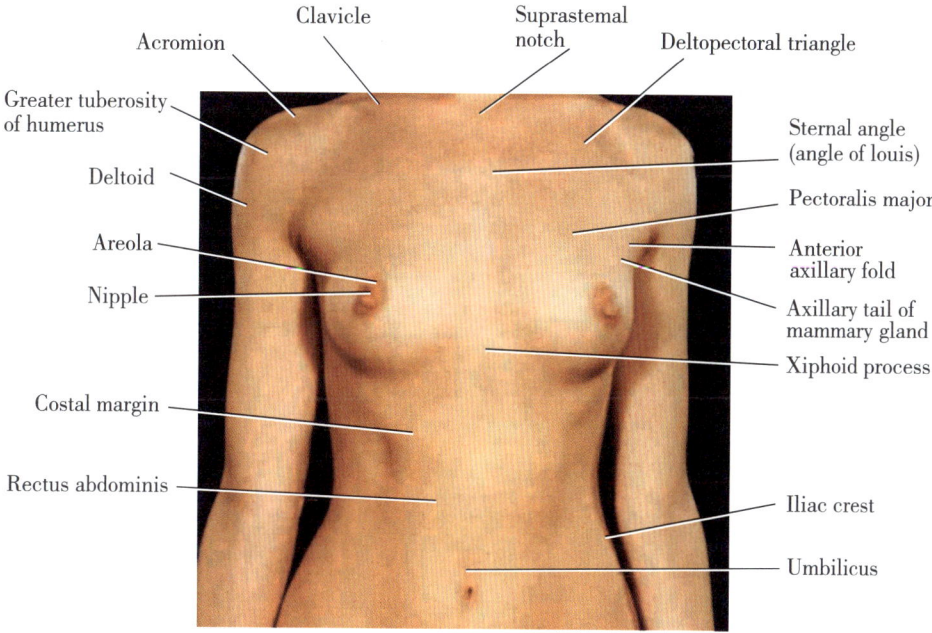

Figure 3-2 Anterior view of the thorax and abdomen of a 29-year-old woman

In young women, it is usually hemispherical and slightly pendulous, overlaps the 2nd to the 6th ribs and their costal cartilages, and extends from the lateral margin of the sternum to the midaxillary line. The greater part of the breast lies in the superficial fascia and can be moved freely in all directions. Its upper lateral edge extends around the lower border of the pectoralis major and enters the axilla, where it comes into close relationship with the axillary vessels. In middle-aged multiparous women, the breast may be large and pendulous, and in older women the breast may be smaller.

In the living subject, the breast is soft, because the fat contained within it is fluid. On careful palpation with the open hand, the breast has a firm, overall lobulated consistency, produced by its glandular tissue.

The nipple projects from the lower half of the breast, but its position in relation to the chest wall varies greatly and depends on the development of the gland. In males and immature females, the nipples are small and usually lie over the fourth intercostal spaces about 10 cm from the midline. The base of the nipple is surrounded by a circular area of pigmented skin called the areola. Pink in color in the young girl, the areola becomes darker in color in the second month of the first pregnancy and never regains its former tint. Tiny tubercles on the areola are produced by the underlying areolar glands(Figure 3-3).

3.2.3 The deep structures

3.2.3.1 The deep fascia

It may be divided into superficial and deep layers.

The superficial layer covering the pectoralis major and serratus anterior is attached to the clavicle superiorly, becomes continuous with the fascia of the abdominal wall inferiorly, and with the periosteum of the sternum medially.

142 Regional Anatomy

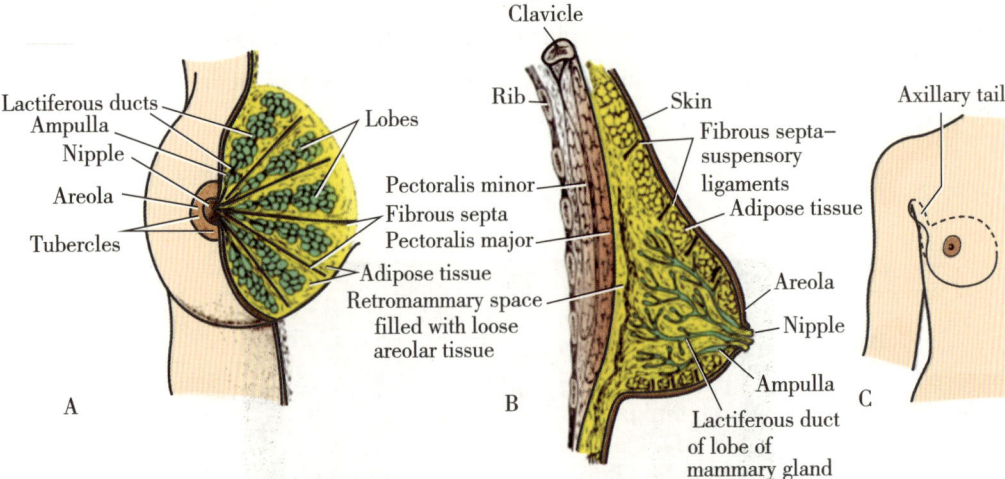

A. Anterior view with skin partially removed to show internal structure; B. Sagittal section; C. The axillary tail, which pierces the deep fascia and extends into the axilla.

Figure 3-3 Mature breast in the female

The deep layer forms the clavipectoral fascia between subclavius and the upper border of the pectoralis minor. It splits downwards into two layers to invest the pectoralis minor and then fuses with the superficial layer to join the axillary facia.

3.2.3.2 The muscles

The most superficial muscle is the pectoralis major, remove the pectoralis major we can see the pectoralis minor. In the lateral thoracic wall, there are the serratus anterior and the external oblique muscle.

3.2.3.3 The intercostal spaces

It contains the intercostal muscles, nerves and vessels (Figure 3-4–Figure 3-6).

(1) The intercostal muscles

There are three layers of muscles from outside to inside in each intercostal space, i.e., external intercostal muscle, internal intercostal muscle and innermost internal intercostal muscle.

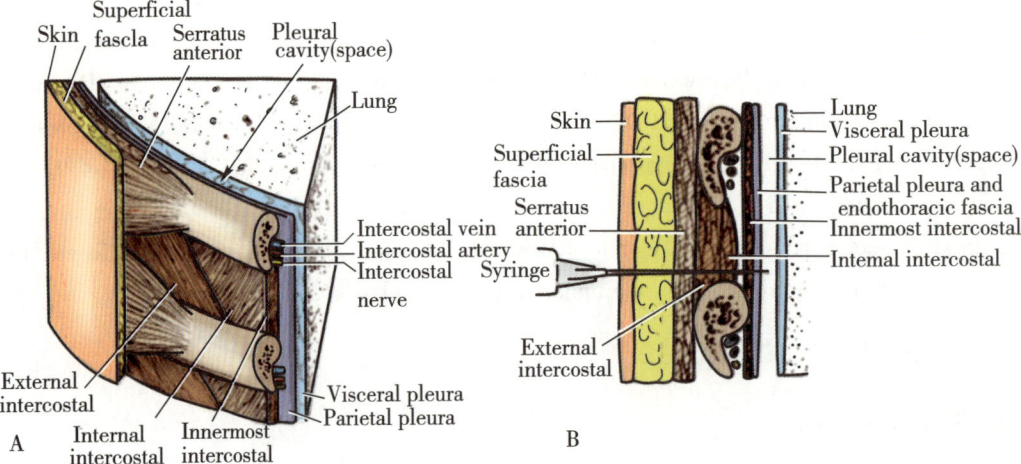

A. Section through an intercostal space; B. Structures penetrated by a needle when it passes from skin surface to pleural cavity.

Figure 3-4 Structures from skin surface to pleural carity

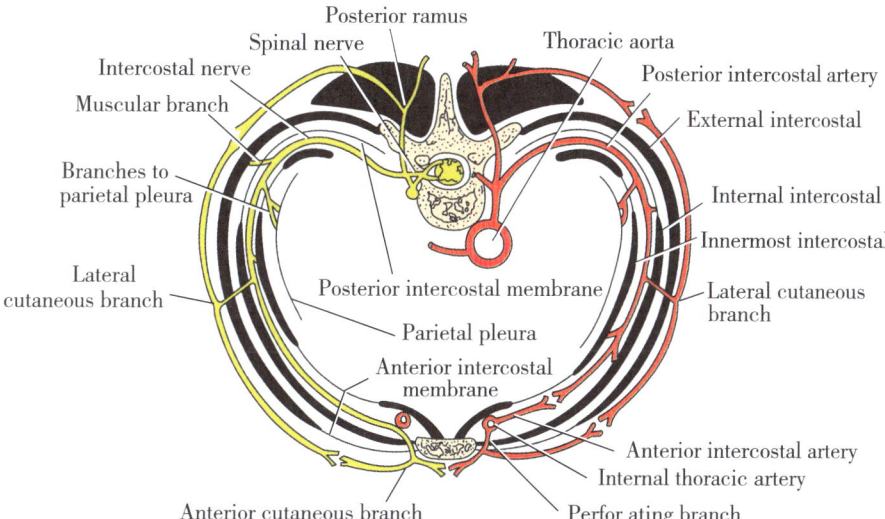

Figure 3-5 Cross section of the thorax showing distribution of a typical intercostal nerve and a posterior and an anterior intercostal atery

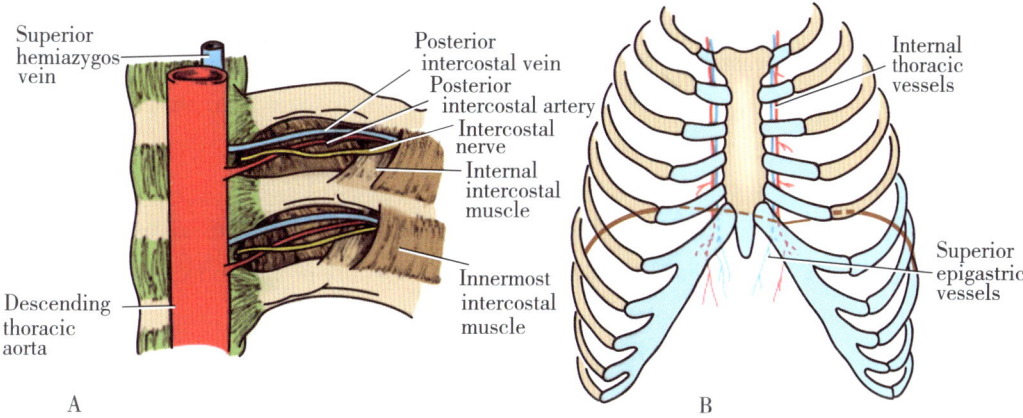

A. Internal view of the posterior end of two typical intercostal spaces, the posterior intercostal membrane has been removed for clarity; B. Anterior view of the chest showing the courses of the internal thoracic vessels. These vessels descend about one fingerbreadth from the lateral margin of the sternum.

Figure 3-6 The courses of the internal thoracic vessels

1) The external intercostal muscle

It arises from the inferior border of the upper rib and inserts to the superior border of the lower rib. Their fibers run downwards, forwards and medially. Anteriorly, the muscles are replaced by the external intercostal membrane. The muscles raise the ribs, enlarge the thoracic cavity and assist in inspiration.

2) The internal intercostal muscle

It arises from the the superior border of the inferior rib and inserts to the inferior border of the superior rib. Their fibers run from anteroinferior to posterosuperior. Posteriorly, the muscles are replaced by the internal intercostal membrane. The muscles depress the ribs, diminishe the thoracic cavity and assist in expiration.

3) The innermost intercostal muscle

It lies at the middle part of each intercostal space. The direction of its fibers is as same as that of the internal intercostal muscle. The both can be differentiated only by the intercostal nerves and vessels between muscle.

(2) The intercostal nerves

There are the twelve pairs of the intercostal nerves are called the subcostal nerves. The intercostal nerves run at first between the parietal pleura and the internal intercostal membrane, then in the costal groove of the corresponding rib, and lie between the internal intercostal muscle and innermost intercostal muscle below the intercostal vessels. The intercostal nerves give off the lateral cutaneous branch near the midaxillary line and the anterior cutaneous branch near the parasternal line.

(3) The intercostal vessels

The posterior intercostals arteries are accompanied by the intercostals nerves. The first two posterior intercostals arteries arise from a branch of the costocervical trunk of the subclavian artery. The other pairs of posterior intercostals artery and the subcostal artery arise from the back of the thoracic aorta. At the costal angle, the posterior intercostal artery gives a collateral branch along the superior margin of the lower rib. The trunk and the collateral branch anastomose with the anterior intercostal branches of the internal thoracic artery.

The posterior intercostal vein accompanies the posterior intercostal artery. The posterior intercostal veins enter the azygos, hemiazygos or accessory hemiazygos veins. Relationship of the intercostal nerves and vessels: before reaching to the costal angle, the intercostal nerves and vessels run in the middle of the space and their arrangement is inconstant; then the trunk lies in the lower margin and the collateral branch lies in the upper margin between the internal intercostal muscle and innermost intercostal muscle, the arrangement from up downwards is the vein, artery and nerve.

(4) The internal thoracic vessels and transversus thoracis

The muscle lies behind the anterior thoracic wall. The internal thoracic artery arises from the subclavian artery, descends into the thorax through the superior aperture of the thorax. Then, this artery runs downwards near the lateral border of the sternum and divides into the superior epigastric and musculophrenic arteries at the level of the 6th intercostal space. The vein accompanies the artery. There are a number of lymph nodes along the internal thoracic vessels, these are called the parasternal lymph nodes.

(5) The endothoracic fascia

It is a thin but dense connective tissue membrane. It lines inner surface of the thoracic wall and upper surface of the diaphragm.

The surgical operation on the pleural cavity must pass through the following layers: skin, superficial fascia, deep fascia and superficial muscles of the thoracic wall, rib and intercostal muscles, endothoracic fascia and parietal pleura.

3.3 The pleura and pleural cavity

3.3.1 Concepts of pleura and pleural carity

(1) The pleura

The pleura is an exceedingly thin layer of serous membrane and possesses excretive and absorptive function. Pleura has two parts, the visceral pleura is adherent to the surface of the lung. The parietal pleura can be subdivided into: ① the costal pleura covers the internal surface of the thoracic wall; ② the diaphragmatic pleura covers the superior surface of the diaphragm; ③ the cupula of the pleura; ④ the mediastinal pleura covers the lateral aspect of the mediastinum (Figure 3-7–Figure 3-9).

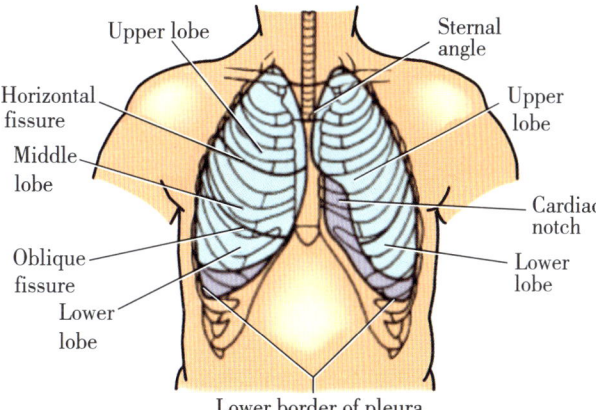

Figure 3-7　Surface markings of the lungs and parietal pleura on the anterior thoracic wall

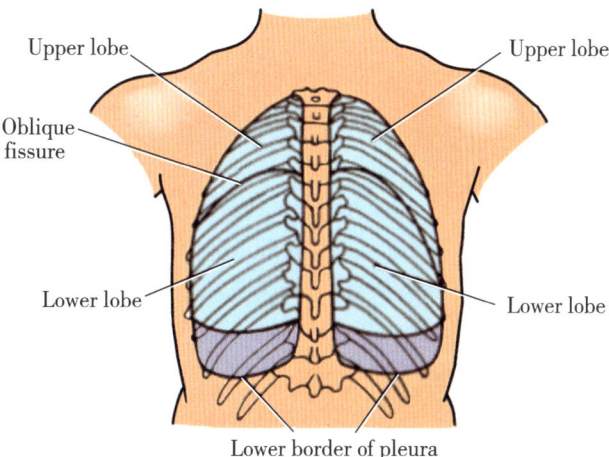

Figure 3-8　Surface markings of the lungs and parietal pleura on the posterior thoracic wall

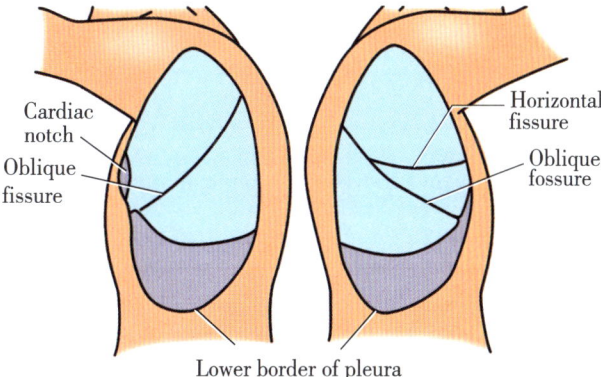

Figure 3-9　Surface markings of the lungs and parietal pleura on the lateral thoracic walls

(2) The pleural cavity

The pleural cavity is only a potential space between the layers of pleura. The cavity contains a layer of serous fluid and presents a negative pressure.

(3) The pleural recesses

The parts of pleural cavity where the lung do not occupy during deep inspiration are called the pleural recess. The largest pleural recess is the costodiaphragmatic recess which is formed by the reflection of the costal and the diaphragmatic pleura. It is the lowest part of the pleural cavity. In certain diseases, various amount of fluid can accumulate in this recess. The costomediastinal recess is formed by the reflection of the costal and the mediastinal pleura, the left recess is larger because of the cardiac notch in the left lung.

(4) The pleural reflection and their projections

The cupula of pleura, the sternal and costal lines of reflection are clinically important.

The cupula of pleura covers the apex of the lung and extends 2 cm above the medial third of the clavicle. Therefore we must pay an attention not to injure the cupula of pleura in operation of the root of the neck.

The sternal reflection descends from the sternoclavicular joints to the midline at the level of the sternal angle. On the right side, the refection continues downwards to the back of the 6th sternocostal joint. On the left side, the reflection passes downwards to the level of the 4th costal cartilage, then, it deviates to the left and descends obliquely to midpoint of the 6th costal cartilage.

Above the sternal angle and below the level of the 4th costal cartilage, the distance between two sternal reflections is larger. The two intervals are called the triangle of thymus and the triangle of pericardium respectively. In the triangle of pericardium, the anterior surface of the pericardium directly contacts with the thoracic wall. Therefore the pericardiocentesis and cardiocentesis can be performed in the 4th and 5th intercostal spaces close to the left margin of the sternum without the damage of pleura.

The costal reflection is where the costal pleura continuous with the diaphragmatic pleura. It passes obliquely across the 8th rib in the midclavicular line, the 10th rib in the midaxillary line, and the 12th rib in the scapular line.

3.3.2 The lungs

The lungs (Figure 3-10, Figure 3-11) are the essential organs of respiration. They are light, soft, spongy and highly elastic. During early life they are pink, but often dark and mottled during late life due to the accumulation of inhaled dust particles. If lungs contain air, they will float in the water. So, the antepartum and postpartum death can be differentiated.

3.3.2.1 The position and shape

The lungs lie in the thoracic cavity and above the diaphragm, meanwhile it is separated from each other by the mediastinum.

Each lung is basically pyramidal, and presents an apex, a base, two surfaces, and three borders. The apex extends into the root of the neck 2 cm above the medial third of the clavicle. The base (diaphragmatic surface) of the lung is concaveand faces the diaphragm. The costal surfaceis large, convex, and in contact with the costal pleura. The mediastinal surfaceis towards the mediastinum. The hilum of the lunglies near the center of this surface. The anterior border is thin and overlaps the pericardium. There is a cardiac notchat the anterior border of the left lung. The posterior border is thick and rounded. The inferior border is thin and descends into costodiaphragmatic recess during inspiration.

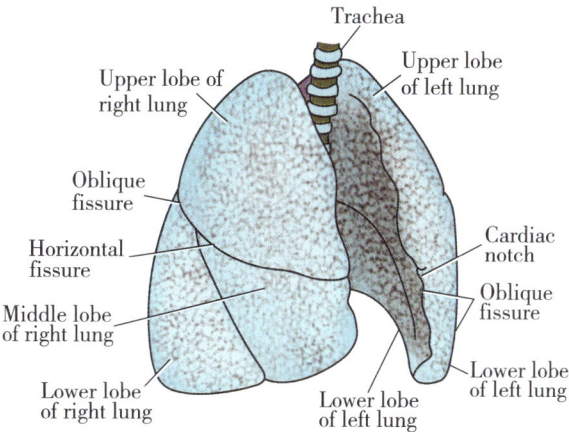

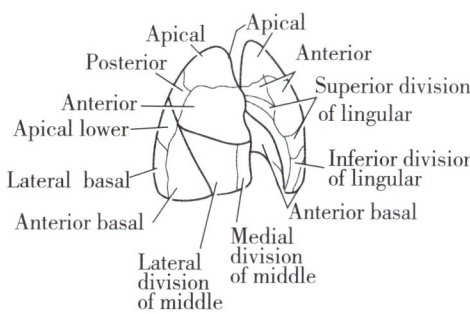

Figure 3-10 Lungs viewed from the right

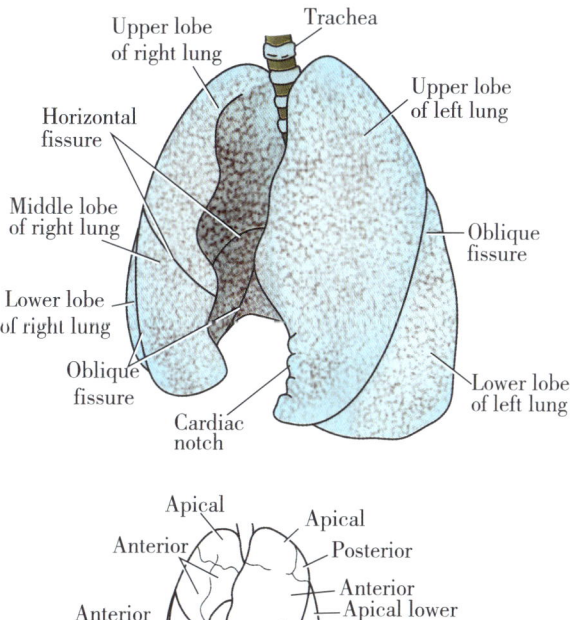

Figure 3-11 Lungs viewed from the left

3.3.2.2 The hilum and root

(1) The pulmonary hilum

The hilum of the lung may be divided into the primary and secondary pulmonary hila. The primary (first) pulmonary hilum usually called pulmonary hilum, lies near the center of the mediastinal surface of the lung, where the bronchi, pulmonary vessels, bronchial vessels, lymph vessels and nerves enter and leave the lung. The secondary pulmonary hilum lies in the depth of the lung where the lobar bronchi, arteries and veins enter and leave the lobe.

(2) The pulmonary root

It is formed by the principal bronchus, the pulmonary artery, the pulmonary veins, the bronchial branches(arteriesand veins), the pulmonary plexuses of nerves and the lymphatic vessels, which are held together by connective tissue and surrounded by the pleura.

Around the root, the parietal and visceral layers of pleura become continuous, below the root, a double layer of pleura is called the pulmonary ligament.

1) The arrangement of the chief structures

The arrangement of the chief structures is same on both sides from before backwards: the pulmonary vein in front, the pulmonary artery in the middle and the bronchus behind. But, from above downwards their arrangement is different on the two sides: on the right, their arrangement is superior lobar bronchus, pulmonary artery, middle and inferior lobar bronchus, and inferior pulmonary vein; on the left side, they are the pulmonary artery, the bronchus, and the lower most structure—the inferior pulmonary vein.

It is remarkable that the vein is always in front and below.

2) The relations of the root of the lungs

In front of the root of the right lung are the superior vena cava and the right atrium, the right phrenic nerves, and pericardiophrenic vessels; above is the azygos vein arch; posterior are the azygos vein and right vagus nerve. In front of the root of the left lung are the left phrenic nerves, and pericardiophrenic vessels; above is the aortic arch; posterior are the thoracic aorta and left vagus nerve.

(3) The bronchopulmonary segments

Each principal bronchus divides into secondary(or lobar) bronchi to the lobes of the lung. The lobar bronchus divides into segmental bronchi.

1) Concept

These segmental bronchi supply sectors of a lobe are called bronchopulmonary segments.

2) Characteristic

Each segment is pyramidal in shape with it's apex towards the pulmonary hilum and the base at the lung surface. It has its own independent segmental bronchus, little anastomose between the segmental arteries. If one segmental bronchus or artery is obstructed, the segmental function will be lost or the segment will be necrosis. Its vein lies between the segments.

Intersegmental veins are the landmark to excise accurately one segment along the boundaries of the segment.

Usually, there are ten segments in the right lung, eight or ten segments in the left lung.

Bronchopulmonary segments have considerable clinical significance for pulmonary radiology, surgery. Bronchial and pulmonary diseases(e. g. , a tumor, an abscess, and tuberculosis) may be localized in one of these segments and may be not remove the other segments or whole lobe and entire lung. But on conditions of malignant tumors and certain infections, surgical resection of several segments, a whole lobe (lobectomy) or an entire lung(pneumonectomy) may be necessary.

3.4 The mediastinum

All the structures and tissues between the mediastinal pleura are called the mediastinum.

The boundaries of the mediastinum are the sternum and costal cartilages in front; the thoracic vertebrae behind; the mediastinal pleura on both sides; the superior thoracic aperture above and the diaphragm below (Figure 3-12).

For descriptive purpose, the mediastinum is divided into superior and inferior medias-tinum by the level of the sternal angle. The superior mediastinum lies above this level. Below this level, the inferior mediastinum is further subdivided into: ①the middle medias-tinum where the pericardium occupies, ②the anterior mediastinum between the pericar-dium and the sternum, and ③the posterior mediastinum between the pericardium and the thoracic vertebrae.

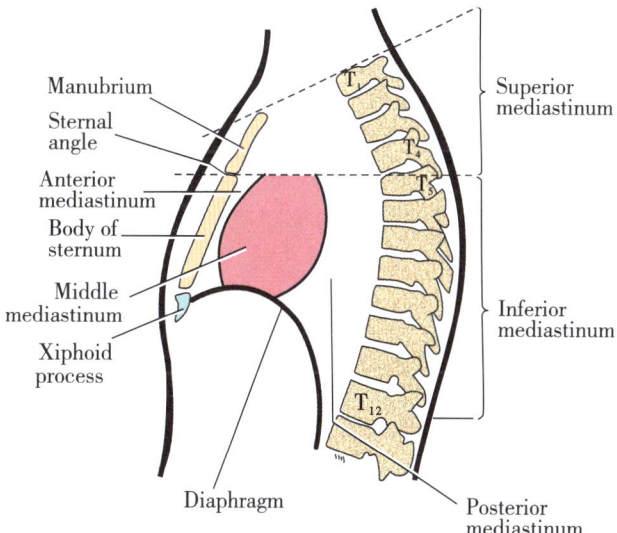

Figure 3-12 Subdivisions of the mediastinum

3.4.1 The superior mediastinum

The main organs from fron backwards are the thymus or its remnant, right and left brachiocephalic veins, superior vena cava, right and left phrenic and vagus nerves, aortic arch and its three branches, trachea, esophagus, thoracic duct, etc.

(1) The thymus

The thymus is a lymphoid organ and its large part lies between the sternum and the trachea, and maybe extends upwards to the inferior border of thyroid, downwards on the anterior surface of pericardium. In fetus and infant, the thymus is large, after puberty the thymus undergoes gradual involution. In adult, it is replaced by the connective tissue.

(2) The superior vena cava and its tributaries

The tributaries are the right and left brachiocephalic veins, they are formed by the union of the internal jugular and subclavian veins behind the sternoclavicular joint. The left brachiocephalic vein is long because it passes from the left to the right side. The right and left brachiocephalic veins unite to form the superior vena cava behind the lower border of the right sternocostal synchondrosis of first rib.

The length of the superior vena cava is about 7 cm. It lies right and lateral to the ascending aorta, runs downwards to the level of the lower border of right third sternocostal joint where it enters the right atrium. Before it enters the heart, the azygos vein crosses over the right root of lung and enters it. The right phrenic nerve descends along the right side of the superior vena cava.

(3) The aortic arch and its branches

This content is an emphasis of the superior mediastenum. The aortic arch lies behind the lower half of manubrium. Its superior border is about at the level of midpoint of the sternal manubrium. In children, the site of the arch lies higher, maybe lies above the jugular notch, therefore attention must be paid in the tracheotomy of the children in the neck. It begins behind the right second sternocostal joint, then arches from right and anterior toward left and posterior, reaches to the left side of the lower border of the fourth thoracic vertebra where it becomes the thoracic aorta.

The aortic arch give off three branches from right to left side at its convexity: the brachiocephalic trunk, the left common carotid and the left subclavian arteries. So above the arch, there are three branches and left brachiocephalic vein. Below the arch is in contact with the bifurcation of the pulmonary trunk, left principal bronchus, arterial ligament, left recurrent laryngeal nerve and superficial cardiac plexus. The left and anterior surface of the arch is adjacent to the left phrenic and left vagus nerve, left mediastinal pleura and lung. The right and posterior surface of the arch is in contact with the superior vena cava, the trachea, esophagus, left recurrent laryngeal nerve, thoracic duct and deep cardiac plexus.

(4) The triangle of arterial duct

The arterial ligament lies between the origin of left pulmonary artery and the inferior surface of the aortic arch. It is the arterial duct in fetus, but it closes to form the ligament after birth. The triangle of arterial duct is encircled by the left pulmonary artery inferiorly, left phrenic nerve anteriorly and left vagus nerve posteriorly. It contains the arterial ligament, the left recurrent laryngeal nerve and the superficial cardiac plexuses. The left recurrent laryngeal nerve is a landmark to find the arterial duct in operation, the arterial ligament lies left to the left recurrent laryngeal nerve.

3.4.2 The middle mediastinum

It lies between the anterior and posterior mediastina. It mainly contains the pericardium and the heart.

3.4.2.1 The pericardium (Figure 3-13)

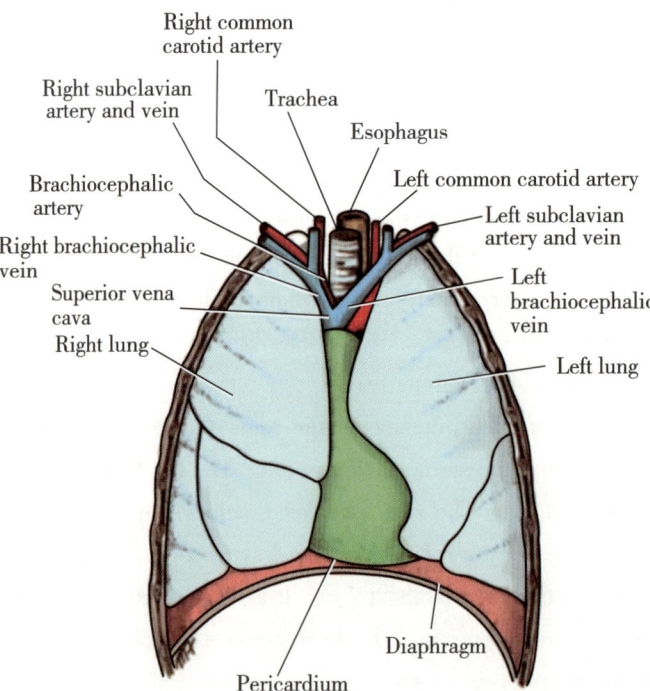

Figure 3-13 The pericardium and the lungs exposed from in front

(1) Composition

It consists of two layers: the outer layer is composed of tough fibrous tissue called the fibrous pericardium, and the inner layer is transparent sac called the serous pericardium.

Inferiorly the fibrous pericardium is fused with the central tendon of the diaphragm. Superiorly it is continuous with the outer membrane of the great blood vessels. The serous pericardium can be divided into parietal and visceral layers. The parietal layer lines the fibrous pericardium and is reflected around the roots of the great vessels to become continuous with the visceral layer. The visceral layer encloses the heart and is often called the epicardium.

The potential space between the parietal and visceral layers is called the pericardial cavity. Normally, the cavity contains a small amount of serous fluid which acts as a lubricant to facilitate movements of the heart.

(2) The sinuses of pericardium

The anteroinferior sinus of the pericardium lies between the anterior and inferior walls of the pericardium. Its position is lower, the excessive pericardial fluid may be accumulated in this sinus in pericarditis, therefore it is the site for pericardiocentesis.

The oblique sinus of the pericardium lies behind the left atrium, between the right and left pulmonary veins. Here the pericardial pus often accumulates.

The transverse sinus of the pericardium lies transversely between the ascending aorta and pulmonary trunk anteriorly and superior vena cava and left atrium posteriorly. The ascending aorta and the pulmonary trunk can be clamped by way of the transverse sinus of pericardium to block the blood stream temporarily in operation of the heart.

(3) Relationships of pericardium (Figure 3-14)

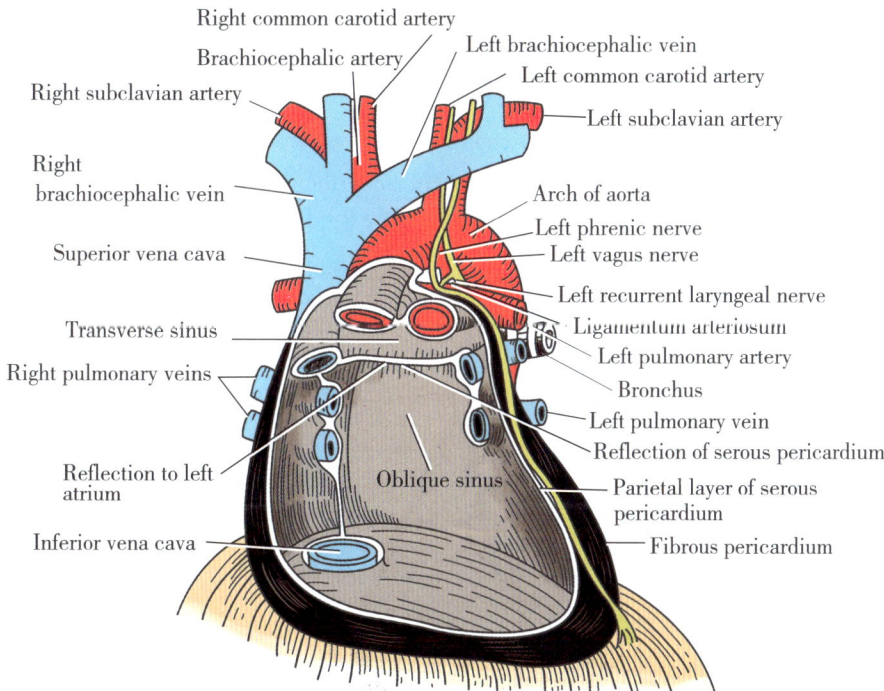

Figure 3-14 The great blood vessels and the interior of the pericardium

Anteriorly, the pericardium is in contact with the sternum costalcartilages, the pleurae, and the bare area of pericardium. Due to the left pleura moves to the left and the pericardium is directly in contact with the anterior wall, this area is called the bare area of pericardium. The pericardiocentesis and cardiocentesis are often performed in this area. Since the left internal thoracic vessels are 1-2 cm apart from the left margin of the sternum, therefore the pericardiocentesis and cardiocentesis can be performed in the 4th and 5th intercostal spaces close to the left margin of the sternum without the damage of pleura and internal thoracic vessels. Laterally, the pericardium is in contact with the mediastinal pleura, the phrenic nerves and the pericardiophrenic vessels. The posterior surface of pericardium is in contact with the thoracic aorta, esophagus, principal bronchi, vagus nerve, azygos vein and thoracic duct. The inferior wall of pericardium fuses with the central tendon of diaphragm and is in contact with the inferior vena cava entering the heart after piercing the diaphragm. The superior surface of the pericardium is continuous with the great vessels entering and leaving the heart.

3.4.2.2 The heart

(1) Surface projection of the heart

Outline of the heart is commonly drawn by four points. ①The left superior point: at the lower border of the second rib in the left and 1.2 cm to the left border of the sternum. ②The right superior point: at the upper border of the third cartilage on the right and 1 cm to the right border of the sternum. ③The right inferior point: at the sixth right sternocostal joint. ④The left inferior point: at the fifth left intercostal space, 7-9 cm to the midline.

(2) Surface projection of the valves

The left atrioventricular valve is at the fourth sternocostal joint on the left. The right atrioventricular valve is in the cross point of the fourth intercostal space and anterior midline. The aortic valve is left to border of sternum at the third intercostal space. The valve of pulmonary trunk is at the third sternocostal joint on the left.

3.4.3 The posterior mediastinum

It lies between the pericardium and lower eight thoracic vertebrae, and contains the following organs: the principal bronchi, thoracic part of esophagus, thoracic aorta, thoracic duct, azygos and hemiazygos veins, vagus nerve, sympathetic trunk (Figure 3-15, Figure 3-16).

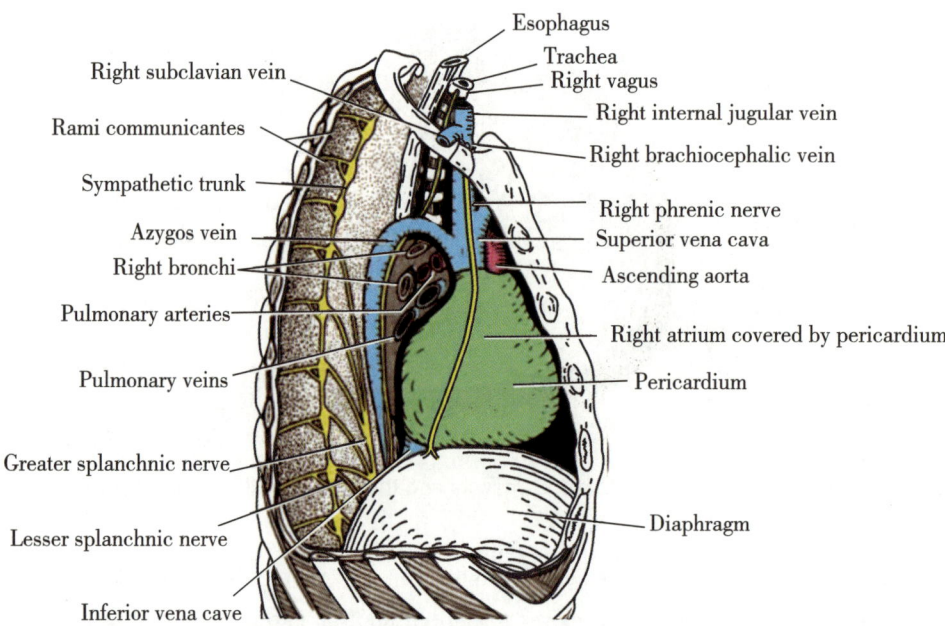

Figure 3-15　Right side of the mediastinum

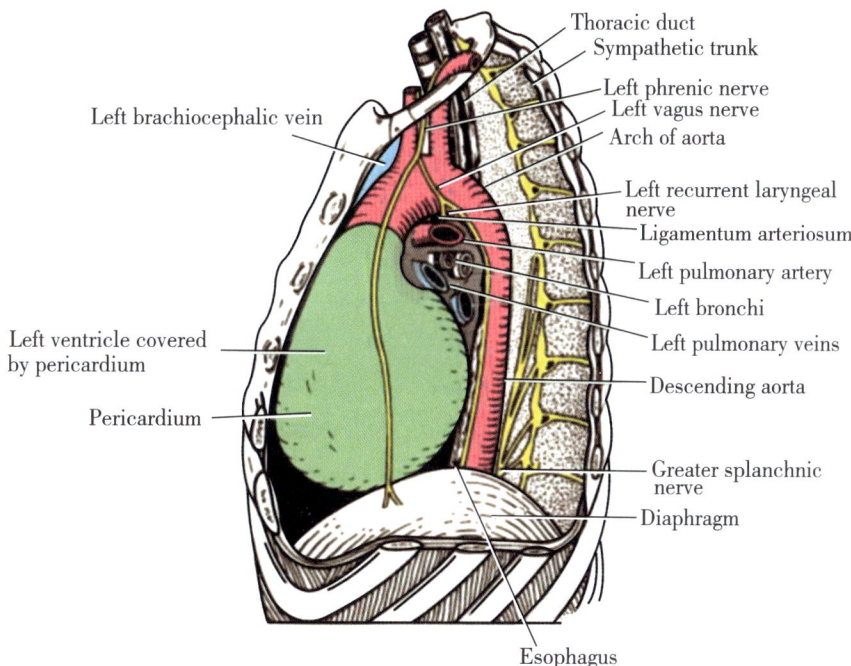

Figure 3-16 Left side of the mediastinum

3.4.3.1 The thoracic aorta

It is the continuation of the aortic arch. It begins on the left side of the lower border of the 4th thoracic vertebra, and descends on the left side of the $5^{th}-12^{th}$ thoracic vertebrae. It lies posterior to the pulmonary root and the pericardium. It terminates at the anterior surface of the 12th thoracic vertebra, enters the abdominal cavity through the aortic hiatus of the diaphragm and becomes continuous with the abdominal aorta.

3.4.3.2 The azygos, hemiazygos and accessory hemiazygos veins

The azygos vein arises from the right ascending lumbar vein in the abdomen, and enters the posterior mediastinum. It ascends on the anterior and right surfaces of the thoracic vertebrae. At the level of the 4th thoracic vertebra, it arches anteriortly and across the root of the right lung, then enters the superior vena cava. The hemiazygos vein arises from the left ascending lumbar vein, enters the thoracic cavity. It ascends on the left side of the thoracic vertebrae, enters azygos vein. The accessory hemiazygos vein enters the hemiazygos vein or enter the azygos vein.

3.4.3.3 The thoracic duct

It arises from the cisterna chyli, passes through the aortic hiatus of the diaphragm to enter the thoracic cavity. It ascends between the thoracic aorta and the azygos vein. At the level of sternal angle, the thoracic duct moves obliquely behind the esophagus to the left side, then ascends between the esophagus and the left pleura to the root of the neck. The thoracic duct should be avoided to injure in operation on the lower lobe of the right lung and the lower segment of the esophagus, the upper lobe of the left lung and the superior segment of the esophagus. Injury of the thoracic duct is followed by achylothorax.

3.4.3.4 The vagus nerve

The left vagus nerve descends to the left side of the aortic arch between the left common carotid and subclavian arteries. At the inferior border of the arch, it gives off the left recurrent laryngeal nerve which rounds the inferior surface of the aortic arch in the left side of the arterial ligament, then the nerve ascends in the groove between the left side of the trachea and esophagus. The main trunk of vagus nerve continually descends behind the root of lung. The left vagus nerve further descends along anterior surface of esophagus, and gives off the branches to form the anterior plexus of the esophagus.

The right vagus nerve descends between the right subclavian artery and vein to the right surface of the trachea, at the inferior border of the artery, it gives off the right recurrent laryngeal nerve. Then descends posterior to the right root of lung. The nerve descends along posterior surface of esophagus to form the posterior plexus of the esophagus. They pierce the esophageal hiatus of the diaphragm to enter the abdominal cavity.

3.4.3.5 The thoracic sympathetic trunk

The upper part of the trunk lies in the heads of ribs; the lower part is in the lateral surface of vertebral bodies. Each sympathetic trunk consists of 10-12 ganglia. The $5^{th}-9^{th}$ ganglia send branches to form the greater splanchnic nerve. The $10^{th}-12^{th}$ ganglia send branches to form the lesser splanchnic nerve. They pass through the diaphragm into the abdomen.

3.4.3.6 The principal bronchi

The trachea divides into the right and left principal bronchi approximately at the level of the sternal angle. The foreign bodies falling into the respiratory tract is common, especially in children. The foreign body often lodges in the trachea or the principal bronchi, seldom in the lobar bronchi (about 56% in the trachea, 32% in the right principal bronchus, 12% in the left principal bronchus). The right principal bronchus is shorter and wider and more vertically than those of the left principal bronchus. This is the anatomical reason of why the foreign bodies are more likely to enter the right principal bronchus.

3.4.3.7 The thoracic part of esophagus

(1) Course

The thoracic part of the esophagus descends in front of the vertebral column, behind the trachea and the pericardium; passes through the superior and posterior mediastina, then through the esophageal hiatus of the diaphragm at the level of 10th thoracic vertebra where it is continuous with the abdominal part of the esophagus. At the thoracic inlet, the esophagus deviates slightly to the left, at the level of tracheal bifurcation, it lies in median plane behind the bifurcation. Behind the pericardium, the esophagus deviates to the right. At the level of the 9th thoracic vertebrae, the esophagus inclines to the left in front of the thoracic aorta.

In the thorax, the esophagus presents three physiological constrictions which are located behind the aortic arch, the left principal bronchus, and passing through the esophageal hiatus of diaphragm. These constrictions are also the common sites of carcinoma of the esophagus.

(2) Relations

Anteriorly, the esophagus is in relation with trachea, left recurrent laryngeal nerve, left principal bronchus, pericardium and diaphragm. Posteriorly, in the retroesophageal space, there are the right posterior intercostal arteries, azygos and hemiazygos veins, thoracic duct and the loose connective tissue. The retroesophageal space is located between the esophagus and the thoracic column, and connects downwards with the retroperitoneal space through the hiatus of the diaphragm and upwards with retropharyngeal space.

On the left side, it is related to the left common carotid artery, left subclavian artery, aortic arch, thoracic aorta, the superior part of thoracic duct, and left mediastinal pleura without the site of the aortic arch. On the right side, there are azygos vein and its arch, and right mediastianal pleura. The esophageal carcinoma is common, its adjacency is very important in operation on the esophageal carcinoma.

(3) Blood supply

The segment of esophagus in the superior mediastinum is supplied by the first, second posterior intercostal arteries and the inferior thyroid artery and the esophageal branches of the aortic arch; the segment in the inferior mediastinum by the esophageal branches and the 4th to 7th posterior intercostal arteries. Although the anastomoses exist between various arteries, but they are not abundant. So, the characteristic of the arterial supply is various origins and segmental distributions. The esophageal fistula and the esophageal diverticulum are easily formed in the esophagus – stomach anastomosis or esophagus – intestines anastomosis after removing the the esophageal carcinoma.

The veins accompany the arteries. The submucous venous plexus of the inferior part of the esophagus anastomoses with the left gastric vein of the portal system. When the portal vein becomes obstructed, the venous blood may enter into the superior vena cava by way of the esophageal venous plexus. Consequently, that results in varicosity of the esophageal veins and hematemesis.

3.5 The diaphragm

The diaphragm separates the thoracic and abdominal cavities. It is composed of a peripheral muscular portion which inserts into a central aponeurosis (Figure 3–17).

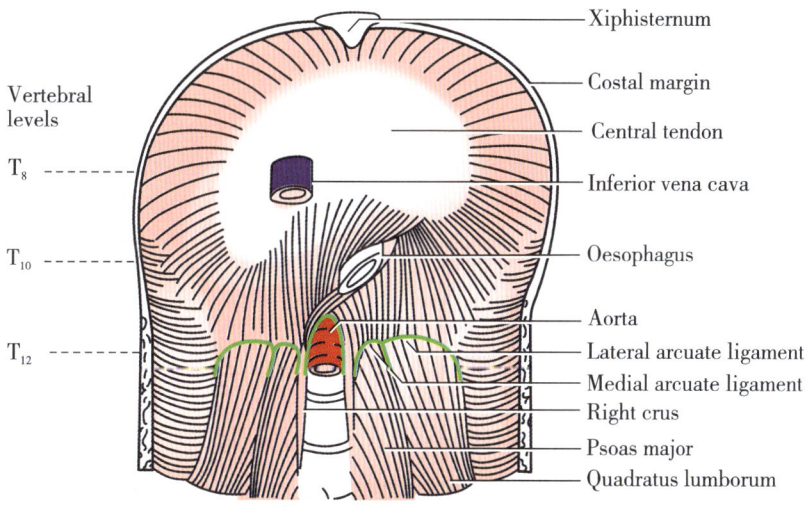

Figure 3–17 Diaphragm (anterior view)

3.5.1 Three component origins of the muscular part

(1) A vertebral part

A vertebral part comprises the crura and arcuate ligaments.

The right crus arises from the front of the L_1–L_3 vertebral bodies and intervening discs. Some fibers from the right crus pass around the lower oesophagus.

The left crus originates from L_1 and L_2 only.

The medial arcuate ligament is made up of thickened fascia which overlies psoas major and is attached medially to the body of L_1 and laterally to the transverse process of L_1. The lateral arcuate ligament is made up of fascia which overlies quadratus lumborum from the transverse process of L_1 medially to the 12th rib laterally.

The median arcuate ligament is a fibrous arch which connects left and right crura.

(2) A costal part—attached to the inner aspects of the lower six ribs.

(3) A sternal part—consists of two small slips arising from the deep surface of the xiphoid process.

3.5.2 Openings in the diaphragm

Structures traverse the diaphragm at different levels to pass from thoracic to abdominal cavities and vice versa. These levels are as follows.

(1) T_8

The opening for the inferior vena cava—transmits the inferior vena cava and right phrenic nerve.

(2) T_{10}

The oesophageal opening—transmits the oesophagus, vagus nerve and branches of the left gastric artery and vein.

(3) T_{12}

The aortic opening—transmits the aorta, thoracic duct and azygos vein.

The left phrenic nerve passes into the diaphragm as a solitary structure.

3.5.3 Nerve supply of the diaphragm

(1) Motor supply

The entire motor supply arises from the phrenic nerves ($C_3 - C_5$). Diaphragmatic contraction is the mainstay of inspiration.

(2) Sensory supply

The periphery of the diaphragm receives sensory fibers from the lower intercostal nerves. The sensory supply from the central part is carried by the phrenic nerves.

3.6 Main contents of the thorax

3.6.1 Pectoral region and breast

Fascial arrangements of pectoral region
Deep fascia

✓ These tissues are very elastic in the pectoral region (allows for chest expansion in inspiration)
✓ Compare against the thick unyielding deep fascia you will see in the arm and forearm
✓ Clavipectoral fascia
    ◊ An example of a deep fascia in the pectoral region that was named by surgeons
    ◊ Hangs from the clavicle—hence the name "clavi"
    ◊ It encases the subclavius muscle, pectoralis major muscle and the pectoralis minor muscle
✓ Costocoracoid membrane
    ◊ Another specific example of a deep fascia in the pectoral region that was named
    ◊ It spans between the upper ribs and coracoid process of the scapula

◊ It is perforated by the cephalic vein, thoracoacromial artery and vein, lateral pectoral nerve, lymphatic channels and lymph nodes and fat

◊ Invests (surrounds and encases) the pectoralis minor muscle

✓ The suspensory ligament of the axilla (armpit)

◊ Is the lowermost, lateral extent of the clavipectoral fascia

◊ When the arm is abducted, the attachments of this fascia cause the hollow of the axilla

◊ In future dissections, you will see how this fascia gives substance and organization to a fatty area that protects all the arteries, veins and nerves that enter/exit the upper extremity

Retromammary bursa

✓ A potential space between deep fascia covering the pectoralis major muscle and overlying (superficial) fascia containing the breast tissue and the skin

✓ In cases of breast cancer, this space is important to both surgeon and patient. Frequently cancer does not travel through this empty space for a time allowing surgeons to do a more limited muscle-sparing type of mastectomy

Superficial fascia, skin and the breast (mammary glands)

Muscles of pectoral region

Muscle	Origin	Insertion	Action	Innervation	Artery	Notes
Pectoralis major	Medial 1/2 of the clavicle, manubrium and body of sternum, costal cartilages of ribs 2-6, sometimes from the rectus sheath of the upper abdominal wall	Crest of the greater tubercle of the humerus	Flexes and adducts the arm, medially rotates the arm	Medial and lateral pectoral nerves (C_5-T_1)	Pectoral branch of the thoracoacromial trunk	The deep fascia on its anterior surface should not be fused to the fascia of the mammary gland—if it is, this is an important clinical sign indicating breast disease (Latin, pectus = breast bone)
Pectoralis minor	Ribs 3-5	Coracoid process of the scapula	Draws the scapula forward, medialward, and downward	Medial pectoral nerve (C_8, T_1)	Pectoral branch of the thoracoacromial trunk	Branches of medial pectoral nerve usually pierce pectoralis minor to reach the pectoralis major muscle (Latin, pectus = breast bone)

Serratus anterior	Ribs 1–8 or 9	Medial border of the scapula on its costal (deep) surface	It draws the scapula forward; the inferior fibers rotate the scapula superiorly	Long thoracic nerve (from ventral rami C_5–C_7)	Lateral thoracic artery	A lesion of long thoracic nerve will cause winging of the scapula (i.e., the medial border of the scapula falls away from the posterior chest wall and looks like an angel's wing) (Latin, serratus = to saw)

Nerve innervations of pectoral and breast region

✓ Medial pectoral nerve
  ◊ This nerve supplies both the pectoralis major and pectoralis minor muscles
  ◊ This nerve originates from the medial cord of the brachial plexus
✓ Lateral pectoral nerve
  ◊ This nerve supplies the pectoralis major muscle
  ◊ This nerve originates from the lateral cord of the brachial plexus
  ◊ The location of these vessels is very confusing to the beginner
✓ Supraclavicular nerves
  ◊ These minor nerves emerge from a cervical plexus in the neck, specifically C_3, C_4
  ◊ These cutaneous nerves provide sensation to skin over the clavicle and upper pectoral area
  ◊ Please wait until November when we dissect the neck region to trace their origins in the lab
✓ Intercostal nerves
  ◊ These nerves arise posteriorly and sweep around laterally from thoracic nerves T_2, T_3, T_4, T_5
  ◊ The tiny sensory branches (encountered today) supply sensation to skin in the pectoral region
  ◊ Each thoracic nerve can be found on the inferior aspect of its rib
    (The T_3 nerve is found inferior to rib 3, the T_4 nerve is found inferior to rib 4, etc.)
  ◊ The T_4 nerve supplies cutaneous sensation to the nipple/areolar region in males/females
  ◊ In female patients with large breasts, the T_4 cutaneous branches travel in the skin and will always innervate the nipple area but may droop far below the inferior portion of rib 4 if the breasts are large

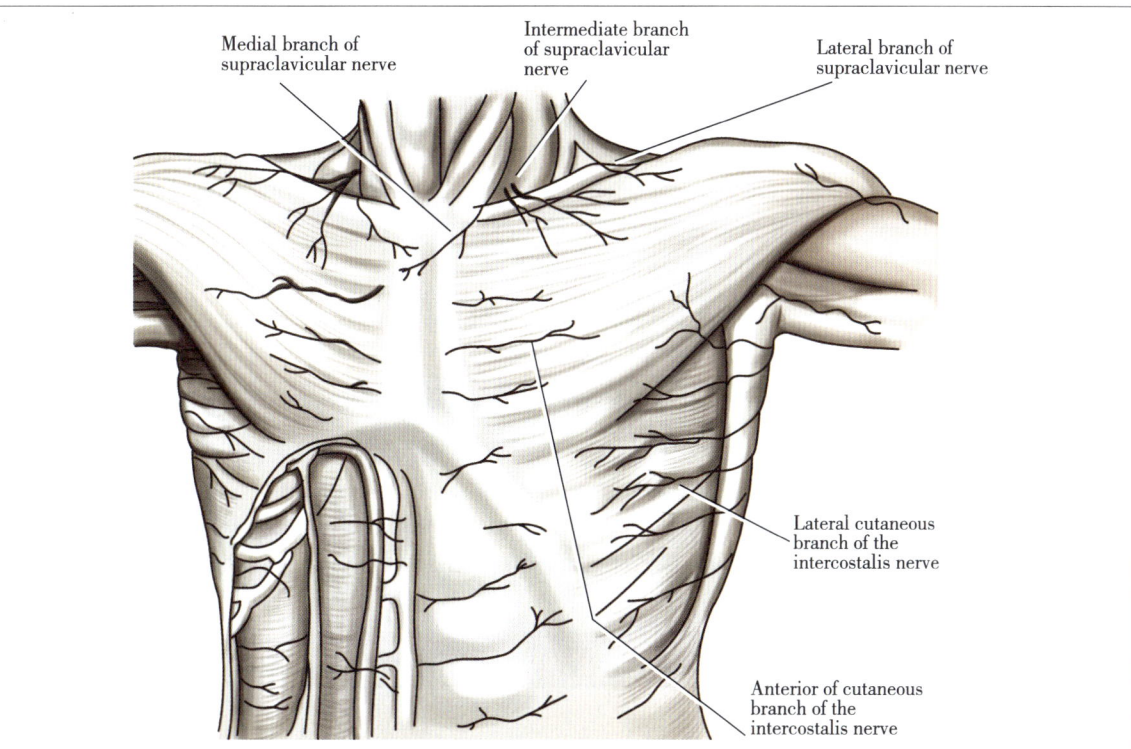

Vascular supply for pectoral region/breast

Arterial supply—axillary artery

✓ The key to locating this major artery is finding the pectoralis minor muscle
  ◊ The 1st portion of the artery is medial to this muscle
  ◊ The 2nd portion of the artery is deep to (behind) this muscle
  ◊ The 3rd portion of the artery is lateral to this muscle

1st portion—superior thoracic artery

✓ Enlarges in lactating females
✓ Is usually very small—don't be distressed if you can't locate it on your cadaver

2nd portion

✓ Thoracoacromial trunk or artery
  ◊ 4 named branches: clavicular, acromial, deltoid, pectoral
✓ Lateral thoracic artery
  ◊ A bit variable in location
  ◊ Anatomical rule: expect variations in cadavers and in future patients
  ◊ Supplies the serratus anterior muscle
  ◊ A major supplier to breast tissue
  ◊ Enlarges during pregnancy/lactation to bring in more fluids for the infant

3rd portion

✓ The branches include:
  ◊ Subscapular artery
  ◊ Anterior circumflex humeral artery

◊ Posterior circumflex humeral artery

Venous supply—axillary vein and tributaries

✓ On the chest wall, this venous network lies anterior to the artery of the same name
✓ Easily distinguished from the artery because of its thinner walls, multiple tributaries, valves
✓ Remember: its flow is reversed in comparison to arteries
✓ This vein (and all others) will return blood toward the heart
✓ The axillary vein changes its name at the lateral border of the 1st rib
✓ It empties into (and becomes) the subclavian vein
✓ One anatomical principle—venous tributaries generally have the same name as the arteries
✓ However, there is one exception in this region
✓ The cephalic vein has no equivalent artery
✓ This exception exists because the cephalic vein is a part of the superficial cutaneous venous drainage pattern (in the future, you, as well as phlebotomists, will search for similar veins to perform venipuncture)

Breast (mammary gland)

Structural organization

Nipple

✓ Found in the T_4 intercostal space—a reliable guide in males and nulliparous females
✓ An unreliable rib guide in multiparous females and large breasted women
✓ Contains the openings for 15–20 lactiferous ducts
✓ Contains circular smooth muscle fibers that contract with stimulation/cold
✓ Develops in the skin along a milk line or ridge as seen in all mammals
✓ Areola—pigmented skin surrounding the nipple
✓ Lactiferous sinuses are located underneath its surface
✓ Darkens with pigment during pregnancy
✓ Montgomery's tubercles—rudimentary milk glands
✓ Breast lobes are pyramidal structures arranged in a radial fashion
✓ Keratinocytes are arranged to drain into lactiferous ducts and into lactiferous sinuses
✓ Stroma—connective tissue—fat, collagen

Suspensory ligaments (Cooper's ligaments)

✓ Are tethered to the surface of the skin
✓ Form defined connective tissue pockets around breast tissue and fat
✓ These fragile ligaments anchor breast tissue to the skin over the pectoral region
✓ These ligaments can easily tear over the course of a lifetime resulting in a progressive drooping when adequate supportive clothing has not been worn

Diagnostic tools of malignancy

✓ Visual
   ◊ Skin dimpling—due to retraction or tension on the suspensory ligaments as a tumor begins to grow and occupy more and more space

- ◊ Nipple retraction—caused by pressure on unyielding (non-elastic) lactiferous ducts
- ◊ Peau d'orange—a change (darkening or roughness in skin texture/color due to edema from blocked lymphatics)
- ✓ Palpation
  - ◊ Ideally, annualannual breast exams are conducted by physicians
  - ◊ Ideally, patients perform monthly breast exams including examination of the
  - ◊ Axillary tail of spence—an extension of the upper lateral quadrant
  - ◊ This portion of the breast pierces through deep fascia and into the axilla
  - ◊ The defect in the deep fascia is known as the Foramen of Langer
- ✓ Radiographic
  - ◊ Mammograms
  - ◊ If cancer is suspected or found, sentinel lymph node mapping is conducted using the lymphoscintigraphy technique
- ✓ Breast is divided into quadrants for descriptive purposes in medical charts: upper outer, upper inner, lower outer, lower inner. The upper outer quadrant is the most frequent site of malignancies

Developmental stages

- ✓ The breast buds (extensions of the surface ectoderm) grow downward into the dermis of the skin and continue to excavate deeper into the superficial fascial layer. Eventually the mammary gland develops into a specially modified sweat gland
- ✓ It is actually a part of the skin; thus it has no capsule to contain it or the spread of neoplastic growth [by contrast, nerves have coverings (epineurium), muscles have coverings (deep fascia)]
- ✓ It should not surprise you that the breast being part of the skin has the same cutaneous nerves as the skin does anywhere else. Fluids in the extracellular space drain into cutaneous lymphatic capillaries, then onto larger channels and eventually into lymph nodes
- ✓ After an initial period of development during gestation, the breast development typically halts until puberty. Extensive ductal development occurs during pregnancy and the volume of breast tissue reaches its high point during lactation
- ✓ Your cadaver specimens are typically post-menopausal and these female breasts have undergone extensive involution, atrophy and replacement with adipose tissue

Anatomic location on chest wall

- ✓ Located purely within the skin and superficial fascia
- ✓ Separated from the underlying musculature by the retromammary bursa and the deep fascia that encases the pectoral muscles

Blood supply—enlarges during pregnancy

- ✓ Superior thoracic artery
- ✓ Lateral thoracic artery
- ✓ Intercostal arteries at the level of T_2, T_3, T_4, T_5
- ✓ Branches off the internal thoracic artery
- ✓ Internal mammary artery is an alternative name frequently used by clinicians

Regional Anatomy

Venous drainage—reverse flow that parallels the arterial flow

Lymphatic drainage (introduction)

✓ Follows the venous drainage
✓ The major flow of lymph and sometimes cancer is directed toward the axilla
✓ Many lymph nodes are present in the axilla and work to impede metastatic advancement
  ◊ Sentinel nodes—are the initial ones along a lymphatic chain where a specific breast region will drain. Sentinel lymph node can be identified by their accumulation of radioactive dye
  ◊ Pectoral nodes—are found along the course of the lateral thoracic vein. These channels drain toward the central group (those that border the axillary vein)
  ◊ Subscapular (posterior) nodes—drain the posterior portions of the thoracic wall and are associated with the axillary tail. They drain toward the central group
  ◊ Central nodes—this group receives lymph from both arm and breast
  ◊ Apical nodes—this group is located high in the cervicoaxillary canal. This is the highway into the lower neck region (under the clavicle but passing over the 1st rib). As these nodes are further along the lymphatic drainage tree, the presence of cancerous cells here indicates that the tumor is spreading (a more advanced stage). Apical node channels drain into the thoracic duct (on the left) or into the lymphatic duct on the right side of the body
  ◊ Infraclavicular nodes penetrate through clavipectoral fascia and drain to the central group
  ◊ Parasternal nodes drain along internal thoracic (mammary) vein and into the chest wall
✓ Abdominal nodes—these drain downward toward the rectus sheath

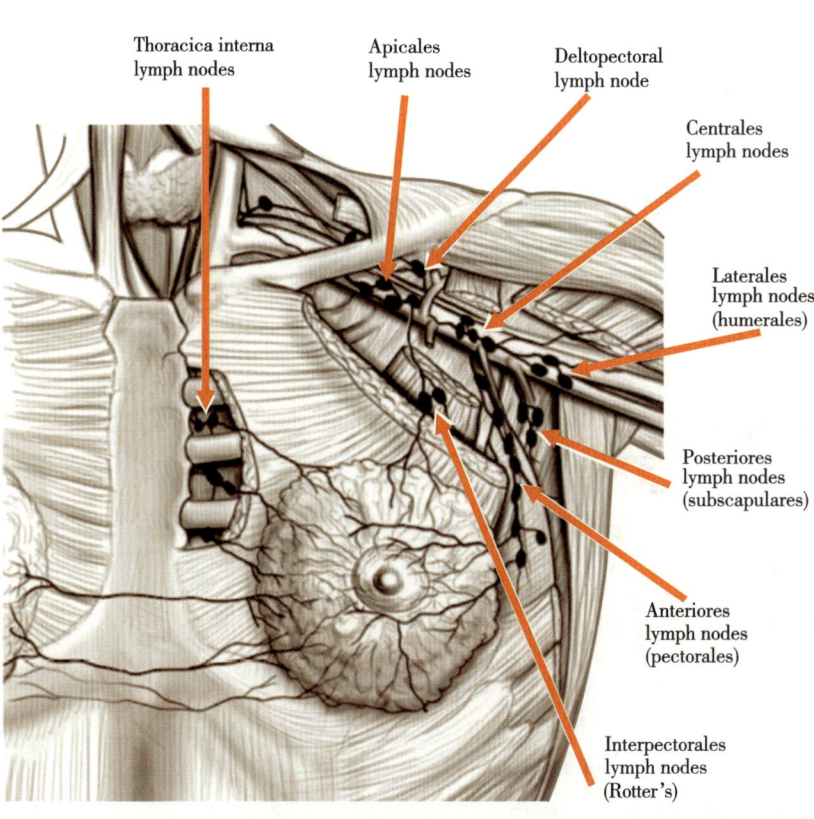

✓ Lymph nodes and lymphatic channels are removed in the axillary region as a surgeon attempts to remove cancerous nodes and stage the cancer (axillary lymph node dissection). The axillary region is often treated with radiation (adjuvant treatment)

✓ Surgical or radiation damage to lymphatic channels in the axilla can interfere with lymphatic drainage from the arm on that side. This condition results in lymphedema (swelling due to accumulation of lymph fluid) of the upper extremity

Clinical breast topics

✓ Gynecomastia—breast enlargement in males (usually during adolescence)
✓ Malignancy—affects 1 out of 8 females during their lifetime
✓ Treatment may be a mastectomy which may or may not be followed by reconstruction
✓ Macromastia—unusually large breasts usually accompanied by side effects such as back problems, ptosis (drooping), ridicule, etc—treatment option (reduction mammoplasty)
✓ Micromastia—may be unilateral side effects may be psychological or aesthetic
✓ Congenital Asymmetry –breast may deformed, unmatched in size/shape
✓ Amastia—the term used to describe the absence of a breast
✓ Polythelia > 2 nipples—located anywhere along the mammalian "milk line"
✓ Polymastia > 2 breasts—an extra lactating breast can become a problem in pregnancy

3.6.2 Intercostal structure

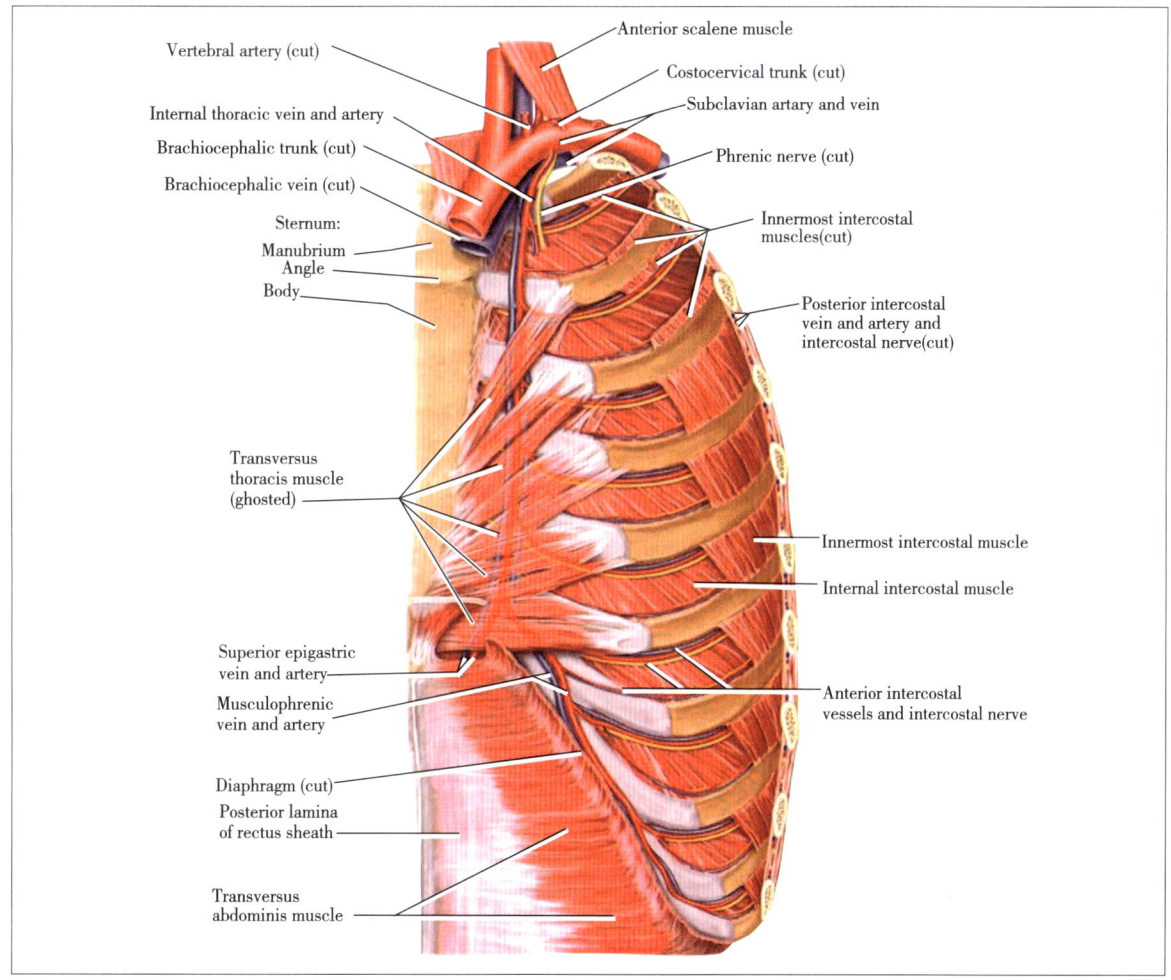

Intercostal muscles
✓ Transverse thoracic muscles: fan-like muscle whose slips spread from the posterior aspect of the lower end of the sternum to the inner surfaces of costal cartilages 2-6 ◊ Muscle slips pass posterior to internal thoracic vessels
Subcostal muscles
✓ Posteriorly placed muscles that span across 2 or more intercostal spaces. ✓ Regarding intercostal muscles in general ◊ Innervated by the corresponding intercostal nerves ◊ Function: muscles of respiration; they fix or approximate the ribs and increase the tonus of intercostal space, resisting especially internal negative/positive pressures
When 1st rib is anchored by the scalene muscles, contraction of intercostal (especially external and intercartilaginous internal) muscles [with the assistance of the levator costae (deep back) muscles] elevates the ribs and raises the sternum. This increase volume of the thoracic cavity, the transverse diameter of the thoracic cage increasing via the "bucket handle" mechanism, and the A-P diameter increasing via the "pump handle" mechanism. The volume increase results in a negative intrathoracic pressure which draws air into the lungs (inspiration) (more importantly, the diaphragm descends simultaneously)
When the lower ribs and inferior costal margin are anchored by the abdominal muscles, contraction of the intercostal muscles (especially the interosseous portion of the internal intercostals) depresses the ribs, decreasing the transverse and A-P diameters, resulting in a positive intrathoracic pressure which pushes air from the lungs (expiration) [contraction of the abdominal muscles, combined with relaxation of the diaphragm, pushes abdominal viscera (and hence the diaphragm) upward—also increasing intrathoracic pressure]
The contraction of the intercostal muscles also adds rigidity to the intercostal spaces during the changes in intrathoracic pressure. In rare cases of congenital absence of intercostal muscle, the intercostal spaces move in and out with respiration
Clinical notes: Intercostal muscles used mostly in forced (active) respiration; the diaphragm is the primary muscle of quiet (at rest) respiration
These movements occur posteriorly at the joints of the heads of the ribs, and the costotransverse joints, with rib elevation and depression occurring primarily via rotation about an axis that traverses the neck of the rib; anteriorly a smaller amount of movement occurs at the sternocostal and interchondral joints. Intercostal neurovascular bundles: pass forward around chest wall in the subcostal groove deep to internal intercostal muscle, superficial to innermost intercostal muscle, endothoracic fascia and pleura When performing a thoracentesis, needle should pass over top of rib to avoid neurovascular bundle
Intercostal arteries
✓ Each space is supplied by a single posterior intercostal artery and paired anterior intercostal arteries ✓ The two lower spaces have only posterior arteries
Posterior intercostal arteries
✓ 1st and 2nd posterior intercostal arteries arise from the superior intercostal artery (a branch of costocervical trunk from subclavian artery)

✓ Remainder arise as direct branches of thoracic aorta

✓ Posterior intercostal arteries of right side longer than those of left since they must cross vertebral column

✓ A small collateral branch arises which runs along superior border of rib below to anastomose with lower of the two anterior intercostal arteries of each space

Anterior intercostal arteries

✓ Those of upper 6 spaces arise from internal thoracic artery

✓ Those of spaces 7–9 arise from musculophrenic artery

✓ Pass laterally to anastomose with posterior intercostal artery and its collateral branch in approximately the anterior axillary line

Clinical notes: The internal thoracic artery arises from the subclavian. It descends just lateral to the sternal border to end at the level of the 6th intercostal space by dividing into the musculophrenic and superior epigastric arteries

✓ The posterior/anterior intercostal arteries and the internal thoracic arteries provide important pathways of collateral circulation in the presence of aortic stenosis

Intercostal veins

✓ Anterior intercostal veins follow retrograde the pattern of the anterior intercostal arteries

✓ Posterior intercostal veins pass in an irregular manner into the brachiocephalic veins (upper intercostal spaces) and the azygos/hemiazygos system of veins (to be discussed with the posterior mediastinum)

Intercostal nerves

✓ Ventral rami of the upper 11 thoracic spinal nerves

✓ Intercostal nerves 7–11 are "thoracoabdominal nerves" since they continue across the subcostal margin to supply the anterolateral abdominal wall (both skin, musculature and peritoneum)

✓ Intercostal nerves have muscular, cutaneous and pleural rami

Thoracic cavity and pleura

Thoracic

✓ Lined by endothoracic fascia and is composed of three completely separated internal divisions or compartments

◊ A central compartment, the mediastinum (Latin: standing in the middle), that contains all other thoracic structures: the heart as well as the thoracic parts of the great vessels, trachea, esophagus, and thymus

◊ Two lateral pulmonary cavities that contain the lungs and are each lined by a collapsed pleural sacs—like inverted, collapsed balloons, with an outer layer (parietal pleura) directly lining the walls of the pulmonary cavity, and an inner layer (visceral pleura) directly lining the lung. The inside of the collapsed sac is essentially "empty but wet", containing only a capillary layer of lubricating pleural fluid

Pleura

Parietal pleura—outer layer of the pleural sac that lines each pulmonary cavity, adhered to the walls by the endothoracic fascia; it is composed of four parts

- ✓ Costal parietal pleura—lines the internal surface of the thoracic wall, but is separated from the thoracic wall by the endothoracic fascia, an extrapleural layer of loose connective tissue that forms an important surgical plane
- ✓ Mediastinal parietal pleura—covers the mediastinum
- ✓ Diaphragmatic parietal pleura—covers the superior surface of the diaphragm
- ✓ Cervical parietal pleura—dome-shaped cap that covers the apex of the lung
  - ◊ Extends superiorly through the superior thoracic aperture
  - ◊ Reinforced by the suprapleural membrane (or Sibson's fascia), a special thickening of the endothoracic fascia

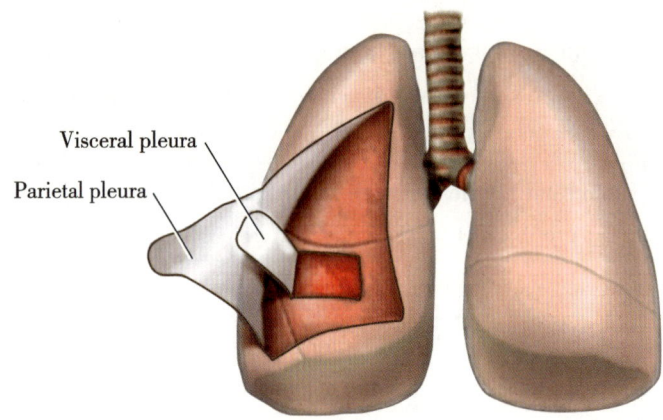

Visceral pleura—inner layer of the pleural sac that invests the lung completely

- ✓ Extends into all of the fissures of the lungs (as well as completely investing them)
- ✓ Provides the lung with a slippery surface that enables it to move freely on the parietal pleura
- ✓ Can not be dissected away from the lung
- ✓ Continuous with the parietal pleura at the hilum of the lung, where the bronchi enter the lung
- ✓ Receives its vascular supply from the bronchial arteries and pulmonary veins

Pleural fluid—lubricating secretion of the pleurae between the two layers

- ✓ Reduces friction as the two layers of pleura move against one another
- ✓ Provides surface tension (keeps the two layers relatively adherent to one another, so when the chest expands, the lungs will also expand)

Lines of pleural reflection—where the parietal pleura changes direction ("turns a corner") as it passes from one wall of the pleural cavity to another

Pleural recesses—potential spaces that are not filled by lungs during normal breathing

Costodiaphragmatic recesses—potential space between the costal and diaphragmatic pleurae that may arise during expiration

Costomediastinal recesses—potential space between the costal and mediastinal parts of the parietal pleura. The left costomediastinal recess is larger due to the cardiac notch in the left lung anterior to the pericardium

> Clinical correlations
>
> ✓ Pleuritis (or pleurisy)—inflammation of the pleura, which makes the visceral and parietal pleura adhere to one another
> ✓ Pneumothorax—entry of air into the pleural (or pulmonary) cavity. This condition results when the continuous pleurae are compromised
> ✓ Hydrothorax—accumulation of fluid in the pleural cavity
> ✓ Hemothorax—accumulation of blood in the pleural cavity
> ✓ Thoracostomy—making a hole in the thoracic wall in order to remove air or fluid from the pleural cavity. This can be accomplished with a wide bore needle or by inserting a drainage tube
> ✓ Thoracentesis—the passage into the pleural cavity with a hypodermic needle for the purpose of removing pathological fluid (blood, pus, pleural effusions). Needle is inserted superior to the rib to avoid damage to the intercostal nerve

3.6.3 Anatomy of lower respiratory tract: lungs and tracheobronchial tree

Gross anatomy of lungs

✓ Essential organs of respiration that oxygenate the blood
✓ Lie free within pulmonary cavity, surrounded by pleural cavity, and attached only by the root of the lung and pulmonary ligaments

Topographical anatomy of the lungs

Common features

✓ Surfaces: ①costal, ②mediastinal, and ③diaphragmatic (base)
✓ Borders: ①anterior, ②posterior, and ③inferior
✓ Features
  ▷ Apices (singular = apex): blunt superior end of the lung extending slightly above 1st rib, or 1.5–2.5 cm above clavicle. Also, the apex of each is posterior to the subclavian vessels

Hilum versus root of the lung

✓ Hilum (plural = hila)—location where structures of the root of the lung enters and exits lung
✓ Root of the lung—all of the structures entering and leaving the lung at the hilum, including bronchi, pulmonary artery and veins, bronchial arteries and veins, lymphatic vessels, and nerves
✓ Superior and inferior lobes, separated by an oblique fissure in each lung
✓ Oblique fissure: begins posteriorly at the level of spinous process of T_3, crosses 5th rib in mid-axillary line, ends at level of 6th costal cartilage
✓ Approximated by lateral border of scapula when arm is fully abducted

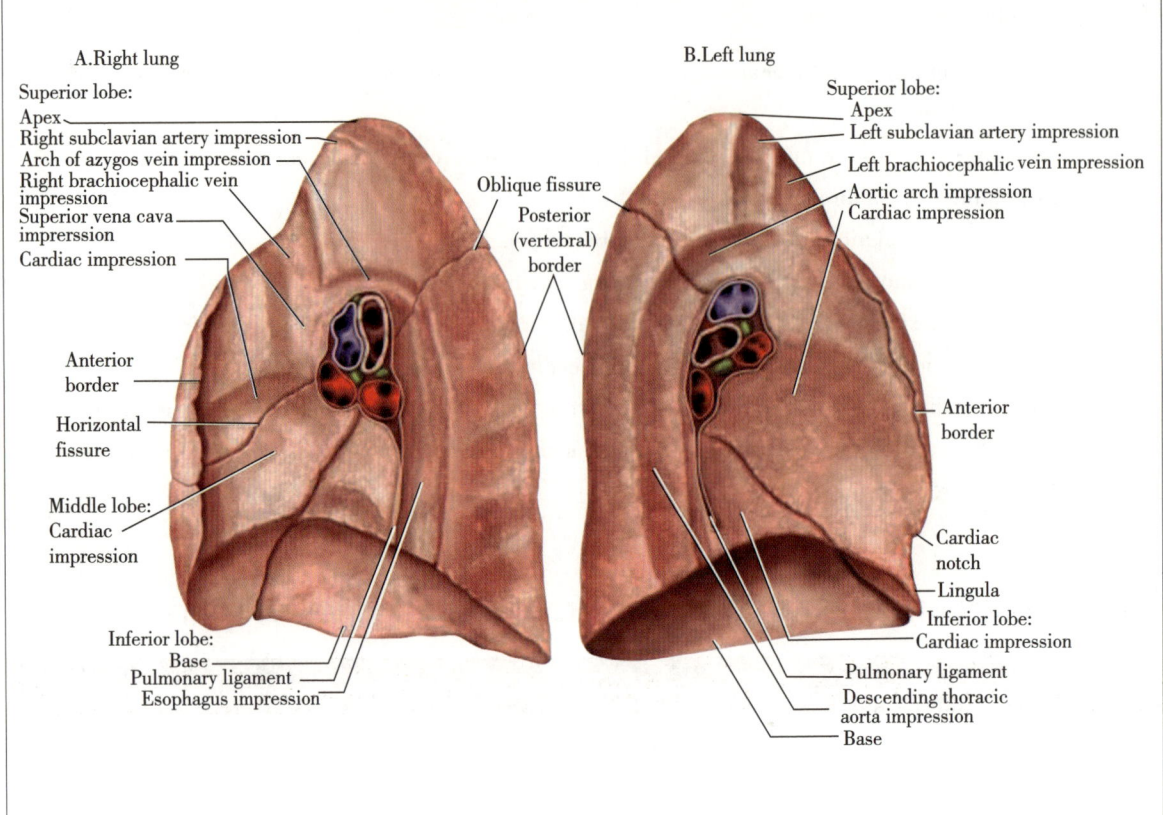

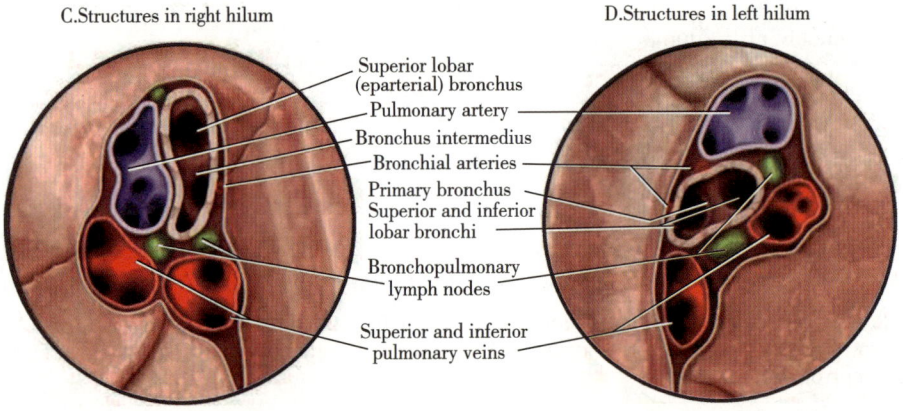

Distinguishing features—lobes and fissures

✓ Right lung has a third (middle) lobe and a horizontal fissure

◊ Visualized in lateral and anterior views

◊ Horizontal fissure follows anterior half of 4th rib

◊ Due to the presence of the liver, right lung is shorter than the left lung, and its base is more concave

◊ Left lung has smaller volume due to left-shift of heart

◊ Heart shift creates a much larger cardiac impression on mediastinal surface, makes cardiac notch in anterior border, and often forms a lingula (or tongue-like extension of the lowermost portion of the superior lobe)

✓ Both lungs have a structure that runs in the vertical plane posterior to their hila, which makes an impression (or groove) in the cadaveric lung: esophagus on right and descending aorta on left

✓ Both lungs have a vessel that arches above their respective hilum that makes an impression in the cadaveric lung: arch of azygos vein on right and arch of aorta on left

Clinical correlation: Most common accessory lobe is the azygos lobe, which appears in the right lung in approximately 1% of people. The azygos lobe occurs when the azygos vein arches over the apex of the right lung, which isolates the medial part of the apex of the right lung creating the azygos lobe

Surface projections of lungs are constantly changing

✓ Anterior borders lie slightly lateral to anterior lines of pleural reflection during expiration, but fill costomediastinal recesses during inspiration

✓ Inferior borders never fully occupy costodiaphragmatic recesses, with the inferior lines of pleural reflection occurring 1-2 rib levels inferior to lung margins

✓ Remember mnemonic devices (number refer to rib levels)
  ◊ Pleura: 2, 4, 6, 8, 10, 12
  ◊ Lungs: 2, 4, 6, 6, 8, 10

Root of lung—connects lung with the heart and trachea

✓ Formed by bronchi, pulmonary artery and veins, bronchial arteries and veins, lymphatic vessels, and nerves—the structures which enter/exit the hilum

✓ Enclosed within the area of continuity between the visceral and parietal pleura called thepleura sleeve (mesopneumonium, or mesentery of the lung), the sleeve being considerably larger than the root, creating a dangling pulmonary ligament (double pleural reflection) like the sleeve of a Chinese robe

✓ Relative positions of structures composing the root of the lung
  ◊ General pattern
    ◆ Pulmonary artery is superior
    ◆ Pulmonary veins are anterior and inferior
    ◆ Bronchi are posterior and central
  ◊ Exception: superior lobar ("eparterial") bronchus of right lung extends above level of right pulmonary artery

Intrapulmonary bronchi

✓ Note: trachea and main bronchi to be covered with superior mediastinum

✓ Bronchi are distinguished by cartilage in walls and filled with air (in life)

Lobar bronchi

✓ Formed at (or immediately lateral to) hilum

✓ Branch into each lobe (thus superior and inferior on left; superior, middle, and inferior on right)

Segmental bronchi

✓ Serve a bronchopulmonary (b. p.) segment (smallest resectable unit of lung)

✓ Right lung = 10 segmental bronchi/bronchopulmonary segments

✓ Left lung = 8 segmental bronchi/bronchopulmonary segments

Intrasegmental bronchi
✓ Approximately 20 generations
Bronchioles (no cartilage)
✓ Distributing, terminal and respiratory (covered in histology)
Clinical correlation 1: Bronchial asthma is a reduction in the caliber of bronchi and bronchioles due to smooth muscle spasm, mucosal edema, and excessive mucus in the lumen of airways. Asthma affects 5% of the population and is a leading cause of disease and disability in children (between ages 2 and 17)   *Clinical correlation* 2: Atelectasis is a decrease or loss of air in (part of) the lung, which results in loss of lung volume
Blood supply of lungs and bronchi
✓ The lungs, like the liver, have a dual blood supply: one system (pulmonary) primarily distributed to the alveoli for gaseous exchange, and a second (bronchial) for supplying the non-alveolar (non-parenchymal or stroma) tissues, such as the structures of the root of the lung, supporting connective tissue, and the visceral pleura
Pulmonary system
Pulmonary arteries
✓ Carry deoxygenated blood from right ventricle   ✓ Each lung is supplied by one large pulmonary artery   ✓ An arterial branch goes to each lobe and bronchopulmonary segment, usually on the anterior   ✓ Aspect of the corresponding bronchus
Pulmonary veins—carry oxygenated blood to left atrium
✓ Each lung has two pulmonary veins draining blood from it   ✓ Intersegmental parts of pulmonary veins lie in the septa of bronchopulmonary segments
Bronchial system
Bronchial arteries
✓ Paired left bronchial arteries arise as initial branches of the descending aorta   ✓ Single right bronchial artery often arises from a superior posterior intercostal artery   ✓ Carry oxygenated blood to non-alveolar tissues
Bronchial veins
✓ Drain only more proximal bronchi and adjacent root structures   ✓ Drain to azygos (on right) and to hemiazygos or left superior intercostal veins (on left)   ✓ Peripheral bronchi and visceral pleura drain into pulmonary veins

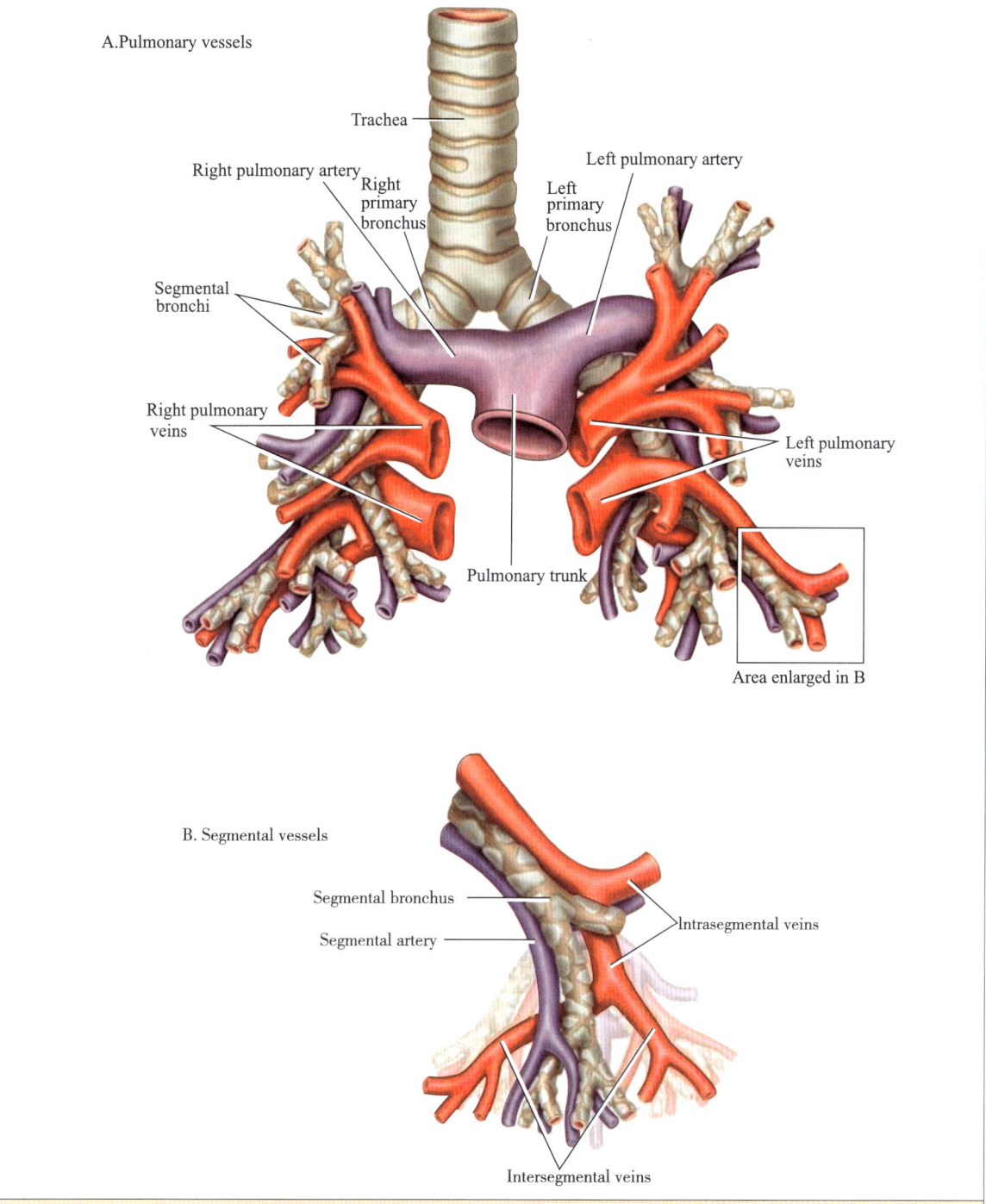

Pattern of branching/relationships

✓ Pulmonary arteries and bronchi are paired, branching simultaneously for intra segmental distribution
  ◊ Bronchial arteries course along bronchi
✓ Pulmonary veins—course independently and inter segmentally

Clinical correlation: Pulmonary thromboembolism (PTE), blockage of a pulmonary artery by an embolus, a foreign body such as a thrombus (a clot formed by constituents of the blood), fat globule, or an air bubble. Therefore, the lung (or a portion of the lung) is ventilated with air but not perfused with blood PTE commonly results in a thrombotic infarct, or an area of dead (necrotic) tissue

Lymphatic drainage of lungs
Superficial (subpleural) and deep (intrapulmonary) plexuses drain toward hilum
✓ Lymph from deep plexus passes through pulmonary (intrapulmonary) nodes ✓ Both subpleural and deep plexuses drain to bronchopulmonary (hilar) lymph nodes ✓ Tracheobronchial nodes receive all lymph from lungs via bronchopulmonary nodes ✓ Inferior tracheobronchial (carinal) lymph nodes receive lymph primarily from inferior lobes ✓ Superior tracheobronchial lymph nodes receive lymph from superior lobes and middle lobe of right side; the right superior tracheobronchial nodes receive most of the drainage from the inferior tracheobronchial (carinal) nodes—consequently, the inferior lobes of the right and (most of the) left lung drain to the right side ✓ Right and left tracheal (paratracheal) lymph nodes receive lymph next as it ascends on each side of the tracheal ✓ Right and left bronchomediastinal lymphatic trunks, which drain to the right and left venous angles, respectively. This chain of nodes also receives drainage from the other thoracic (mediastinal) viscera (heart, esophagus)

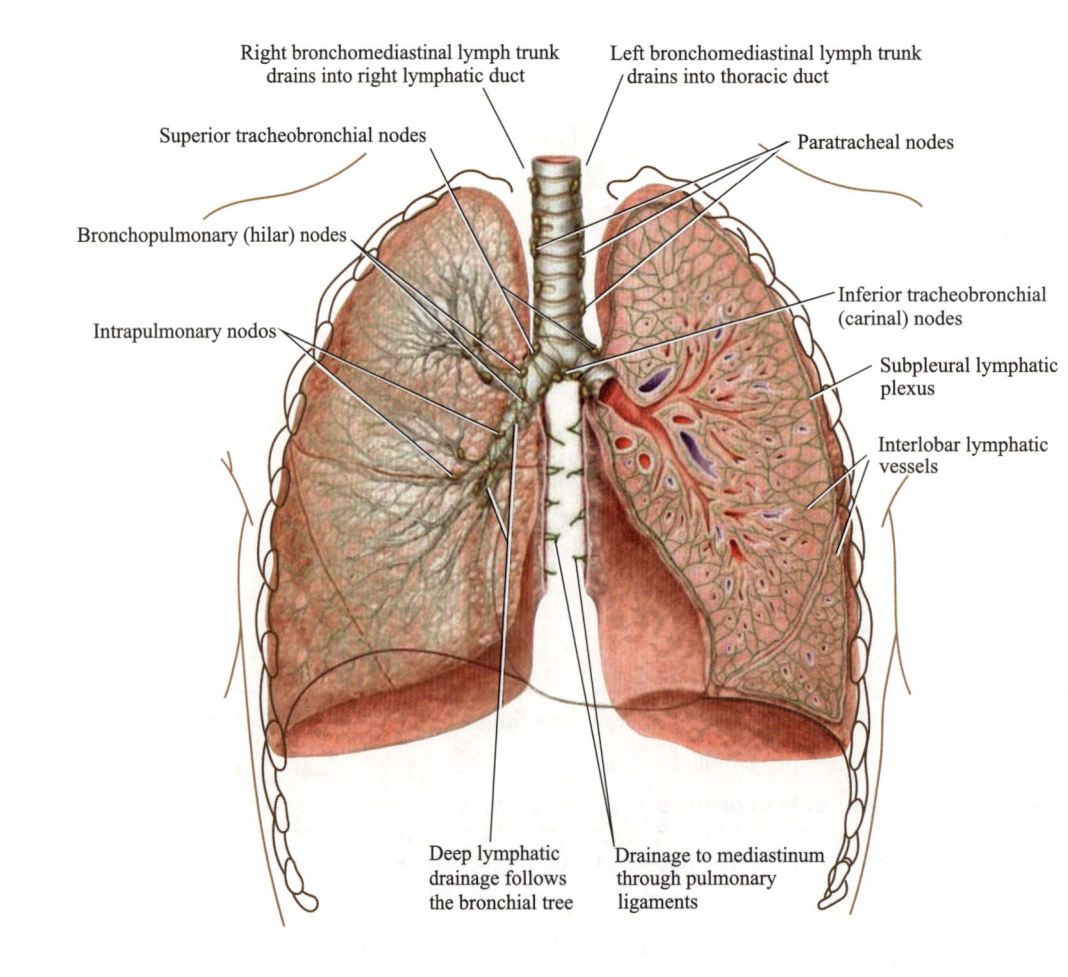

Innervation of lungs
Pulmonary nerve plexuses, which lie mainly on the posterior (but also on the anterior) aspects of the primary bronchi and their derivatives, provide innervation. The plexuses convey:

✓ Parasympathetic innervation from branches of the vagus nerve (CN X), which pass posterior to the root of the lung; the vagus nerves provide:
  ◊ Motor fibers to smooth muscle of bronchial tree (bronchoconstriction)
 Note: excessive stimulation of these motor fibers, via inhaled irritants, airborne allergens, exercise, stress, or other factors, may produce asthma
  ◊ Inhibitory fibers that inhibit vasoconstriction by the sympathetic system (i.e., they indirectly cause vasodilation of constricted vessels)
  ◊ Reflex afferent fibers from stretch receptors conveying information regarding distension from tactile/irritant/cough receptors in respiratory mucosa
 ✓ Sympathetic innervation from cardiopulmonary splanchnic nerves (visceral branches of the sympathetic trunks); the splanchnic nerves provide:
  ◊ Vasomotor fibers producing vasoconstriction
  ◊ Inhibitory fibers that inhibit bronchoconstriction by parasympathetic system
  ◊ Secretomotor fibers to bronchial glands

Clinical notes: The autonomic innervation is not extensive; all effects are relatively mild. However, sympathomimetic drugs can be helpful in inhibiting the spasmodic contraction of the bronchiolar smooth muscle during an asthma attack

Radiographs and cross-sectional anatomy
✓ Normal chest film: apices, costal margins, costodiaphragmatic recesses, domes of diaphragms, cardiophrenic angle, cardiac silhouette, shadow of root of lung   ✓ Transverse cross-sections: apices in sections of lower neck, costal surface (note vertebral part, posterior to root), mediastinal surface with cardiac impressions causing lung to be found anterior and posterior to heart, inferior border in costodiaphragmatic recesses in "abdominal" cross section

3.6.4 Autonomic innervations of thorax

Overview
✓ For purposes of study and description, the body's nervous system can be divided and subdivided in a number of different ways. The nervous system is not, in fact, separable into components; it is one continuous, very interactive structure and any and all schemes for segmenting it are artificial devices for conceptual purposes. Nonetheless, such schemes are most useful in understanding the structure and function of this complex and miraculous system

Central nervous system (CNS)
A hollow tube in a dark, bony cave
✓ Brain   ◊ Housed inside cranium (skull)

- ✓ Spinal cord
  - ◊ Housed inside the spine (vertebral column)
  - ◊ Gray matter vs. white matter
  - ◊ Gray matter central, butterfly-shaped on X-section
  - ◊ Largely consists of neuron cell bodies
  - ◊ Posterior horn, anterior horn and [between T_1–L_2(L_3)] lateral horn
  - ◊ White matter peripheral
  - ◊ Largely consists of nerve fibers (axons) and myelin

Peripheral nervous system (PNS)

Nerve fibers, neurons and nerve terminals outside of brain and spinal cord (and, generally, their bony encasements)

- ✓ Cranial nerves
  - ◊ 12 pairs
- ✓ Spinal nerves
  - ◊ All exit in relationship to the spinal (vertebral) column
  - ◊ 31 pairs

Sensory (afferent) nervous system vs. motor (efferent) nervous system

The sensory (afferent) nervous system

Unipolar neurons
- ✓ Cell bodies located outside of (but close to) CNS
  - ◊ Posterior root (spinal) ganglia
  - ◊ Sensory ganglia of cranial nerves
- ✓ Have one process, which almost immediately divides into:
  - ◊ A peripheral process (dendrite)—sensory end-organ
  - ◊ A central process (axon)—CNS (via a posterior root in the case of spinal nerves)

The motor (efferent) nervous system

Bipolar neurons
- ✓ Cell bodies of fibers exiting the CNS located in gray matter
- ✓ Fibers (axons conducting impulses peripherally) exit CNS via anterior roots of spinal nerves or via cranial nerves

The motor (efferent) nervous system

The somatic motor system

"Somatic": relating to the wall of the body cavities (includes limbs)

- ✓ Organization: only 1 neuron between CNS and the end-organ
  - ◊ The cell body of this one and only neuron is located within the gray matter of the CNS (in the case of spinal nerves, within the anterior horn of gray matter), and now we have learned that the same fiber which exits the CNS extends all the way to—and terminates upon—the structure being innervated, regardless of the distance involved

▷ I. e., no cell bodies of somatic motor fibers are located outside the CNS
✓ End-organ: always skeletal (striated, voluntary) muscle
▷ I. e., structures which we normally willfully (voluntarily) control

The visceral motor system

✓ The organs of the body cavities; in this case, the definition is extended to include blood vessels and glands which lie outside body cavities

Organization: 2 neurons between CNS and end-organ

Presynaptic (preganglionic) neuron

✓ Its fibers exit the CNS, thus its cell body must be located within the gray matter of the CNS
✓ The axon leaving the CNS terminates only within an autonomic ganglion upon the cell body

Postsynaptic (postganglionic) neuron

✓ "Ganglion": a collection of nerve cell bodies (or, in some cases, a single nerve—cell body) located outside the CNS
✓ Thus, by definition, these cell bodies are located outside the CNS (further from the CNS than the afferent cell bodies of sensory ganglia) and constitute autonomic ganglia
✓ Axon terminates upon the end-organ

End-organs (must be one of these)

✓ Smooth (non-striated, "involuntary") muscle: blood vessels, hollow organs and ducts, arrector pili muscles, intrinsic eye muscle
✓ Glands: sweat, salivary, lacrimal
✓ Modified cardiac muscle: SA and AV nodes

Subdivisions

Two subdivisions are normally described

✓ Common features
　▷ Both share previously-mentioned features of the visceral motor system
　▷ Both have 2 neurons (pre- and postsynaptic) between the CNS and end-organ
　▷ Both innervate structures over which we normally do not exert willful control (smooth muscle, glands, etc.)
✓ Distinctions
　▷ The two subdivisions may be distinguished in several ways

(1) Anatomic distinction

✓ Based upon the location of the cell body of the presynaptic neuron, and the level at which the presynaptic fibers exit the CNS
✓ Presynaptic cell bodies are only found in certain, distinct locations within the CNS
　▷ Within cranium (gray matter of brain) associated with motor nuclei of certain cranial nerves (Ⅲ, Ⅶ, Ⅸ and Ⅹ)
　▷ Within gray matter of thoracic and upper lumbar spinal cord segments $[T_1-L_2(L_3)]$
　▷ Within gray matter of the middle sacral spinal cord segments (S_2-S_4)

(2) Pharmacological distinctions

A clinically-important distinction is that the transmitter substance of the postsynaptic neurons of the two subdivision differ in their pharmacology. We will not concern ourselves with this distinction here

✓ Certain drugs selectively mimic the effects of stimulation by one subdivision or the other
✓ Other drugs selectively suppress or block the effects of stimulation by one subdivision or the other
✓ E. g. , "beta blockers" block effects of the sympathetic nerve system on the heart; atropine blocks acetylcholine effects (e. g. , suppresses secretions)—parasympathetic system blocked

(3) The two subdivisions are also distinguished on the basis of the relative lengths of the pre- and postsynaptic fibers, and functional distinctions

The thoracolumbar (sympathetic) nervous system

Presynaptic neurons

Cell bodies

✓ Collectively, the cell bodies of presynaptic sympathetic neurons form a column of cells which extend the length of the thoracic and upper lumbar portions of the spinal cord = the intermediolateral cell column (IML). When observed in a transverse section of the spinal cord, the IML appears as the lateral horn of gray matter
✓ The IML is the only place presynaptic sympathetic cell bodies are found
✓ The IML, then, extends from T_1 to $L_2(T_3)$ spinal cord segments
✓ The IML is somatopically arranged (i. e. , portions concerned with innervation of the head located superiorly, portions concerned with innervation of feet located inferiorly)
✓ Thus, we can specifically locate cell bodies within the IML concerned with innervating the smooth muscle or glands contained within a given area of the body
- ▷ T_1-T_6 portions of IML
    - ◆ Head and neck
    - ◆ Chest
    - ◆ Upper limb
    - ◆ Gastrointestinal tract to diaphragm
- ▷ T_7-T_{11} portions of IML
    - ◆ Abdomen
    - ◆ Wall of trunk
    - ◆ Gastrointestinal tract from gastroesophageal junction to rectosigmoid junction
- ▷ $T_{12}-L_2(T_3)$ portion of IML
    - ◆ Lower limb
    - ◆ Pelvic viscera
    - ◆ Rectum/anal canal

Nerve fibers (axons)

✓ Exit CNS via anterior roots (they are motor fibers)
✓ Become components of the mixed spinal nerve as roots join
✓ Enter the anterior ramus

- ✓ Exit the spinal nerve via a communicating branch (called a white ramus communicans, since most presynaptic fibers are myelinated)
- ✓ Enters the paravertebral (chain) ganglia or sympathetic trunks

Clinical notes: All presynaptic sympathetic fibers follow the path above. Presynaptic sympathetic fibers are never found in spinal nerves distal to the white rami communicans

White rami communicans

- ✓ Are very short branches of the anterior rami of spinal nerves T_1–L_2(L_3)
- ✓ Do not exist in association with any other spinal nerves
- ✓ Are the only means by which presynaptic fibers reach the sympathetic trunks
- ✓ Also convey peripheral processes of afferent neurons located in the posterior root ganglia of T_1–L_2(L_3)
- ✓ These fibers are conducting sensory (pain) information from the viscera to the CNS
- ✓ The visceral afferent fibers are not part of the autonomic nervous system, they merely "hitch a ride" with it
- ✓ The ANS is a purely motor system

Sympathetic trunks (paravertebral ganglia)

Paired structures lying on the lateral and anterior aspects of the vertebral column, extending nearly its entire length (from vertebra L_1 at base of skull to tip of sacrum)

- ✓ Like a string of beads in appearance
- ✓ "Beads" = autonomic (sympathetic) ganglia
- ✓ "String" = interganglionic connections (see below)
- ✓ Not segmental (only 3 cervical ganglia)

Returning to the course of the presynaptic sympathetic fibers, while all fibers have followed the same course thus far, upon reaching the sympathetic trunk the presynaptic fibers may do one of four things

- ✓ Terminate in the first ganglion encountered
- ✓ Ascend to a higher ganglion to terminate
- ✓ Descend to a lower ganglion to terminate
- ✓ Traverse the sympathetic trunk without terminating

(The latter phenomenon applies only to presynaptic fibers involved in the innervation of abdominopelvic viscera—i.e., body cavity viscera located below the diaphragm. Presynaptic fibers involved in the innervation of all other parts of the body terminate within the sympathetic trunks)

Only the presynaptic fibers initially conveyed by spinal nerves T_7–T_{11} concerned with the innervation of structures lying within dermatomes T_7–T_{11} (and some of the presynaptic fibers initially conveyed by spinal nerves T_3–T_6 concerned with the innervation of thoracic viscera) synapse at the level of their parent spinal nerve. Otherwise, all other presynaptic fibers must ascend or descend to ganglia at levels other than their level of entrance before they terminate

- ✓ Above nerve T_1 (the highest white ramus communicans), in the cervical portion of the trunk, all fibers are ascending
- ✓ Below nerve L_2 (the lowest white ramus communicans), all fibers are descending
- ✓ In between T_1 and L_2, the trunk contains both ascending and descending fibers

It is, of course, only via ascending and descending fibers that the cervical, lower lumbar and sacral portions of the trunk could receive presynaptic fibers, since those portions of the trunk have no rami communicans associated with them

It should be apparent now that the interganglionic connections of the paravertebral ganglia consist of ascending and descending presynaptic sympathetic fibers [plus visceral afferent fibers running in the opposite direction to reach posterior root ganglia of $T_1-L_2(T_3)$]

Of course, when the presynaptic fibers terminate, they can only terminate by synapsing with a postsynaptic neuron within an autonomic ganglion

Branches of the sympathetic trunk/distribution of sympathetic innervation

Two sets of branches arise from the sympathetic trunks: parietal and visceral

Parietal branches

✓ Gray rami communicans
  ▷ Run laterally from the ganglia of the trunk
  ▷ Convey postsynaptic fibers (unmyelinated) arising from postsynaptic cell bodies located in the ganglion from which the gray ramus extends
  ▷ Generality: postsynaptic fibers do not ascend or descend within the sympathetic trunk, but exit from the trunk at the level of the synapse between pre- and postsynaptic neuron
  ▷ Extend to the anterior rami of all 31 pairs of spinal nerves
  ▷ Postsynaptic fibers enter into both the posterior and anterior rami of each spinal nerve, and all branches of all spinal nerves will include some postsynaptic fibers
  ▷ Thus spinal nerves and their associated gray rami communicans are the means by which postsynaptic fibers reach all parts of the neck, body wall and limbs. However, since spinal nerves are not distributed to the head, another means is provided for distribution there

✓ Cephalic arterial rami
  ▷ Arise from the inferior, middle and superior cervical ganglia
  ▷ Join vertebral, external and internal carotid arteries (respectively) about which they form periarterial sympathetic plexuses which follow the arteries and their branches
  ▷ Most postsynaptic fibers reach their destination in the head (arteries and skin, mostly), although a few leave the periarterial plexuses to join branches of cranial nerves to reach their final destination
  ▷ The gray rami communicans and the cephalic arterial rami are thus the means of parietal distribution of sympathetic innervation, in which postsynaptic fibers are conveyed to the head, neck, body wall and limbs, where they produce:
    ◆ Vasomotion (the primary function of the sympathetic nerve system)
    ◆ Pilomotion ("goose bumps")
    ◆ Sudomotion (sweating)
(Some additional functions are served in the head in relation to the eye)

Clinical notes: Since postsynaptic sympathetic fibers are responsible for the innervation of the smooth muscle of blood vessels, they are distributed to all parts of the body, except for the avascular structures (epidermis, cartilage, cornea, nails, hair, etc.)

Visceral branches (splanchnic nerves): a splanchnic nerve is a nerve which passes to and innervates the viscera of the body cavities

Clinical notes: Although all the visceral (vs. parietal) branches of the sympathetic trunks are splanchnic nerves, not all splanchnic nerves are branches of the trunks. The term "splanchnic nerve" in itself is not specific as to the type of fibers contained. Pre- and postsynaptic sympathetic, parasympathetic and afferent fibers are all found in various splanchnic nerves. The term "splanchnic nerve" merely tells us that the nerve is bound for the viscera of the body cavities, and thus the fibers contained are "visceral" (visceral efferent and visceral afferent) fibers

There are three basic varieties of splanchnic nerves:
✓ Cardiopulmonary splanchnics
✓ Abdominopelvic splanchnics
✓ Pelvic splanchnics
(Since the pelvic splanchnics are neither associated with the sympathetic trunks nor involved in conveying sympathetic fibers (pre- or postsynaptic), we shall not be further concerned with them at this time)

Splanchnic nerves conveying sympathetic fibers:
✓ Run medially from the sympathetic trunks
✓ Account for the majority of splanchnic nerves
✓ Include:
  ◊ Cardiopulmonary splanchnics: arise from the cervical and upper thoracic sympathetic trunks
    ◆ Convey postsynaptic fibers (as well as visceral afferents)
    ◆ Postsynaptic cell bodies located at the cervical and upper thoracic portions of the trunks
    ◆ Note: the cell bodies of the presynaptic neurons associated with these postsynaptic fibers are located in the T_1-T_6 portions of the IML cell column of gray matter. Likewise, the visceral afferent fibers conveyed by the cardiopulmonary splanchnics have their cell bodies located in the posterior root ganglia of spinal nerves T_1-T_6
    ◆ Run mostly to the cardiac and (anterior) pulmonary plexuses
    ◆ Nerve plexuses which do not include ganglia, since fibers are already postsynaptic
    ◆ Serve the viscera of the thoracic cavity—viscera located superior to the level of the diaphragm
  ◊ Abdominopelvic splanchnics: arise from lower thoracic and lumbar portions of trunks
    ◆ Include greater, lesser, least, lumbar and sacral splanchnics
    ◆ Convey presynaptic sympathetic fibers (cell bodies located in the IML cell column, $T_7-L_2(T_3)$) that have traversed the trunks without synapsing [as well as visceral afferent fibers with cell bodies located in the posterior root ganglia of spinal nerves $T_7-L_2(T_3)$]
    ◆ Run to the para-aortic plexus of nerves surrounding the abdominal aorta, where the presynaptic fibers will synapse in autonomic ganglia (prevertebral or collateral ganglia) located mainly around the origins of the major (visceral) branches of the aorta (i.e., celiac, superior mesenteric, renal ganglia)
    ◆ The postsynaptic fibers arising in the prevertebral ganglia following the arteries with which the ganglia are associated (in the form of periarterial plexuses) to reach their end organs (blood vessels and intrinsic nerve plexuses of the gut)

> ◆Note: the cells of the adrenal medulla are directly stimulated by presynaptic sympathetic fibers which traverse both the paravertebral and prevertebral ganglia without synapsing. The cells of the adrenal medulla, derived from migrating neural crest cells (their development is similar to that of the postsynaptic neuron), actually function as the postsynaptic neurons, their neurotransmitter substance being released into the blood stream for a generalized sympathetic response

> General rule: presynaptic sympathetic fibers involved in the innervation of structures outside the abdominopelvic cavity will synapse in the paravertebral ganglia (sympathetic trunks)

3.6.5 Superior and posterior mediastinum

Mediastinum

✓ "Standing in the middle" between the two pleural sacs, completely separating them
✓ Contains all the structures in the thorax except the lungs and pleura
✓ Extends from the superior thoracic aperture to the diaphragm inferiorly and from the sternum and costal cartilages anteriorly to the vertebral bodies posteriorly
✓ In life, it is a soft, pliable dynamic structure, not the hard, rigid structure encountered in cadaver
  ↳ Lower structures move with motion of heart, respiration, swallowing
  ↳ Influenced by gravity
    ◆Sags to the left when one is lying on their left side
    ◆Structures lie lower when standing, slightly higher when lying supine
  ↳ If thoracic wall is punctured, pneumothorax may result in lung collapse (atelectasis) and an open "sucking wound" and reversing mediastinal shift
  ↳ If punctured by a slit-like wound (e.g., a diagonal knife wound), the wound may function as a valve: air enters pleural cavity during inspiration, cannot escape during expiration → tension pneumothorax with one-way mediastinal shift

Subdivisions

Superior mediastinum

✓ Extends from superior thoracic aperture to the transverse thoracic plane
✓ A horizontal plane passing through the sternal angle and T_4/T_5 intervertebral disc
✓ Contents include upper part of thymus/thymic remnant; brachiocephalic veins and upper half of superior vena cave (SVC); aortic arch and branches; trachea; esophagus; thoracic duct; phrenic, vagus, and left recurrent laryngeal nerves; and the superior tracheobronchial, paratracheal and brachiocephalic lymph nodes

Inferior mediastinum

✓ Between the transverse thoracic plane and the diaphragm
✓ Subdivided into:
  ↳ Anterior mediastinum
    ◆Smallest subdivision
    ◆Posterior to the sternum and transverse thoracic muscles
    ◆Anterior to the pericardium

◆ Contains the lower part of the thymus or thymic remnants, sternopericardial ligaments
◊ Middle mediastinum
   ◆ Essentially conterminous with the fibrous pericardium plus the mediastinal portion of the roots of the lungs
   ◆ Contains the heart, phrenic nerves, main bronchi, and the origins/terminations of the great arteries and veins, including:
      • Ascending aorta
      • Pulmonary trunk, right and left pulmonary arteries
      • Inferior half of SVC
      • Terminations of IVC, pulmonary veins and azygos veins
   ◆ Most important compartment clinically
◊ Posterior mediastinum
   ◆ Located posterior to pericardium and diaphragm and anterior to the inferior 8 thoracic vertebrae
   ◆ Contents include the esophagus, vagi, descending (thoracic) aorta, thoracic duct, azygos venous system, and posterior mediastinal lymph nodes

Superior mediastinum

Major contents (from anterior to posterior): gland, veins, arteries, airway, food passage, lymph duct

Thymus

✓ Prominent in infancy
✓ Plays an important role in the development and maintenance of the immune system

Great vessels and nerves of mediastinum

Brachiocephalic veins: valveless

✓ Formed by the union of the internal jugular and subclavian veins (venous angle)
   ◊ Venous angles receive major lymphatic trunks of body
✓ Unite to form SVC
✓ Right brachiocephalic vein
   ◊ Short vein formed posterior to sternoclavicular joint by union of right subclavian and internal jugular veins (right venous angle)
   ◊ Paralleled by two major nerves: right phrenic nerve lays posterolateral to vein and right vagus nerve lies posteromedial to vein
✓ Left brachiocephalic vein
   ◊ Large vein formed posterior to sternoclavicular joint by union of left subclavian and internal jugular veins
   ◊ Twice as long as the right because it crosses midline to merge with right brachiocephalic vein to form SVC on right side
   ◊ Crosses left vagus nerve, left common carotid artery, and brachiocephalic trunk
   ◊ Receives the left superior intercostal vein, inferior thyroid vein(s) and thymic veins

Superior vena cava

✓ Formed on right side of the superior mediastinum by merger of brachiocephalic veins
✓ Drains blood from all structures superior to the diaphragm (except lungs and heart)

- ✓ Anterolateral to the trachea and posterolateral to the ascending aorta
- ✓ Right phrenic nerve runs on right side of SVC, between SVC and mediastinal pleura
- ✓ Terminal half of the SVC is in the middle mediastinum, where it lies beside the ascending aorta, entering right atrium level of 3rd costal cartilage

Vagus (X) nerves

- ✓ Descend from the neck posterolateral to the common carotid arteries, anterior to subclavian arteries
- ✓ Enter superior mediastinum posterior to sternoclavicular joints and brachiocephalic veins
- ✓ Pass posterior to roots of lungs
- ✓ Right vagus nerve
  - ◊ As it passes anterior to right subclavian artery, gives off right recurrent laryngeal nerve
  - ◊ Runs posteroinferiorly on the right side of the trachea
- ✓ Left vagus nerve
  - ◊ As it descends lateral to aortic arch, gives off left recurrent laryngeal nerve—loops under arch, passing posterior to ligament arteriosum, then ascends to larynx
  - ◊ Right and left vagi break up into branches. That contribute to:
    - ◆ Right pulmonary plexus (posterior to root of the right lung)
    - ◆ Esophageal plexus (surrounds esophagus)
    - ◆ Cardiac plexus (between ascending aorta and bifurcation of trachea)

Phrenic nerves

- ✓ Arise from ventral rami from C_3, C_4 and C_5
- ✓ Enter superior mediastinum between the subclavian arteries and origin of brachiocephalic veins
- ✓ Pass anterior to roots of lungs
- ✓ Sole motor nerves of diaphragm (also supply most of sensory innervation), ramifying on its inferior (abdominal) surface after penetrating it
- ✓ Right phrenic nerve
  - ◊ Descends on right side of brachiocephalic vein, SVC and pericardium over right atrium
  - ◊ Descends to the right of IVC to penetrate diaphragm (may traverse hiatus of IVC)
- ✓ Left phrenic nerve
  - ◊ Descends on left surface of arch of the aorta, anterior to the right vagus nerve
  - ◊ Runs along the pericardium, penetrating diaphragm independently

Arch of aorta

- ✓ Curved continuation of ascending aorta
- ✓ Lies posterior to the 2nd left sternocostal joint (level of the sternal angle)
- ✓ Arches superoposteriorly and to the left, but its main direction is posterior (nearly lies in sagittal plane)
- ✓ Passes to left side of trachea and esophagus as it arches over the root of the left lung. Becomes thoracic (descending) aorta posterior to root of left lung
- ✓ Can be visualized on radiographs as the "aortic knob"
- ✓ Ligamentum arteriosum passes between root of the left pulmonary artery and the arch of aorta
  - ◊ Remnant of embryonic ductus arteriosus that shunted blood from the left pulmonary artery to aorta
- ✓ Left recurrent laryngeal nerve hooks under arch of the aorta posterior to ligament arteriosum
  - ◊ Ascends to larynx between the trachea and esophagus

Branches of arch of aorta

- ✓ Brachiocephalic (arterial) trunk
  - ◊ First and largest branch
  - ◊ Divides into the right subclavian and right common carotid arteries
- ✓ Left common carotid artery
  - ◊ Arises from arch posterior and to left of brachiocephalic trunk
  - ◊ Ascends anterior to left subclavian artery
- ✓ Left subclavian artery
  - ◊ Initially ascends with (but posterior to) left common carotid through superior mediastinum
  - ◊ Indents left lung/pleural sac as it passes laterally to exit superior thoracic aperture

Clinical considerations

- ✓ Aneurysm of arch of the aorta
  - ◊ Pressure may be exerted on trachea and esophagus causing difficulty with breathing and swallowing
- ✓ Congenital anomalies of aortic arch
  - ◊ Patent ductus arteriosus
    - ◆ Usually small, producing few symptoms in early childhood
    - ◆ If large, young child may develop congestive heart failure
    - ◆ Symptoms similar to ventricular septal defect, but hearts sounds are distinct
    - ◆ Easily treated via surgical ligation

Right aortic arch

- ✓ Arches over the root of the right lung
- ✓ Must pass posterior to the esophagus for thoracic aorta to continue in its usual position on left side

Double aortic arch

- ✓ Forms a vascular ring around the esophagus and trachea
- ✓ Retroesophageal right subclavian artery
  - ◊ Instead of arising as a terminal branch of the brachiocephalic trunk, the right subclavian arises as a 4th branch of arch and then crosses posterior to the esophagus to reach the right upper limb
  - ◊ May compress the esophagus and cause difficulty in swallowing (dysphagia)
- ✓ Coarctation of the aorta
  - ◊ Aorta constricted or stenotic
  - ◊ If coarctation is distal to the ligamentum arteriosum, a good collateral circulation usually develops by way of intercostal and internal thoracic arteries carrying blood around the coarctation to the descending aorta distal to the stenosis

Trachea

- ✓ Wide fibrocartilaginous tube for conducting from upper respiratory tract to lungs
- ✓ Begins in the neck atcricoid cartilage (level of vertebra C_6)
- ✓ Descends into superior mediastinum anterior to esophagus deviating slightly to the right
- ✓ Posterior surface is flat where applied to the esophagus
- ✓ Patency is maintained by C-shaped tracheal cartilages in anterolateral walls

- ✓ Terminates at level of sternal angle, bifurcating into the right and left main bronchi
  - ▷ Keel-like cartilage (carina) is internal landmark of bifurcation
  - ▷ Tracheobronchial lymph nodes occur at bifurcation
    - ◆ Superior tracheobronchial nodes lie superior to origin of main bronchi
    - ◆ Inferior tracheobronchial (carinal) nodes lie inferior to origin of main bronchi
- ✓ Widening or distortion of the carina results from invasion and enlargement of inferior tracheobronchial lymph nodes in bronchiogenic carcinoma
- ✓ Can be directly observed via mediastinoscopy or thoracoscopy
  - ▷ Ascending aorta lies anterior bifurcation of trachea; arch passes on its left side

Esophagus

- ✓ Narrow fibromuscular tube
- ✓ Connects the pharynx with the stomach
- ✓ Has cervical, thoracic and abdominal parts
- ✓ Superior mediastinal part (of thoracic part) lies between the trachea and vertebral column

Posterior mediastinum

- ✓ Posterior to heart
- ✓ Contents of posterior mediastinum (anterior to posterior)
  - ▷ Esophagus and vagus nerves
  - ▷ Thoracic (descending) aorta
  - ▷ Thoracic duct
  - ▷ Azygos/hemiazygos system of veins
- ✓ Esophagus trachea (anterior to superior mediastinal part of esophagus) terminates at level of sternal angle
  - ▷ Primary anterior relationship of posterior mediastinal part of esophagus = left atrium of heart
    - ◆ Separated from it by oblique pericardial sinus
  - ▷ Posterior relationships = bodies of vertebrae T_5–T_7/thoracic aorta
  - ▷ Thoracic aorta located to left superiorly, but soon comes to lie posterior to esophagus.
  - ▷ Esophageal "constrictions"—3 areas of narrowing normally visible under contrast radiography that must be distinguished from pathology
    - ◆ Pharyngoesophageal constriction/junction—superior esophageal sphincter—C_6 level
      - • Narrowest, at beginning of esophagus
    - ◆ Thoracic (broncho-aortic) constriction—arch of aorta/left bronchus—T_4/T_5 level
      - • Actually two separate indentations
      - • Aortic is slightly higher, observed in an AP view
      - • Bronchial slightly lower, observed in a lateral view
    - ◆ Diaphragmatic constriction—esophageal hiatus of the diaphragm (inferior esophageal sphincter)—T_{10} level

Blood vessels (of entire esophagus)

Arteries of esophagus

- ✓ Cervical esophagus : inferior thyroid artery
- ✓ Superior mediastinal esophagus : superior intercostal and bronchial arteries
- ✓ Posterior mediastinal esophagus : direct esophageal branches of thoracic aorta
- ✓ Abdominal (cardial) esophagus : esophageal branch of left gastric artery

Veins of esophagus

- ✓ Cervical esophagus : middle thyroid vein
- ✓ Superior mediastinal esophagus : superior intercostal and bronchial veins
- ✓ Posterior mediastinal esophagus : esophageal veins
- ✓ Abdominal (cardial) esophagus : esophageal branch of left gastric artery

Innervation of esophagus

- ✓ Upper 1/3 of esophagus is composed of striated (voluntary) muscle
    - ◊ Innervation of upper part is by recurrent laryngeal nerves (from vagus)
- ✓ Lower 1/3 of esophagus is composed of smooth (involuntary) muscle
- ✓ Middle 1/3 of esophagus is composed of mixed striated and smooth muscle
    - ◊ Lower 2/3 of esophagus is supplied by esophageal plexus of nerves formed
        - ◆ Mainly by the right and left vagus nerves (somatic and parasympathetic fibers)
        - ◆ With contributions from the right and left sympathetic trunks (cardiopulmonary splanchnic nerves)

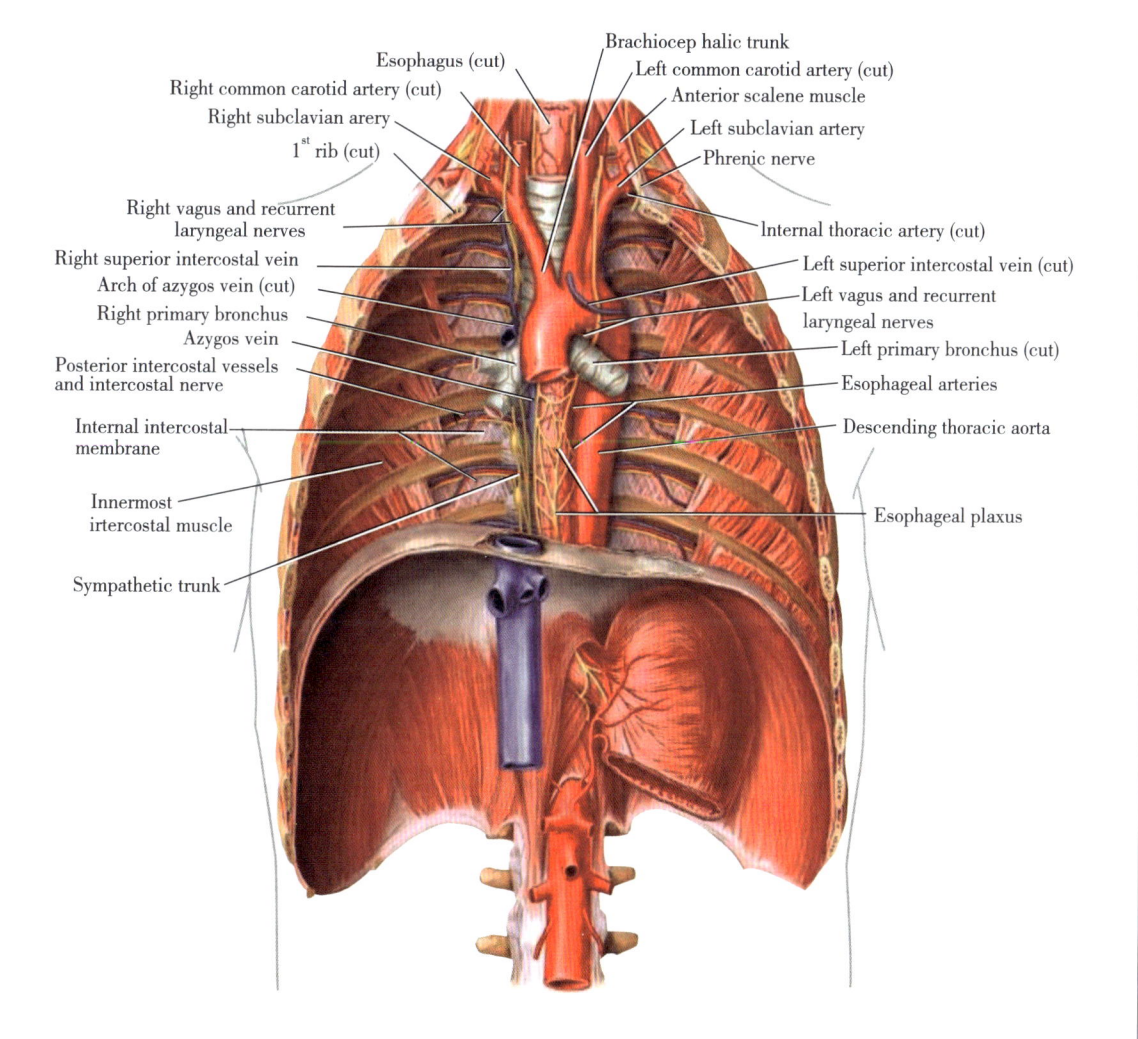

Vagus nerves

- Right vagus nerve
  - After sending branches to pulmonary plexus, passes to posterior aspect of esophagus
  - Ramifies, mingling with branches of left vagus to form esophageal plexus, temporarily losing identity
  - Reforms prior to passage through esophageal hiatus (diaphragm) into posterior esophageal trunk
- Left vagus nerve
  - Similar to right vagus (above), but passes to anterior aspect of esophagus
  - After losing identity in esophageal plexus, reforms into anterior vagal trunk

Thoracic aorta

- Continuation of the arch of the aorta at level of vertebra T_4
- Lies to the left of the vertebral column superiorly, and then it approaches the median plane inferiorly
- Passes through the diaphragm at the aortic hiatus at level of vertebra T_{12}

Branches

- Anterior unpaired visceral branches
  - Pericardial: to the posterior aspect of the pericardium
  - Esophageal: from the front of the aorta
  - Mediastinal: supply lymph nodes and posterior mediastinum
- Lateral paired visceral branches
  - Bronchial: 1 right and 2 left. Only left arteries arise from the aorta
- Posterolateral paired parietal branches
  - Posterior intercostal arteries and subcostal artery
  - Superior phrenic: from the lowermost part of the thoracic aorta

Thoracic duct

The largest lymphatic channel of the body

- Returns lymph and chyle to the bloodstream from all of body below the diaphragm and from the left half of the body above the diaphragm
- Arises from the chyle cistern
  - Lies anterior to body of vertebra L_2 posterior to abdominal aorta, in crevasse between aorta and right crus of the diaphragm
    - Receives lymphatic trunks draining GI tract which carry absorbed fat (chyle)
    - Receives right and left lumbar trunks from the lower limbs and pelvis
- Course of thoracic duct
  - Passes through the aortic hiatus of diaphragm
  - Approximately at the level of vertebra T_5 (sternal angle) inclines to left side of median plane
  - Ascends posterior to aortic arch and on left side of the esophagus to traverse superior thoracic aperture
  - Arches laterally and then inferiorly, anterior to subclavian artery to enter left venous angle
- Accidental rupture or surgical section of this channel allows spilling into the thoracic cage with resulting pressure on the lungs and heart (chylothorax)
- Blockage of lymph flow (e.g., by tumor or parasites) → accumulation, especially in gravity-dependent lower limbs, scrotum = lymphedema

Azygos system of veins: non-symmetrical system

√ Venous counterpart thoracic aorta
√ Valveless—blood can flow backward (to IVC/left renal vein) if blocked

Azygos vein

√ Ascending, valveless longitudinal venous channel of right side
√ Formed at the level of median arcuate ligament of diaphragm by the junction of:
  ◊ lateral root of azygos vein
    ◆ Formed by junction of right ascending lumbar vein and the right subcostal vein
  ◊ Medial root of azygos vein
    ◆ Communication with IVC at the level of renal veins (remnant of the continuity of the right supracardinal vein of the embryo)
    ◆ Ascends along the right side of the vertebral column
    ◆ Overlies the posterior intercostal arteries
    ◆ Usually located to right of aorta—often on the middle of the thoracic vertebral bodies
    ◆ At the level of vertebra L_4, arches anteriorly over root of right lung
    ◆ Enters posterior aspect of SVC just before it pierces the pericardium receives
      • 11th through 5th right posterior intercostal veins
      • Right superior intercostal vein—formed by merging of 2th–4th right posterior intercostal veins
      • Hemiazygos and accessory hemiazygos veins—may cross midline independently or form a common trunk
      • Esophageal veins
      • Mediastinal, pericardial and right bronchial veins

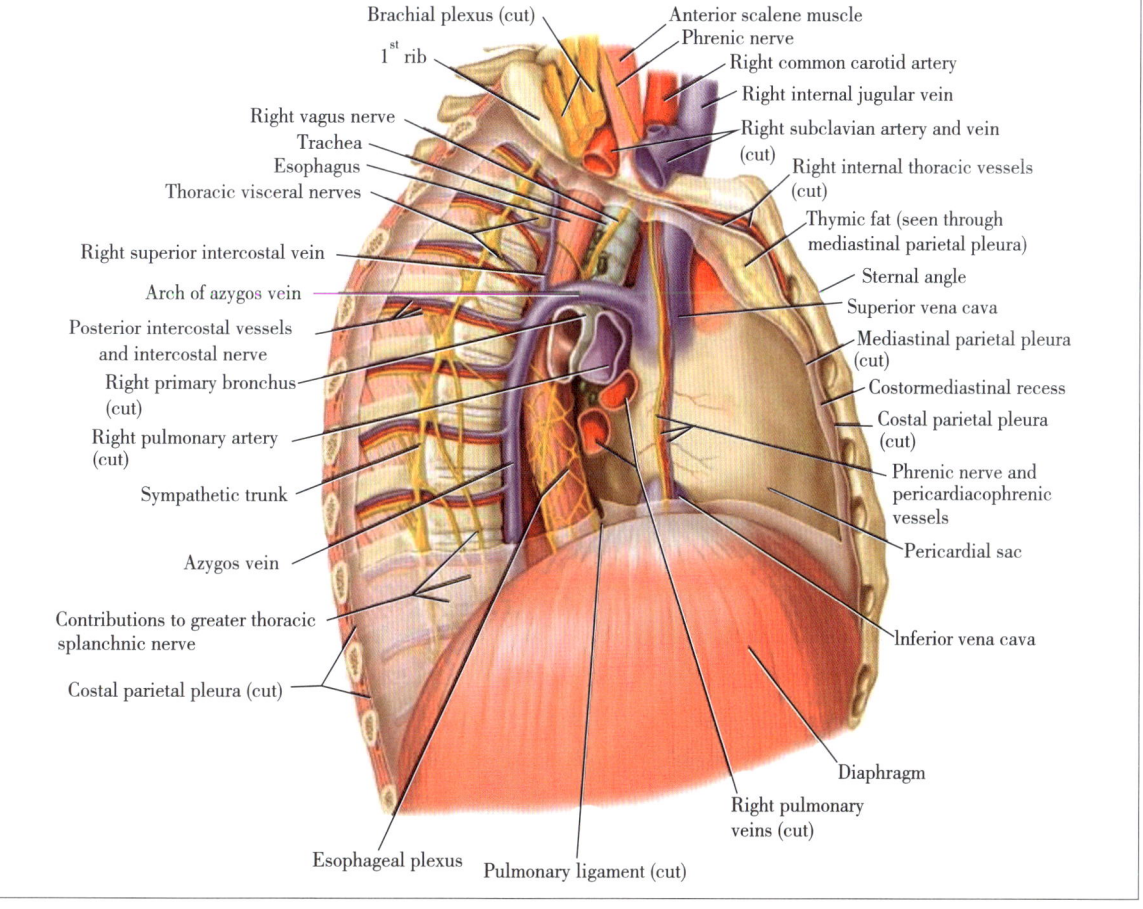

Hemiazygos vein

✓ Ascending, valveless longitudinal venous channel of left side
✓ Formed at the level of median arcuate ligament of diaphragm by the junction of:
　◊ Lateral root of hemiazygos vein
　　◆ Formed by junction of left ascending lumbar vein and the left subcostal vein
　◊ Medial root of hemiazygos vein
　　◆ Communication with left renal vein at the renal level (remnant of the continuity of the left supracardinal vein of the embryo)
　　◆ Ascends on the left side of vertebral bodies and posterior to thoracic aorta as high as vertebral T_9
　　◆ Passes to right across midline, anterior to vertebral column and posterior to aorta, esophagus, and thoracic duct
　　◆ Empties into azygos vein
　　◆ Receives:
　　　• Lower 4 or 5 left posterior intercostal veins from spaces 7, 8, 9, 10, and 11
　　　• Lower esophageal veins

Accessory hemiazygos vein

✓ Valveless, descending longitudinal venous channel in the place of the hemiazygos vein in the upper portion of the chest on the left side
✓ Interposed between the upper end of hemiazygos and left superior intercostal veins
✓ Descends superficial to the posterior intercostal arteries
✓ At level of vertebra T_8 it turns right, passes posterior to aorta, thoracic duct and esophagus
✓ Empties into the azygos vein
✓ Receives:
　◊ Posterior intercostal—spaces 5–7 or 8
　◊ Left bronchial veins
✓ May communicate with left superior intercostal vein
✓ Note that the 1st posterior intercostal veins drain directly into the brachiocephalic veins, and right posterior intercostal veins 2–4 drain via a common trunk (right superior intercostal vein) into the azygos vein; left posterior intercostal veins 2–4 drain via the left superior intercostal vein into the left brachiocephalic vein

3.6.6　The heart

The pericardium

✓ As an overview, take a minute to marvel over the functionality (purpose) of the pericardial sac and the pericardial cavity. This organ must dangle within sufficient space to allow it to undergo the wringing and squeezing movements associated with about 72 beats per minute for a lifetime. Thus the pericardial cavity containing the heart tube develops within a tough fibrous compartment that is lined with a delicate serous layer that lubricates itself and diminishes friction

Adult pericardial sac contains the heart and is comprised of 2 portions

✓ Outer layer of fibrous pericardium
  ◊ Is continuous with the adventitia (outer histological layer) of inflow and outflow vessels
  ◊ Completely partitions the inferior portion of the middle mediastinum from the abdominal cavity
  ◊ Is fused inferiorly to the central tendon of the diaphragm
  ◊ Is entirely unyielding (non-elastic)—this anatomical circumstance can be responsible for a potentially lethal condition—cardiac tamponade
  ◊ If the pericardial sac fills with fluid (pericardial effusion), it compresses the heart. To compensate, the heart beats faster and faster—tachycardia (in this instance) is an ineffective life-threatening response. Pericardiocentesis is an intervention whereby a needle is introduced into the pericardial sac and excessive fluid is aspirated. This is a risky procedure, since one must know the boundaries of the "bare area" of the heart where there is no intervening pleural sac. To puncture the pleural sac and deflate a lung would further endanger the patient
✓ The serous pericardium forms an inner lining within the tough fibrous pericardium and is further divided into
  ◊ A parietal layer
    ◆ This layer forms the lining of the pericardial sac
    ◆ This layer is a single transparent layer of serous secreting mesothelial cells
    ◆ This layer is tightly adherent to the fibrous pericardium
    ◆ At the locations where great vessels enter and leave the surface of the heart, this continuous layer coats the surface of these vessels and covers the surface of the heart
  ◊ A visceral layer
    ◆ Where this layer covers the surface of the heart, it is also known as the epicardial layer—immediately beneath this single layer of cells, one will note the accumulation of considerable fat. This is the anatomic region where one finds the coronary vessels
  ◊ Pericarditis—an acute inflammatory condition that causes these serous cells to secrete excessive fluid

Right and left phrenic nerves

✓ Functions
  ◊ Provide sensory innervation to:
    ◆ The central tendon of the diaphragm
    ◆ The mediastinal pleura
    ◆ The diaphragmatic pleura
    ◆ The pericardial sac (fibrous portion and parietal portion)
  ◊ Provide motor innervation to the posterior and central portions of the diaphragm
✓ These nerves are made of contributions from the cervical spinal cord at C_3, C_4, C_5
✓ These nerves pass through the neck (cervical) region and are considered a part of the cervical plexus

Embryological considerations

✓ These nerves migrated into the diaphragmatic muscles and established motor end plates during a very early stage of development
✓ In other words, these muscles became innervated when the mesoderm of the septum transversum was passing through the neck region during folding of the embryo

Mature location after developmental phases are completed
✓ Phrenic nerves became embedded on the outside surface of the fibrous pericardium
✓ These nerves are plastered (trapped) between the medially positioned fibrous pericardium and the laterally positioned parietal (mediastinal) pleura
✓ Phrenic nerves pass ventral (anterior) to the root of the lung
✓ Right phrenic nerve—in its course downward through the thoracic regions, it hugs the lateral surfaces of the right brachiocephalic vein, the superior vena cava, and the right atrium
✓ Left phrenic nerve—proceeds down the left side of the pericardium
Introduction to referred pain using the phrenic nerve as an example
✓ In addition to the phrenic nerves, other nerves also transmit sensory data back to the spinal cord segments at $C_3 - C_5$. These other sensory nerve territories for C_3, C_4, C_5 are found in the skin of the cervical region. The area of skin that is supplied by a specific spinal cord segment is known as a dermatome. Whenever a painful stimulus originates anywhere within the sensory distribution for C_3, the messages travel to the dorsal root ganglion cells at the C_3 level of the spinal cord. The brain which does not have a somatotopic map for visceral regions such as the pericardial sac and inner regions of the pleura or diaphragm then "senses" that there is a pain originating in the neck region along the C_3 nerve distribution. The inability of the brain to pinpoint exactly where the pain is originating produces a phenomenon known as referred pain
✓ Some examples of referred pain associated with the phrenic nerves
◊ A pain in the neck or upper shoulder region frequently occurs when CO_2 gas is introduced into the peritoneal cavity. This is a common procedure when surgeons are performing laproscopic procedures as they do during gall bladder surgery (cholecystecomy). After surgery some residual gas may remain. When a patient sits up in bed or begins to ambulate, gas rises along the inferior surface of the diaphragm where it irritates and can produce a temporary "pain the neck" that has nothing to do with muscular strain
◊ When there is a breach in the integrity of the digestive system and gastric contents, or pancreatic enzymes or pus accumulate on the inferior surface of the diaphragm, this too irritates the phrenic nerve and causes a "pain in the neck"
◊ When there is an accumulation of blood or infectious agents in the pericardium or in the pleura (supplied by the phrenic nerve), this is another cause for a refered pain in the neck or upper shoulder
Blood supply to the pericardial sac
Parietal layer
✓ Pericardiacophrenic arteries and veins. These are the main branches and are multiple
✓ These are branches from the right and left internal thoracic arteries and veins
◊ Small branches in the mediastinum provide secondary sources of blood and fluids. These spring from the bronchial, esophageal and superior phrenic arteries and veins
✓ Visceral layer (epicardium of the heart) is supplied/drained by coronary arteries and cardiac veins
Adult pericardial cavity
✓ A potential space between the visceral and parietal layers of serous pericardium
✓ Usually contains a small amount of fluid useful for reducing friction
✓ Once the pericardium is opened, 2 sinuses or recesses can be located

Pericardial sinuses

✓ Understanding of these is based on the embryological pattern of development. An understanding of these aids cardiac surgeons

Transverse sinus in the adult

✓ If at the upper end of the pericardial sac, you pass the index finger of your left hand anterior to the svc and curve it downward and push it toward the left. Your finger will pass posterior to the aorta and pulmonary artery and will appear on the left side of the pericardial sac. Your finger will be in the transverse sinus

✓ This circumstance occurs because the inflow and outflow vessels for the heart enter and exit from the fibrous pericardial sac at a fixed point. During development, the elongating heart tube is forced to twist and turn as it expands with the confines of the fibrous pericardial sac. Thus the outflow side of the heart tube (aorta + pulmonary trunk) comes to lies adjacent to one of the inflow vessels (superior vena cava). However close in proximity the final position of the inflow vessels and outflow channels come to each other, they always remain independent of each other and are coated with their original layer of serous or visceral pericardium

✓ This is a great spot to place a clamp on outflow vessels if you desire to pursue a career as a cardiothoracic surgeon. One day in the distant future, you may want to "cross-clamp" the aorta to stop the backflow of blood and remove the heart for a transplant or repair a traumatic hole or repair a dissecting aortic aneurisym. You may save a life if you remember this embryological oddity

◊ In the dissecting lab, you can reach into the transverse sinus, grab the outflow vessels and cut across them when you are ready to remove the heart for study purposes

Oblique sinus in the adult

✓ If you pass your hand under and upward behind the base of the heart like you were going to grasp and remove the heart, as your fingers touch the back wall of the pericardial sac, they will encounter the rest of the inflow vessels known as the pulmonary veins and inferior vena cava. This region is a cul-de-sac (in other words, your fingers won't pass through to the other side of the heart, because this is a blind ending)

✓ This is also one of those locations where the parietal pericardial layer becomes continuous with the vessels that enter the heart and changes its name to visceral pericardium

◊ In the dissecting lab, you will place a scalpel in the oblique sinus, sever the pulmonary veins and inferior vena cava as they run into the heart. The heart will fall into your hands and you can remove it from your cadaver for more in-depth study and dissection

Spatial boundaries of pericardial sac in the adult

The superior boundary (top of the pericardial sac)

✓ Is located at thesternal angle (this the junction between the manubrium and body of the sternum
✓ It is a radiographic landmark area at T_2—anteriorly
✓ If you take a transverse section at this horizontal level, it will intersect the disk space between T_4 and T_5 posteriorly

Lower boundary of the pericardial sac is permanently fused to the diaphragm

✓ This radiographic landmark is located at the T_8 level of the spinal column
✓ The pericardial sac at this level is pierced by the inferior vena cava

◊ Anterior surface of the pericardial sac
- ◆ Between the levels of T_2–T_4, the right and left parietal pleura is sandwiched behind the sternum and the anterior wall of the pericardial sac
- ◆ Thus if an assailant fired a bullet (made a sagittal entry wound) or a surgeon cut through the sternum with a bone saw, the right and left pleura sacs could be cut. This would introduce air into the pleural cavity and deflate the lungs before reaching the fibrous pericardial layer beneath
- ◆ Below T_4, the left pleural sac is pushed laterally by the large space occupied by the pericardium. This leaves a bare area of the pericardium, where there is no anterior overlap by the parietal pleura
- ◆ This is the region where the pericardial sac is entered during cardiac surgery or pierced during a pericardiocentesis procedure

◊ Posterior surface
- ◆ There will be another lecture on the contents of the posterior mediastinum
- ◆ The back wall of the pericardial sac contacts structures in the post mediastinum

◊ The contents of the pericardial sac
- ◆ The lower half of the superior vena cava—where the ascending aorta (contained within the pericardial cavity) exits the pericardial cavity, enters the superior mediastinum and becomes known as the aortic arch

External anatomy of the heart

✓ Apex—directed to the left, deep to the 5th left intercostal space at the mid-clavicular line
✓ Base—where the roots of the inflow vessels enter on the posterior aspect at T_5–T_8

Sternocostal (anterior) surface and borders

✓ When viewed from the front, the right ventricle makes up most of the anterior surface of the heart
✓ Posterior surface
  ◊ The left atrium and left ventricle make up most of the posterior aspect of the heart
✓ Diaphragmatic surface
  ◊ Is comprised of about 2/3 of the left ventricle and $1/3^{rd}$ of the right ventricle

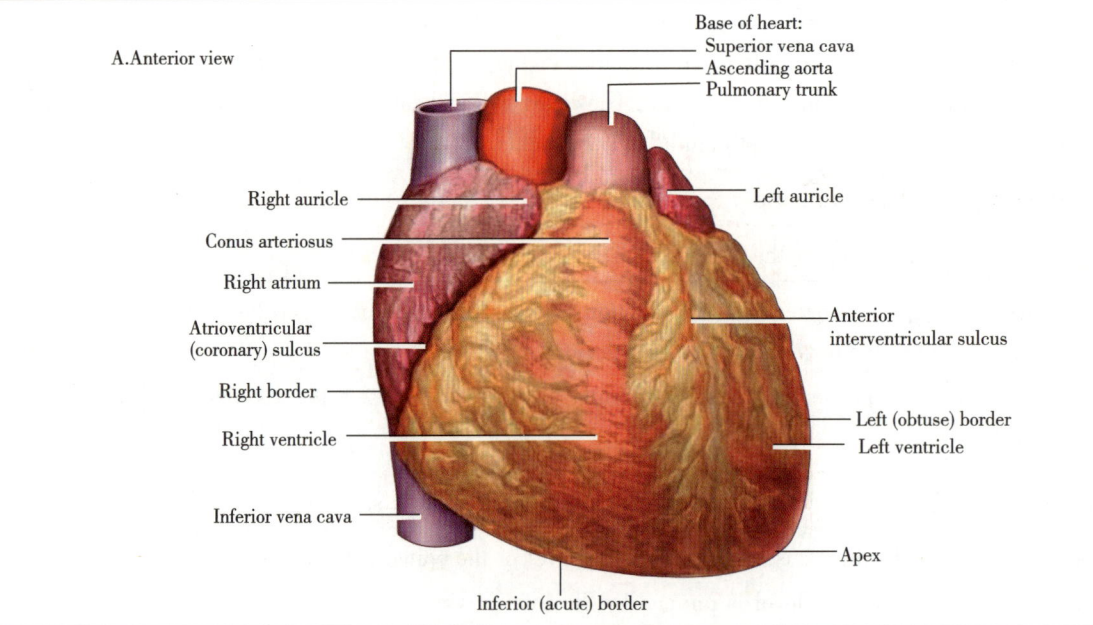

A. Anterior view

Base of heart:
- Superior vena cava
- Ascending aorta
- Pulmonary trunk

Right auricle
Conus arteriosus
Right atrium
Atrioventricular (coronary) sulcus
Right border
Right ventricle
Inferior vena cava
Inferior (acute) border
Left auricle
Anterior interventricular sulcus
Left (obtuse) border
Left ventricle
Apex

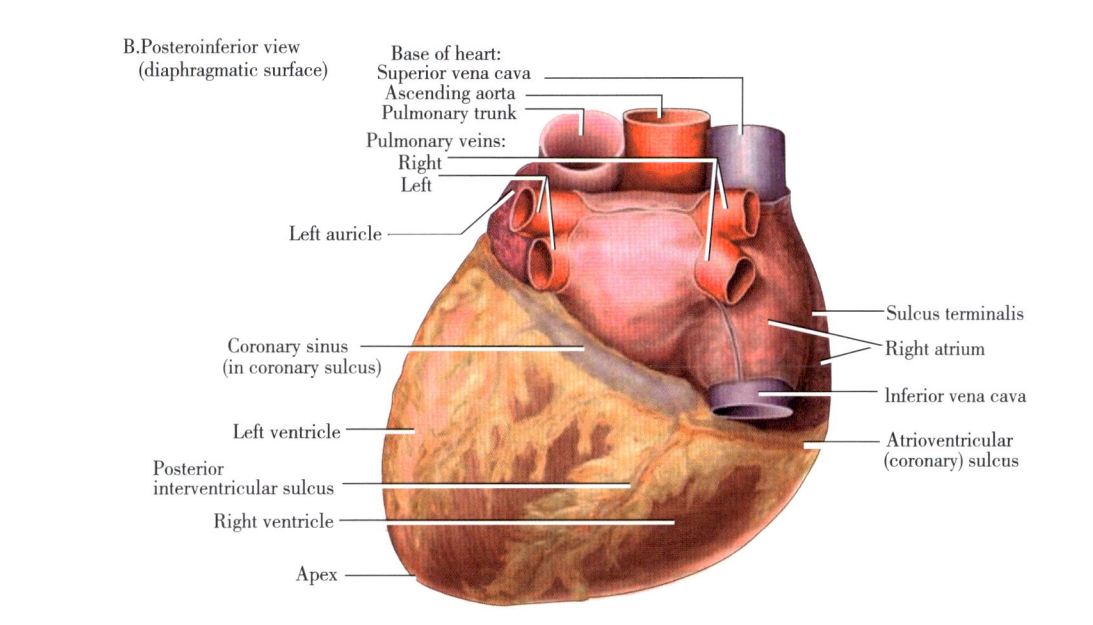

Atrioventricular sulcus or coronary sulcus

✓ Visualize a crown (left corona) around the heart
✓ Both atria are positioned above this sulcus (groove)
✓ Both ventricles are positioned below this sulcus
✓ This marks the separation between the superior atria and inferior ventricles
✓ Visualize where the original heart tube buckled and indented as it twisted
✓ This atrioventricular sulcus (deep groove) holds the right coronary artery, left coronary artery, circumflex artery and coronary sinus
✓ On the internal aspect of the heart, if you slice away the overlying atria and look at the interior of the heart you will note that all 4 heart valves are positioned on the same plane that is in the same plane as the atrioventricular sulcus

Interventricular sulcus

✓ The anterior portion of the sulcus continues as a posterior sulcus
✓ This is an external line of separation between the right and left ventricles
✓ It is formed as the original muscular septum grows upward separating a single ventricular chamber into 2 chambers, a right and left ventricle
✓ This groove holds the left anterior descending artery, great cardiac vein, middle cardiac vein
✓ These external surface features are not immediately visible on a cadaver heart. You will have to probe through considerable fat that obscures the coronary vessels. During life, this fat is at body temperature and is considerably more transparent and less rigid and fixed

Positional abnormalities

✓ The heart tube sometimes loops in the opposite direction to the normal pattern
✓ If this happens, the heart can be reversed in its location and the middle mediastinum protrudes more into the right side of the thorax. This condition is known as situs inversus

✓ Imagine how perplexed you would be as a pediatrician trying to listen to the heart and its valves in such a patient and only hearing air rushing in and out of the lungs. This is one of the reasons for knowing a bit of cardiac embryology

Vasculature of the heart

Arterial supply

Right coronary artery

✓ Begins in the coronary sinus of the ascending aorta immediately superior to the right aortic cusp
✓ Backfills from the ascending aorta during diastole when the myocardium is in a relaxed state and the aortic cusps are closed
✓ Note that it could not possibly fill during systole, because the right aortic cusp is flattened against the opening
✓ This vessel runs around the right side of the heart in the atrioventricular groove along with considerable fat and buried underneath the transparent visceral pericardial layer
✓ The artery to the sinuatrial node (sa node) is typically the first branch
   ▷ Occlusion in this vessel leads to ischemic damage to the heart's natural pacemaker cells
✓ Marginal branch—runs along the diaphragmatic surface where it typically supplies the right ventricular myocardium
✓ Posterior interventricular artery
   ▷ Is a continuation of the right coronary artery
   ▷ Sends off a branch supplying the av node in 85% of patients; thus this is another location where coronary artery occlusion can have a negative impact on heart rate
   ▷ Runs in the posterior interventricular groove, supplies the myocardium of the posterior right ventricle, frequently the atrioventricular node and the interventricular septum

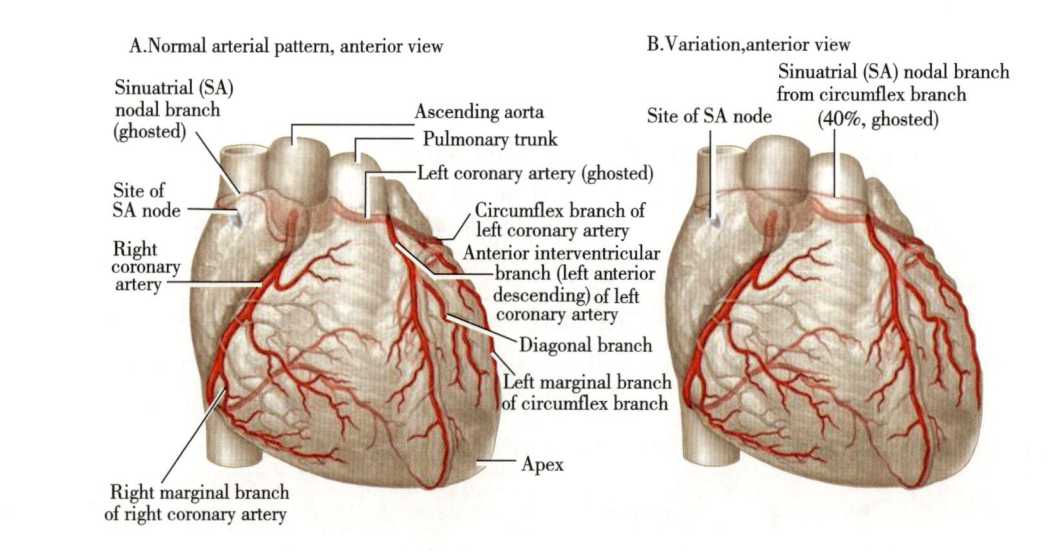

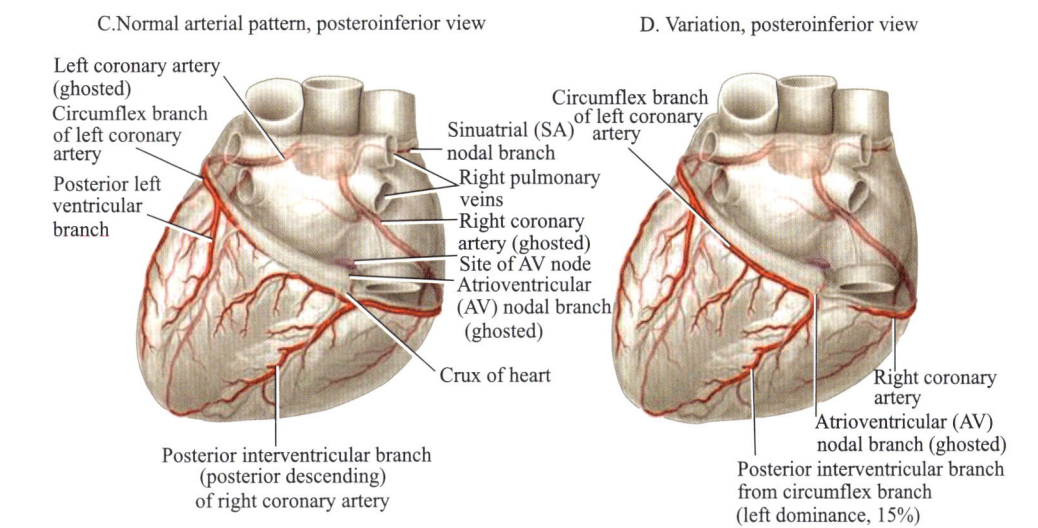

Left coronary artery

✓ Typically has 2 major branches
✓ Begins in the coronary sinus at the base of the ascending aorta immediately superior to the left aortic cusp
✓ Backfills from the ascending aorta during diastole when the myocardium is in a relaxed state and the aortic cusps are closed
✓ Left (anterior) interventricular artery or left anterior descending
  ◊ Supplies most of myocardium of the left ventricle, 2/3 of the interventricular wall
✓ Circumflex branch
  ◊ Encircles posteriorly in the atrioventricular (coronary) sulcus

Common sites of occlusion—leading to ischemia—myocardial infarction (MI)

✓ The most frequent site of coronary artery occlusion is the left anterior descending artery
  ◊ This vessel is a critical site since it supplies the left ventricle and interventricular septa
  ◊ This vessel is also critical since it supplies the crura of the atrioventricular bundle of his
✓ The second most common site of coronary artery disease is the right coronary artery
  ◊ This is also a critical vessel since it usually supplies the SA and AV nodes not to mention the right ventricular muscle

Common clinical cardiac procedures

✓ Angiographic studies—balloon angioplasty to remove plaque with or without stent placement
✓ Coronary artery bypass (abbreviated cab)
✓ Vascular grafts are typically harvested from saphenous veins, left internal mammary artery or radial artery
✓ Transesophageal echocardiograms. A probe is placed in the esophagus and dynamic videos of heart structure and function are obtained

Venous drainage of the heart itself—coronary sinus

✓ This is the largest vessel in the coronary drainage system
✓ This large collecting sinus empties into the right atrium

✓ This channel receives almost all the veins (except anterior cardiac veins, thebesian veins)
✓ This is a remnant of the left common cardinal vein from the embryo
✓ This is the embryological equivalent to the left superior vena cava. During development it typically regresses in size
✓ Sometimes it remains enlarged due the failure of the left brachiocephalic vein to develop a shunt returning blood toward the right side of the heart and into the typical adult svc (the right one)

Great cardiac vein

✓ Runs alongside the left anterior descending artery (LAD)
✓ This blood arrives in this area from the LAD and this is the outflowing drainage pattern for this arterial bed
✓ This large vein is embedded deep in the anterior interventricular sulcus

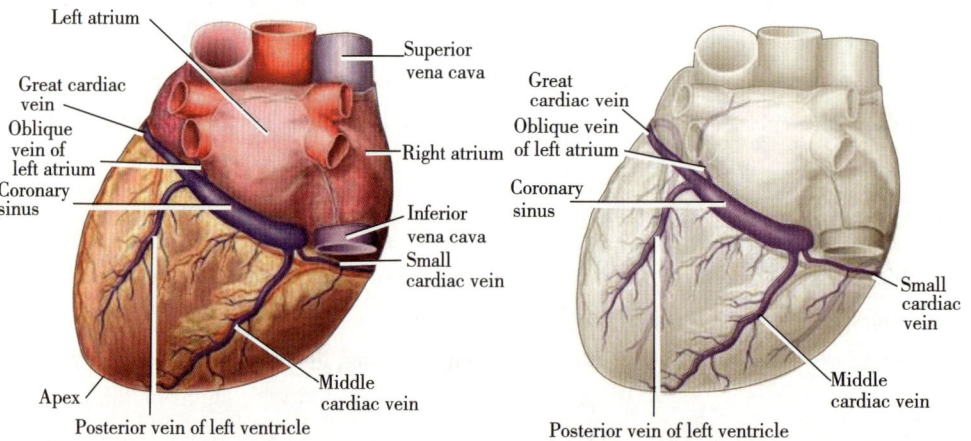

Middle cardiac vein

✓ Runs in posterior interventricular sulcus
✓ Drains the posterior ventricular structures
✓ Drains directly into the coronary sinus

Small cardiac veins

✓ Begin near the apex of the heart on the sternocostal surface
✓ Run posteriorly with the right coronary artery

Oblique vein (of marshall) on left atrium

✓ An embryological remnant of the left superior cardinal vein
✓ In lab look for its ligamentous connection with the left superior intercostal vein
✓ In rare cases, it remains a large vessel returning considerable blood volumes downward into the coronary sinus

The besian veins—venae cordis minimi—drain from the myocardium directly into the heart's chambers

✓ Have no valves
✓ Provide an important alternative route for coronary blood flow
✓ If a systemic artery (such as the left internal thoracic artery) is anastomosed into the coronary sinus, arterial blood can retrogradely flow into cardiac veins (since veins have no valves) and back into capillaries and thus nourish the myocardium. Venous blood can then mostly drain from the heart wall by the thebesian system which directly empties into the heart chambers and is carried away
  ◊ Anterior cardiac veins
✓ Also drain blood from the right ventricle directly into the right atrial chamber

Intermediate portions of the heart

Musculature of the heart

Myocardium

✓ The arrangement of the myocardial fibers is helical. There are 2 simple loops that were determined by unwinding the heart to resemble its early origins as a simple tube
✓ Myocardial cells in the atria have an intrinsic rate of contraction that differs from the myocardial cells found in the ventricles
✓ Myocardium takes its origin (attachments) from the skeleton of the heart
✓ The left side of the heart in the adult is the high pressure side; thus the musculature of the left ventricle is thicker and of greater mass

Specializations of cardiac muscle

✓ Pectinate muscles—restricted in location to the atria
✓ Trabecula carneae—restricted in location to the ventricles
✓ Papillary muscle—restricted in location to the ventricles
  ◊ This is a type of trabeculae
  ◊ A control mechanism that opens the tricuspid and mitral valves
  ◊ Receive direct innervation from the intrinsic system of the heart
  ◊ Arise from the ventricular wall (from the surface of the trabeculae carnae)
  ◊ Attach to the free edge of the valve leaflets by strong fibrous tissue bands known as the chordae tendineae

◆ Chordae tendineae cardiac muscle differentiates into a fibrous cord of connective tissue during the development of the heart
　　◆ These are like the cords of a parachute, with the leaflets of the valve being the parachute
　　◆ The chordae tendineae from the papillary muscle attach to the lateral edges of two adjacent leaflets
　　◆ After blood enters the ventricle through the atrioventricular valve, the ventricle will contract to increase the intraventricular pressure and thus "squeeze" the blood out either the aortic or pulmonary outlets. The increasing intraventricular pressure causes a backflow to accumulate against the underside of the leaflets, causing them to "snap" shut. The pressure continue to increase and would evert the leaflets into the atria (much like a cheap umbrella that gets destroyed in the wind) if it were not for the chordae tendineae attached to their free edges resisting such eversion. Those chordae tendineae that arise from papillary muscles produce active resistance since the papillary muscles contract as the ventricle contracts

Skeleton of the heart—fibrous trigone—annuli fibrosa

Composition

✓ Consists of fibrous connective tissue in the child. In later life this may become fibrocartilaginous tissue
✓ This material is ring-shaped and these rings are collectively known as annuli fibrosa
✓ There are 4 of these rings

Functions

✓ Keep the atrioventricular and semilunar ostia (openings) patent
✓ Prevent the collapse of these openings
✓ Provide attachment sites for the leaflets and cusps of the heart valves; hence all the valves are suspended from these 4 tough, fibrous rings of connective tissue
✓ Note their similarity to the plastic rings that hold together a 6-pack of drinks
✓ This skeleton serves as the origin and insertion for the myocardial fibers
✓ Function as electrical insulators, separating the electrical impulses that flow downward through the atrial myocardium from those that pass through the ventricular myocardium. Thus the atrial chambers contract slightly before the ventricles
✓ Provide passage for the atrioventricular bundles exiting from the atrioventricular node to carry the atrial conducting impulses to the ventricles

Internal anatomy of the heart

Right adult atrium

✓ The superior point of entry into this chamber is from the SVC (which contains no valves)
✓ Blood flow is directed downward into the right ventricle
✓ The sulcus terminalis is a groove on the outer surface of this chamber
✓ The crista terminalis is a raised internal ridge of myocardium that separates the smooth internal portion of the right atrium from the roughened pectinate muscles in the auricle
✓ Both of these structures mark the position of the original sinuatrial valve that developed in the heart tube between the sinus of the veins (sinus venosum) and the primitive atrium
✓ Sinus venarum—smooth part of the right atrium, embryological remnant of sinus venosum

✓ Auricle—rough area inside the right atrium, was the original atrium in the days of the original heart tube before it started buckling and twisting and remodeling itself

✓ Pectinate muscles [comb-like ridges of myocardium inside the original atrium (auricle)]

✓ Interatrial septum

  ◊ The left atrium is located on the other side of this rather thin septum

  ◊ The composition of the right and left side of this wall of tissue differ in their embryological origins

✓ The fossa ovalis is a depression in the interatrial septum

  ◊ The limbus fossa ovalis is a sharp crescent-shaped edge of the fossa ovalis that is also on the right side of the interatrial septum

  ◊ In the embryo, the right and left atria have a direct communication to each other

  ◊ At birth, the two flaps of the interatrial wall (the embryological remnants of the septum primum and the septum secundum) are pressed together by the increase in blood pressure. This obliterates the communication between the right and left atria

  ◊ In adults, a probe can be easily passed between these walls of tissue. This condition is called a patent fossa ovalis. It is present in 25% of cadavers in the laboratory

  ◊ When the interatrial septum is defective, this is known as anatrial septal defect (ASD). This allows for thrombi (which would normally be filtered in the pulmonary capillary beds) to enter the systemic circulation and travel to the brain causing a stroke

Valves of the right atrium

✓ Eustachian valve

  ◊ This is a flap of tissue (or valve of the IVC)

  ◊ It is an incomplete valve marking the opening of the inferior vena cava into the right atrium

  ◊ It is an embryological remnant of the valve of the sinus venosus

  ◊ In the embryo, it formerly directed blood toward the fossa ovalis and into the left atrium

✓ The besian valve

  ◊ Found at the opening of coronary sinus into the right atrium

  ◊ It is also a remnant of sinuatrial valve in the embryo

Sinuatrial node (sa node)

✓ The intrinsic pacemaker of the heart

✓ It is located near the cephalic end of the crista terminalis

✓ It is embedded in the heart wall near the junction of the auricle and the SVC

Right adult ventricle

✓ Right ventricle forms 2/3 of the sternocostal surface of the heart

✓ It has a thinner wall than the left ventricle

✓ Inflow into this chamber is conducted past the atrioventricular opening

✓ The opening into this chamber is guarded by a valve

Right atrioventricular valve—the tricuspid valve

✓ This valve is suspended from one of the annuli fibrosi

✓ You will observe the suspension of 3 bits of tissue attaching to this sturdy lip

- ✓ A posterior cusp of connective tissue
- ✓ A septal cusp of connective tissue (locted on the interventricular septum)
- ✓ An anterior cusp that is attached to the anterior wall of the right ventricle
- ✓ What is purpose of valves? (to keep blood from flowing back into the atrium)
- ✓ When do the valves close? (during ventricular systole)
- ✓ The closing (approximation) of atrioventricular valves produces a heart sound—the "lub" of lub-dub

Chordae tendineae—strings or cords of tough connective tissue that attach or tether the cusps to either papillary muscles or the intermuscular septum in the case of the septal cusp. If chordae were absent or didn't form, the cusps would blow back into the right atrium when the right ventricle contracts. Strings keep the valves tethered when the papillary muscle contracts

Septomarginal trabecula is also known as the moderator band. This bundle of myocardium quickly conducts nerve impulses to the anterior papillary muscle. This is a great design plan—it allows for the more distant anterior papillary muscle to be ready to contract in synchrony with remainder of the right ventricular myocardium

Trabeculae carneae—ridges of myocardium within the ventricles

Supraventricular crest

- ✓ Muscular ridge leading into the conus arteriosus outflow tract of the heart. This is located where the ridged muscular ventricular wall becomes a smooth pulmonary outflow tract
- ✓ The outflow pathway from the right ventricle above this area is guarded bysemilunar valves that lead into the pulmonary trunk
- ✓ Semilunar valves are 3 in number. There is an anterior cusp, a right cusp and a left cusp
- ✓ The leaflets of each cusp are semicircular pieces of connective tissue known as alunula
- ✓ The central portion of these cusps are thickened into nodules
- ✓ The semilunar valves close (fill like pockets) during diastole by the backflowing of blood
- ✓ The ventricles fill with blood during myocardial relaxation (diastole)

Pulmonary trunk

- ✓ This is the low resistance outflow tract from the right ventricle
- ✓ Blood is carried upward and digresses to either the right or left pulmonary artery
- ✓ Deoxygenated blood passes through this pathway on its way to the pulmonary capillary bed
- ✓ Dislodged clots from deep venous thrombosis (DVT) are trapped along this circuit
- ✓ If the thrombosis is large enough, it may wedge itself in the pulmonary trunk and the patient will die on the spot, because this will halt blood flow in the circulatory system

Clinical notes: Pulmonary valve stenosis or valvular incompetence. This condition results in a heart murmur due to turbulent blood flow. Stenosis eventually leads to hypertrophy of the right ventricle due to the extra work it must perform. If prolonged, the heart becomes inefficient in its stroke volume and congestive heart failure ensues

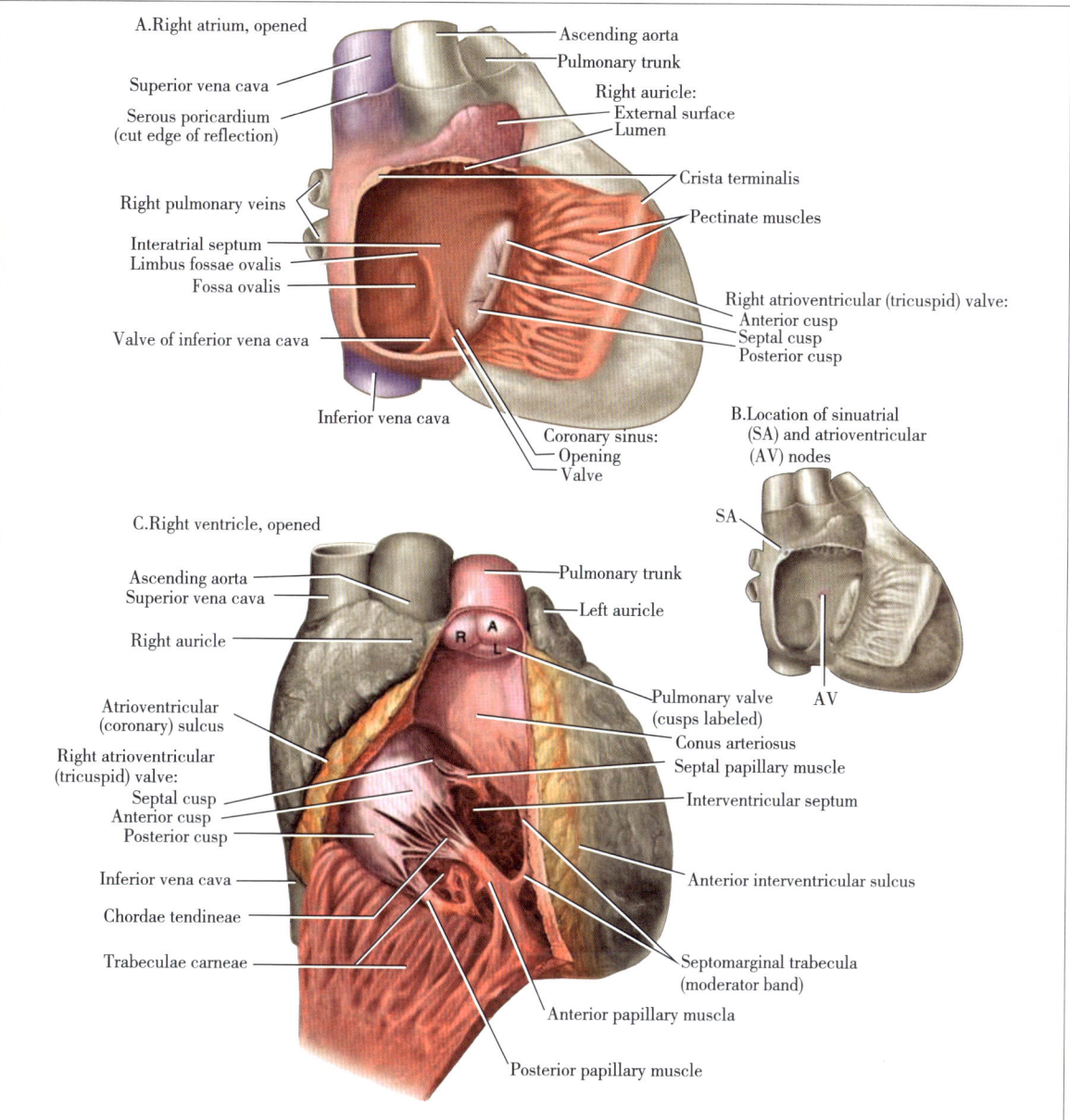

Left atrium

Auricle

✓ Pectinate muscles—identify the rough portion of the original atrium during the heart tube stage
✓ Smooth portion is where the pulmonary veins were incorporated into the heart wall
✓ This chamber rests up against the esophagus

Interatrial septa

✓ Thin area over fossa ovalis, this is where ASD are located due to the frequent failures due to the complex partitioning pattern of the original single atrium
✓ At birth, when a baby takes its first breath, the pulmonary resistance decreases, blood flows into the lungs and returns into the left atrium. Thus left atrial pressure ↑ and the thin septum primum is shoved up against the septum secundum. This serves as a shut-off valve between the right and left atrium
✓ The clinical consequences of ASD are many. Ex: if blood clots from the legs (from deep venous thrombosis) are returned toward the heart, normally they become clogged in the progressively smaller pulmonary arteries. If an ASD is present, clots slip directly from the right atrium into the left atrium and

then the left ventricle. They are likely to be transported upward to the brain resulting in a cerebrovascular accident (stroke)

Left ventricle

✓ Has the thickest wall (myocardium) of all the chambers
✓ Blood enters by passing through the left atrioventricular opening that guards the opening between the left atrium and left ventricle
✓ This opening can be closed by the action of the mitral valve
  ◊ The mitral valve is a bicuspid valve (anterior and post cusps)
  ◊ It is the valve that is most likely to be affected by disease
  ◊ Mitral valve stenosis or insufficiency can be repaired by placement of a porcine graft or replacement with a valve prosthesis

Chordae tendineae—each attach to a papillary muscle

Trabeculae carneae—randomly patterned raised myocardium inside the chamber

Interventricular septum

✓ Structure forms the walls between the right and left ventricles
✓ It contains thick muscular and thin membranous portions
✓ There is an embryological basis for this anatomical curiosity
✓ Pars muscularis or muscular portion is the thick inferior portion and was derived from the original interventricular septal material
✓ Pars membranacea is the thinner portion that develops at a much later time during the development of the heart. It is subject to frequent congenital malformations known as ventricular septal defects
  ◊ There are two further regions to the membraneous area within the center of the heart. This thin portion is interpositioned and forms a small part of the lower right atrium, upper right ventricle and upper left ventricle. One can take a flashlight and shine it in the upper left ventricle wall and see the glow of the light through either the right atrium (or the right upper ventricle)

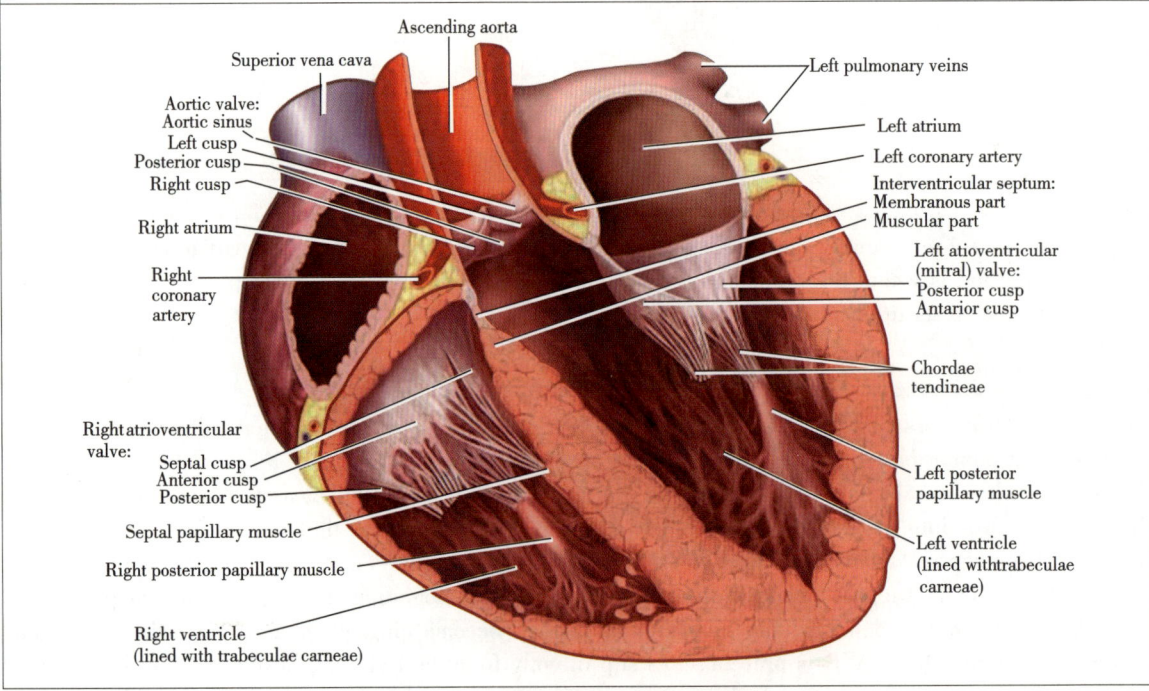

Aortic vestibule—a superior outflow tract that is smooth walled and leads into the aorta (a vestibule is the anteroom before entering the house)
- Aortic orifice
  - Is surrounded by another fibrous ring of the annulus fibrosus
  - The 3 semilunar valves (cusps) are located at this spot
- Aortic sinuses
  - When the blood rushes back during diastole and gets trapped in the cusps of the semilunar valves, the pressure causes dilation in the aortic wall above each cusp that is known as an aortic sinus

Ascending aorta

- Begins at the aortic orifice and continues upward as the aorta passes outside of the pericardial sac. At this point the vessels become known as the arch of the aorta
- This portion of the aorta is exposed to the strongest pressures and is a frequent site for an aortic aneurysm. If this ruptures through the aortic wall, the pericardial sac instantly fills with blood, the pumping action of the heart is hindered, blood pressure plummets and the patient dies

Innervation of the heart

- Intrinsic system
  - Cardiac muscle has the ability to contract when grown under in vitro conditions
  - The myocytes in each chamber develop their own intrinsic contraction rate
  - I.e., the atrial muscle cells contract at a different rate than the ventricular muscle cells
  - During fibrillation, the normal coordinated contraction pattern is replaced with a rapid irregular twitching that does not maintain the normal circulatory output
- The conducting system
  - Begins in the sinuatrial node
    - This region is called the pacemaker of the heart
    - These cells have an intrinsic set rhythm
    - They cannot be visualized in the gross anatomy laboratory
    - Electrical currents are propagated from these cells downward through the atrial wall to the atrioventricular (AV) node
  - The atrioventricular node—located in the floor of the right atrium
    - Specifically, it is embedded in the cardiac tissue above the opening to the coronary sinus and above the opening to the right ventricle
    - Fibers exiting the AV node skirt the border of the membranous septum
    - These fibers pierce the right trigone region of the annulus fibrosus
    - These fibers proceed downward as theatrioventricular bundle of his

Clinical notes: Cardiac surgeons must take special care to avoid placing a suture through this conducting pathway during a VSD repair

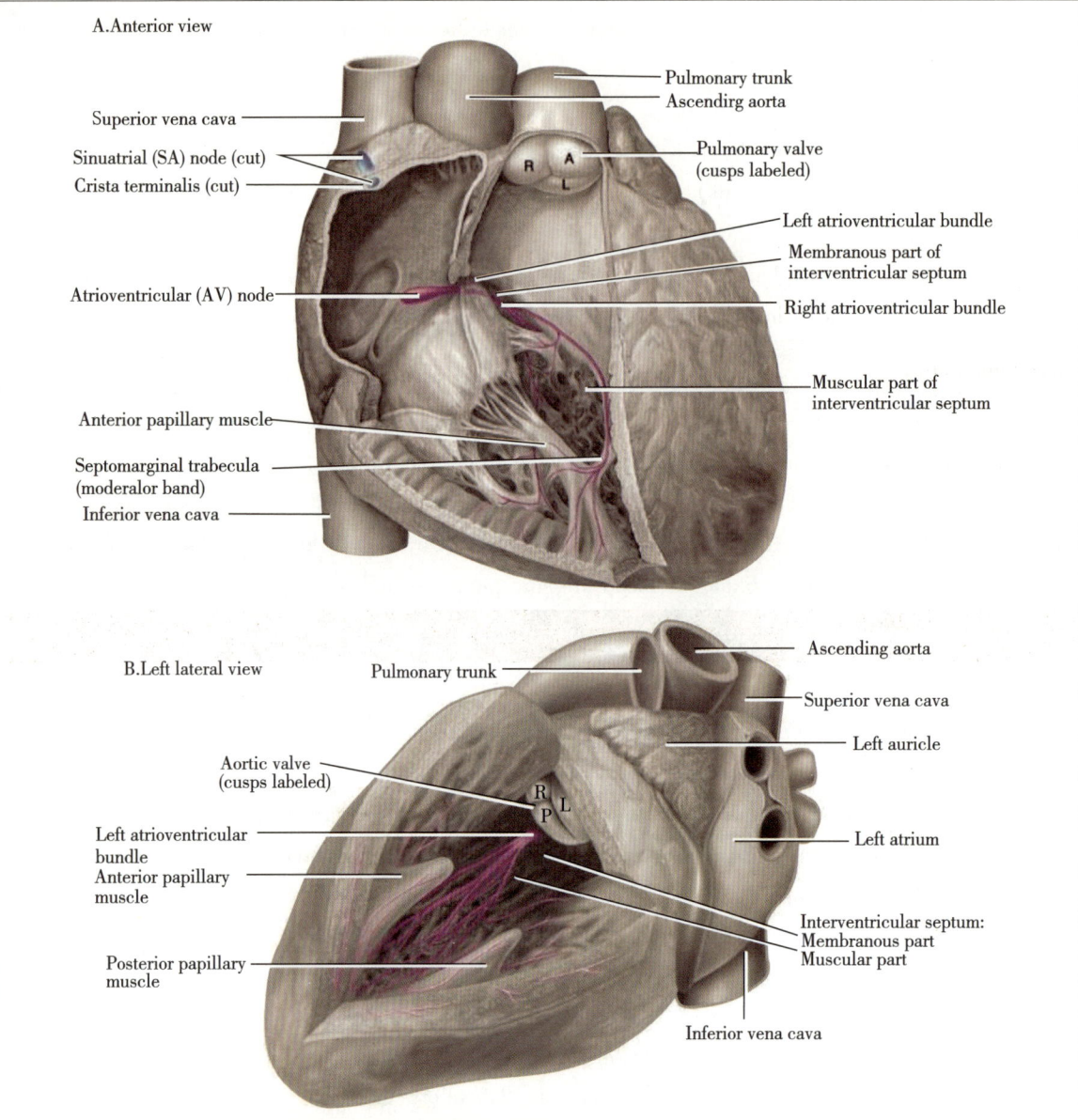

A. Anterior view
B. Left lateral view

The atrioventricular bundle fibers

✓ Branch into right and left crura (legs) that run through the interventricular septum
✓ The right crus transmits the electrical current to the right ventricular muscle and
✓ The left crus transmits the electrical current to the left ventricular muscle
✓ In the right ventricle an additional band can be noted
✓ This is the so called moderator band orseptomarginal trabecula
✓ This particular trabecula is enlarged and was judged by anatomists to be worthy of naming. It extends as a free bundle across the right ventricular cavity near the apex and contains a special bundle of fibers
✓ This is a great design plan. It allows for anterior papillary muscles to be ready to contract simultaneously in coordination with the whole of the ventricular musculature

Purkinje cells (or subendocardial branches of the av bundle)

✓ These are the terminal cells in the conducting system
✓ The atrioventricular bundle fibers branch and give rise to these

✓ They are too tiny to see with the naked eye on your cadaver
✓ They are distributed throughout the ventricular wall

Extrinsic system (autonomic input)

Sympathetic system

✓ Sympathetic input arrives at the heart from a variety of directions

✓ Cervical contributions

◊ Cervical cardiac branches are grey rami that descend through the neck region

◊ Their preganglionic cell bodies reside in the IML at T_1–T_6

◊ Their postganglionic cell bodies reside in the cervical sympathetic ganglion at either the superior, middle or inferior cervical sympathetic ganglion

◊ Once synapses occur, this fine meshwork of nerves travel downward as the superior, middle and inferior cervical cardiac branches

◊ These autonomic connections synapse on the sinuatrial node as well as on the major arteries in the thorax

✓ Thoracic contributions

◊ Cardiopulmonary splanchnic nerves

◊ Their preganglionic cell bodies reside in the IML at T_1–T_6

◊ They travel outward through the ventral root and continue into sympathetic ganglia

◊ After synapsing the postganglionic fibers travel toward the viscera and become part of the cardiac and pulmonary plexi

✓ Systemic contributions

◊ Arrive through the bloodstream in the form of the circulating hormones known as epinephrine and norepinephrine

◊ The preganglionic cell bodies reside in the IML at T_5–T_9

◊ The fibers travel out through ventral roots and do not stop to synapse on the sympathetic ganglion cells in the region

◊ Instead they continue downward as greater splanchnic nerves that pierce through the diaphragm and synapse on chromaffin cells in the adrenal medulla

◊ These cells release adrenaline into the venous circulation and immediately return to the heart through the inferior vena cava pass through the heart and out and bind to receptors on smooth muscle and on the sinuatrial node

◊ This is the only mechanism by which heart transplant patients can increase their heart rate when they are planning to exercise. They have to play some mind games to stimulate the adrenal medulla to release these circulating levels. Otherwise, their cardiac output will not increase in response to exercise and they will faint

Parasympathetic system

✓ Right and left vagus nerves are the sole suppliers for this contrasting part of the autonomic nervous system in the thorax

✓ These nerves are part of the craniosacral outflow system

✓ Specifically the cell bodies for the vagus nerves arise in the brainstem

✓ These nerves (the presynapatic fibers) pass down through the neck and thorax to their final destination on small ganglia (postsynaptic cell bodies) along the upper 2/3 of the gastrointestinal tract

✓ As they pass through the thoracic region they emit superior and inferior cardiac (presynaptic fibers) nn as well as one or more thoracic branches to other structures in this region

✓ These presynaptic neurons (that are quite lengthy) then synapse on clusters of postsynaptic cell bodies that reside within the walls of the great vessels, coronary vessels and on the sinuatrial node. Thus postsynaptic neurons in the parasympathetic system are typically short in length

Sensory input and the visceral afferent messages from the heart

When the myocardium does not receive sufficient oxygen, it becomes ischemic and noxious stimuli travel back to the spinal cord like any other sensory stimuli

✓ These afferent (sensory) messages from the viscera (heart and great vessels) travel back to spinal cord segments along the various sympathetic nerve routes

✓ Once these sensory messages converge on the dorsal root ganglion (for example: the T_1 spinal cord level), they become mixed with sensory messages from the T_1 cutaneous (dermatome) distribution

✓ The brain doesn't have a somatotopic map for the heart. Amazingly there is no place in your brain to interpret a pain in the heart! Thus, no patient will be able to tell you that they have a pain in the left coronary artery and that this vessels is occluded or in spasm

✓ However, people who are experiencing transient ischemia in the heart muscle usually experience a pain in the skin over their left chest wall, down the medial side of their arm (an ulnar distribution), and sometimes in the left cervical region and mandible. If this pain subsides when the patient rests for a few minutes or when they swallow a nitroglycerin tablet to dilate their coronary arteries, this pain is called angina pectoris

✓ If the patient experiences a crushing and unremitting pain in this same cutaneous distribution that does not subside in a few minutes, the patient is experiencing a serious myocardial infarction and is likely having a heart attack

✓ The cutaneous distribution of the pain is yet another example of a referred pain. The noxious sensory information is confused by the brain and is "felt" by the patient in the region of dermatomes T_1-T_4

✓ While you are learning the classical pain symptoms associated with a myocardial infarction (MI), please also learn that there is a wide variation in the pain response mechanism. For some reason which is unknown at this time, women who are experiencing an MI do not always display these classic signs and may only report a shortness of breath and a general feeling of malaise. There are also some minor cross-over connections in some patients and their pain will be experienced on the right side or on the back

✓ Human variation is the norm. This is a major anatomical principle that is as important to learn as the host of specifics

Chen Yiyong, Cheng Jiamao, Zhang Yanru

Chapter 4

The Abdomen

4.1 Introduction

The abdomen is the middle portion of the trunk between the thorax and the pelvis. It consists of three parts, i.e., the abdominal wall, the peritoneum and the abdominal organs.

4.1.1 The boundaries of the abdomen

On the surface of the trunk, the abdomen is bounded superiorly by the lower margin of the thoracic cage, and inferiorly, by the upper margin of the bony pelvis roughly (Figure 4-1).

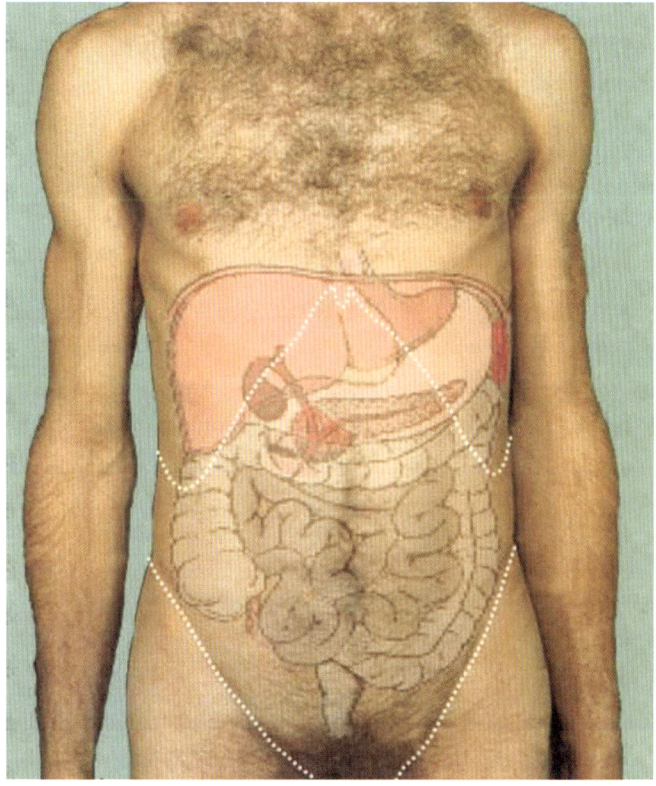

Figure 4-1 The boundaries of the abdomen

Internally, the abdominal cavity is separated from the thoracic cavity by the diaphragm. The diaphragm is a dome-like flat muscle. Its peripheral part attaches along the lower margin of the thoracic cage, but its central part extends superiorly into the thoracic cage and reaches the level of the 5th rib. Thus the roof of the abdominal cavity is, in fact, higher than the external boundary of the abdomen. For this reason, several abdominal organs beneath the diaphragm, such as the liver, the spleen, and the kidneys, are completely or partly located within the thoracic cage. This is clinically important because in some cases of violence-caused thoracic injuries, these abdominal organs may be involved. For example, a rib fracture in the left thoracic wall may injure not only the pleura and the left lung, but also the spleen, leading to severe dyspnea and intra-abdominal bleeding.

4.1.2 The regions of the abdomen

Topographical divisions of the abdomen are used to describe the location of the abdominal organs and the pain associated with abdominal problems. The two schemes most often used are a four-quadrant pattern, and a nine-region pattern (Figure 4-2).

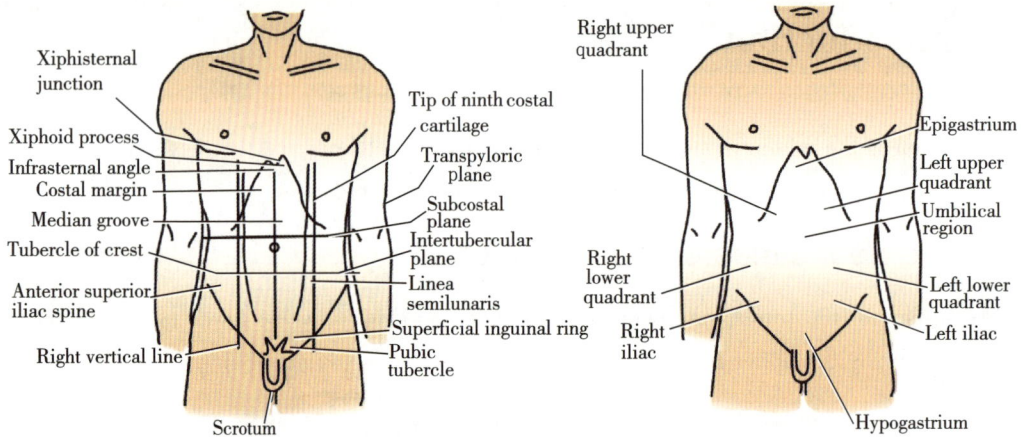

Figure 4-2 Body landmarks and regions of the anterior abdominal wall

(1) Nine-region pattern

For the descriptive purpose, the abdomen is sub-divided into nine regions by four planes (two transverse and two sagittal). One of the two transverse planes passes through the lowest points of the costal arches and is called the subcostal plane. Note, however, that sometimes the thanspyloric plane, halfway between the jugular notch and the symphysis pubis or halfway between the umbilicus and the inferior end of the body of the sternum, intersecting with the costal margin at the ends of the ninth costal cartilages, is used instead. The other transverse plane passes through the two iliac tubercles, called the intertubercular plane. The two sagittal planes pass through the mid-point of the inguinal ligament on ether sides. Between the two sagittal planes, there are three regions. From above downwards, they are defined as the epigastric, umbilical and hypogastric regions, respectively; lateral to each sagittal plane and from above downwards, are the right or left hypochondriac, lumbar and iliac regions.

(2) Four-quadrant pattern

A horizontal transumbilical plane passing through the umbilicus and intersecting with the vertical median plane divides the abdomen into four quadrants: the right upper, left upper, right lower, and left lower quadrants.

4.1.3 Surface anatomy of the abdomen

On the surface of the abdomen, there are several important landmarks, including bony landmarks and soft landmarks (Figure 4-3). You should identify them on the cadaver before the dissection.

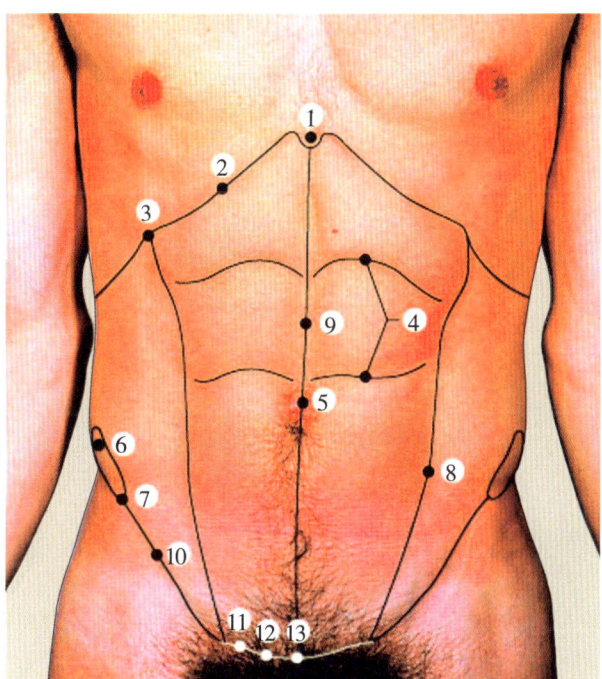

1—xiphoid process; 2—costal arches or costal margins; 3—9th costal cartilage; 4—the tendinous intersections; 5—umbilicus; 6—tubercle of the iliac crest; 7—anterosuperior iliac spine; 8—linea semilunaris; 9—linea alba; 10—inguinal fold; 11—pubic tubercle; 12—pubic crest; 13—pubic symphysis.

Figure 4-3 Surface anatomy of the abdomen

4.1.3.1 Bony landmarks

(1) Xiphoid process

It lies in a depression at the apex of the subcostal angle, opposite the level of T_9.

(2) Pubic symphysis

It connects the symphysial surfaces of the pubis of both sides, lying at the level of the coccyx.

(3) Costal arches or costal margins

They are formed by the 7th-10th costal cartilages, respectively, and reach their lowest level (10th costal cartilage) in the midaxillary line.

(4) Infrasternal or subcostal angle

It is formed between the right and left costal margins.

(5) Iliac crest

It forms the lower limit of the abdominal wall at the side. Its highest point lies at the level of L_4 slightly below the normal level of umbilicus.

(6) Anterosuperior iliac spine

It is the anterior end of the iliac crest, lying at the level of the sacral promontory.

(7) Tubercle of the iliac crest

It is situated on the outer lip of the iliac crest about 5 cm behind the anterior superior iliac spine.

4.1.3.2 Soft landmarks

(1) Inguinal fold

It extends from the anterior superior iliac spine to the pubic tubercle, placed at the junction of the anterior abdominal wall with the front of thigh, overlying the inguinal ligament.

(2) Linea alba

It is marked by a vertical groove (median furrow) which divides the anterior abdominal wall into the right and left halves.

(3) Umbilicus

It lies a little below the middle of the median furrow at the level of the junction between the third and fourth lumbar vertebrae.

(4) Linea semilunaris

It is a few centimeters lateral to the median furrow, showing a curved vertical groove, extending from the costal margin at the tip of 9th costal cartilage to the pubic tubercle. It corresponds to the lateral margin of the rectus abdominis.

(5) Three transverse furrows

They may be seen crossing the upper part of the rectus abdominis, and correspond to the tendinous intersections of the muscle. One lies opposite the umbilicus, the other opposite the free end of xiphoid process, and the third lies midway between the former two.

(6) McBurney's point

It lies at the junction of lateral one-third and medial two-thirds of the line joining the right anterior superior iliac spine to the umbilicus, corresponding, roughly, to the position of the base of appendix.

4.2　The anterolateral abdominal wall and the inguinal region

For descriptive purpose, the abdominal wall is divided into two parts by two post-axillary lines. The front part is called the anterolateral abdominal wall and the back part, the posterior abdominal wall. In comparison to the posterior wall, the anterolateral abdominal wall is much thinner and devoid of bony structures. Therefore it provides a convenient approach to access the abdominal organs in surgery.

4.2.1　The anterolateral abdominal wall

The anterolateral abdominal wall consists of six layers with different tissue components (Figure 4-4). From superficial to deep, they are the skin, the superficial fascia, the muscular layer, the transverse fascia, the extraperitoneal fascia and the parietal peritoneum. The superficial fascia is composed of loose connective tissues rich in the fat, so it is also called the "subcutaneous fatty tissue". The muscular layer is formed by four pairs of flat muscles. In each side the rectus abdominis muscle lies along the median line, and lateral to it are three flat muscles, the external oblique, the internal oblique and the transversus abdominis muscles. The fascia transversalis is a part of the endoabdominal fascia, which lines the inner surface of the muscular layer. The extraperitoneal fascia is not a layer of membrane; it is, in fact, a potential space between the transverse fascia and the parietal peritoneum, and is filled by a thin layer of cotton-like loose connective tissue. Therefore in surgery, it is usually called the "extraperitoneal space". The parietal peritoneum is a serous membrane that forms the innermost layer of the abdominal wall.

Among these six layers, the superficial fascia and the muscular layer contain important blood vessels and nerves, and their components vary upon different areas. These are key factors in selection of an abdominal incision for operations. Thus, in this section, we'll focus on these two layers.

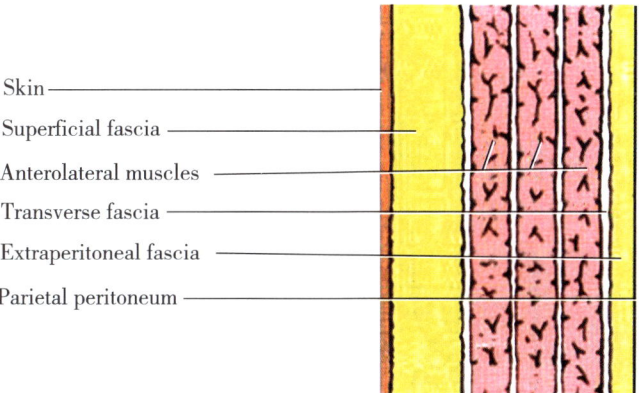

Figure 4-4 Layers of the anterolateral abdominal wall

4.2.1.1 Superficial structures

(1) The skin

The skin of the anterolateral abdominal wall contains more elastic fibers. Surgeons use the skin flap with vessels for plastic surgery.

(2) The superficial fascia

The superficial fascia is composed of loose connective tissues rich in fat. That is why surgeons usually call it "the subcutaneous fatty tissue". In this layer, there are numerous superficial veins, small arteries and cutaneous nerves that supply both the superficial fascia and the skin.

1) Features of the superficial fascia below the umbilicus

A very important feature of the superficial fascia in the anterolateral abdominal wall is that below the level of umbilicus, the fascia is divided into two layers: a superficial fatty layer called Camper's fascia, and a deep membranous layer called Scarpa's fascia (Figure 4-5). The Camper's fascia is a part of the subcutaneous fatty tissue all over the body. However, a membranous layer of the superficial fascia in human body appears only in a few regions. In addition to the lower part of the anterolateral abdominal wall, the membranous layer can be seen in the penis, the scrotum and the perineum. In each of these regions, the membranous layer has its own special name. In the lower part of the anterolateral abdominal wall, as mentioned above, it is called Scarpa's fascia; in the penis, it is called the superficial fascia of penis; in the scrotum, it is termed as the dartos scrotum because the membrane contains sparsely distributed smooth muscle cells; and in the perineum, it is called Colle's fascia (superficial perineal fascia). The membraneous layers of the superficial fasia in all of these regions are continuous. In the median plane of the trunk, we can see that the Scarpa's fascia continues with the superficial fascia of the penis, and the latter, with the scrotal dartos that extends posteriorly, becoming the Colle's fascia.

In dissection, there is a very important step to verify the continuation of Scarpa's fascia. You can cut the two layers of the superficial fascia transversely at the level 5 cm below the umbilicus; insert one of your finger deep to Scarpa's fascia and then push your finger inferiorly along deep surface of the Scarpa's fascia, you will find that your fingers can reach the scrotum, because the Scarpa's fascia and the scrotal dartos are continuous. But if you change the direction of your finger and go towards the thigh, your fingers can reach only 1 or 2 cm below the inguinal ligament. This is because the Scarpa's fascia is fused into the fascia lata at this level. The continuation of Scarpa's fascia are clinically important in diagnosis of the injury to the bulbar part of the urethra. You have learned that the posterior end of the sponge or penile part of urethra is slightly expanded and called the urethral bulb. It is located in a fascial space called the superficial perineal pouch that is just deep to Colle's fascia. If the urethra in the bulb is injured, the urine leaks directly into the pouch. And then conducted by the continuous membranous layer, the urine extends into the scrotum, the penis, and the lower part of the anterior abdominal wall. This causes obvious edema in the areas involved— a special sign for the injury to the bulb of the urethra.

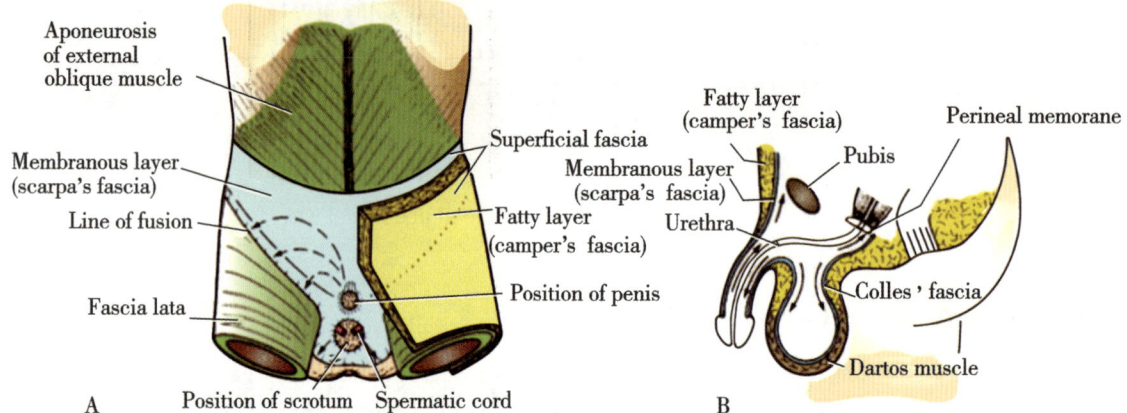

A. Note the line of fusion between the membranous layer and the deep fascia of the thigh or the fascia lata; B. Note the attachment of the membranous layer to the posterior margin of the perineal membrane. Arrows indicate paths taken by the urine in cases of ruptured urethra.

Figure 4-5 Arrangement of the fatty layer and the membranous layer of the superficial fascia in the lower part of the anterior abdominal wall

2) Superficial veins

When the skin is removed, you can see numerous superficial veins in the exposed fatty tissue. These veins run tortuously and anastomose to form a network around the umbilicus. This network is called the periumbilical venous plexus (Figure 4-6). Superiorly, the periumbilical venous plexus drains into the axillary vein through the thoracoepigastric and then the lateral thoracic veins; inferiorly, the plexus is drained by two tributaries of the greater saphenous vein: the superficial epigastric vein and the superficial circumflex iliac vein. As you have already learned, the axillary vein belongs to the superior vena cava system and the greater saphenous vein, to the inferior vena cava system. Thus, the periumbilical venous plexus is one of the most important communicating pathways between the two venous systems. In addition, the periumbilical venous plexus is drained by the paraumbilical vein to the hepatic portal vein. So the plexus is one of the important sites for the porto-systemic anastomosis.

3) Superficial arteries

Most of the arteries in the superficial fascia of the anterolateral abdominal wall are very small and are not accompanied by veins. So they are not easy to be recognized by naked eye in a cadaver. However, in the lower part of the wall, there are two arteries: the superficial epigastric artery that runs superomedially towards the umbilicus, and the superficial circumflex iliac artery that distributes along the inguinal ligament. Both arteries are the branches of the femoral artery and are accompanied by the same-named

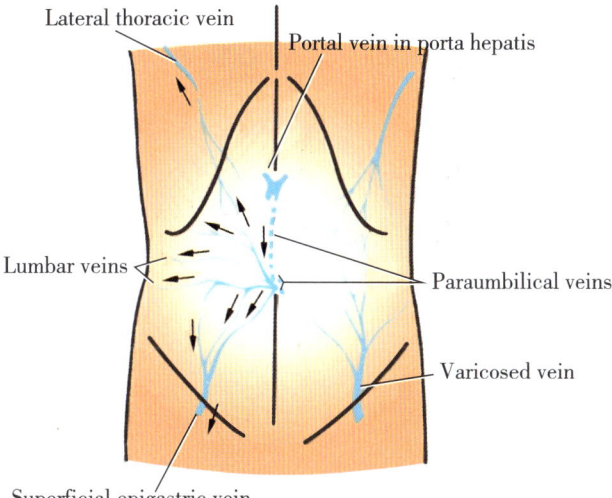

Figure 4-6 Superficial veins of the anterior abdominal wall

(On the right are anastomoses between systemic veins and the portal vein via paraumbilical veins. Arrows indicate the direction taken by venous blood when the portal vein is obstructed. On the left is an enlarged anastomosis between the lateral thoracic vein and the superficial epigastric vein. This occurs if either the superior or the interior vena cava is obstructed)

veins, the superficial epigastric vein and the superficial circumflex iliac vein. So they can be recognized with their accompanying veins as reference. You know, the lower part of the anterolateral abdominal wall is a private part of the body, and you just learned that its skin is supplied by the arteries with accompanying veins. For the two reasons, the lower part of the anterolateral abdominal wall is a perfect donor area for the skin flaps with pedicle in plastic surgery.

4) Superficial lymphatics

Above the level of the umbilicus, the lymphatics run upwards to drain into the axillary lymph nodes. Below the level of the umbilicus, they run downwards to drain into the superficial inguinal lymph nodes.

5) Cutaneous nerves

The nerves in the superficial fascia of the anterolateral abdominal wall are the cutaneous branches from the $7^{th}-12^{th}$ thoracic nerves and the 1st lumbar nerve (Figure 4-7). These branches are distributed over the abdominal wall in a "segmental manner". Here, the segmental manner means that each pair of the cutaneous branches supply a band-like area, and all the areas are arranged one by one from above downwards; but there are some degree of overlap between the adjacent bands. Usually, the cutaneous branches of the 6th thoracic nerve are distributed over a band-like area at the level of the xiphoid process, those of the 8th thoracic nerve, at the level of the costal arch, and those of the 10th thoracic nerve, at the level of the umbilicus. The cutaneous branches of the 1st lumbar nerve are distributed just above the inguinal ligament or at the level of the pubic symphysis. Because the areas supplied by the adjacent nerves are partly overlapped, an injury of one or two cutaneous nerves during the abdominal operations does not obviously affect the sensations of the skin.

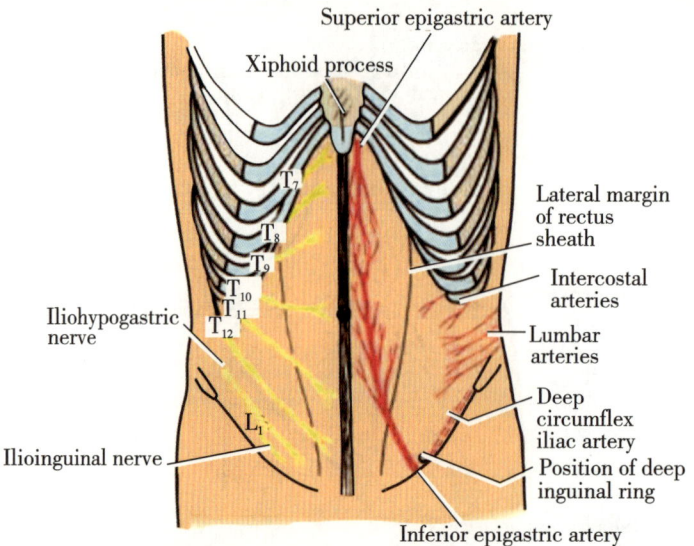

Figure 4-7 Segmental innervation of the anterior abdominal wall (right) and arterial supply to the anterior abdominal wall (left)

4.2.1.2 The muscular layer and deep vessels and nerves

(1) Muscles of the anterolateral abdominal wall

The muscular layer of the anterolateral abdominal wall is composed of four muscles on each side, i. e., the rectus abdominis, the external oblique, the internal oblique and the transversus abdominis muscles (Table 4-1).

(2) The rectus abdominis muscle and the rectus sheath

The rectus abdominis muscle has a long strip-like shape with three or four tendinous intersections (Figure 4-8). And lateral to it are three flat muscles. From surperficial to deep, they are the external oblique, the internal oblique and the transversus abdominis muscles. Near the lateral margin of the rectus abdominis muscle, all of these three flat muscles become aponeuroses that enclose the rectus muscle to form a sheath called the rectus abdominis sheath.

The anterior wall of the rectus abdominis sheath is complete and is firmly adherent to the tendinous intersections of the rectus muscle, while its posterior wall is incomplete above the costal margin and below the arcuate line (Figure 4-9). As you can see in the transverse section of the abdominal wall above the umbilicus, the external oblique aponeurosis contributes to the anterior wall of the sheath, the transverse abdominal aponeurosis, to the posterior wall; while the internal oblique aponeurosis splits at the lateral border of the rectus muscle and contributes to both the anterior and posterior walls. However, if we make a transverse section of the anterior abdominal wall above the costal margin, we will find that the anterior wall of the sheath is formed by the external oblique aponeurosis, but the posterior wall is deficient. The rectus muscle rests directly on the 5th, 6th and 7th costal cartilages. If we make a transverse section through the lower part of the anterolateral abdominal wall, we will find that all of the three aponeuroses pass over the anterior surface of the rectus muscle. This means the posterior wall of the rectus abdominis sheath disappears. Usually, at the level of 3 to 4 cm below the umbilicus, we can see the free lower edge of the posterior wall of the rectus abdominis sheeth, called the arcuate line.

Table 4-1 Muscles of the anterior abdominal wall

Muscle	Origin	Insertion	Innervation	Actions
External oblique	Muscular slips from the outer surfaces of the lower eight ribs	Outer lip of iliac crest; aponeurosis ending in the xiphoid process, linea alba, pubic symphysis, pubic crest, and pectineal line of pubis	Anterior rami of lower six thoracic nerves (T_7–T_{12})	Support for abdominal viscera; compress abdominal contents and thus help in all expulsive acts (micturition, defaecation, parturition, vomiting, etc.); flexion of the trunk or lumbar spine, lateral flexion of the trunk, rotation of the trunk
Internal oblique	Lateral 2/3 of inguinal ligament, intermediate area of iliac crest, thoracolumbar fascia	Lower three or four ribs, aponeurosis ending in the xiphoid process, linea alba, pubic crest, and pectineal line of pubis	Anterior rami of lower six thoracic nerves (T_7–T_{12}) and L_1	
Transversus abdominis	Lateral 1/3 of inguinal ligament, inner lip of iliac crest, thoracolumbar fascia, lower six costal cartilages	Aponeurosis ending in the xiphoid process, linea alba, pubic crest, and pectineal line of pubis	Anterior rami of lower six thoracic nerves (T_7–T_{12}) and L_1	
Rectus abdominis	pubic symphysis, pubic crest, pubic tubercle	Xiphoid process, 5th–7th costal cartilages	Anterior rami of lower six or seven thoracic nerves (T_7–T_{12})	
Pyramidalis	Body of pubis, pubic symphysis	Linea alba	Subcostal nerve	Tenses the linea alba

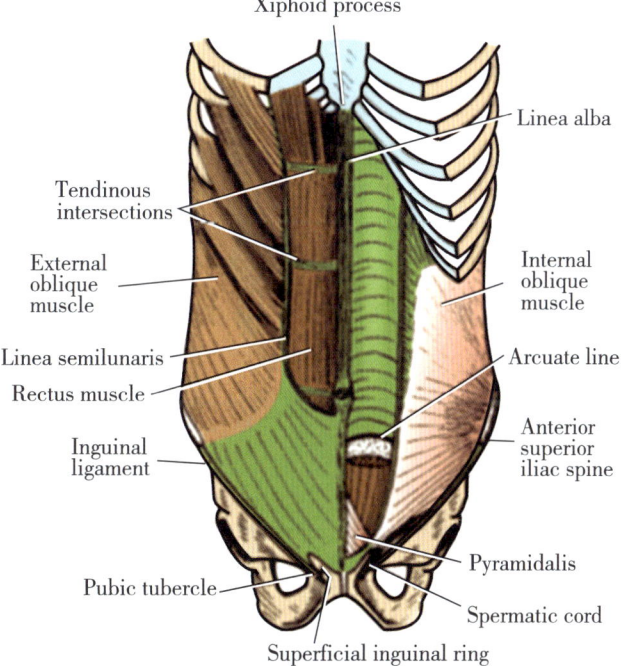

Figure 4-8 Anterior view of the rectus abdominis muscle and the rectus sheath
(On the right side, the anterior wall of the sheath has been partly removed, revealing the rectus muscle with its tendinous intersections. On the left, the posterior wall of the rectus sheath is shown. The edge of the arcuate line is shown at the level of the anterior superior iliac spine)

In addition to the arcuate line, there are other two important structures. Thelinea alba is a white median line running from the xiphoid process to the pubic symphysis. It is formed by densely interlacing of the aponeurotic fibers. The linea semilunaris is a curved line representing the lateral margin of the rectus abdominis muscle.

The rectus abdominis is the chief and largest content, the pyramidalis lies in front of the lower part of the rectus abdominis. In addition, the superior epigastric vessels, the inferior epigastric vessels, and the terminal parts of the lower six thoracic nerves.

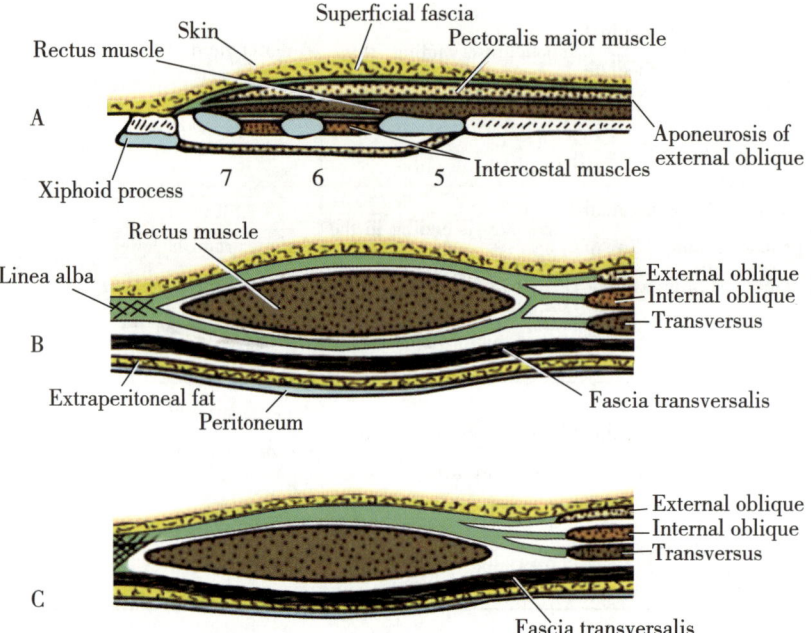

A. Above the costal margin; B. Between the costal margin and the level of the anterior superior iliac spine; C. Below the level of the anterior superior iliac spine and above the pubis.

Figure 4-9 Transverse sections of the rectus sheath seen at three levels

(3) Deep blood vessels and nerves

The four pairs of abdominal muscles are innervated by the anterior branches from the lower 6 pairs of the thoracic nerves and the first lumbar nerve. They are the $7^{th}-11^{th}$ intercostal nerves, the subcostal nerve, the iliohypogastric and the ilioinguinal nerves. These nerves run mainly between the internal oblique and the transversus abdominis muscles and except for the iliohypogastric and ilioinguinal nerves, all of them are accompanied by the related blood vessels, the $7^{th}-11^{th}$ posterior intercostal vessels and the subcostal vessels.

There are other two important arteries running within the rectus sheath: the superior epigastric artery from the internal thoracic artery, and the inferior epigastric artery that is a branch of the external iliac artery. These two arteries run along the posterior wall of rectus abdominis sheath and penetrate the rectus abdominis muscle to supply it.

4.2.2 The inguinal region

In the lower part of the anterolateral abdominal wall, there is a triangular area in each side, which is bounded inferiorly by the inguinal ligament, medially by the lower part of the lateral margin of the rectus abdominis muscle, and superiorly by a horizontal line from the anterosuperior iliac spine to the lateral margin of the rectus abdominis muscle. This triangular area is called the inguinal region. The inguinal region is clinically important, because it is a common site of abdominal hernia. It refers to a protrusion of any anatomical structures from its normal position.

4.2.2.1 Anatomical features of different layers of the inguinal region

(1) External oblique aponeurosis

The lower edge of the external oblique aponeurosis attaches laterally to the anterosuperior iliac spine, and medially to the pubic tubercle, forming a slightly thickened band called the inguinal ligament. In other words, the inguinal ligament is the thickened lower edge of the external oblique aponeurosis spanning between the anterosuperior iliac spine and the pubic tubercle (Figure 4-10). Some fibers from the medial part of the ligament extend posteriorly and attach to the pecten pubis, forming a small and curved fibrous band called the lacunar ligament. The fibers from the lacunar ligament extend laterally along the pecten pubis, becoming a thickened fiberous band on the bony surface, this is called the pectineal ligament. There are also some fibers from the medial part of the inguinal ligament which extend medially to join the anterior wall of the rectus abdominis sheath, forming the reflected ligament. Another important structure in the external oblique aponeurosis is a triangular shaped slit located lateral and a little superior to the pubic tubercle. We call it superficial inguinal ring. It must be emphasized that the superficial inguinal ring is not a natural slit or opening. If it is intact, it is just a ring-like boundary that represents the extension of the external oblique aponeurosis onto the spermatic cord to form the external spermatic fascia.

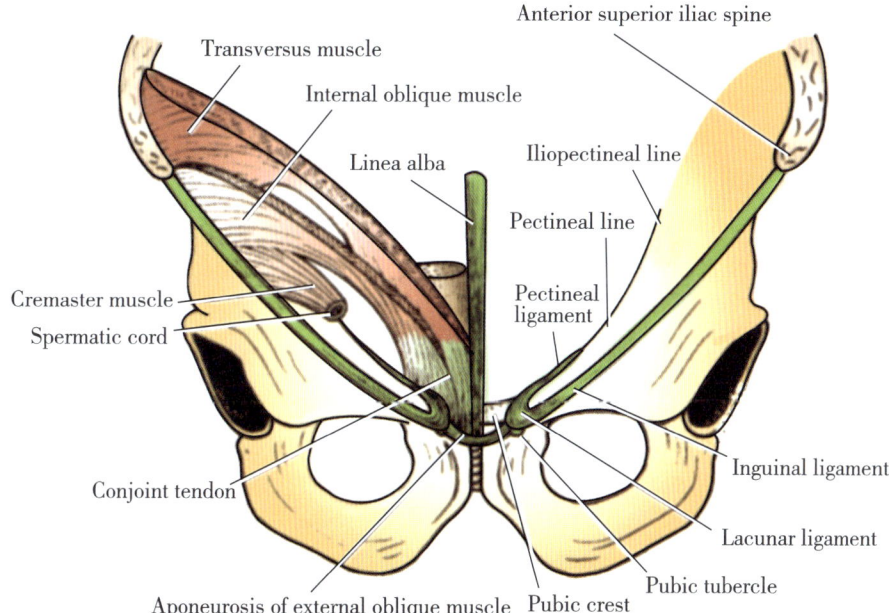

Figure 4-10   Anterior view of the pelvis showing the attachment of the conjoint tendon to the pubic crest and the adjoining part of the pectineal line

(2) Internal oblique and transversus abdominis muscles

The lower part of the internal oblique and transversus abdominis muscles originate from the lateral portion of the inguinal ligament. The origin of the internal oblique muscle occupies the lateral half or two thirds of the ligament, and that of the transversus abdominis muscle takes the lateral one third. Then the lower fibers of the two muscles form an arcuate muscular edge and finally join into a common tendon to insert into the pubic tubercle. This common tendon is called the conjoint tendon or inguinal falx. In addition, there are a small amount of muscular fibers of the internal oblique and transversus abdominis muscles which extend along the spermatic cord into the scrotum. These delicate muscular fibers cover the spermatic cord and hold the testis, forming the cremaster (suspensory muscle of the testis).

(3) Fascia transversalis

Above the midpoint of the inguinal ligament, the fascia transversalis forms an opening through which the spermatic cord comes out. This opening is called the deep inguinal ring. Similar to the superficial inguinal ring, the deep inguinal ring is not a natural opening. It is just a ring-like boundary between the transverse fascia and the internal spermatic fascia.

(4) Extraperitoneal fascia

You have learned that the extraperitoneal fascia is, in fact, a potential space between the transverse fascia and the parietal peritoneum. In the inguinal region, this space contains several ligaments and blood vessels, including a very important artery, the inferior epigastric artery. The inferior epigastric artery originates from the external iliac artery. It runs superomedially to enter the rectus abdominis sheath.

4.2.2.2 The inguinal canal

The inguinal canal is an oblique inter-muscular passage located above the medial part of the inguinal ligament. It has two openings and four walls (Figure 4-11). The internal opening or the entrance of the canal is the deep inguinal ring in the fascia transversalis, and it's external opening or exit is the superficial inguinal ring in the external oblique aponeurosis. The superior wall of the canal is the arcuate lower edge of the internal oblique and the transversus abdominis muscles, and the inferior wall is the medial part of the inguinal ligament. The anterior wall of the inguinal canal is formed by the external oblique aponeurosis and reinforced laterally by the origin part of the internal oblique abdominis muscle, and its posterior wall is the transverse fascia, reinforced medially by the inguinal falx.

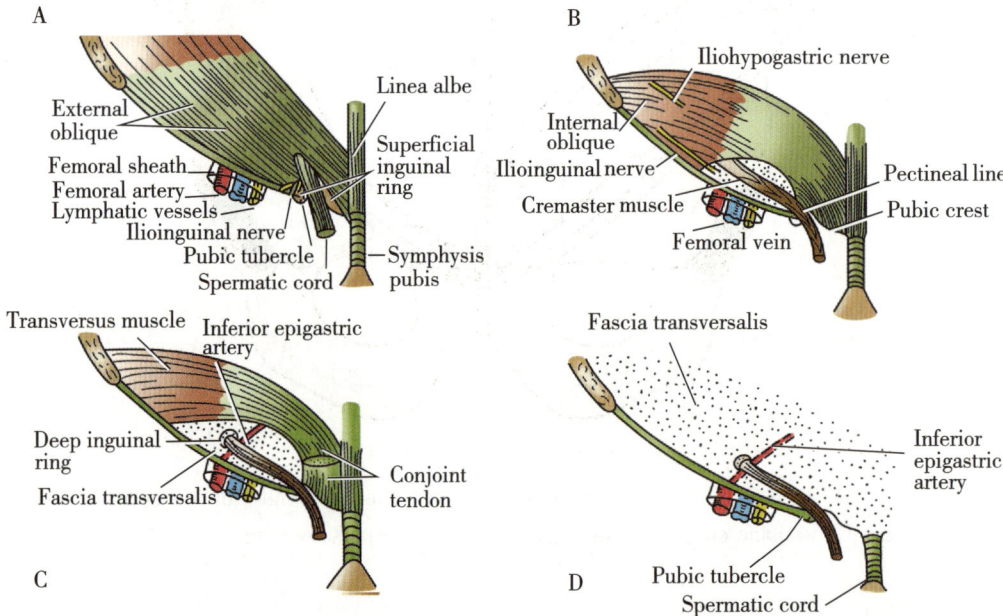

Figure 4-11 Inguinal canal showing the arrangement of the external oblique muscle (A), the internal oblique muscle (B), the transversus abdominis muscle (C), and the fascia transversalis (D)

Note that the anterior wall of the canal is formed by the external oblique, and the internal oblique, and the posterior wall is formed by the fascia transversalis and the conjoint tendon. The deep inguinal ring lies lateral to the inferior epigastric artery.

The inguinal canal transmits the spermatic cord in male or the round ligament of uterus in female. In both sexes the ilioinguinal nerve and the genital branch of genitofemoral nerve pass through it. However, the two nerves enter the canal along with the cremaster rather than passing through the deep inguinal ring.

The inguinal canal is clinically important, because it is a potential passage between the abdominal cavity and the scrotum in male. In some conditions, such as a chronic increase of the endo-abdominal pressure or poor development of the abdominal muscles, the contents of the abdominal cavity, for example an intestinal loop, may protrude through the deep inguinal ring into the canal, or even more, pass through the canal into the scrotum. If this happens, it is called the oblique (or indirect) inguinal hernia.

4.2.2.3 Hesselbach triangle

On the internal aspect of the lower part of the anterior abdominal wall, there is a very small triangular area bounded laterally by the inferior epigastric vessels, inferiorly by the medial part of the inguinal ligament and medially by the lateral margin of the rectus abdominis muscle. This area is called the Hesselbach triangle or the inguinal triangle.

The Hesselbach triangle is clinically important, because it is another common site of abdominal hernia. In the lower part of the triangle (below the arcuate lower edge of the internal oblique and transversus abdominis muscles), there are no muscular coverings and the superficial inguinal ring is located here. Thus, contents of the abdominal cavity, such as an intestinal loop, may protrude anteriorly through this weak area and emerge from the superficial inguinal ring. If this happens, it is called the direct inguinal hernia.

You have already learned that below the medial part of the inguinal ligament, there is another important structure, the femoral ring, bounded anteriorly by the inguinal ligament, medially by the lacunar ligament, posteriorly by the pectineal ligament and laterally by the femoral vein. The femoral ring is the opening of the femoral canal and the site of femoral hernia.

Note that: located superiorly and inferiorly along the medial part of the inguinal ligament, there are three special anatomical structures potentially related to the abdominal herniation. The Hesselbach triangle is related to the direct inguinal hernia; the ingunal canal, to the oblique inguinal hernia; and the femoral ring, to the femoral hernia. Clinically, the inguinal hernias (including the direct and oblique) are more common in male; and the femoral hernia usually appears in female.

4.2.2.4 Testis descent and vaginal process evolvement during embryonic development

The testis in the early embryo is located in the posterior abdominal wall, outside the parietal peritoneum. With development of the embryo, the testis, guided by the gubernaculum, gradually descends along the posterior abdominal wall and reaches the inguinal region at the time of 3-4 months. Then the testis passes through the preformed inguinal canal and finally reaches the scrotum at the time around birth. Before the arrival of the testis, a very small peritoneal diverticulum or pouch, called the vaginal process has been formed. It gradually protrudes and inferomedially to push the layers of the anterior abdominal wall to form the scrotum. Thus a passage between the abdominal cavity and the scrotum is established and this is the original inguinal canal. After then, the arrival testis with its appendix gradually passes through the canal, but outside the vaginal process, into the scrotum. Once the testis reaches the scrotum, the vaginal process gradually closes from its origin downwards. Finally its proximal major part becomes a very slender cord, called the vaginal ligament; and its distal part remains as a sac of serous membrane that covers the anterior surface of the testis. This serous sheath on the surface of the testis is called the tunica vaginalis of testis. The vaginal ligament, together with the components of the appendix of the testis including the ductus deferens, the testicular artery, the pampiniform plexus, and the lymphatics and nerves to the testis, constitute the spermatic cord that extends from the deep inguinal ring to the root of the scrotum. The inner three layers of the anterior abdominal wall that had been pushed down to the scrotum become three coverings on the spermatic cord and the testis: the internal spermatic fascia that comes from the transverse fascia, the cremaster, from the internal oblique and the transversus abdominis muscles, and the external spermatic fascia, from the external oblique aponeurosis (Figure 4-12).

If the proximal part of the vaginal process fails to close after birth, the tunica vaginalis remains open to the peritoneal cavity. Thus, when the endo-abdominal pressure lifts, for example when the newborn baby is loudly crying, serous fluid in the peritoneal cavity leaks into the tunica vaginalis, leading to expansion of the scrotum. When the baby falls asleep, the enlarged scrotum shrinks to its normal size. This condition is called the communicating hydrocele of tunica vaginalis. Even more, an intestinal loop may also pass through the unclosed vaginal process into the scrotum, leading to the congenital oblique inguinal hernia.

If the testis fails to descend into the scrotum after birth, but staying at anywhere in its descending way, it is called the cryptorchidism or undescended testis.

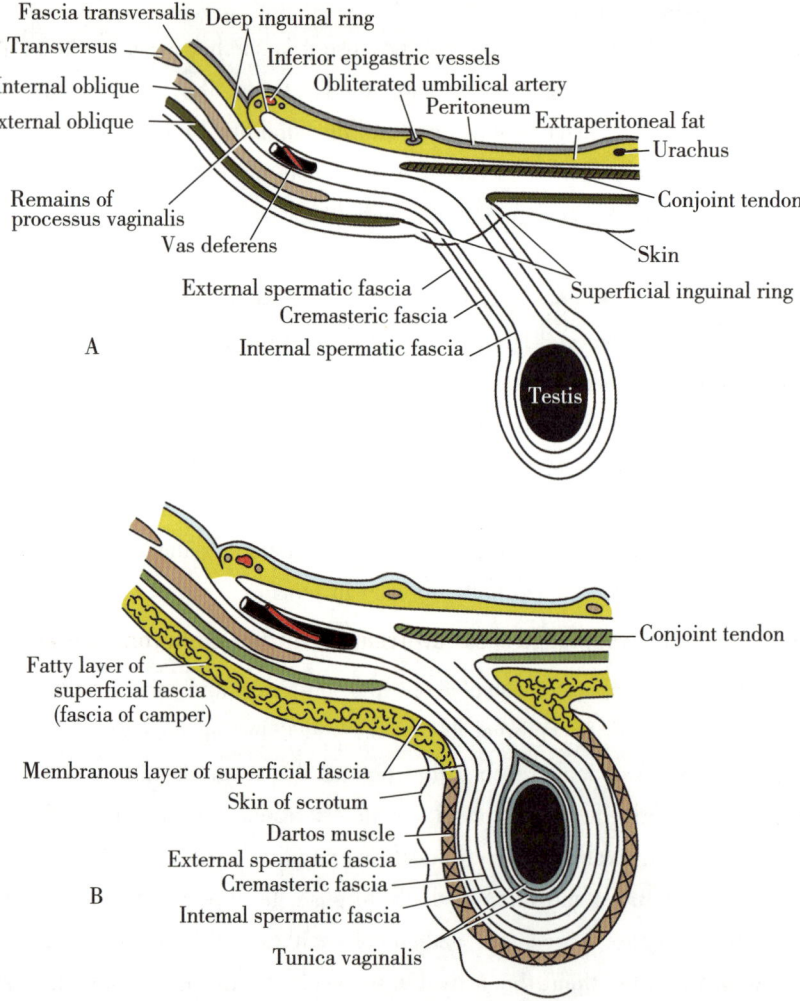

A. Continuity of the different layers of the anterior abdominal wall with coverings of the spermatic cord; B. The skin and superficial fascia of the abdominal wall and scrotum have been included, and the tunica vaginalis is shown.

Figure 4-12　Coverings on the spermatic cord and the testis

4.3 The peritoneum and peritoneal cavity

4.3.1 Introduction to the peritoneum

The peritoneum is the serous membrane in the abdominal cavity. It includes two layers: the parietal peritoneum that lines the inner surface of the abdominal and pelvic walls and the lower surface of the diaphragm, and the visceral peritoneum that covers most abdominal organs (Figure 4-13).

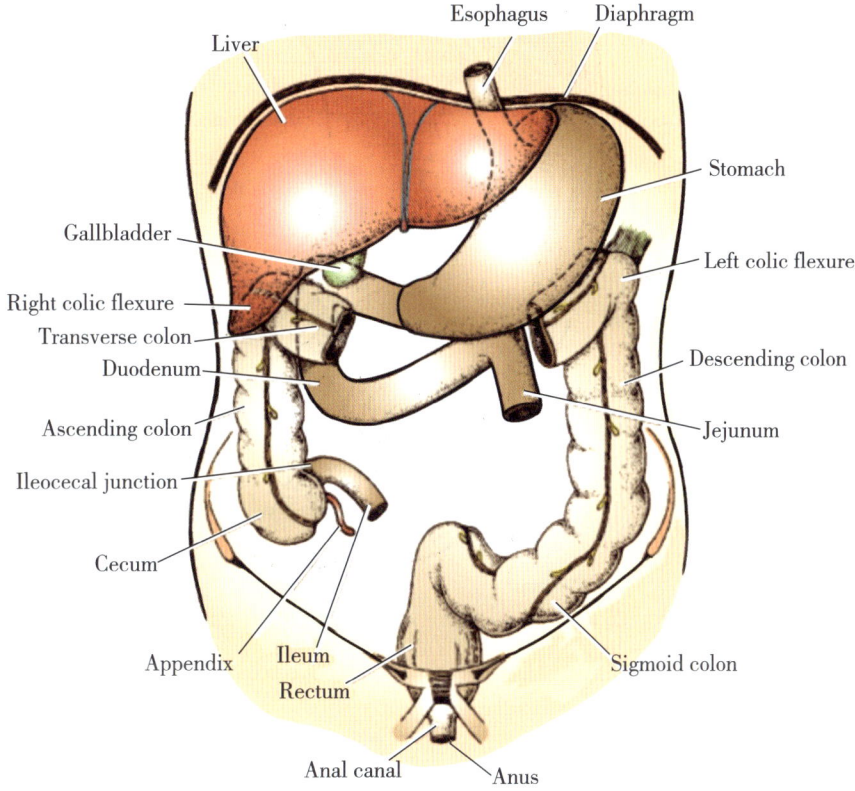

Figure 4-13　General arrangement of abdominal viscera

The two layers of peritoneum are continuous, they enclose a potential space called the peritoneal cavity. In male, the peritoneal cavity is completely closed; but in female it is potentially open to the external environment through the uterine tubes, uterus and vagina. Thus, a retrograde infection of the genital tract in female may cause inflammation of the pelvic peritoneum.

The peritoneal cavity is divided broadly into two parts, the lesser sac or the omental bursa that is situated behind the stomach, lesser omentum and the liver, and the greater sac that is the main larger part except for the lesser sac. Two sacs communicate with each other through the epiploic foramen or foramen of Winslow.

Abdominal cavity is bounded by the diaphragm, the abdominal and pelvic wall, and the pelvic diaphragm, which is divided by the plane of pelvic inlet into the abdominal cavity proper, a larger upper part, and the pelvic cavity, a smaller lower part.

4.3.2 Structures formed by the peritoneum

When reflecting from the inner surface of abdominal cavity to an organ or extending from one organ to another, the peritoneum forms various structures such as the omenta, the mesenteries, the peritoneal ligaments, and the recesses or pouches (Figure 4-14).

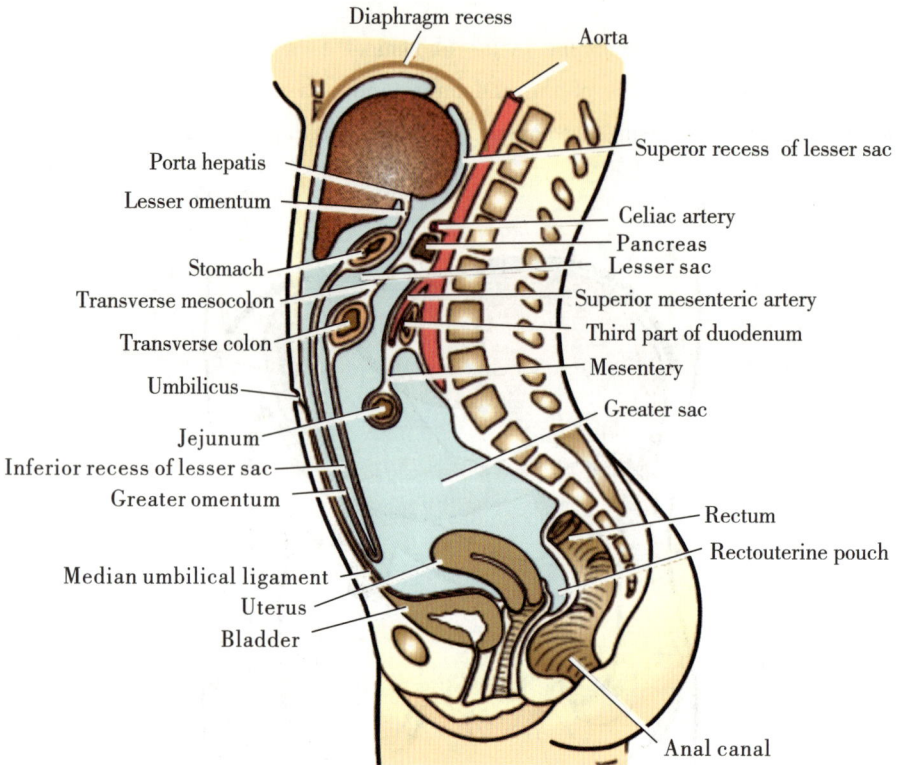

Figure 4-14 Sagittal section of the female abdomen showing the arrangement of the peritoneum

4.3.2.1 The omenta

The omenta are double or multi-layered large peritoneal sheets extending from the stomach to nearby organs.

(1) Greater omentum

It is a large four-layered fold of peritoneum. Anterior two layers descend from the greater curvature of stomach and the superior part of the duodenum to a variable extent, fold upon themselves to form the posterior two layers. Posterior two layers ascend to the anterior surface of the head, and the anterior border of the body of pancreas. Gastrocolic ligament is the upper part of the anterior two layers of greater omentum, extending between the stomach and the transverse colon.

The right and left gastroepiploic vessels anastomose with each other in the interval between the first two layers of the greater omentum a little below the greater curvature of the stomach.

(2) Lesser omentum

It is a two-layered fold of peritoneum, extending from the lesser curvature of the stomach and the first part of the duodenum to the liver (porta hepatis). It consists of two parts: the hepatogastric ligament, which is the portion of the lesser omentum between the stomach and the liver, and the hepatoduodenal ligament, the portion between the duodenum and the liver.

Along the lesser curvature of stomach and the upper border of the adjoining part of the duodenum, the lesser omentum contains the right gastric vessels and the left gastric vessels. The right margin of lesser omentum is free and contains the hepatic artery proper, the common bile duct, the hepatic portal vein, lymph nodes and lymphatics, hepatic plexus of nerves.

(3) Lesser sac or omental bursa

It is a large recess of the peritoneal cavity behind the stomach, lesser omentum and the liver, and in front of the peritoneum on the posterior abdominal wall (Figure 4-15). Its anterior wall is formed, from above downwards, by the caudate lobe of the liver, the lesser omentum. The stomach, and the anterior two layers of the greater omentum. The posterior wall is formed, from down upwards, by the posterior two layers of the greater omentum, the structures forming the stomach bed (the transverse colon and transverse mesocolon, the peritoneum covering the pancreas, the left kidney and the left suprarenal gland) (Figure 4-16). The upper border is formed by the peritoneum on the inferior surface of the diaphragm and the caudate lobe of the liver. The left border is closed by the gastrosplenic ligament, the spleen, and the lienorenal or splenicorenal ligament. The right border communicates with the greater sac through the epiploic foramen at its upper part.

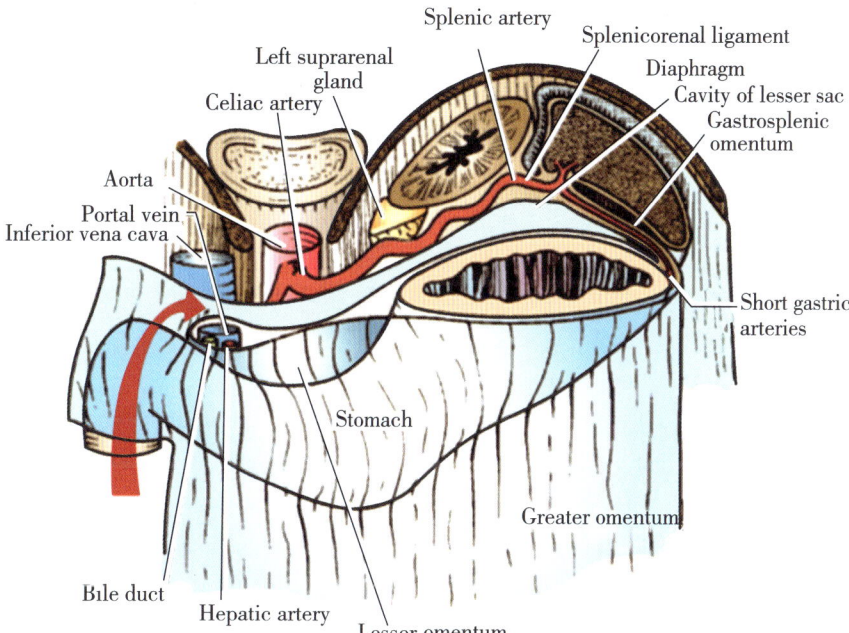

Figure 4-15 Transverse section of the lesser sac showing the arrangement of the peritoneum in the formation of the lesser omentum, the gastrosplenic ligament, and the lienorenal ligament (arrow indicates the position of the opening of the lesser sac)

(4) The omental foramen or Winslow foramen

It is a vertical slit-like opening through which the lesser sac communicates with the greater sac. It is situated in front of $T_{12}-L_2$ vertebrae, and is bounded anteriorly by the right free margin of the lesser omentum (hepatoduodenal ligament), containing the hepatic artery, bile duct and the portal vein; posteriorly by the peritonium on the inferior vena cava; superiorly by the caudate lobe of the liver, inferiorly by the upper part of duodenum. It can lodge one or two fingers.

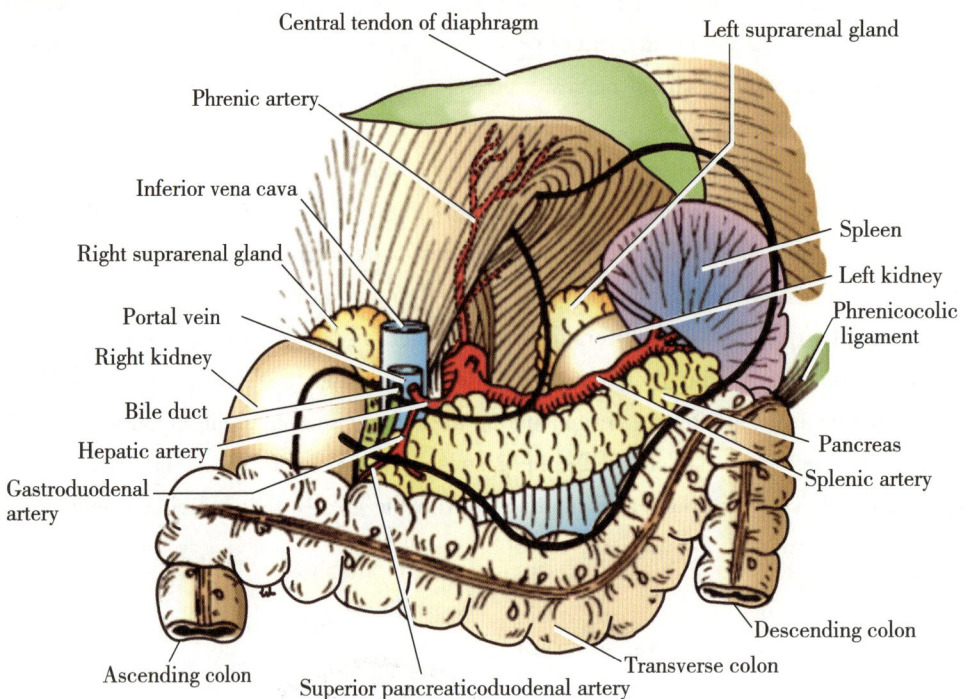

Figure 4–16 Structures situated on the posterior abdominal wall behind the stomach

4.3.2.2　The mesenteries

The mesenteries are double layered peritoneal sheets that suspend the intestines to the posterior abdominal wall.

(1) Mesentery of small intestine or mesentery proper

It is a broad, fan-shaped fold of peritoneum, suspending the coils of jejunum and ileum to the posterior abdominal wall. Its attached border, or root of the mesentery is 15 cm long, extending from the duodenojejunal flexure on the left side of vertebra L_2 to the right sacroiliac joint, crossing over the duodenum, the abdominal aorta, the inferior vena cava, the right ureter, and so on. It contains the jejunal and ileal branches of the superior mesenteric artery and the accompanying veins, lymphatics, lymph nodes, and the autonomic nerve plexuses.

(2) Mesoappendix

It is a small, triangular fold of peritoneum, suspending the vermiform appendix to the lower end of the mesentery close to the ileocaecal junction. It contains vessels, nerves, lymph nodes and lymphatics of the appendix. The appendicular artery runs in its free margin.

(3) Transverse mesocolon

It is a broad fold of peritoneum, suspending the transverse colon to the posterior abdominal wall. Its root is attached to the pancreas. The transverse mesocolon contains the middle colic vessels, the nerves, lymph nodes and lymphatics of the transverse colon.

(4) Sigmoid mesocolon

It is a triangular fold of peritoneum, suspending the sigmoid colon to the pelvic wall. It contains the sigmoid and superior rectal vessels, nerves, lymph nodes and lymphatics.

4.3.2.3　The ligaments

The ligaments are double-layered peritoneal folds connecting an organ to the abdominal wall or spaning between adjacent organs.

(1) Ligaments of the liver

1) Falciform ligament of liver

It is a sickle-shaped fold of peritoneum (double layers), connecting the anterosuperior surface of liver to the anterior abdominal wall and to the undersurface of the diaphragm.

2) Ligamentum teres hepatis

It is in the free border of the falciform ligament, extending from the umbilicus to the inferior border and inferior surface of the liver. It is formed by the obliterated umbilical vein, and contains the paraumbilical veins.

3) Coronary ligament

It is formed by the reflection of the peritoneum from the diaphragm to the liver. The area between the upper and lower (or anterior and posterior) layers of the coronary ligament is the bare area of live, this area is devoid of peritoneum and lies in contract with diaphragm.

4) Left and right triangular ligaments

They are formed by the right extremity of coronary ligament and left leaf of falciform ligament, respectively.

(2) Ligaments of the stomach

1) Gastrosplenic ligament

A double layers of peritoneum that connects the fundus of stomach to the hilum of spleen. In this double layers of peritoneum are the short gastric and left gastroepiploic vessels.

2) Gastrophrenic ligament

It extends between the cardia of the stomach to the diaphragm.

3) Gastropancrestic ligament

It connects the pyloric part of the stomach to the pancreas.

(3) Ligaments of the spleen

1) Lienorenal ligament

It extends between the hilum of spleen and anterior aspect of left kidney. The splenic vessels, nerves, lymphatics, as well as the tail of pancreas, lies within this ligament.

2) Splenophrenic ligament

It extends between the posterior end of the spleen to the diaphragm.

3) Splenocolic ligament

It connects the spleen and the left colic flexure.

(4) Phrenicocolic ligament

It is continued from the left colic flexure to the diaphrgam opposite the 10th and 11th ribs.

4.3.2.4 Folds, fossae or recesses, and pouches of the peritoneum

The folds are peritoneal elevations often overlying the blood vessels. Peritoneal fossae or recesses are small pockets of the peritoneal cavity enclosed by small, inconstant folds of peritoneum, while pouches are large constant peritoneal depressions usually located between adjacent pelvic organs.

(1) Peritoneal folds and recesses of the posterior abdominal wall

1) Superior duodenal and inferior duodenal folds

The superior duodenal fold is situated on the left side of the ascending part of the duodenum at the level of vertebra L_2. It is semilunar in shape with a free lower border. The inferior duodenal fold extends between the ascending part of the duodenum and the abdominal aorta at the level of vertebra L_3, and is triangular in shape with a free upper border.

2) Superior duodenal and inferior duodenal recesses

The former is present deep to the superior duodenal fold with its orifice looking downwards, the latter lies deep to the inferior duodenal fold with its orifice looking upwards.

3) Retrocaecal recess

It lies behind the caecum and often contains the appendix. Its orifice looks downwards.

4) Intersigmoid recess

It is constantly present in the foetus and in early infancy, but may disappear with age. It lies left posterior to the sigmoid mesocolon, and is infundibular in shape with its orifice looking downwards.

5) Hepatorenal recess

It is the right subhepatic space, lying between the right lobe of liver, the right kidney and suprarenal gland, and the right colic flexure. This space is the lowest part of the abdominal cavity proper when the body is supine.

(2) Peritoneal folds and fossae of the anterior abdominal wall

On the back of the anterior abdominal wall below the umbilicus, there are a number of peritoneal folds and fossae.

1) Starting from the median plane these are five peritoneal folds.

Median umbilical fold: It contains the median umbilical ligament formed by the remnant of the urachus in the median line, connecting the umbilicus with the apex of the urinary bladder.

Medial umbilical folds: They are, one on each side of the median umbilical fold, raised by the medial umbilical ligaments formed by the obliterated umbilical arteries.

Lateral umbilical folds: They are lateral to the medial umbilical folds, raised by the inferior epigastric vessels.

2) From the median plane, above the inguinal ligament, there are also three pairs of peritoneal fossae.

Supravesical fossae: They are located one on each side of the median umbilical fold.

Medial inguinal fossae: They are located between the medial umbilical folds and the lateral umbilical folds, respectively, corresponding to the inguinal triangle.

Lateral inguinal fossae: They are located lateral to the lateral umbilical folds, respectively, corresponding to the deep inguinal ring.

(3) Peritoneal pouches of the pelvis

1) Rectovesical pouch

It is located between the rectum and the urinary bladder in male pelvis.

2) Rectouterine or Douglas pouch

It is located between the rectum and the uterus in female pelvis, and has a close relation to the posterior vaginal fornix.

3) Vesicouterine pouch

It is located between the urinary bladder and the uterus in female pelvis.

4.3.3 Exploration of the peritoneal cavity

The extension and relationship of these peritoneal structures are difficult to display by images or describe by language. Thus, the best way to study the peritoneum is exploring the opened peritoneal cavity on a cadaver. This section just outlines the important peritoneal structures. The rests will be described when the related organs are studied in later sections.

As shown in the median plane of the body, the peritoneum on the inferior surface of the diaphragm reflects onto the upper surface of the liver, forming a double-layer peritoneal fold called the coronary ligament of liver. After enclosing the liver, the two layers of peritoneum extend inferiorly to the lesser curvature of stomach. Thus a double-layered peritoneal sheet is formed between the liver and the stomach. It is called the lesser omentum. The lesser omentum is usually divided into two parts. Its left major part that spans between the inferior surface of the liver and the lesser curvature of stomach is called the hepatogastric ligament. The right part that connects the superior part of the duodenum to the porta hepatis is called the hepatoduodenal ligament. The right edge of the lesser omentum is free, and the hepatoduodenal ligament surrounds three important structures (the common bile duct, the hepatic artery proper and the hepatic portal vein) that run up into the porta hepatis.

The layers of peritoneum on the anterior and posterior surfaces of the stomach meet at the greater curvature, and extend inferiorly to form a large and apron-shaped peritoneal sheet, called greater omentum. The lower edge of the greater omentum is free because the two layers of the peritoneum fold back and ascend to invest the transverse colon. Thus, the major part of the greater omentum is, in fact, a four-layer sheet. However, its upper part spanning between the transverse colon and the greater curvature of stomach is only double-layered, and we call this double-layered narrow part the gastrocolic ligament.

After investing the transverse colon, the peritoneum extends to the inner surface of the posterior abdominal wall, forming a double-layered peritoneal sheet that suspends the transverse colon to the posterior abdominal wall. We call this sheet the transverse mesocolon. Below the root of the transverse mesocolon, the peritoneum on the posterior abdominal wall raises a double-layered and folded sheet to suspend the small intestine. This folded sheet is the so called mesentery of small intestine.

Among these peritoneal structures, the greater omentum is movable in the abdominal cavity. Its lower and two lateral edges are free, so that its distal part can quickly move and adhere to an infected organ to wrap it. This can prevent the spreading of a local inflammation in the abdominal cavity. In addition, the greater omentum is rich in small blood vessels. These vessels have a strong ability to regenerate and can quickly grow into an injured tissue after the omentum adheres to it. Therefore, in surgery, the omental flaps or strips are perfect transplantation materials to be used in treatment of an indolent wound.

The peritoneal cavity can be divided into two parts. One is a space behind the stomach and lesser omentum, and is enclosed by the posterior layer of the coronary ligament, the liver, the lesser omentum, the posterior wall of the stomach, the gastrocolic ligament, the transverse colon and its mesocolon, and the peritoneum on the upper part of the posterior abdominal wall and the inferior surface of the diaphragm. This space is called the lesser sac or the omental bursa. The rest of the peritoneal cavity is called the greater sac. The passage between the two sacs is the omental foramen that is located behind the hepatoduodenal ligament. In today's dissection, you can insert one or two of your fingers into the foramen to detect its boundaries.

4.3.4 Divisions of the peritoneal cavity

In the *Regional Anatomy*, the peritoneal cavity is usually divided into asupracolic and an infracolic compartments by the transverse colon and its mesocolon (Figure 4-17). The supracolic compartment is also called the subphrenic space, because it is located just below the diaphragm.

(1) Supracolic compartment

In the supracolic compartment, there are several peritoneal spaces that are clinically important. Between the inferior surface, the diaphragm and the superior surface of the liver is the suprahepatic space.

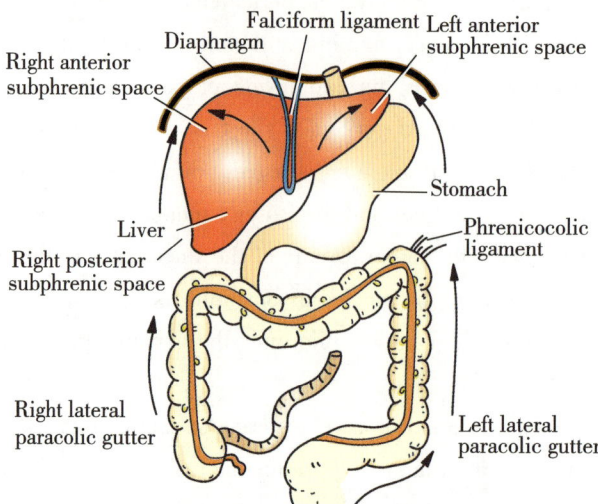

Figure 4-17 Normal direction of flow of the peritoneal fluid from different parts of the peritoneal cavity to the subphrenic spaces

This space is bounded posteriorly by the coronary ligament and is subdivided by the falciform ligament into two parts: the right and the left suprahepatic spaces. Between the low surface of the liver and the transverse mesocolon is the subhepatic space. This space is divided into three parts with two that are important. The first one is the omental bursa located behind the stomach and lesser omentum. The other is called the hepatorenal recess that lies right to the free edge of the lesser omentum and extends between the the liver, and the the right kidney to the posterior abdominal wall.

The hepatorenal recess communicates superiorly with the right suprahepatic space and to the left with the omental bursa through the omental foramen. More importantly, it is the lowest portion of the peritoneal cavity when a person lies in supine position. For this reason, it is the commonest site of a subphrenic abscess, which may be caused by the spread of infection from the gall bladder, the appendix, or other organs in the region, and is one of the commonly used sites for draining an inflamed peritoneal cavity. The inflammation of the peritoneum is called peritonitis. It is a dangerous condition usually caused by an opening injury of the abdomen or a perforating gastric ulcer that leaks gastric juice into the peritoneal cavity. An emergency treatment for this condition is washing the infected peritoneal cavity and administering large doses of antibiotics. After the operation, a drainage tube is usually inserted through the posterior abdominal wall into the hepatorenal recess to drain off the excessive exudate from the peritoneum.

(2) Infracolic compartment

In the infracolic compartment, there are two important longitudinal peritoneal grooves. One is located lateral to the ascending colon and is called the right paracolic gutter. The other, located lateral to the descending colon, is the left paracolic gutter. Inferiorly, these two grooves communicate with the pelvic cavity; but superiorly, the left paracolic gutter is blocked by the phrenicocolic ligament, a double-layered peritoneal fold spanning between the diaphragm and the left colic flexure. The right paracolic gutter communicates superiorly with the right hepatorenal recess. Thus, in a patient with perforating appendicitis, pus may leak downwards into the pelvic cavity or upwards into the hepatorenal recess through the right paracolic gutter; and even more, the pus may spread into the right suprahepatic space, leading to a generalized peritonitis.

Surrounded by the ascending, transverse, descending and sigmoid colons, there are two peritoneal spaces separated by the root of the mesentery of small intestine. The right one is called the right mesenteric sinus, which is bounded by the ascending colon, the right part of the transverse mesocolon and the root of the mesentery of small intestine. The left one is called the left mesenteric sinus, which is incompletely bounded by the root of the mesentery of small intestine, the left part of the transverse mesocolon, and the descending and sigmoid colons. The left mesenteric sinus opens inferiorly to the pelvic cavity.

Zhang Bensi

4.4 Organs in the supracolic compartment

4.4.1 Stomach

The stomach is the most dilated part of the digestive tract between the esophagus and duodenum. Its position varies considerably upon different body shapes. But in general, it is located partly in the left hypochondriac region and partly in the epigastric region. The stomach is a saclike organ with two openings. Its entrance is called the cardia, which connects to the esophagus. The exit of the stomach is called the pylorus that continues to the duodenum. The upper or the right edge of the stomach is called the lesser curvature. Near its distal one third, there is a sharp notch, called the angular incisure. The lower or the left edge of the stomach is termed the greater curvature, which ends superiorly at the cardiac notch.

(1) Division

Upon its morphology, the stomach is divided into four parts. The cardiac part is a ring-shaped zone surrounding the cardiac orifice. The fundus is its dome-like uppermost part. The body is the major part in the middle, and the pyloric part is its distal portion. Usually the pyloric part is subdivided into a funnel-shaped pyloric antrum and a tube-like pyloric canal. The circular smooth muscles in the wall of the pyloric canal are thickened to form the pyloric sphincter.

Functionally, the superior major parts of the stomach, including the cardiac part, the fundus and the body, are called the digestive part because the glands in the mucosal membrane of these three parts secrete more than 70% amount of hydrochloric acid and pepsin. These secretions help the stomach to digest food into chyme. The pyloric part is termed the emptying part in which the contraction of the pyloric antrum advances chyme into the duodenum and the pyloric sphincter prevents the backflow of chyme into the stomach.

(2) Relations

Superiorly, the uppermost part of the stomach is related to the diaphragm with the cardia below the esophageal hiatus. Thus in some conditions, such as a chronic increase in abdominal pressure and poor development of the esophageal hiatus, the cardiac part or the fundus of stomach may protrude through the hiatus into the thorax. This disease is called the hiatus hernia (Belching, epigastric fullness and burn feeling). Anteriorly, the upper part of the anterior wall of the stomach is covered partly by the liver and partly the diaphragm, and the lower part directly contacts the inner surface of the anterolateral abdominal wall. Posteriorly, the stomach is related to the spleen, the omental bursa and the organs behind the bursa, including the left kidney, the left suprarenal gland, the pancreas, the transverse colon and the transverse mesocolon. All of these organs or structures are together called the stomach bed. The posterior relations of the stomach are clinically important. For example, a perforating gastric ulcer in the posterior wall of the stomach may leak gastric juice into the omental bursa, leading to a severe chemical peritonitis. Sometimes a chronic and indolent gastric ulcer in the posterior wall of the stomach may cause adhesion of the stomach to pancreas, thus the ulcer may gradually penetrate the posterior wall of the stomach and invade the pancreatic tissue. This is called penetrating gastric ulcer.

(3) Ligaments

The peritoneum on the surface of the stomach extends onto the diaphragm and nearby organs, forming several important ligaments, including: ① the hepatogastric ligament that is the left part of the lesser omentum spanning between the liver and the lesser curvature of stomach; ② the gastrocolic ligament that is the double-layered upper part of the greater omentum spanning between the greater curvature of stomach and the transverse colon; ③ the gastrosplenic ligament that extends from the fundus of the stomach to the hilum of the spleen; ④ the gastrophrenic ligament which connects the cardiac part of the stomach to the diaphragm. These peritoneal ligaments are important. They fix the stomach in place and protect its blood vessels (the vessels of the stomach usually run between the two layers of the ligaments).

(4) Blood supply

The arteries to the stomach are all derived from the celiac trunk or its branches (Figure 4-18). The celiac trunk originates from the abdominal aorta about 1 cm below the aortic hiatus of diaphragm. It is a short arterial trunk that divides into three major branches: the left gastric artery, the splenic artery and the common hepatic artery. In today's dissection, you must identify the trunk and carefully trace its branches to the stomach.

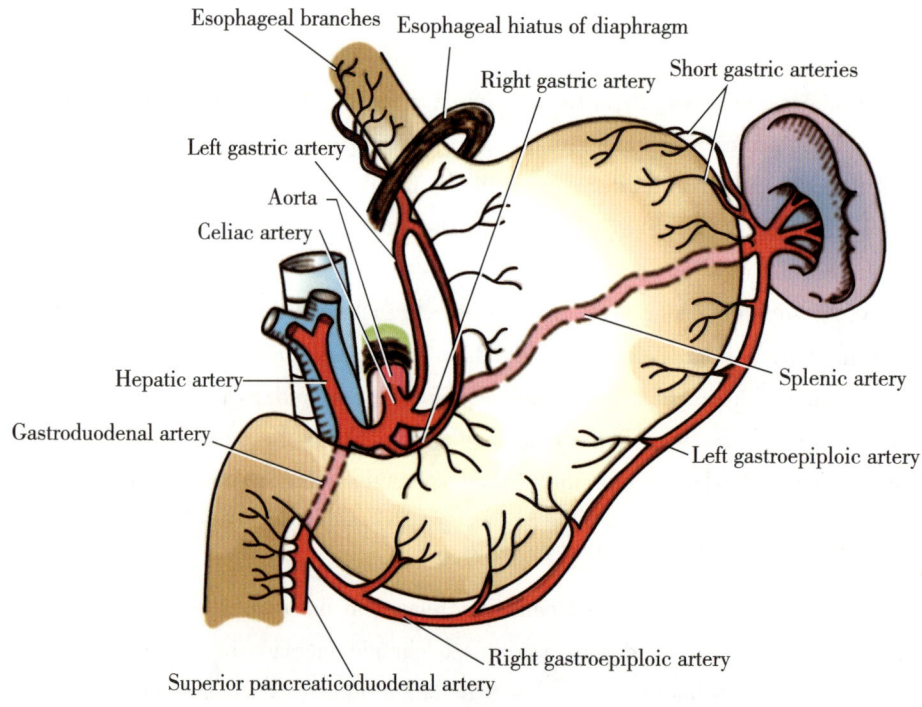

Figure 4-18 Arteries that supply the stomach
(Note that all the arteries are derived from branches of the celiac artery)

Along the lesser curvature of stomach, there are two arteries: the left gastric artery that directly originates from the celiac trunk and the right gastric artery usually from the proper hepatic artery. These two arteries run between the two layers of the hepatogastric ligament and anastomose to form an arterial arch which gives off small branches to supply the upper part of the stomach. Along the greater curvature of stomach there are also two arteries: the left gastroepiploic artery that originates from the splenic artery and the right gastroepiploic artery that is a branch of the gastroduodenal artery. These two arteries run between the two layers of the gastrocolic ligament and anastomose to form an arterial arch that gives off small branches superiorly to the stomach and inferiorly to the greater omentum. Several small branches from the splenic artery near the hilum of the spleen run superiorly to the fundus of stomach, these are called the short gastric arteries. In some individuals, there is a small branch of the splenic artery that runs superiorly along the posterior abdominal wall and reaches the upper part of the posterior wall of stomach through the gastrophrenic ligament. If exist, this artery is called the posterior gastric artery and it should be protected from injuring during the partial gastrectomy.

All arteries of the stomach are accompanied by related veins with the same name, and these veins are finally drained into thehepatic portal vein.

(5) Lymphatic drainage

As a general pattern, the deep lymphatic nodes in the body are distributed along with arteries, so similar to the veins, the majority of local lymph nodes are named after the arteries they accompany. Please keep this in your mind, it helps you to remember the names and locations of most local lymph nodes. You have just learned four major arteries to the stomach, the right and left gastric arteries, and the right and left gastroepiploic arteries. Distributed along these arteries are four major groups of local lymph nodes, the right and left gastric lymph nodes, and the right and left gastroepiploic lymph nodes(Figure 4-19). Each group of the lymph nodes drains the area of the stomach where its related artery supplies. Near the hilum of the spleen, there are several lymph nodes called the splenic lymph nodes that collect lymph from the spleen and the fundus of the stomach. In addition, there are two groups of lymph nodes located above and beneath the pylorus, which are called the supra-pyloric and the sub-pyloric lymph nodes, respectively. These lymph nodes collect lymph from the pylorus of stomach and the superior part of duodenum. All of the lymph nodes of the stomach are drained into the celiac lymph nodes that are located around the root of the celiac trunk and finally drained into the thoracic duct.

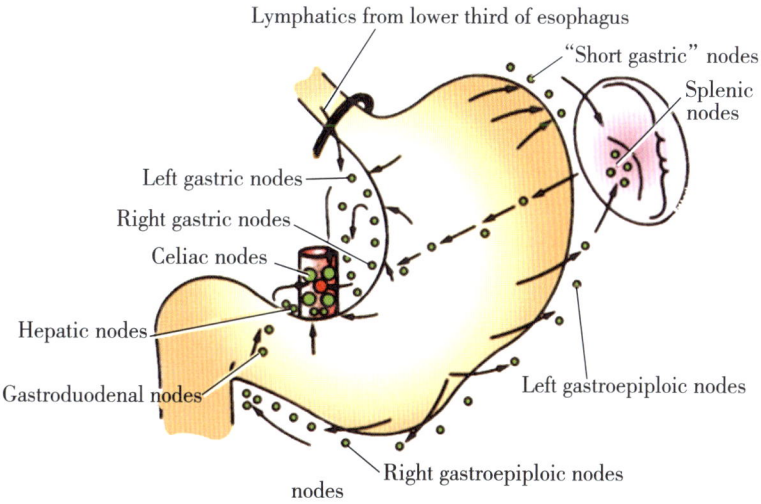

Figure 4-19 Lymph drainage of the stomach
(Note that all the lymph eventually passes through the celiac lymph nodes)

(6) Nerves

The stomach is innervated by both sympathetic and parasympathetic nerves (Figure 4-20). The sympathetic nerve inhibits the function of the stomach, while the parasympathetic nerves enhance its peristalsis (vermicular movement) and secretions of gastric juice. The sympathetic fibers come from the celiac plexus. These fibers are very slender and are distributed as plexus along the arteries to the stomach. The parasympathetic fibers come from the anterior and posterior vagal trunks. Both trunks are formed by reorganization of the esophageal plexus. The anterior vagal trunk enters the abdominal cavity along the anterior surface of the esophagus. Near the cardia of the stomach, it divides into two branches. One is called the hepatic branch that joins hepatic plexus to innervate the liver and bile ducts; and the other, the anterior gastric branch that descends along the lesser curvature of stomach. In its course, the anterior gastric branch gives off a number of tiny branches to the anterior wall of the major part of the stomach and a group of terminal branches that innervate the pyloric part. The posterior vagal trunk enters the abdominal cavity along the posterior surface of the esophagus, it also splits into two branches: a celiac branch that joins the celiac plexus and a posterior gastric branch that descends along the lesser curvature. Similarly, the posterior gastric branch also gives off tiny branches to the posterior wall of the major part of the stomach, and terminal branches to the pyloric part.

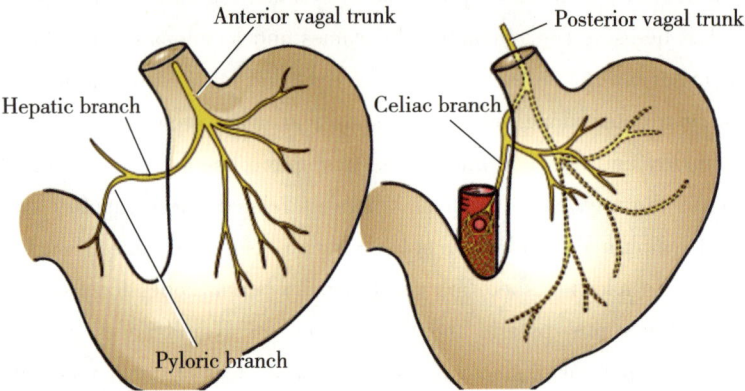

Figure 4-20　Distribution of the anterior and posterior vagal trunks within the abdomen

(Note that the celiac branch of the posterior vagal trunk is distributed with the sympathetic nerves as far down the intestinal tract as the left colic flexure)

4.4.2　Duodenum

The duodenum is the first part of the small intestine. It is located on the posterior abdominal wall, surrounding the head of pancreas. According to its course, the duodenum is divided into four parts:
- The superior part that is the beginning part of the duodenum extended from the pylorus of stomach.
- The descending part that descends along the right side of the pancreatic head.
- The horizontal part that crosses transversely over the vertebral column at the level of 3rd lumbar vertebra.
- The ascending part that ascends obliquely to the level of the second lumbar vertebra and continues to the jejunum by forming the duodenojejunal flexure.

Here, you should note that the proximal half of the superior part of duodenum is relatively dilated and its wall is slightly thinner. This proximal part is called the duodenal ampulla. The duodenal ampulla is a common site of peptic ulceration. The end of the duodenum, the duodenojejunal flexure, is fixed by a fibromuscular band extending from the right crus of diaphragm. This fibromuscular band is called the suspensory muscle of duodenum or the ligament of Treitz. The ligament of Treitz is an anatomical marker for the beginning of the jejunum.

The duodenum is supplied by two arteries: the superior and the inferior pancreaticoduodenal arteries. There are two superior pancreaticoduodenal arteries: the anterior and the posterior (Figure 4-21, Figure 4-22). Both originate from the gastrodoudenal artery and descend on the anterior or posterior surface of the pancreatic head along the duodenum. They anastomose with the anterior or posterior branches of the inferior pancreaticoduodenal artery that arises from the superior mesenteric artery. These arteries supply not only the duodenum, but also the pancreatic head.

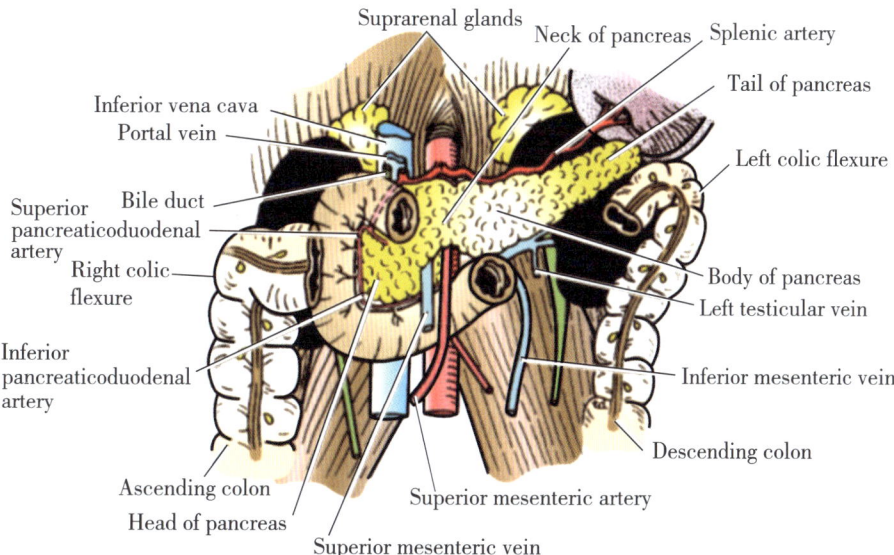

Figure 4-21　Pancreas and anterior relations of the kidneys

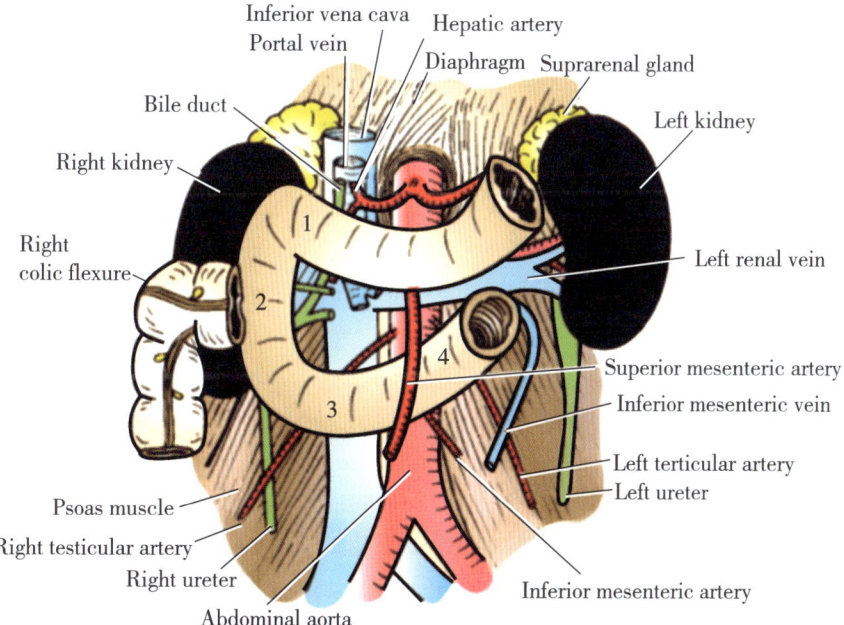

Figure 4-22　Posterior relations of the duodenum and the pancreas
(The numbers represent the four parts of the duodenum)

4.4.3 Liver

(1) Position

The liver is the largest digestive gland in the human body. It is located mostly in the right hypochondriac region and partly in the epigastric region and the left hypochondriac region. Usually, its superior surface reaches the level of the 5th rib. Its lower edge, in the right hypochondriac region, corresponds to the costal arch, but in epigastric region it is 2-3 cm below the xiphoid process. The liver is fixed on the inferior surface of the diaphragm, so during respiration it slightly moves up and down periodically along with the diaphragm.

(2) Relations

Superiorly, the liver is covered by the diaphragm. Inferiorly, the liver is related to the right colic flexure, the right kidney, the right suprarenal gland, the superior part of the duodenum and the stomach.

(3) Ligaments

The liver is fixed in place by its peritoneal ligaments. The peritoneum on the inferior surface of the diaphragm reflects onto the upper surface of the liver, forming the double layered coronary ligament. The posterosuperior surface of the liver between the anterior and posterior layers of the coronary ligament is not covered by the peritoneum, and is therefore called the bare area of liver. The potential space between the bare area of live and lower surface of the diaphragm is called the subphrenic extraperitoneal space. At the right and left angles of the bare area, the anterior and posterior layers of the coronary ligament form two angular peritoneal folds that are called the right and left triangular ligaments, respectively. The middle part of anterior layer of the coronary ligament folds and extends inferiorly to form a double-layered longitudinal band that links the liver to diaphragm and the anterior abdominal wall. This peritoneal band is called the falciform ligament. The lower edge of the falciform ligament is free. It encloses a connective tissue cord that extends downward to the umbilicus. This cord is called the round ligament of liver or ligamentum teres hepatis. It is the remains of the embryonic umbilical vein.

(4) Shape

The liver is a wedge-shaped organ with a convex superior surface and a flat inferior surface (Figure 4-23). On its inferior surface, there are three deep grooves: a right longitudinal groove, a left longitudinal groove and a short transverse groove. The transverse groove is also called the porta hepatis because several important structures pass through it to enter or leave the liver. The right and the left hepatic ducts leave the porta hepatis to form the common hepatic duct which then unites the cystic duct to form the common bile duct. Both proper hepatic artery and the the hepatic portal vein split into a right and a left branches that pass through the porta pepatis to enter the liver. These three structures, the common bile duct, the proper hepatic artery and the hepatic portal vein, together with the nerves and lymphatic vessels of the liver are tightly packed by the hepatoduodenal ligament to form the hepatic pedicle.

The anterior half of the right longitudinal groove holds the gallbladder and is therefore called the fossa for gallbladder. The posterior half of the groove is called the vena cava sulcus, because the inferior vena cava extends superiorly along it. The upper part of the sulcus is called the second porta hepatis, in which three major hepatic veins (the right, the intermediate and the left hepatic veins) leave the liver to join the inferior vena cava. The lower part of the sulcus is called the third porta hepatis where several small short hepatic veins leave the liver and drain into the inferior vena cava.

(5) Division

You have already learned that the liver is divided into four lobes according to its superficial features.

On its superior surface the falciform ligament divides the liver into the right and the left lobes; and in its inferior surface, there are two additional lobes between the right and left longitudinal grooves: the quadrate lobe anterior to the porta hepatis and the caudate lobe posterior to it. This traditional division of the liver upon its superficial features looks naturally, but it does not reflect the characteristics of the organ's interior structures—the organization of the intra-hepatic tubular systems.

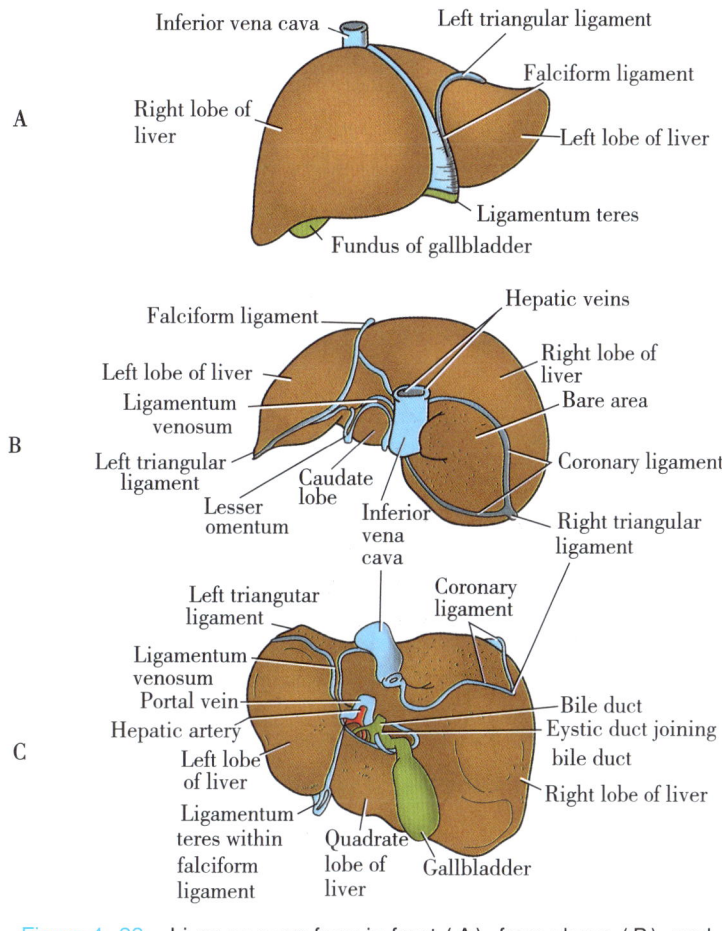

Figure 4-23　Liver as seen from in front (A), from above (B), and from behind (C)

(Note the position of the peritoneal reflections, the bare areas, and the peritoneal ligaments)

By using the cast liver specimen and the technology of 3-dimentional reconstruction from the images of sectional anatomy, it is demonstrated that two tubular systems exist in the liver. The intra-hepatic bile ducts and the branches of both hepatic portal vein and proper hepatic artery are distributed in the hepatic tissue in the same way and they are bounded together by a connective tissue sheath, thus they constitute a common tubular system in the liver, called Glisson System. The tributaries of the hepatic veins constitute another intra-hepatic tubular system; these tributaries run between the major branches of the Glisson System. Each major branch of the Glisson System, together with its associated hepatic tissue, forms a relatively independent unit. This unit is called a hepatic segment, and each segment is roughly bounded by the tributaries of the hepatic veins. Upon this, the liver can be divided into two halves, five lobes and eight segments. In surgery, the hepatic segment is the minimal resectable unit of the liver.

4.4.4 The extrahepatic bile ducts

(1) Composition

The extrahepatic bile ducts include the hepatic ducts, the common hepatic duct, the gallbladder, the cystic duct and the common bile duct that finally unites the pancreatic duct to open into the duodenum at the major duodenal papilla (Figure 4-24). In a living body, bile is secreted continuously by the liver and flows through the hepatic ducts, the common hepatic duct and the cystic duct into the gallbladder, where it is stored and concentrated. When stimulated, e.g., after a meal, the gallbladder contracts and forces the bile flowing through the cystic and the common bile ducts into the duodenum. Where the bile mixes with the pancreatic juice from the pancreatic duct and activates the pancreatic enzymes (the pancreatic enzymes are in form of proenzyme, and must be activated by the components of bile to obtain the digestive activities).

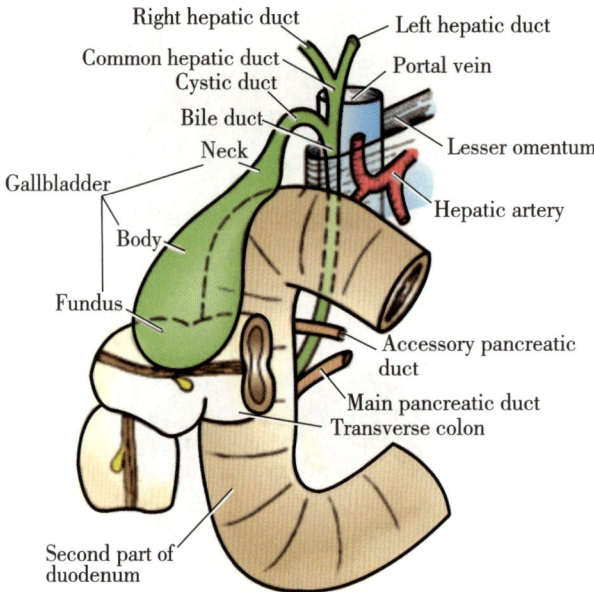

Figure 4-24 The bile ducts and the gallbladder

(Note the relation of the gallbladder to the transverse colon and the duodenum)

(2) Divisions

The gallbladder is a long pear-shaped sac. It is divided into three parts. Its distal part, which protrudes beyond the anterior edge of the liver is the fundus; its proximal part that becomes constrictive is the neck; and the part between the fundus and the neck is the body.

The common bile duct is divided into four segments according to its course and relations. The first segment, which runs in the hepatoduodenal ligament is called the supraduodenal part, because it is located above the superior part of the duodenum; the second that descends behind the superior part of the duodenum is called the retroduodenal part; then, the common bile duct passes through the head of the pancreas and is embedded in the pancreatic tissue, this segment is the pancreatic part; and finally the duct penetrates obliquely through the posteromedial wall of the descending part of the duodenum, this segment is called the intraduodenal part. It is this part that unites the pancreatic duct.

(3) Clinically important features

The fundus of the gallbladder protrudes beyond the anterior edge of the liver. Thus it directly contacts the inner surface of the anterior abdominal wall at the site where the lower egde of the right costal arch intersects the linea semilunaris (the lateral margin of the rectus abdominis muscle). This intersection point is called Murphy point. The Murphy point is clinically useful in diagnosis of disorders of gallbladder. For example, if you gently press with you finger at the Murphy point in a patient with inflammation of gallbladder (cholecystitis), and ask the patient to take a deep breath, a tenderness will appear during inspiration. This is clinically called the Murphy sign.

The neck of the gallbladder, at its junction with the body, usually forms a very small sac, called Hartmann pouch; on the inner surface of the cystic duct, the mucosal membrane forms several spiral folds, called Heister valves. These structures sometimes block the passing of tiny gallstones, leading to a spasm of the gallbladder. This will cause a severe pain in the right upper part of the abdomen, which is clinically called biliary colic.

The gallbladder is supplied by a very tiny artery called the cystic artery. It is usually a branch of the right hepatic artery, but its origin varies considerably. For example, it may arise from the proper hepatic artery or from the left hepatic artery; and even more, the right hepatic artery, which gives off the cystic artery, may arise from the superior mesenteric artery. Although its origin is inconstant, the cystic artery usually (61.67%) reaches the gallbladder by passing through a triangle, which is bounded by the porta hepatis, the common hepatic duct and cystic duct. This is called Calot Triangle. It is a useful mark to identify and ligate the cystic artery in the operation to resect the gallbladder (cholecystectomy).

The supraduodenal part of the common bile duct is closely related to two important structures, the proper hepatic artery on its the left and the hepatic portal vein behind it. These three structures are tightly packed by the hepatoduodenal ligament. In an operation of common bile duct, caution must be taken to avoid injury of any one of these two blood vessels. The pancreatic part of the common bile duct is embedded in the pancreatic tissue or passes behind the posterior surface of the pancreatic head. Therefore, in a patient with the cancer of pancreatic head, the growing tumor may compress the common bile duct, thus blocking the flow of bile. This will cause the obstructive jaundice (a yellowish staining of the skin and sclera due to increased level of bile pigments in blood). The intraduodenal part of the common bile duct obliquely passes through the wall of the duodenum, where it unites the pancreatic duct to form a small bulb called the Vater ampulla (hepatopancreatic ampulla). The Vater ampulla finally opens into the duodenum at the major duodenal papilla. Surrounding the Vater ampulla, and the distal ends of both common bile and pancreatic ducts, there are layers of circular smooth muscles, called the Oddi sphincter. Functionally the Oddi sphincter controls the release of both bile and pancreatic juice into the duodenum. Heavy drink of wine, particularly hard liquor, is not good for health. One reason for this is that alcohol may cause edema of the major duodenal papilla and spasm of the Oddi sphincter. In this condition, a contraction of the gallbladder may force the bile flowing into the pancreatic duct and activate the pancreatic enzymes, leading to an autodigestion of the pancreatic tissues. This is a type of acute pancreatitis.

In Chinese, there are about 70% of the population whose common bile duct is united with the pancreatic duct.

4.4.5 Pancreas

(1) Position

The pancreas is located in the retroperitoneal space. Its major part attaches on the posterior abdominal wall at the level of the 1st-2nd lumbar vertebrae.

(2) Division

The pancreas can be divided into four parts (Figure 4-25). Its right part surrounded by the duodenum is the head. Its major part in middle is the body and the junction between the head and the body is the neck. The left part that extends towards the spleen and does not tightly attach on the posterior abdominal wall is the tail of the pancreas.

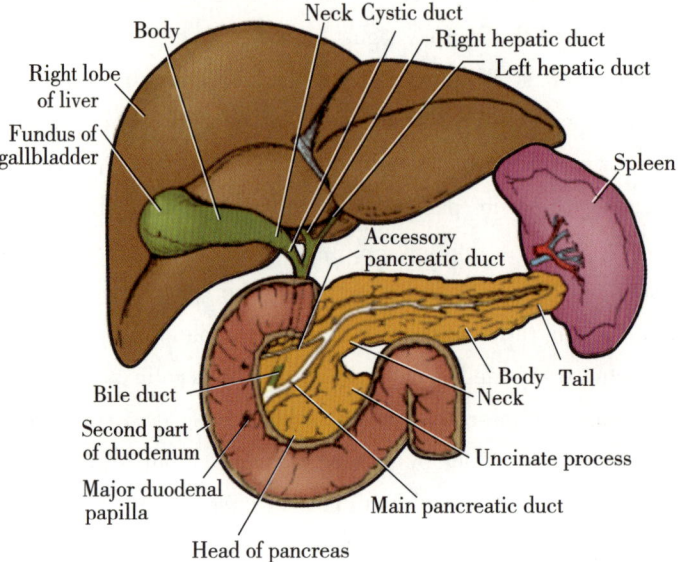

Figure 4-25　Different parts of the pancreas dissected to reveal the duct system

(3) Blood supply

The pancreatic head is supplied by the superior and inferior pancreaticoduodenal arteries. The other parts of the pancreas are supplied mainly by the pancreatic branches of splenic artery.

4.4.6　Spleen

(1) Position

The spleen is located in the left hypochondriac region, between the fundus of the stomach and the diaphragm. Usually its long axis corresponds to the left 10th rib.

(2) Shape and relations

The spleen has a blunt posterior edge and a sharp anterior edge with several incisures called the splenic notches (Figure 4-26). The lateral (diaphragmatic) surface of the spleen is convex, fitting the lower surface of the diaphragm. Its medial (visceral) surface is a little concave, related to the fundus of the stomach, the left kidney and the tail of the pancreas. A longitudinal cleft in the center of the medial surface is called the splenic hilum, through which the splenic artery, the splenic vein, and nerves and lymphatic vessels enter or leave the spleen. These structures are bounded by connective tissue to form the splenic pedicle. In living bodies, the spleen is very fragile, so it is easy to be broken by violence. If the spleen is injured, it bleeds badly. In this case, an emergency resection of the spleen may be lifesaving.

In some individuals, one or more small and round nodules may be found near the splenic hilum. If exist, they are called the accessory spleens. The accessory spleens have the same tissue structure and function with the spleen. Thus, in a surgical treatment for the hypersplennism, not only the spleen, but also accessory spleens must be removed.

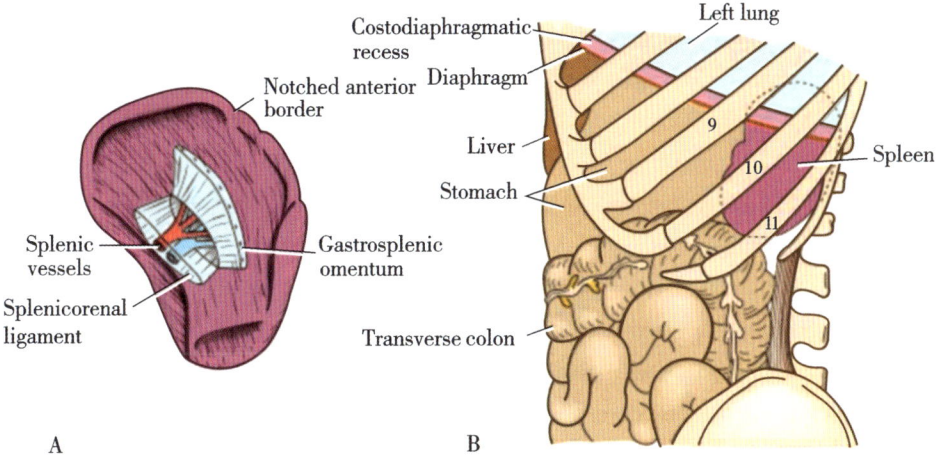

A. It is oval shaped and has a notched anterior border; B. Shows relation of spleen to adjacent structures.

Figure 4-26 Spleen

4.5 Organs in the infracolic compartment

The infracolic compartment is occupied by the major part of the lower digestive tract, including the jejunum, the ileum, the cecum with the appendix, and the colon. The colon is subdivided into the ascending colon, the transverse colon, the descending colon, and the sigmoid colon.

The jejunum and ileum are together 6-7 m long. They are convoluted in the abdominal cavity and are suspended by the mesentery of small intestine to the posterior abdominal wall. Therefore, they are also called the mesenteric small intestine. The mesentery of small intestine is a double-layer peritoneal sheet. Its intestinal edge matches the full length of mesenteric small intestine, but its root is only about 15 cm long, extending along the posterior abdominal wall from the end of the duodenum to the right iliac fossa. Thus, the mesentery is folded in the abdominal cavity and if fully spread, it has a fan-like shape. The ascending and descending colons are tightly attached on the posterior abdominal wall, but the transverse and sigmoid colons are suspended by their own mesenteries, the transverse mesocolon and the sigmoid mesocolon. So that in the abdominal cavity the ascending and descending colons are immovable, while the jejunum, the ileum, the transverse and sigmoid colons that are suspended by mesenteries are movable. These movable intestines sometimes may undergo an abnormal twisting that is called the volvulus. Clinically, a volvulus usually takes place in the jejunum and ileum, or sometimes in the sigmoid colon, but seldom in transverse colon. This is because the mesenteric small intestine and sigmoid colon have a shorter mesenteric root in comparison to their length.

4.5.1 Blood vessels, lymphatics and nerves of organs in infracolic compartment

(1) Arteries

The organs in the infracolic compartment are supplied by two arteries: the superior mesenteric artery and the inferior mesenteric artery.

The superior mesenteric artery originates from the abdominal aorta at the level of the 1st lumbar vertebra, behind the neck of the pancreas. By crossing over the anterior surface of the horizontal part of the duodenum, it enters the root of the mesentery of small intestine and runs to the right iliac fossa. Before crossing over the duodenum, It gives off a small inferior pancreaticoduodenal artery to the duodenum and the head of the pancreas. In its course, it sends 15-18 jejunal and ileal arteries that run between the two layers of the mesentery and finally supply the jejunum and ileum. The superior mesenteric artery also gives off three colic branches. The first one is the ileocolic artery which runs along the posterior abdominal wall to the right iliac fossa, where it divides into a colic branch to the lower part of the ascending colon, an ileal branch to the terminal part of the ileum, and an anterior and a posterior cecal arteries to the cecum. The ileocolic artery also gives off a very small branch to the appendix, called the appendicular artery. The origin of the appendicular artery is inconstant; it may originate from the colic branch, the ileal branch or the posterior cecal artery. The other two colic branches of the superior mesenteric artery are the right and middle colic arteries. The right colic artery supplies the upper part of the ascending colon, and the middle colic artery enters the transverse mesocolon and supplies the major part of the transverse colon (Figure 4-27).

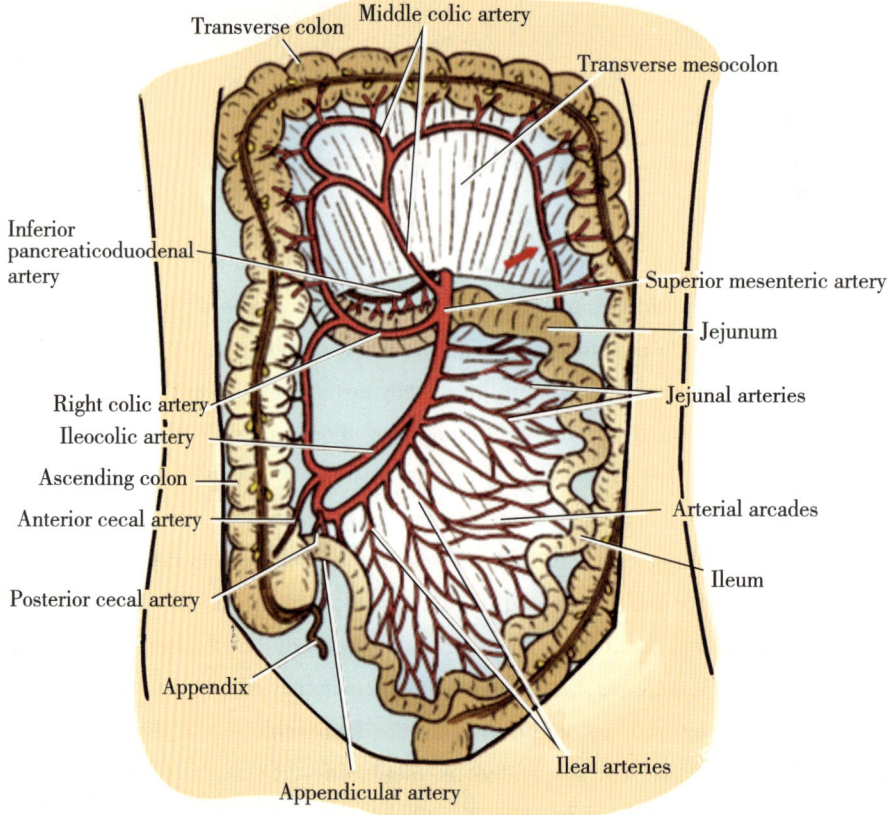

Figure 4-27 Superior mesenteric artery and its branches

[Note that this artery supplies blood to the gut from halfway down the second part of the duodenum to the distal third of the transverse colon (arrow)]

Because the mesentery of small intestine has a fan-like shape, the jejunal and ileal arteries run between its two layers in a radiate way. Near the intestinal edge of the mesentery, these arteries anastomose to form a series of arterial arches. From the distal arcades, small and straight branches arise to supply the intestinal wall. These small branches are called the vasa recta (straight arteries) and they are the terminal arteries (no longer anastomose with the others). Because the jejunal and ileal arteries are distributed in a radiate way and the vasa recta are the terminal arteries, in the operation to remove part of small intestine, a

V-shaped incision should be made on the mesentery with an increased angle of 20°-30° through the intestinal wall. This is the so called wedge-shaped resection of small intestine. It can prevent the anastomosed ends of the intestine from ischemic necrosis.

The inferior mesenteric artery arises from the abdominal aorta at the level of L_3. It gives off a number of branches. The first is called the left colic artery that supplies the left 1/3 of the transverse colon and the descending colon; the second are 3-4 sigmoid arteries that enter the sigmoid mesocolon and supply the sigmoid colon; the last one is called the superior rectal artery that runs inferiorly along the posterior abdominal wall to the pelvic cavity, where it supplies the upper part of the rectum.

The colic branches of the superior and inferior mesenteric arteries anastomose to form a complete arterial arcade along the margin of the colon from the ileocecum to the sigmoid colon. This arcade is called the colic marginal artery, which then gives off longer and shorter branches to supply the colon wall.

(2) Veins, lymphatics and nerves

The superior and inferior mesenteric arteries and all their branches are accompanied by the veins with the same name and these veins finally drain into the hepatic portal vein. In addition, superior and inferior mesenteric arteries are also accompanied by lymph nodes and autonomic nervous plexuses. These lymph nodes and nervous plexuses are also named after their related arteries. The superior and inferior mesenteric lymph nodes, together with the celiac lymph nodes, drain into the thoracic duct. The superior and inferior mesenteric plexuses are distributed along with the arteries to the related organs. In today's dissection, when you trace the arteries, you should identify all of these structures.

4.5.2 Hepatic portal system

(1) Hepatic portal vein and its tributaries

The main trunk of the hepatic portal system (HPS) is the hepatic portal vein. It is formed by confluence of the superior mesenteric and the splenic veins above the pancreas. The hepatic portal vein runs superiorly in the hepatoduodenal ligament to the porta hepatis, where it splits into a right and a left branches to enter the liver (Figure 4-28). In addition to the superior mesenteric and the splenic veins, the hepatic portal vein has other five major tributaries. The first one is the inferior mesenteric vein that usually drains into the splenic vein. The second three are the cystic vein, and the right and left gastric veins which all drain directly into the hepatic portal vein. The last two are a pair of paraumbilical veins that originate from the periumbilical venous plexus, run in the round ligament of liver and are finally drained into the left branch of the hepatic portal vein. Except for the splenic and the paraumbilical veins, the tributaries of the hepatic portal vein collect blood from the digestive tract, the blood contains high levels of nutrient molecules and these molecules are delivered to the liver and processed by the hepatocytes, becoming more absorbable or nontoxic to the body. This is one of the important functions of the liver, called biotransformation. In this context, the hepatic portal vein is the functional vessel of the liver.

(2) Characteristics of the hepatic portal system

To fit its functions, the hepatic portal system has two important characteristics.

The two ends of the hepatic portal system connect to the capillaries. At its distal end, its tributaries connect to the capillaries; at the other end, the branches of the hepatic portal vein in the liver finally connect to the hepatic sinusoids, a kind of enlarged capillaries.

The tributaries of the hepatic portal system have little valves. Thus, in some hepatic diseases such as the cirrhosis, the portal circulation through the liver may be blocked or restricted, leading to an increased blood in the hepatic portal vein. This is called portal hypertension. In this conditions, blood in the hepatic

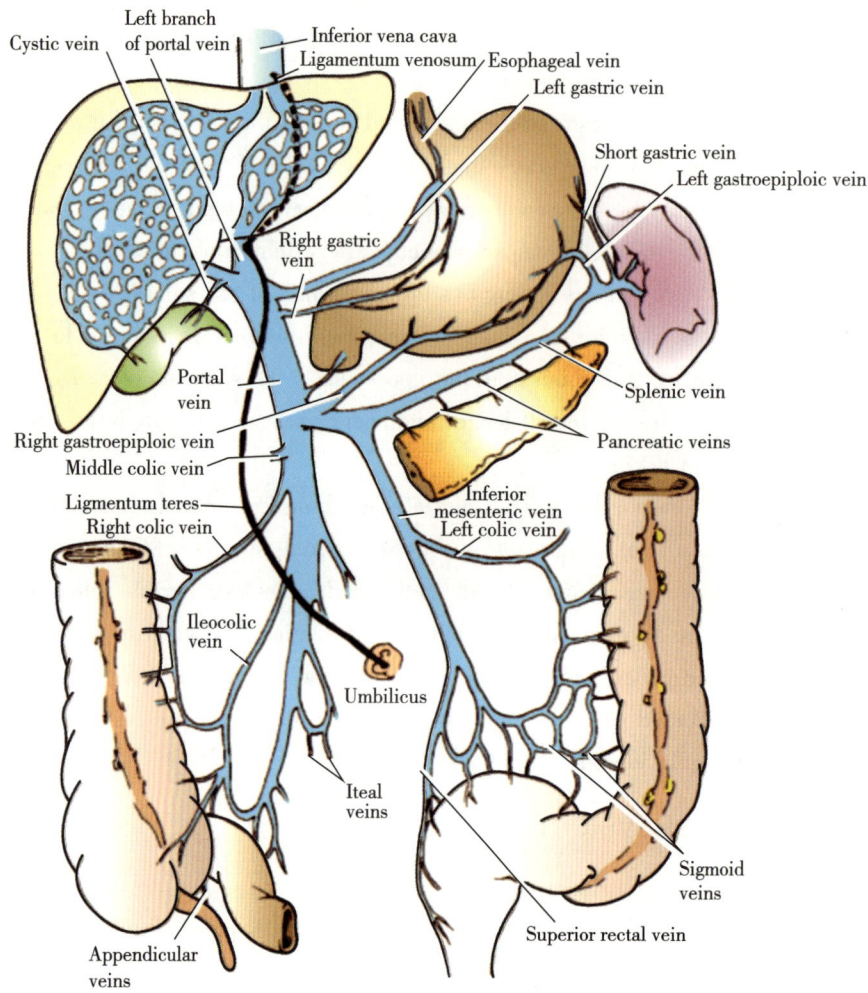

Figure 4-28 Tributaries of the portal vein

portal system will flow in a reverse direction through the portosystemic anastomoses into the superior and inferior vena cava systems.

(3) Portosystemic anastomoses

In the human body, the tributaries of hepatic portal system and systemic venous system (the superior and the inferior vena cava) anastomose at four major sites: the lower part of the esophagus, the umbilical region of the anterior abdominal wall, the lower part of the rectum and the retroperitoneal space in the posterior abdominal wall.

In the lower part of the esophageal wall, the submucosal layer has numerous small veins which anastomose to form the esophageal venous plexus. The upper part of plexus is drained via the esophageal vein and then the azygos vein into the superior vena cava, and the lower part of the plexus drains through the left gastric vein into the hepatic portal vein.

In the umbilical region, the periumbilical venous plexus is drained superiorly and inferiorly by the superficial and deep veins in the anterior abdominal wall into the superior and inferior vena cava. Internally, the plexus is drained through the paraumbilical veins into the hepatic portal vein (Figure 4-29).

In the lower part of the rectum, there are numerous small veins in its submucosal layer and around its surface. These small veins anastomose to form therectal venous plexus that is drained superiorly through the superior rectal vein and then the inferior mesenteric vein into the hepatic portal vein; and inferiorly it is drained through the inferior rectal and anal veins into the inferior vena cava system.

In the retroperitoneal space of the posterior abdominal wall, there are extensive anastomoses between small tributaries of the hepatic portal vein and inferior vena cava. These venous anastomoses are together called Retzius veins.

When a portal hypertension appears (for example in the patients with cirrhosis), the increased blood pressure may produce varices (the veins become extremely dilated) at the portosystemic anastomoses. The esophageal varices is the most dangerous because the dilated submucosal veins are very superficial and therefore may be damaged by solid food, leading to massive bleeding. The bleeding of esophageal varices is difficult to stop and is therefore aleading cause for the death of the patients.

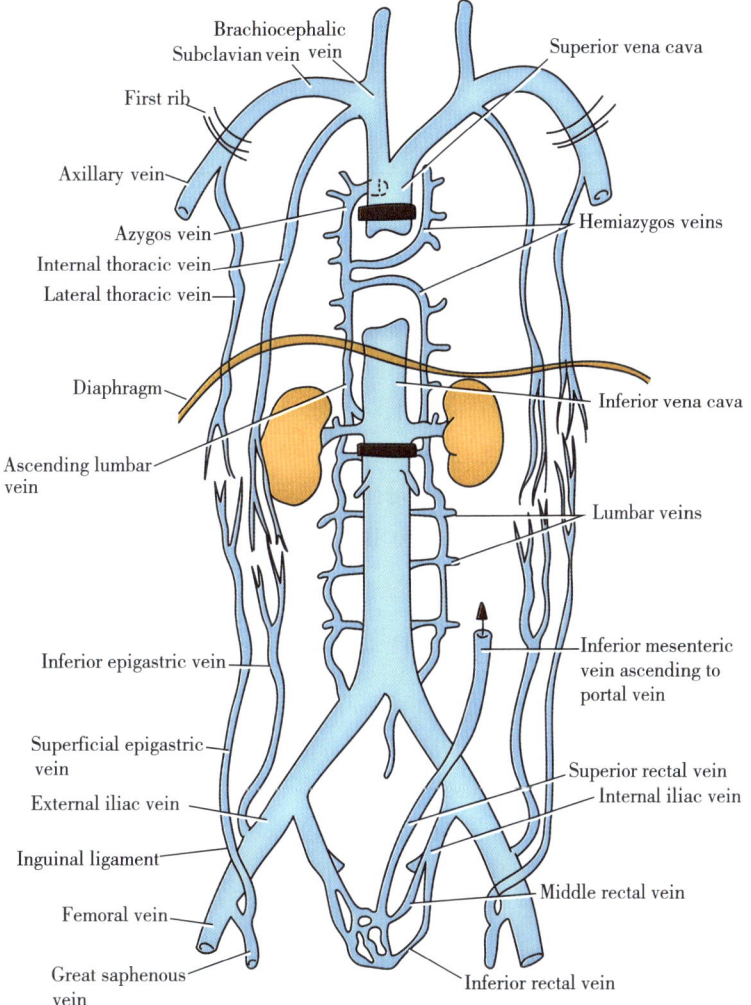

Figure 4-29 The possible collateral circulations of the superior and inferior venae cava
[Note the alternative pathways that exist for blood to return to the right atrium of the heart if the superior vena cava becomes blocked below the entrance of the azygos vein (upper black bar). Similar pathways exist if the inferior vena cava becomes blocked below the renal veins (lower black bar). Note also the connections that exist between the portal circulation and systemic veins in the anal canal]

4.5.3 Jejunum and Ileum

Jejunum and ileum constitute the major part of the small intestine between the duodenum and the cecum. They are together 6-7 m long. Usually, the jejunum contributes to the proximal 2/5 of the length and the ileum, to the remainder. But between them, there is no distinctive boundary. The Table 4-2 lists the major characteristics of the jejunum and the ileum, which are useful for you to distinguish these two intestinal segments.

Table 4-2 The characteristics of the jejunum and the ileum

Characteristic	Jejunum	Ileum
Position	Upper 2/5	Lower 3/5
Diameter	Greater	Less
Wall	Thicker	Thin
Circular folds	Larger, numerous and large villi	Fewer, smaller and less abundant villi
Vascularity	Greater	Less
Vasa recta	Long	Short
Colour	Deeper red	Paler pink
Lymphatic follicles	Solitary	Aggregated
Fat in mesentery	Less	More

In general, the jejunum is located in the left upper quadrant of the abdomen, while the ileum in the right lower part with a few of loops descending into the pelvic cavity. In living bodies, the jejunum is relatively red in color, and the ileum, a little pale and pink. The wall of the jejunum is thicker, and on its inner surface, there are much more circular mucosal folds. The submucosal lymphatic tissues in the jejunum are dispersedly distributed as independent tiny nodules called the solitary lymphatic follicles; while in the ileum, particularly in its distal portion, the independent nodules sometimes aggregate into long oval-shaped patches, called the aggregated lymphatic follicles or Peyer patches. The jejunal arteries form less arterial arches, usually only 1-2 tiers. But the arcades are bigger and their vasa recta are relatively longer than those formed by the ileal arteries.

4.5.4 Characteristics of the colon

The colon has three distinctive structures, the colic bands (teniae coli), the haustra coli and the epiploic appendices. The colic bands are three thickened muscular ribbons in the wall of the colon. They are formed by longitudinally arranged smooth muscles. Because of the tonic contraction of the smooth muscles (tonic contraction: in living body, there are always a small amount of muscles that maintain contraction to keep the shape or posture of an organ or a body part), the colic bands are shorter than the length of the colon. This endows the colon a typical shape of tucks and pouches. The haustra coli are the pouches of the colon wall between the tucks. The epiploic appendices are the peritoneal protrusions on the surface of the colon filled with fatty tissue. These distinctive structures sometimes can be used to distinguish the colon from the small intestine, particularly in a radiograph.

4.5.5 Cecum

The cecum is the beginning part of the large intestine located in the right iliac fossa. It is a blind intestinal pouch and is almost entirely covered by the peritoneum. But it has no mesentery. The distal end of the ileum invaginates into the cecum in its posteromedial wall, forming a superior and an inferior mucosal lips that are called the ileocecal valve. Functionally, the ileocecal valve can prevent the backflow of feces from the cecum into the ileum. About 2 cm below the ileocecal valve, there is an orifice that is the opening of the appendix.

4.5.6 Appendix

(1) Shape of appendix

The appendix is a small intestinal protrusion from the posteromedial wall of the cecum. It is worm-shaped and usually 5-7 cm long. The base of the appendix is located at the convergent point of three colic bands, and its distal end is blind and free. The appendix is invested by the peritoneum that forms a small triangular-shaped mesentery called the mesoappendix. The appendicular artery runs between the two layers of the mesoappendix along its free edge. In the operation to resect the inflamed appendix (appendectomy), you can find and ligate the artery at the root of the mesoappendix.

(2) Common positions of appendix

The appendix is located in the right iliac region. On the surface of the body, we can use two points to roughly locate its position. One is the McBurney point that is located at the lateral one third of the line from the right anterosuperior iliac spine to the umbilicus. The second is the Lanz point located at the right one third of the line connecting the two anterosuperior iliac spines. The two points are clinically useful in diagnosis of acute appendicitis. The appendicitis is an inflammation the appendix. It usually begins with an indistinctive abdominal pain in the periumbilical region. So in its early stage, it is not easy to diagnose. In this case, you can slightly press with a finger at the McBurney or the Lanz point and then quickly withdraw your finger to release the pressure. If a deep tenderness appears when you press at any one of these two points and a rebound tenderness appears when you withdraw your finger, that is a reliable sign for this disease.

Although the base of the appendix is fixed on the cecum, its distal end is movable. Therefore the appendix may vary in its position. In Chinese population, there are five common positions of the appendix.

- Retro-cecal position: the appendix is located behind the cecum.
- Pelvic position: the distal end of the appendix is close to or over the margin of the pelvic cavity.
- Sub-cecal position: the appendix lies below the cecum.
- Pre-ileal position: the appendix lies in front of the ileum.
- Retro-ileal position: the appendix lies behind the ileum.

The appendix in different positions has different relations, which may cause misdiagnosis of acute appendicitis. For example, the distal end of a pelvic appendix in female may be closely related to the uterine tube. In this case, an inflammation of the appendix may be misdiagnosed as the rupture of tubal pregnancy (the tubal pregnancy refers to the development of a fertilized ovum in the uterine tube). In the retro-ileal position, the distal end of the appendix is closely related to the ureter. Thus, an inflammation of the appendix may irritate the ureter, leading to pyuria, hematuria (pus and red blood cells appear in patient's urine) and even more ureteric colic. In this case, the appendicitis may be misdiagnosed as the ureteritis or the ureteric obstruction.

(3) Unusual positions of appendix

Sometimes the appendix may have an unusual position due to an abnormal location of the cecum during the embryonic development. In the early stage of the embryo, the cecum is originally located in the right upper part of the abdomen. With the development, it gradually descends to the right iliac fossa. If the cecum fails to fully descend, the appendix will be located higher than its normal position. This condition is called the undescended appendix. An inflammation of an undescended appendix may be difficult to be distinguished from the cholecystitis, especially when the appendix is located just beneath the liver. If the cecum is over-descended, the appendix will be located in the pelvic cavity. This is called the over-descended appendix. In rare cases, the cecum and the appendix may be located in the left iliac fossa due to an abnormal rotation of the midgut during the embryonic development. This is called the left appendix. Sometimes the appendix may be located between the psoas major muscle and the cecum, or even more, it may be embedded in the posterior wall of the cecum. In this condition, the appendix is not covered by the peritoneum and is therefore called the extraperitoneal appendix. An inflamed extraperitoneal appendix may be difficult to find during the operation; in this case, you should follow one of the three colic bands to their convergent point to locate the base of the appendix.

4.6 Retroperitoneal space

The retroperitoneal space is a potential space in the posterior abdominal wall, between the parietal peritoneum and the endoabdominal fascia. It is the continuation of the extraperitoneal fascia in the anterolateral abdominal wall. Superiorly it communicates with the loose connective tissues in the posterior mediastinum through the lumbocostal triangles, and inferiorly it extends to the retrorectal space. Thus an inflammation in the retroperitoneal space may spread upwards to the mediastinum and downwards to the pelvis.

The retroperitoneal space is important because it contains the major trunks of blood vessels, some important nervous and lymphatic structures, and paired abdominal organs.

(1) The abdominal aorta

The abdominal aorta is the continuation of the thoracic aorta. It begins at the aortic hiatus of the diaphragm and descends along the anterior surface of the vertebral column. At the level of the 4th lumbar vertebra, it divides into two common iliac arteries. In its course, the abdominal aorta gives off three un-paired visceral branches that supply the organs in the supra-colic and infra-colic compartments. It also gives off paired parietal and visceral branches to the diaphragm, the abdominal wall and the pared abdominal organs in the retroperitoneal space. These branches include the inferior phrenic arteries that supply the diaphragm, the middle suprarenal arteries to the suprarenal glands, the renal arteries to the kidneys, the testicular arteries in male or ovarian arteries in female which supply the testes or ovaries, and four pairs of the lumbar arteries to the lower part of the abdominal wall.

(2) The inferior vena cava

The inferior vena cava is formed by confluence of two common iliac veins. It runs superiorly along the right side of the abdominal aorta. Its tributaries in the retroperitoneal space basically accompany the related branches of the abdominal aorta.

(3) The lumbar sympathetic trunks

The lumbar sympathetic trunks are the continuations of the thoracic sympathetic trunks. They run inferiorly between the lateral side vertebral column and the origin of the psoas major muscle. Each lumbar sympathetic trunk consists of 3-4 lumbar sympathetic ganglia which are linked by the interganglionic fibers.

(4) The celiac plexus

The celiac plexus is the biggest and most complex autonomic nervous plexus in the human body. It is located on the anterior surface of the upper part of the abdominal aorta, surrounding the origins of the celiac trunk and the superior mesenteric artery. The plexus contains a number of sympathetic ganglia. The paired celiac ganglia are located near the origin of the celiac trunk and receive the preganglionic fibers from the greater splanchnic nerve. Near the origin of the renal arteries, you may find the paired aorticorenal ganglia that receive the preganglionic fibers from the lesser splanchnic nerve. However, in the majority of Chinese population, the aorticorenal ganglia are merged into the celiac ganglia. Inferiorly, the celiac plexus extends on the surface of the lower part of the abdominal aorta, forming the abdominal aortic plexus. The fibers of both celiac plexus and abdominal aortic plexus surround the branches of the abdominal aorta, forming the secondary plexuses such as the superior mesenteric plexus and the renal plexus and the inferior mesenteric plexus. These plexuses are distributed along with the arteries to innervate the organs they supply.

(5) The lumbar lymph nodes

Along the abdominal aorta and the inferior vena cava, there are a number of longitudinally arranged lymph nodes, called the lumbar lymph nodes. The final efferent vessels of the lymph nodes form the right and left lumbar trunks which drain into the chyle cistern. The chyle cistern is the dilated beginning part of the thoracic duct located beneath the aortic hiatus of the diaphragm.

(6) The suprarenal glands

The suprarenal glands are located above the upper end of the kidney in each side.

(7) The kidneys and the ureters

The kidneys and the abdominal part of the ureters are commonly involved in diseases of the urinary system and will be described in detail in the following sections.

4.6.1 Kidneys

(1) Position

The kidneys are located on the posterior abdominal wall lateral to each sides of the vertebral column (Figure 4-30). Their upper ends usually reach the level of T_{11} and the lower ends, at the level of L_3 vertebra, but the right kidney is slightly lower than the left due to the large size of the liver.

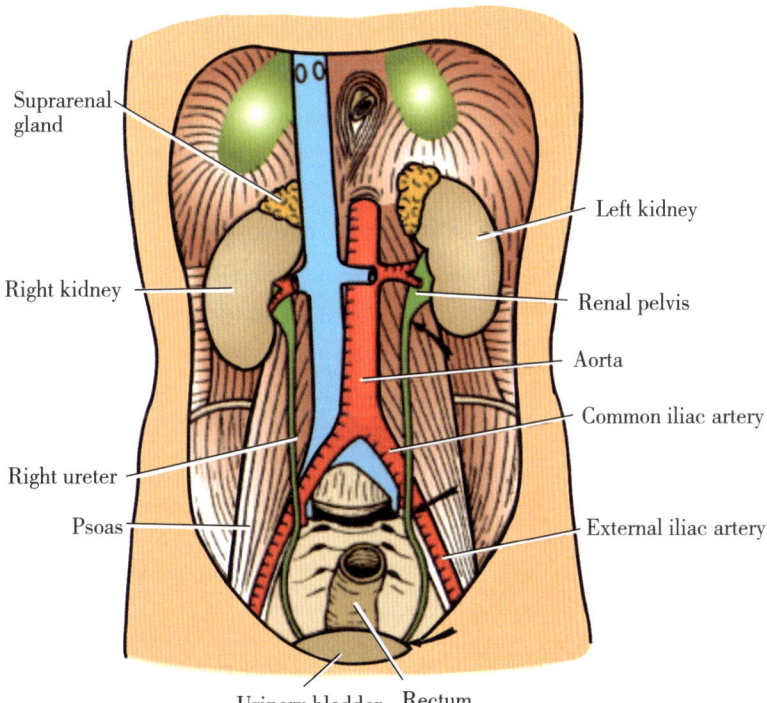

Figure 4-30 Posterior abdominal wall showing the kidneys and the ureters in situ

(Arrows indicate three sites where the ureter is narrowed)

On the outer surface of the posterior abdominal wall, we can roughly locate the position of the kidney with a superficial mark called the renal angle, which is formed by intersecting of the lateral margin of the erector spinal muscle and the lower edge of 12th rib. The renal angle is clinically useful in diagnosis of some renal diseases. For example, in the patient with chronic nephritis or renal calculus, a slight percussion on the apex of the angle causes deep internal pain.

(2) Relations

Superiorly, the upper end of the kidney on each side is related to the suprarenal gland. Medially, the left kidney is related to the abdominal aorta and the right, to the inferior vena cava; for both kidneys, the renal vessels and renal pelvis pass through their hilums. Posteriorly, the upper part of the posterior surface of the kidney is related to the diaphragm, the costodiaphragmatic recess, the 12th rib, and the subcostal nerve and vessels; the middle and lower part of the posterior surface of the kidney is related to the psoas major muscle, the quadratus lumborum and the transverse abdominis muscle. In addition, the iliohypogastric and ilioinguinal nerves also pass obliquely along the posterior surface of the kidney. The posterior relations of the kidney are clinically important because the operations on this organ are usually taken through a back approach (make incision on the posterior abdominal wall). Therefore, when opening the posterior abdominal wall to expose the kidney, caution must be taken to avoid injuries of these important structures, particularly the iliohypogastric and ilioinguinal nerves.

(3) Shape

The kidneys are bean shaped. Each has an anterior and a posterior surfaces, a superior and an inferior poles, and a lateral and a medial margins. In its medial margin, there is a vertical cleft called the renal hilum. The renal hilum extends interiorly and expands to form a central cavity in the kidney, called the renal sinus. The renal hilum is a passage through which the renal vessels, renal pelvis, lymphatic vessels and nerves enter or leave the kidney. All of these structures are together wrapped by loose connective tissues, forming the renal pedicle. The three major structures of the renal pedicle, the renal artery, renal vein and renal pelvis are arranged in an order from superior downwards, while the renal vein, the renal artery and the renal pelvis, from anterior to posterior.

Some common congenital anomalies of the kidney are seen in Firgure 4-31.

(4) Renal arteries and segments of kidney

Near the renal hilum, each of the renal arteries splits into an anterior and a posterior branches. The anterior branch is subdivided into four segmental arteries: the superior segmental artery to the upper pole of the kidney, the anterosuperior and the anteroinferior segmental arteries to the middle part of the anterior half of the kidney, and the inferior segmental artery to the lower pole (Figure 4-32). The posterior branch of the renal artery extends into the renal sinus, where it continues as the posterior segmental artery to supply the middle part of the posterior half of the kidney. All the segmental arteries are the terminal arteries that do not anastomose with each other. Therefore, each segmental artery supplies a relatively independent part of renal tissue, called a segment of kidney. Thus, each kidney can be divided into five segments: the superior, the inferior, the posterior, the anterosuperior and the anteroinferior segments. If a segmental artery is damaged, the related segment will undergo ischemic necrosis. In some individuals, the superior or the inferior segmental artery may have an origin far away from the kidney. They may originate from the midway of the renal artery or from the abdominal aorta. These variational vessels are called the superior polar artery or the inferior polar artery and they should be protected during the operation.

Chapter 4   The Abdomen   249

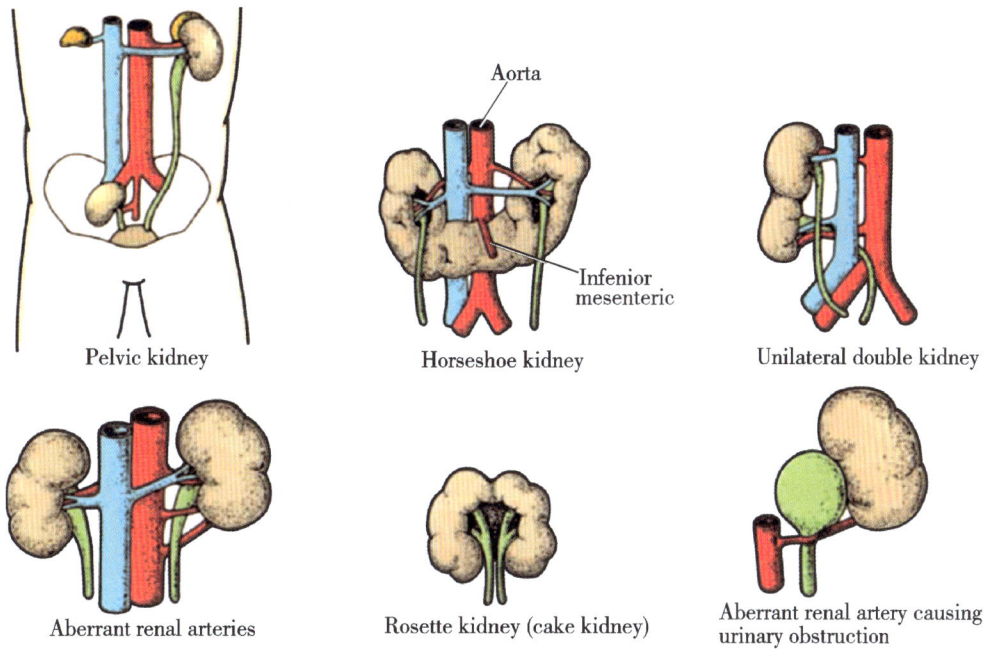

Figure 4-31   Some common congenital anomalies of the kidney

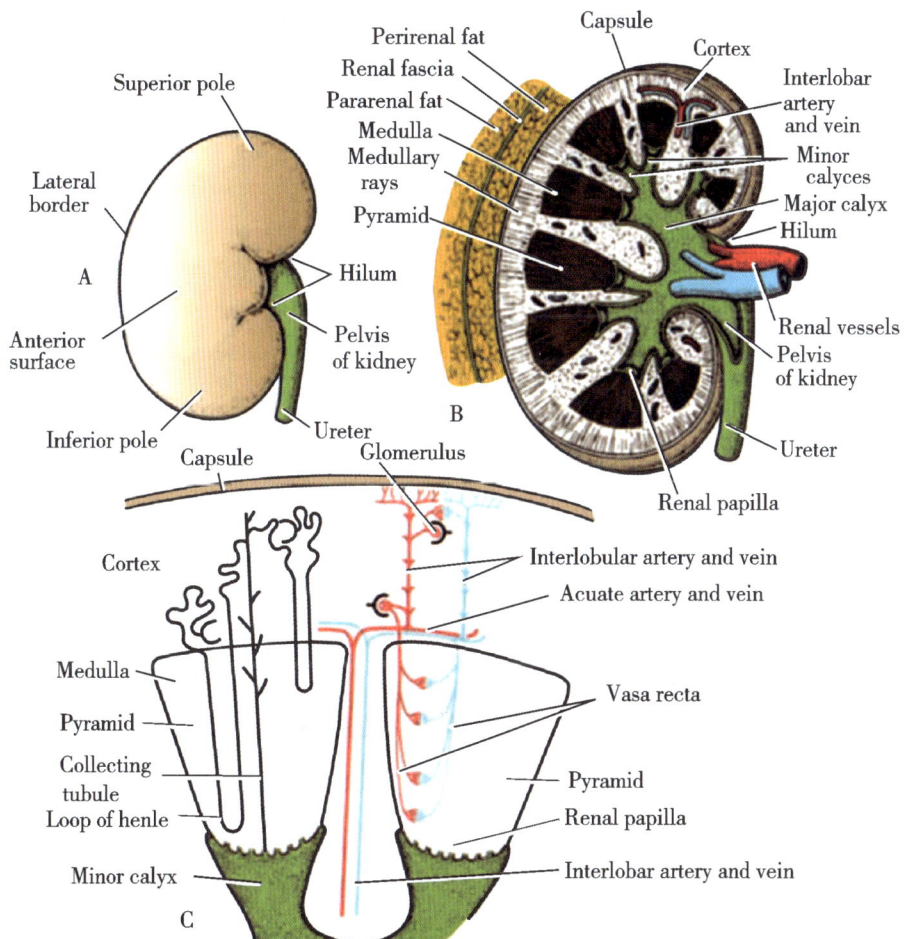

A. Right kidney, anterior surface. B. Right kidney, coronal section showing the cortex, medulla, pyramids, renal papillae, and calyces. C. Section of the kidney showing the position of the nephrons and the arrangement of the blood vessels within the kidney.

Figure 4-32   Right kidney and it's blood vessels

(5) Capsules of kidney

The kidney is surrounded by three coverings. From inner outwards, they are the fibrous capsule, the perirenal fat capsule and the renal fascia. The fibrous capsule is a connective tissue membrane covering the surface of the kidney. It is thin, transparent, and easy to be peeled off from the surface of the kidney in a living body. The perirenal fat capsule is a layer of fatty tissue surrounding the kidney outside the fibrous capsule. In a fat person, this layer of fatty tissue may be very thick and extends into the renal sinus. The renal fascia is derived from the endoabdominal fascia that splits into an anterior and a posterior layers to envelope both the kidney and the suprarenal gland. Superiorly, the anterior and posterior layers of the renal fascia merge into the diaphragmatic fascia. Inferiorly, however, the two layers of the renal fascia do not merge, but gradually replaced by loose connective tissues. Thus the renal fascia is open inferiorly. For this reason, in some individuals, especially the person who is very thin, the kidney may descend to a relatively lower position. This is called the nephroptosis. External to the renal fascia, especially behind its posterior layer, there is an aggregation of fatty tissue, called pararenal fat.

4.6.2 Abdominal part of ureter

The ureters are a pair of muscular tubes that conduct urine from the kidneys to the urinary bladder. On each side, the ureter begins at the end of the renal pelvis. The junction is at the level of the lower pole of the kidney. Then it descends along the surface of the psoas major muscle and crosses over the external iliac vessels into the pelvic cavity. The wall of the ureter is thick and its lumen, very narrow with an internal diameter of 2-7 mm. Thus, in the operation of ureter anastomosis, the two ends should be anastomosed in a diagonal plane to prevent anastomotic stenosis.

In its course, the ureter has three physiological constrictions with two in its abdominal part; one is at its beginning (the pelvoureteric junction), usually at the level of the lower end of kidney. This constriction has an internal diameter about 2 mm. The second is at its segment crossing over the external iliac vessels. In the patients with the renal or ureteric calculus, these constricted sites sometimes block the passing of tiny stones, leading to the spasm of the ureter, which causes a sharp abdominal pain along the course of the ureter, called the ureteric colic.

Tan Jianguo

4.7 Main contents of the abdomen

Overview

Chinical notes: Weak areas are the superficial and deep inguinal rings→ herniation

Indirect inguinal hernia	Direct inguinal hernia
✓ Viscera enter deep inguinal ring and travel along canal ✓ Emerge from superficial ring and into scrotum ✓ Accompanied by sac of peritoneum	✓ Viscera protrude anteriorly ✓ Usually passes through inguinal (Hassalbach's) triangle

Relations of posterior abdominal wall

✓ The posterior abdominal wall is composed of the bodies and discs of the five lumbar vertebra centrally
✓ On each side (from medial to lateral)
- ▷ Psoas major
- ▷ Psoas minor
- ▷ Quadratus lumborum
- ▷ Ilium
- ▷ Iliacus

✓ The diaphragm also contributes to the upper part of the wall

Relations

✓ Posterior relations
- ▷ Erector spinae lies behind the quadratus lumborum
- ▷ More superficially = lateral dorsi
- ▷ Thoracolumbar fascia

✓ Lateral relations
- ▷ Origins of internal oblique and trannsversus abdomen from thoracolumbar fascia lie at lateral edge of quadratus lumborum

✓ Anterior relations
- ▷ Related to structures in abdominal cavity
  - ◆ Aorta
  - ◆ Inferior vena cave (IVC)
- ▷ These lie on the front of the vertebral bodies, with psoas minor at their sides
  - ◆ Crura of diaphragm partly cover the upper LV
  - ◆ Medial arcuate ligament of diaphragm bridges psoas major
  - ◆ Lateral arcuate ligament of diaphragm bridges quadratus lumborum
  - ◆ Abdomial part of sympathetic trunk passes behind medial arcuate ligament
  - ◆ Lumbar plexus lies in psoas major
  - ◆ Cisterna chyli lies in front of L_1 and L_2 (on right side of aorta)
  - ◆ Kidneys and suprarenal glands lie below the arcuate ligament
  - ◆ Lower down
     Right = cecum and ascending colon
     Left = descending colon
- ▷ Elsewhere the wall is line by parietal peritoneum

Lesser sac

✓ The lesser sac is a large bursa which facilitate the movements of the stomach

Location and extent

✓ Lies behind the lesser omentum and the caudate lobe of liver
✓ Passes downwards behind stomach then between the two anterior and two posterior layers of greater omentum

Subdivision

✓ The chief subdivisions are the superior and inferior recesses

✓ These are separated from each other by a constricted area (vestibule) which lie between the left and right gastropancreatic folds
✓ An extension of the sac towards the hulum of the spleen is called the splenic recess

Superior recess	Inferior recess	Splenic recess
✓ Lies behind lesser omentum and caudate lobe of liver	✓ Lies behind stomach and between the layers of greater omentum	✓ Lies between gastrosplenic ligament in front and lieno-renal ligament behind

Relations

✓ Anteriorly
- ◊ Lesser omentum
- ◊ Caudate lobe of liver
- ◊ Posterior surface of stomach
- ◊ Anterior 2 layers of greater omentum

✓ Posteriorly
- ◊ Aorta and branch
- ◊ Diaphragm
- ◊ Left kidney
- ◊ Pancreas
- ◊ Posterior two layers of greater omentum

✓ Left
- ◊ Left margin of greater omentum
- ◊ Ligaments : gastrosplenic
    - ◆ Gastrohepatic
    - ◆ Lienorenal

✓ Right
- ◊ Peritoneal reflection from caudate lobe of liver to posterior abdominal wall
- ◊ Right margin of greater omentum

✓ Inferiorly
- ◊ Lower margin of greater omentum

Openings

✓ The part of the lesser sac behind the lesser omentum communicates with the greater sac via the epiploic foramen (foramen of winslow)

✓ Boundaries of epiploic formen (of winslow)
- ◊ Anteriorly
    - ◆ The free border of lesser omentum, containing bile duct, hepatic duct, portal vein behind
- ◊ Posteriorly
    - ◆ IVC (covered with peritoneum)
- ◊ Superiorly
    - ◆ Caudate process from caudate lobe of liver
- ◊ Inferiorly
    - ◆ 1st part of duodenum

Chapter 4　The Abdomen　253

Chinical notes：①Intra-abdominal herniation of intestine through epiploic foramen；②spread of infections and fluids/accumulation of fluids

Stomach

Parts and peritoneum

- ✓ The stomach is situated in the upper part of the abdomen
- ✓ Extending from left hypochondrium to epigastric and umbilical regions

Shape

It is roughly J-shaped, with 2 curvatures

Lesser curvature	Greater curvature
✓ Forms right border of stomach ✓ Concave ✓ Extends from cardiac orifice to pylorus ✓ Near pylorus, notch=incisura angularis	✓ Forms left border of stomach ✓ Covex ✓ Extends from left of cardiac orifice→over fundus→inferior part of pylorus

Openings

Cardiac orifice	Entry of esophagus
✓ Pyloric orifice (pylorus)	✓ Opens into duodemum ✓ Controlled by pyloric sphincter around pyloric canal

Divisions/Parts

✓ The stomach is divided into a fundus, body and a pyloric part

Fundus	✓ Dome-shaped ✓ Projects upward and to the left from cardiac orifice ✓ Separated from body by horizontal line ✓ Joining cardiac orifice to greater curvature ✓ Usually full of gas
Body	✓ Extends from level of cardiac orifice to level of incisura angularis
Pyloric part	✓ Subdivided into 　◊ Pyloric antrum=proximal part 　◊ Pyloric canal=distal part=thick wall→pyloric sphincter

Peritoneal relations

- ✓ Lesser omentum descends from liver to lesser curvature of stomach, called gastrohepatic ligament
- ✓ At lesser curvature, the two layers of lesser omentum separate to cover anterior and posterior surface
- ✓ Except "bare area" near cardiac orifice where it is in direct contact with left crus of diaphragm
- ✓ On left upper part of greater curvature, the two layers meet and continue to diaphragm and spleen
   ◊ Gastrophrenic ligament
   ◊ Gastrosplenic ligament
- ✓ On lower part of greater curvature, the two layers meet and continues downwards as anterior two layers of greater omentum

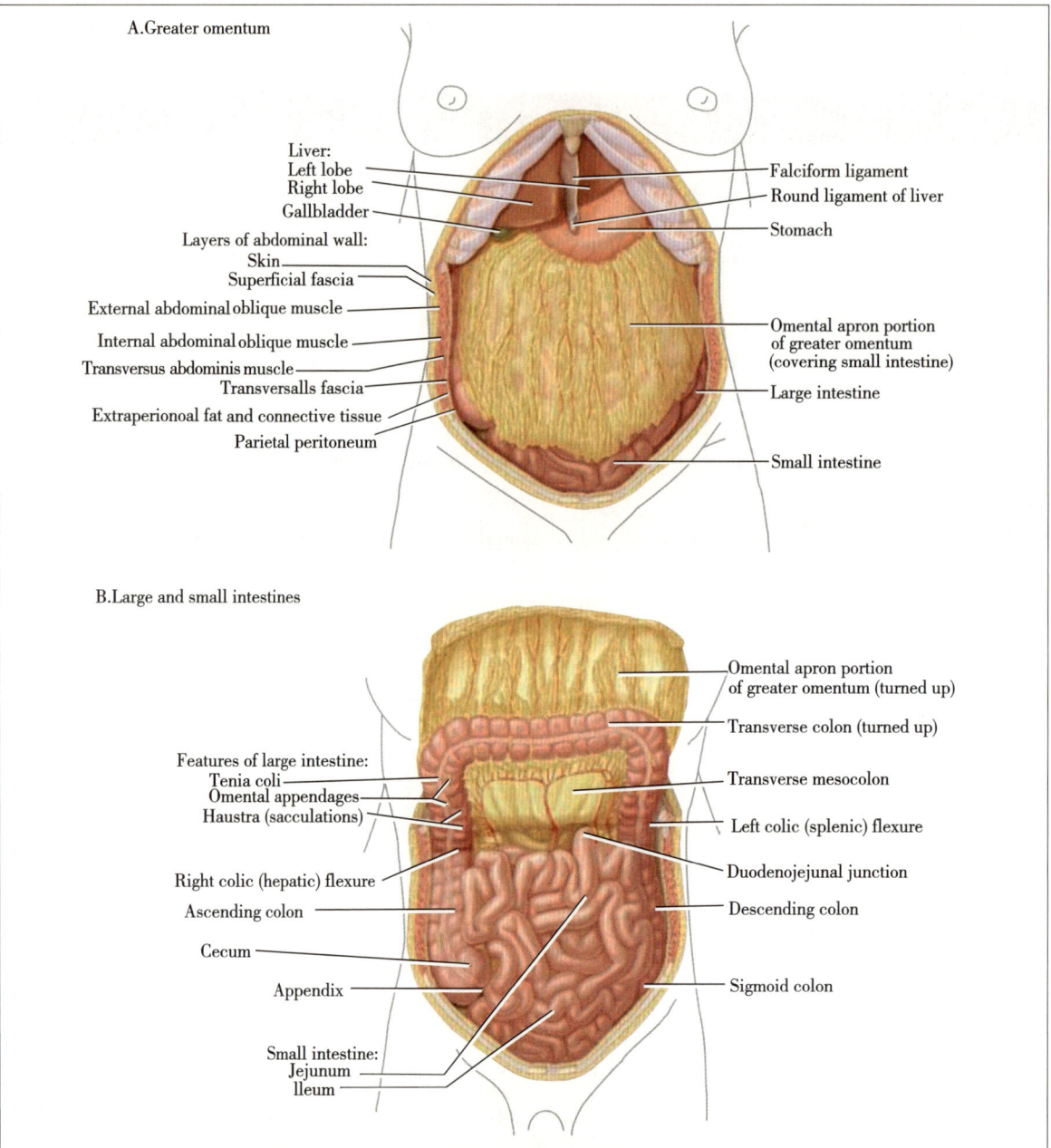

A. Greater omentum

B. Large and small intestines

Chinical notes
✓ Fundus contains air, percussion will produce tympany. Thus dullness over this area means enlarged left lobe of liver, enlarged spleen, left pleural effusion
✓ Porto-systemic anatomosis at lower end of esophagus and near cardiac opening
◊ Esophageal varices may occur
✓ Congenital pyloric stenosis
◊ Hypertrophy of pyloric sphincter
✓ Greater omentum "walls off" sites of infection

Stomach relations
✓ The stomach is situated in upper part of abdomen, extending from left hypochondrium to epigastric and umbilical regions

✓ The stomach is relatively mobile (except at cardiac orifice) and its position may vary
✓ The relations described are thus the more typical ones

Anterior relations	Posterior relations
✓ Inferior surface of left lobe of liver; overlaps lesser curvature ✓ Left half of diaphragm; related to fundus and part of body ✓ Left lung and pleura; anterior to diaphragm ✓ Left costal margin ✓ Anteruir abdominal wall ✓ Transverse colon (especially when stomach is empty) ✓ Note: part of greater sac may intervene between stomach and these structures	✓ Diaphragm ◊ Related to fundus of stomach ✓ Left lung and pleura ◊ Posterior to diaphragm ✓ Spleen ◊ Related to fundus as well as body ◊ Separated from stomach by greater sac ✓ Left kidney ◊ Retroperitoneal ✓ Letf adrenal gland ◊ Retroperitoneal ✓ Desc aorta ◊ Slightly to right of midline ◊ Related to pylorus ✓ Pancreas ◊ Related to pylorus and body ✓ Mesocolon ◊ Related to lower part of body of stomach ◊ Stretches from hepatic flexure to splenic flexure ✓ Middle colic artery ◊ Between layers of mesocolon ✓ Transverse colon ◊ Variable ◊ May be related to greater curvature ◊ Splenic flexure

Chinical notes

✓ Perforation of posterior wall of stomach caused by ulcer can cause perforation of splenic artery → bleeding
✓ Fluid accumulation in lesser sac → forward displacement of stomach

Stomach: blood supply

✓ The blood supply of the stomach is derived from all 3 branches of the celiac trunk
　◊ Left gastric artery
　◊ Hepatic artery
　◊ Splenic artery
✓ The venous drainage is mainly through the superior mesenteric, splenic and portal veins

Arterial supply

The gastric arteries

Left gastric artery	Right gastric artery
✓ Arises from celiac trunk ✓ Desc along lesser curvature of stomach	✓ Arises from hepatic artery at upper border of pylorus ✓ Runs to the left along lesser curvature
✓ The 2 arteries anastomse to forma double channel ✓ Along lesser curvature and supplies it ✓ They lie in the lesser omentum and send branches through the muscles and submucosa to supply the mucosa directly	

The gastro-epiploic arterires

Left gastro-epiploic artery	Right gastro-epiploic artery
✓ Arises from splenic artery ✓ Runs along gastrosplenic ligament and to the right along greater curvature	✓ Arises from gastroduod artery (branch of hepatic artery) ✓ Runs to the left along greater curvature
✓ The 2 arteries anastomose to form a channel along the greater curvature and supply it ✓ They lie in the greater omentum, about 1 cm from greater curvature ✓ They send branches into the anterior and posterior walls of the stomach and these may anatomose with branches from lesser curvature	

Short gastric arteries

✓ Arise from splenic artery
✓ Run along gastrosplenic ligament
✓ Supply fundus of stomach

Venous drainage

✓ The veins arise from a superficial network of capillaries which form a plexus in the submucosa
✓ The veins terminate as follows
   ▷ Left and right gastric veins drain into portal vein
   ▷ Left gastro-epiplocic and short gastric veins drain into splenic vein
   ▷ Right gastro-epiploic vein drains into superior mesenteric vein

Chinical notes

✓ The extensive anastomosis provides good collat circulation
✓ Thus ligation of one of the major arteries will not have a great effect on the circulation

Stomach: lymphatic drainage

✓ Lymphatic cap arising from mucosa form a submucous plexus from which LV arise to follow BV

Zones of drainage

✓ The zones of drainage are indicated thus:
   ▷ A line drawn from highest part of fundus to pylorus
   ▷ The lower part is subdivided into left and right halves
✓ Thus there are 3 zones
   ▷ Zone I = upper 2/3

◊ Zone Ⅱ = lower right half
◊ Zone Ⅲ = lower left half

Lymph nodes

✓ Zone Ⅰ
　◊ Drain into left gastric nodes (along left gastric vessels)
　◊ Some drain into hepatic nodes
　◊ Small minority around pyloric region drain into right gastric nodes
✓ Zone Ⅱ
　◊ Drain into right gastro-epiploic nodes
　◊ Some drain into pyloric nodes
✓ Zone Ⅲ
　◊ Drain into pancreatico-splenic nodes

All 3 zones ultimately drain into celiac nodes

Clinical notes: Spread of cancer

Stomach: nerve supply

✓ The stomach receives both sympathetic and parasympathetic nerve supply
　◊ Sympathetic arteric supply: celiac plexus
　◊ Parasympathetic supply: vagus nerve

Sympathetic supply

✓ PreGN fibres
　◊ Arise from T_6-T_{12} segments of spine cord from ILN (lateral horn)
　◊ Leaves spine cord along ventral roots of spinal nerve
　◊ Enter sympathetic trunk via WRC
　◊ Without synapsing, leave sympathetic trunk via splanchnic nerve
　◊ Synapse at celiac ganglia with post-synaptic neurons
✓ PGN fibres
　◊ From celiac ganglia, follow branches of celiac trunk
　◊ Enter stomach tog with branches of vagi
　◊ Terminate in myenteric and submucosal plexuses

Parasympathetic supply

✓ Anterior (left) vagal trunk
　◊ Enter abdomen in front of esophagus
　◊ Gives off hepatic branches
　◊ From which pyloric branches may arise to supply pyloric region
　◊ The trunk then divides into branches which supply body of stomach
✓ Posterior (right) vagal trunk
　◊ Enters abdomen behind esophagus
　◊ Divides into branches which supply body of stomach
　◊ Large branch passes to celiac plexus where its branches are distributed as far as splenic flexure of colon and pancreas

Chinical notes

✓ Pain fibres accompany sympathetic fibres
   ▷ Thus sympathectomy may be performed to relieve pain
✓ Pain is referred to epigastrium
✓ Vagotomy may be performed to lower secretion of acid
   ▷ Especially when peptic ulcer present

Duodenum

✓ The duodenum is the proximal part of the small intestine
✓ It is also the shortest and most fixed part

Course

✓ Extends from pylorus to duod-jejunum flexure
✓ About 25 cm
✓ Forms a C-shape, the concavity of which is occupied by the pancreas
✓ Its course can be described in 4 parts: superior, descending, horizontal, ascending

1st (superior) part

✓ About 5 cm long
✓ Begins at level of LV_1 to the right of midline
✓ Lies on transpyloric plane

Relations

Anteriorly	Posteriorly	Superiorly	Inferiorly
✓ Quadrate lobe of liver ✓ Gallbladder	✓ Lesser sac ✓ Gastroduod artery ✓ Common bile duct and portal vein ✓ IVC	✓ Epiploci foramen ✓ Right gastropancreatic fold	✓ Head of pancreas ✓ Superior pancreatico-duod vessels

2nd (descending) part

✓ 8 cm long
✓ Runs down vertically to right of LV_2 and LV_3

Relations

Anteriorly	Posteriorly	Superiorly	Inferiorly
✓ Fundus of GB ✓ Right lobe of liver ✓ Transverse colon ✓ Coils of SI	✓ Hilus of right kidney ✓ Commencement of right ureter	✓ Asc colon ✓ Right colic (hep) flexure ✓ Right lobe of liver	✓ Head of pancreas ✓ Bile duct and main pancreatic duct pierce the wall about halfway down posterior medial aspect ✓ Accessory pancreatic duct

3rd (horizontal) part

- ✓ About 8 cm long
- ✓ Runs to the left at/below subcostal plane (across LV_3)

Relations

Anteriorly	Posteriorly	Superiorly	Inferiorly
✓ Roots of mesentry ✓ Superior mes vessels in it (root of mesentery) ✓ Coils of SI	✓ Right ureter ✓ Right psoas muscle ✓ IVC ✓ Aorta	✓ Head of uncinate process of pancreas	✓ Coils of jejunum

4th (ascending) part

- ✓ About 5 cm long
- ✓ Runs upwards and to the left
- ✓ Ends at duodeno-jejunal flexure at level of LV_2
- ✓ Note: ligament of Treitz holds it in postion

Relations

Anteriorly	Posteriorly
✓ Beginning of root of mesentery ✓ Coils of jejunum	✓ Left margin of aorta ✓ Medial border of left psoas muscle

Blood supply

✓ Proximal part (to opening of bile duct) ✓ Superior pancreaticoduodenal artery from gastroduod artery)	✓ Distal part ✓ Inferior pancreaticoduodenal artery from superior mesenteric artery)

Lymphatic drainage

Upwards	Downwards
✓ Superior pancreaticoduodenal nodes ✓ Gastroduod nodes ✓ And thence into celiac nodes	✓ Inferior pancreaticoduodenal nodes ✓ And thence to superior mesenteric nodes ✓ Into pyloric nodes from 1st part of duodenum

Venous drainage

- ✓ Veins correspond to arteries
  - ▷ Superior veins drains into portal vein
  - ▷ Inferior veins drains into superior mesenteric vein
- ✓ Thus the venous drainage is ultimately into the portal vein
- ✓ Veins correspond to arteries
  - ▷ Superior veins drains into portal vein
  - ▷ Inferior veins drains into superior mesenteric vein
- ✓ Thus the venous drainage is ultimately into the portal vein

Nerve supply

✓ Sympathetic and parasympathetic fibres from celiac and superior mesenteric plexuses

Chinical notes

✓ Duodenal ulcer produced by acid chyme from stomach
  ♦ Especially on anterolat wall of 1st part of duodenum
✓ Ulcer on posterior wall of 1st part of duodenum may erode gastroduodenal artery
  ♦ Hemorrhage

Jejunum and ileum

✓ These parts of the small intestine extend from duodenojejunal(DJ) junction to ileocecal junction
✓ They are suspended by mesentery and are thus free mobile
✓ The upper 2/5 is arbitrarily designated jejunum, here being no clear-cut distinction

Comparison of jejunum and ileum

Jejunum	Ileum
✓ Lies in upper part of peritoneal cavity	✓ Lies in lower part of peritoneal cavity and in pelvis
♦ Below left side of transverse mesocolon	✓ Narrower bore
✓ Wider bore	♦ Thinner wall
♦ Thicker wall	♦ Less red
♦ Redder (more vascular)	✓ Plicae circulares smaller, fewer and widely separate
✓ Mucous membrane folded→ plicae circulares	♦ In lower ileum, absent
♦ Folds are larger, more numerous and closely set	✓ Ileal mesentery attached to lower part of posterior abdominal wall and to the right of aorta
✓ Jejunal mesentery attached to posterior abdominal wall and to the left of aorta	✓ Blood supply: several arcades
✓ Blood supply: fewer arcades	♦ Numerous short branches
♦ Long infreq branches	✓ Fat deposits: throughout mesentery
✓ Fat deposits: mostly near root, scanty near intestinal wall	♦ Mesentery is opaque
♦ "Clear windows" in mesentery	✓ Aggregation of lymphoid tissue
✓ No Peyer's patches	♦ Peyer's patches present in mucous membrane found along ant-mesenteric border

Blood supply

✓ The blood supply is from the superior mesenteric artery, which is the artery to the midgut
✓ Branches—superior mesenteric artery lies between the folds of the mesentery; 15-20 jejunal and ileal branches arise from its convex left side and runs towards the intestinal wall
✓ Arcades—each branch divides into 2 unite with adj branches to from a series of arcades
  ♦ Branches from the arcades divide and form a series of arcades
  ♦ Less arcades in jejunum, more in ileum
  ♦ From the terminal arcades, small straight branches (vasa recta) runs towards the intestinal wall and supply it
  ♦ Longer, less freq terminal branches in jejunum shorter, more numerous terminal branches in ileum
  ♦ Lowest part of the ileum is also supplied by the ileocolic arteries

Venous drainage
✓ The veins correspond to the branches of the superior mesenteric artery
✓ They drain mainly into the superior mesenteric vein

Chinical notes
✓ Identification of jejunum and ileum is very impartant during surgery
✓ Thrombosis of superior mesenteric artery will cut off blood supply to midgut→ ischemia, may result in death due to intestinal obstruction

Transverse colon

✓ The transverse colon is part of the large intestine

Position and extent
✓ 40–50 cm long
✓ Runs across upper abdomen from right to left from hepatic flexure to splenic flexure
✓ Occupies umbilical and hypogastric regions

Appearance	
External	Internal
✓ Long muscle aggregated into 3 bands: taeniae coli ✓ The wall is sacculated i.e., haustrations ✓ Finger-like evaginations of serous coat containing fat ▷ Appendices epiploicae	✓ Absence of mucosal folds (plicae circulares) ✓ Absence of villi ✓ Absence of Peyer's patches

Mesentery
✓ Well-defined mesentery = transverse mesocolon
✓ Attached to superior border of transverse colon
✓ Longest part in the middle, shortest part at the flexures
✓ Thus flexures are relatively fixed whereas rest of transverse colon are mobile

Flexures	
Left colic flexure (splenic flexure)	Right colic flexure (hepatic flexure)
✓ More acute ✓ At higher level than right colic flexure ✓ It is suspended from the diaphragm by phrenico-colic ligament	✓ Less acute ✓ At lower level than left colic flexure (because of greater size of right lobe of liver)

Relations	
Anteriorly	Posteriorly
✓ Greater omentum ✓ Anterior abdominal wall	✓ 2nd part of duodenum ✓ Head of pancreas ✓ Coils of jejunum and ileum

Blood supply, venous drainage, lymphatic drainage and nerve supply		
	Proximal 2/3	Distal 1/3
Blood supply	✓ Middle colic artery (from superior mesenteric artery)	✓ Left colic artert (from inferior mesenteric artery)
Venous drainage (veins accompany artery)	✓ Middle colic vein (into superior mesenteric vein)	✓ Left colic vein (into inferior mesenteric vein)
Lymphatic drainage (LV drain into nodes along the colic vessels)	✓ Superior mesenteric nodes	✓ Inferior mesenteric nodes
Nerve supply ✓ Sympathetic fibres ✓ Parasympathetic fibres	✓ Superior mesenteric plexuses ✓ Vagus nerve	✓ Inferior mesenteric plexuses ✓ Pelvic splanchnic nerve (sacral outflow)

Chinical notes: Ancer of the colon; colostomy
I. e., colon is brought to the surface through an incision of anterior abdominal wall

Superior mesenteric artery

Origin

✓ Arises from ventral aspect of aorta
✓ At level of LV_1

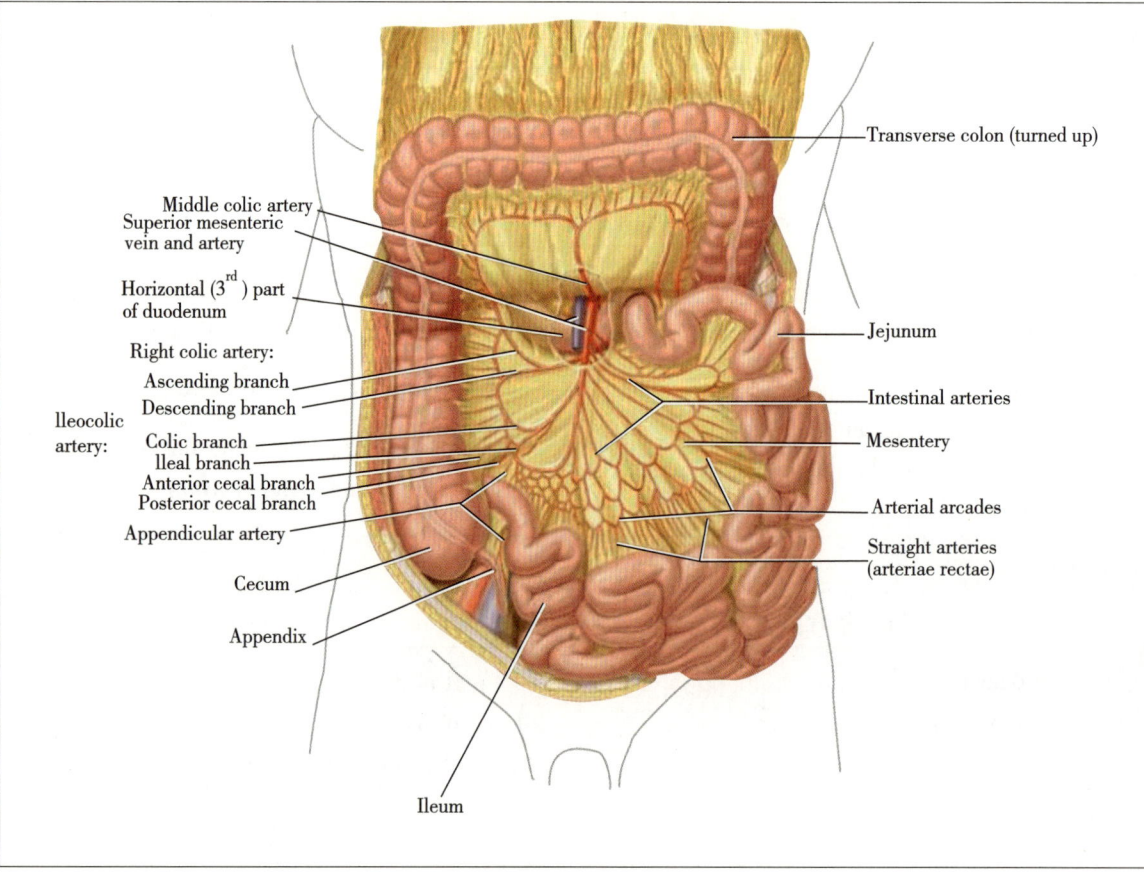

Course	
✓ Runs downward and to the right behind neck of pancreas ✓ In front of 3rd part of duodenum, left renal vein and uncinate process of pancreas ✓ Enters root of mesentery before giving off its branches ✓ Runs downward and to the right between the layers of the mesentery ✓ Ends by anastomosing with the ileal branch of its own ileocolic branch	
Branches	
Inferior pancreatico-duod artery	✓ Passes to the right (can be single/double) ✓ Along upper border of 3rd part of duodenum ✓ Supplies pancreas and the part of duodenum after entry of bile duct
Middle colic artery	✓ Runs forward in transverse mesocolon ✓ Divides into left and right branches ✓ Supplies transverse colon
Right colic artery	✓ Passes to the right ✓ Divides into ascending and descending branches ✓ Supplies ascending colon
Ileocolic artery	✓ Passes downward and to the right ✓ Gives off 　◊ Superior branch: anastomose with right colic artery 　◊ Inferior branch: anastomose with superior mesenteric artery: gives off anterior and posterior cecal arttery
Jejunal and ileal branches	✓ 15-20 in number ✓ Arise from left (convex) side of artery ✓ Form arcades from which terminal straight branches arise to supply jejunum and ileum
Area of supply	
✓ The superior mesenteric artery is the artery of the midgut ✓ Thus its area of supply extends from the duodenum below the entry of the common bile duct to the proximal 2/3 of the transverse colon	
Chinical notes	
✓ Occlusion of a series of branches results in poor nutrition of affected part of intestine 　◊ No (rare) ischemia due to abundant anastomoses ✓ Occlusion of artery will affect a large part of gut→ ischemia 　◊ Death occurs due to intestinal obstruction	

Portal vein

✓ The portal vein is a valveless vein about 8 cm long
✓ It drains blood from the GIT in the abdomen and most of the GIT in pelvis
✓ Is also receives blood from the pancreas, spleen and gallbladder

Origin	
✓ Formed by the union of the superior mesenteric vein and splenic vein ✓ Behind neck of pancreas at level of LV_1	
Course	
✓ Runs upward and to the right ✓ Posterior to 1st part of duodenum ✓ Reach free border of lesser omentum and enters hepatoduod ligament ✓ Lies in front of epiploic foramen ✓ Asc to the porta hepatis, lying behind hepatic artery and bile duct ✓ Breaks up into right and left terminal branches which lie behind the corresponding branches of the hepatic artery ✓ The portal vein is peculiar in that it behaves like an artery ✓ I. e., breaks up into cap in the liver and unites again to form the hepatic veins	
Tributaries	
Auperior mesenteric vein	✓ Begins in right iliac fossa ✓ Asc in the mesentery ✓ Joins splenic vein→ portal vein
Aplenic vein	✓ Begins at hilum of spleen ✓ Runs in lienorenal ligament ✓ Then runs behind body of pancreas (lying below splenic artery) ✓ Joins superior mesenteric vein→ portal vein
Inferior mesenteric vein	✓ Upward continuation of superior rectal vein ✓ Asc lateral to inferior mesenteric artery ✓ Enters splenic vein just before formation of portal vein → does not drain directly into portal vein
Chinical notes	
✓ Wide angle of union between superior mesenteric and splenic vein leads to streaming of blood flow in portal vein ✓ I. e., right lobe of liver receives blood mainly from intestines, left lobe, caudate and quadrate lobes receive blood mainly from stomach and spleen, thus, this is important in the spread of infectious growths ✓ Portal hypertension causes blood to be diverted via the portal-systemic anastomoses into systemic circulation (may cause varicosities)	
Portal-systemic anastomoses	
✓ Under normal conditions, portal venous blood→ liver → IVC ✓ The portal-systemic anastomoses provide an alternative route for returning blood to the IVC should the above route be blocked	

Regions of anastomoses	
Regions	Veins involved
Lower 1/2 of esophagus	✓ Esophageal branches of left gastric vein (portal) ✓ Esophageal vein (systemic)
Anal canal	✓ Auperior rectal vein (portal) ✓ Middle and inferior rectal veins (systemic)
Paraumbilical region	✓ Paraumbilical veins in falciform ligament (portal) ✓ Superficial veins of anterior abdomen wall (systemic)
Retroperitoneal region	✓ Veins of ascending and descending colon, duodenum, pancreas and liver (portal) ✓ Renal, lumbar and phrenic veins (systemic)

Chinical notes

✓ Portal hypertension: blood diverted via these anastomoses to systemic circulation and hence return to heart
✓ Portal-cava shunts
  ◊ I. e., direct connection between portal vein and IVC may be created to treat portal hypertension

Common bile duct

✓ The common bile duct averages about 8 cm in length
✓ Its main function is to transmit bile into the duodenum

Origin

✓ Formed by the union of the cystic and common hepatic duct
✓ Position of the junction is variable

Course

Its course can be divided into supraduod, retroduod and infraduod (pancreatic) parts

✓ Supraduod part
  ◊ Desc along right free margin of lesser omentum
  ◊ Encircled by LN at its commencement
  ◊ Relations: left = hepatic artery
              posterior = portal vein, epiploic foramen, IVC
✓ Retroduod part
  ◊ Desc behind 1st part of duodenum
  ◊ Relations: left = gastroduod artery
              posterior = portal vein and IVC
✓ Infraduod part (pancreatic part)
  ◊ Begins at upper limit of head of pancreas and descending behind it
  ◊ Terminates by piercing posteromedial aspect of the middle of descending (2nd) part of duodenum
  ◊ At this part → usually joined by main pancreatic duct
  ◊ Form an ampulla in duodenal wall = ampulla of Vater
  ◊ Opens in duodenum by means of duodenal papilla

Note: the ampulla is surrounded by a sphincter = sphincter of Oddi

◊ Relations: anterior = head of pancreas
　　　　　　 posterior = IVC
　　　　　　 left = main pancreatic duct
　　　　　　 right = 2nd part of duodenum

Blood supply, venous drainage, lymphatic drainage

	Upper part	Lower part
Blood supply	✓ Cystic artery	✓ Posterior/superior pancreaticoduodenal artery
Venous drainage	✓ Enter liver	✓ Portal vein
Lymphatic drainage	✓ Cystic nodes	✓ Hepatic nodes → celiac nodes

Nerve supply

✓ Sympathetic and parasympathetic fibres from hepatic plexus

Chinical notes: ① Presence of gallstones → blockage of bile duct (cholecystitis). ② This may lead to obstructive jaundice

Pancreas

✓ The pancreas is situated retroperitoneally in the epigastric and hypochondriac regions
✓ It extends from the concavity of the duodenum to the hilum of the spleen
✓ It can be divided into a head, neck, body and tail

A. Surface features

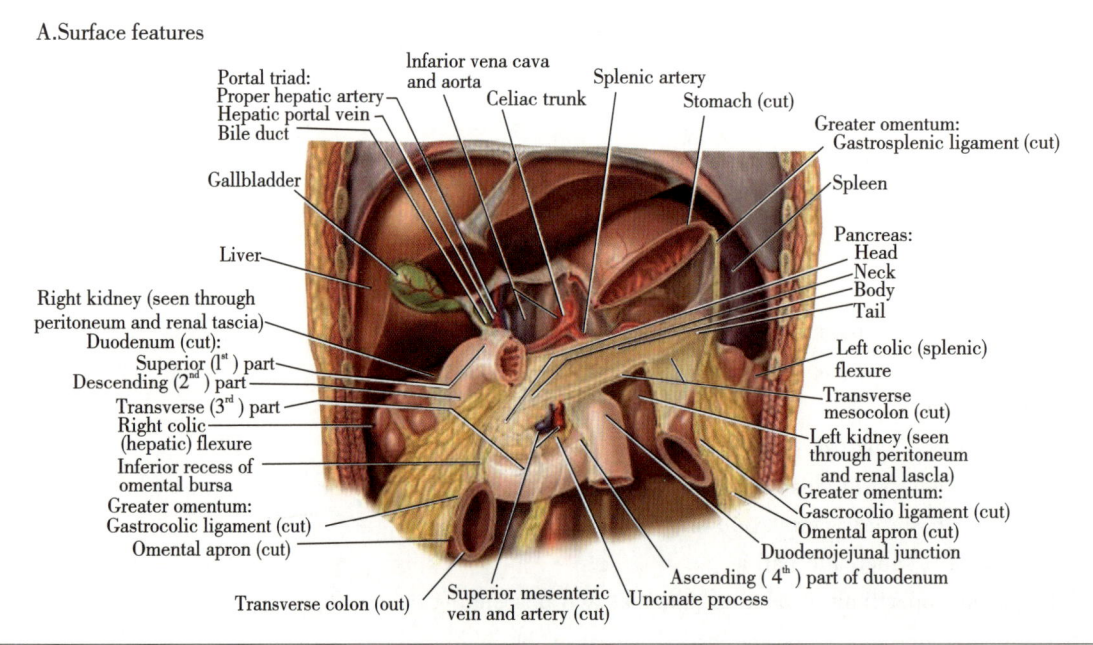

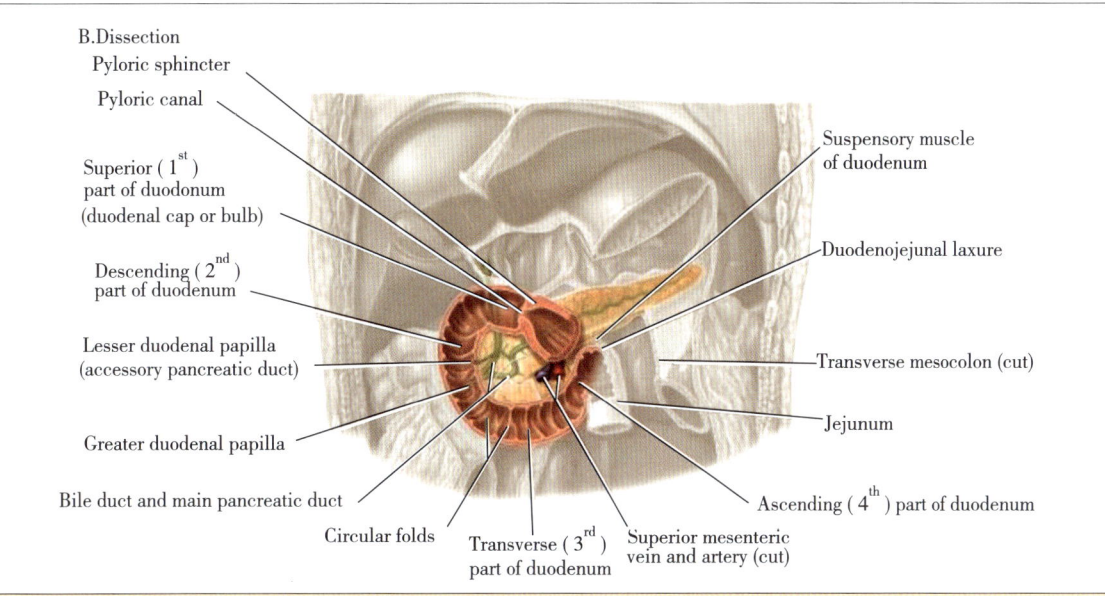

B. Dissection

Relations

(1) Of the head—situated within concavity of duodenum

Anteriorly	Posteriorly
✓ Proximal end of transverse colon ✓ Transverse mesocolon ✓ Posterior wall of lesser sac ✓ Coils of jejunum	✓ Medial border of right kidney ✓ Right renal vessels ✓ IVC ✓ Termination of left renal vein ✓ Right crus of diaphragm ✓ Infraduod (pancreatic) part of common bile duct

(2) Of the neck—joins the head to body of pancreas

Anteriorly	Posteriorly
✓ Covered with peritoneum ↓ Posterior wall of lesser sac ✓ Gastroduod artery ✓ Superior pancreaticoduodenum artery	✓ Superior mesenteric vein ✓ Splenic vein ✓ These 2 veins join to form portal vein

(3) Of the body

Anteriorly	✓ Covered with peritoneum ↓ Posterior wall of lesser sac ✓ Stomach ✓ The peritoneum on anterior surface is continuous with ascending layers of greater omentum
Posteriorly	✓ Splenic vein ✓ Aorta and origin of superior mesenteric artery ✓ Left crus of diaphragm ✓ Left suprarenal gland ✓ Left kidney ✓ Left renal vessels

Inferiorly	✓ Duodenojejunal flexures
	✓ Coils of jejunum
Superiorly	✓ Projection (omental tuberosity)
(4) Of the tail	

✓ Lies within lieno-renal ligament
✓ Closely related to splenic vessels
✓ In contact with hilum of inferior part of gastric surface of spleen

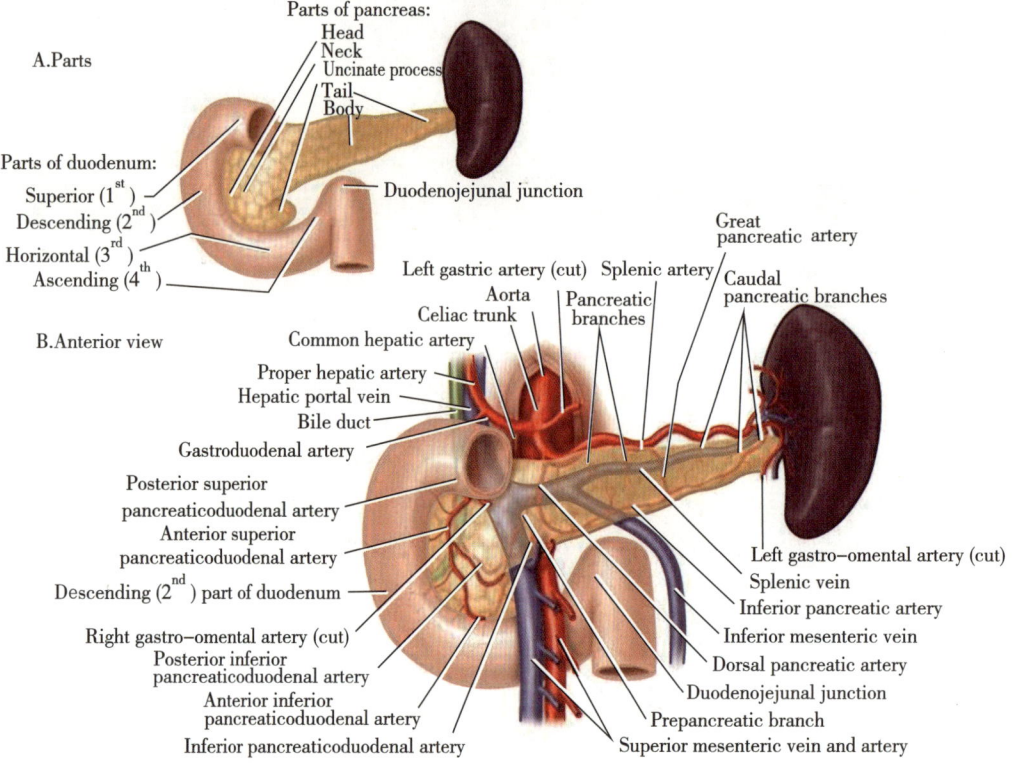

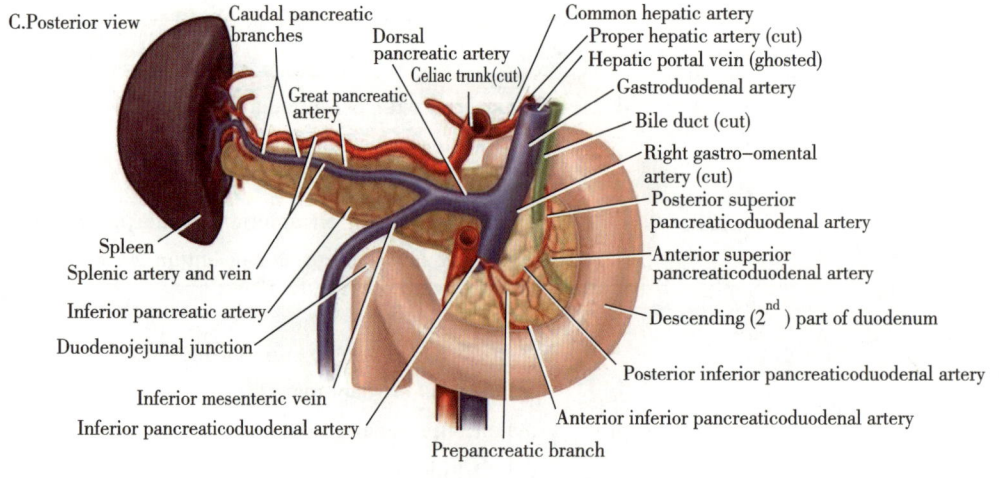

Blood supply
✓ Branches from superior and inferior pancreatico-duodenal arteries
✓ Branches from splenic artery

Lymphatic drainage
✓ Head and body
◊ Superior and inferior pancreatico-duodenal nodes celiac and superior mesenteric nodes
✓ Tail
◊ Pancretico-lienal nodes (in hilum of spleen)

Chinical notes
✓ Gland is deeply situated → diagnosis of disease difficult
✓ Common site of cancer = head of pancreas
◊ This may lead to obstruction of common bile duct → obstructive jaundice
✓ Perforating ulcers of posterior gastric wall may penetrate the pancreas
◊ Cause leakage of digestive juices

Spleen

- ✓ The spleen is a lymphoid organ
- ✓ It functions
   - ◊ As a site of immune response
   - ◊ As a filter, i.e., remove old red blood cells
   - ◊ As a blood reservoir

Position
✓ It occupies the left hypochondium
✓ Its long axis follows the shaft of the 10th rib
✓ Extend forward from scapular line to mid-axillary line

Relations	
Anterior (visceral) surface	Posterior surface
✓ The related viscera produce impressions on this surface ✓ Stomach ✓ Tail of pancreas ✓ Left colic flexure ✓ Left kidney	✓ Diaphragm ✓ Left pleura (left costodiaphragmatic recess) ✓ Left lung ✓ $9^{th}, 10^{th}$ and 11th ribs

Peritoneum	
Spleen is surrounded by peritoneum	
Gastrosplenic ligament	Lienorenal ligament
✓ Passes from hilus to fundus of stomach ✓ Carry short gastric and left gastroepiploic vessels	✓ Passes from hilus to front of left kidney ✓ Carry splenic vessels, tail of pancreas

Hilus of spleen

Transmits splenic vessels, lyphatics and autonomic nerves

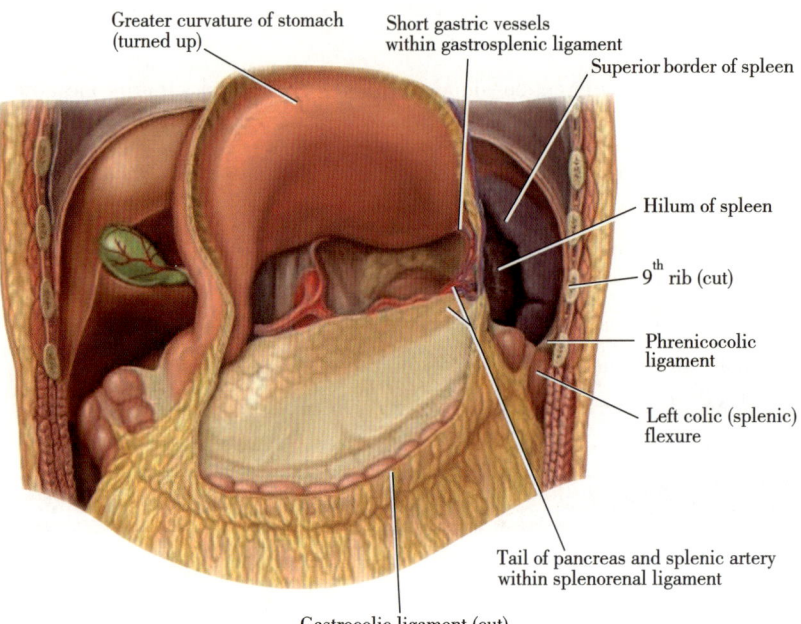

A. Dissection

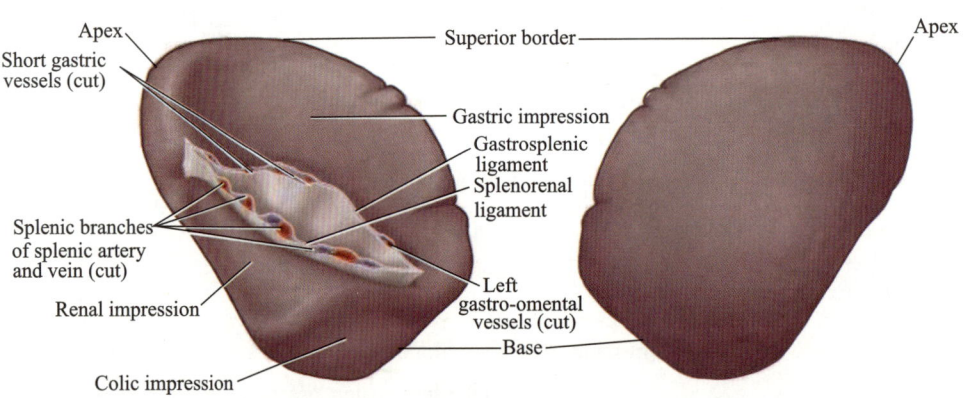

B. Visceral surface

C. Diaphragmatic surface

Blood supply

✓ Splicen artery (branch of celiac trunk)
  ⬦ Runs along upper border of pancreas
  ⬦ Divides into 5 or 6 branches at hilus and enters the spleen

Venous drainage

✓ Splenic vein
  ⬦ Leaves hilus and runs behind body of pancreas
  ⬦ Joins superior mesenteric veins to form portal vein

Lymphatic drainage
✓ Emerge from hilus
✓ Drain into pancreatico-duodenal nodes→ celiac node
Nerve supply
✓ Derived from celiac plexus
✓ Accompany splenic artery and enters hilus
Chinical notes
✓ Fracture of left lower ribs may result in ruptured spleen
✓ Infection→ enlargement of spleen

Suprarenal glands

✓ These are yellowish retroperitoneal bodies lying on the upper poles of each kidney
✓ They are surrounded by renal fascia but are seperated from kidneys by peri-renal fat
✓ They secrete hormones
　♢ Cortex : glucocorticoids, minerocorticoids, and sex hormones
　♢ Medulla adrenalin and noradrenalin

Relations

	Right suprarenal	Left suprarenal
Shape	✓ Pyramindal	✓ Semilunar
Anteriorly	✓ IVC ✓ Bare area of liver ✓ Posterior surface of right lobe of liver	✓ Postero-inferior surface of stomach ✓ Pancreas ✓ Splenic vessels
Posteriorly	✓ Diaphragm ✓ Kidney	✓ Left crus of diaphragm
Medially	✓ Right inferior phrenic artery ✓ Celiac ganglion	✓ Inferior phrenic artery ✓ Left gastric artery ✓ Left celiac ganglion

Blood supply

Artery	Originate from
Superior suprarenal artery	✓ Inferior phrenic artery
Middle suprarenal artery	✓ Aorta
Inferior suprarenal artery	✓ Renal artery
Venous drainage	
✓ Right suprarenal→ IVC ✓ Left suprarenal→left renal vein	

Lymphatic drainage
✓ Into para-aortic nodes

Nerve supply
✓ PreGN sympathetic fibres from T_8–T_{11}, via greater and lesser splanchnic nerve
✓ No parasympathetic supply

Chinical notes
✓ Disease/atrophy→insufficiency of mineralocorticoids and glucorticoids, results in Addison's disease
✓ Hyperactiviy→hermaphroditism→Cushing's syndrome

Kidneys

✓ The kidneys are retroperitoneal
✓ They lie on either side of the vertebral bodies occupying the paravertebral gutters of the posterior abdominal wall
✓ The right kidney is lower than the left kidney

Right kidney

✓ Anterior surface
  ◊ Right suprarenal gland
  ◊ Right lobe of liver
  ◊ 2nd part of duodenum
  ◊ Hepatic flexure of colon
  ◊ Coils of small intestine
  ◊ Area related to liver and small intestine covered by peritoneum
✓ Posterior surface
  ◊ The diaphragm separates upper pole from pleura and costodiaphragmatic recess
  ◊ 12th rib and last i/c space
  ◊ Medial and lateral arcuate ligament
  ◊ Below these, from medial to lateral
  ◊ Tips of transverse processes of LV_1 and LV_2
  ◊ Psoas major
  ◊ Quaratus lumborum
  ◊ Tranversus abdominis
  ◊ Intervening between kidney and quadratus lumborum from above downwards
  ◊ Subcostal nerve
  ◊ Iliohypogastric nerve
  ◊ Ilioinguinal nerve

Left kidney

✓ Anterior surface
  ◊ Left suprarenal gland
  ◊ Spleen
  ◊ Posterior surface of stomach

- ◊ Body of pancreas
- ◊ Splenic vessels
- ◊ Splenic flexure of colon, i. e., left colic flexure
- ◊ Coils of jejunum
- ◊ Left colic vessels
- ◊ Area related to stomach, spleen, jejunum covered with peritoneum
- ◊ The rest are devoid of peritoneum
- ✓ Posterior surface
  - ◊ The diaphragm separates upper pole from pleura and costodiaphragmatic recess
  - ◊ 11th and 12th ribs and last i/c space
  - ◊ Medial and lateral arcuate ligament
  - ◊ Below these, from medial and lateral
  - ◊ Tips of transverse processes of LV$_1$ and LV$_2$
  - ◊ Psoas major
  - ◊ Quadratus lumborum
  - ◊ Transversus abdominis
  - ◊ Intervening between kidney and quadratus lumborum from above downwards
  - ◊ Subcostal nerve
  - ◊ Iliohypogastric nerve
  - ◊ Ilioinguinal nerve

Ureter

- ✓ The ureter is about 25 cm. It is partly in the abdomen and partly in the pelvis
- ✓ Throughout its course it is retroperitoneal

Origin

- ✓ Begins as the renal pelvis
- ✓ At medial border of kidneys

Constriction

- ✓ At junction with renal pelvis
- ✓ At brim of lesser pelvis (pelvic brim)
- ✓ Passage through bladder wall

Course

- ✓ Passes downwards and medially
- ✓ Runs on psoas major
- ✓ Crosses in front of bifurcation of common iliac artery
- ✓ Enters pelvis
- ✓ Runs downwards and backwards
- ✓ Then opposite ischial spine it turns forward and medially
- ✓ Reaches bladder obliquely

Relations of right ureter

- ✓ At renal pelvis

- ◊ Branches of renal vessels lie both in front and behind
- ◊ Duod lies in front
- ◊ Psoas major is posterior
- ✓ Abdominal
  - ◊ Anteriorly
    - ◆ 3rd part of duodenum
    - ◆ Right colic vessels
    - ◆ Ileocolic vessels
    - ◆ Right gonadal vessels
    - ◆ Root of mesentery
    - ◆ Terminal part of ileum
  - ◊ Posteriorly
    - ◆ Psoas major
    - ◆ Tips of lumbar transverse processes
    - ◆ Genitofemoral nerve
    - ◆ Bifurcation of right common iliac artery
  - ◊ Medially
    - ◆ IVC

Pelvic part

	Female	Male
Posteriorly	✓ Internal iliac artery and vein ✓ Lumbosacral trunk ✓ Sacroiliac joint	✓ Internal iliac artery and vein ✓ Lumbosacral trunk ✓ Sacroiliac joint
Laterally	✓ Fascia covering obturator internus ✓ Branches of internal iliac artery ✓ It forms the posterior boundary of ovarian fossa	✓ Fascia covering obturator internus ✓ Branches of internal iliac artery
As it turns forward towards the bladder	✓ Lies slightly above lateral fornix of vagina ✓ Uterine artery crosses it from lateral to medial side	✓ Ductus deferens crosses it superior from lateral to medial ✓ Seminal vesicle lies below and behind it

- ✓ Intravesical part
  - ◊ Enters the bladder obliquely and acts as a valve to prevent backflow of urine

Relations of left ureter

- ✓ At renal pelvis
  - ◊ Branches of renal vessels lie both in front and behind
  - ◊ Pancreas and coils of small intestine in front
  - ◊ Psoas major is posterior
- ✓ Abdominal
  - ◊ Anteriorly
  - ◊ Left gonadal vessels

- ◊ Left colic vessels
- ◊ Sigmoid colon
- ◊ Sigmoid mesocolon
- ✓ Posteriorly
  - ◊ Psoas major
  - ◊ Tips of lumbar transverse processes
  - ◊ Genitofemoral nerve
  - ◊ Bifurcation of left common iliac artery
- ✓ Medially
  - ◊ Inferior mesenteric vessels
- ✓ Pelvic part and intravesical part
  - ◊ Same as for right ureter

Blood supply

- ✓ Renal artery
- ✓ Aorta
- ✓ Common iliac artery
- ✓ Vesical artery

Venous drainage

- ✓ Corresponds to blood supply

Lymphatic drainage

Part of the ureter	Drains into
Upper 1/3	✓ Nodes around renal artery
Middle 1/3	✓ Common iliac nodes
Lower 1/3	✓ Common, internal and external iliac nodes

Nerve supply

- ✓ Sympathetic supply from T_{10} to L_1
- ✓ Via renal, hypogastric and pelvic plexuses

Clinical notes

- ✓ Renal stones may cause obstruction of ureter
  - ◊ Most common sites of lodging of stones are at the constrictions
- ✓ Renal colic : referred pain which passes from loin to groin
  - ◊ I. e., T_{11} to L_2 segments

Inferior vena cava

Origin

- ✓ Formed by union of the 2 common iliac veins
- ✓ On right side of lower border of LV_5

Course

- ✓ Asc in front of lower LV
- ✓ On right side of abdomen aorta
- ✓ In front of right crus of diaphragm and right suprarenal gland
- ✓ Enters thorax via caval opeing in diaphragm at level of TV_8
- ✓ Pierces pericardium
- ✓ Opens into RA

Relations

Anteriorly	Posteriorly
✓ Root of mesentery	✓ Right sympathetic trunk
✓ Right gonadal artery	✓ Right crus of diaphragm
✓ Duodenum and pancreas	✓ Right suprarenal gland
✓ Portal vein and liver	✓ Right celiac ganglion

Tributaries

- ✓ Common iliac veins (left and right)
- ✓ Lumbar veins
- ✓ Left and right renal veins
- ✓ Jepatic veins
- ✓ Right gonadal vein
- ✓ Right suprarenal vein (left veins empty into left renal vein→ IVC)
- ✓ Right inferior phrenic vein

Chinical notes: Occlusion of IVC→ blood will still reach RA via porto-systemic anastomoses

Lumbar sympathetic trunks

✓ The sympathetic trunks are 2 ganglionated nerve cords situated on either side of vertebral column, extending from base of skull to coccyx

✓ In front of coccyx, the 2 trunks end in a single terminal ganglion known as ganglion impar

Course of lumbar sympathetic trunk

- ✓ Continuation of thoracic part of sympathetic trunk
- ✓ Enters abdomen behind medial arcuate ligament
- ✓ Desc in front of LV bodies
- ✓ Along medial border of psoas major
- ✓ Right trunk: overlapped by IVC
- ✓ Left trunk: lies to the left of aorta
- ✓ Desc into pelvis medial to lumbosacral trunk and behind common iliac vessels

Ganglia

- ✓ Possess 4 segmentally arranged ganglia
- ✓ 1st and 2nd often fused together
- ✓ They (1st and 2nd) also receive WRC from L_1 and L_2

Branches

✓ GRC—to the lumbar spinal nerve
  ◊ Distributed to arrector pili muscles, BV and sweat glands of skin
✓ Fibres to sympathetic plexuses on abdominal aorta and its branches
  ◊ E. g. , celiac plexuses, superior and inferior mesenteric plexuses
✓ Fibres which pass down into pelvis to hypogastric plexus

Chinical notes: Lumbar sympathectomy→ produces cutaneous vasodilation

Zhang Bensi, Sun Chenyou, Chen Hao

Chapter 5

The Pelvis and Perineum

5.1 Introduction

The pelvis lies below and behind the abdomen and is where the trunk communicates with the lower limbs. It is enclosed by bony, muscular, and ligamentous walls. The bony pelvis is formed by the two hip bones and the sacrum and coccyx. It has an upper part, the greater pelvis, flanked by the iliac bones, and a lower part, the lesser pelvis. The greater and lesser pelvis meet at the pelvic brim(Figure 5-1). The pelvic cavity is continuous with the abdominal cavity and is therefore lined by the peritoneum of the greater peritoneal sac. The peritoneum passes down the alimentary tract, the bladder, and the internal reproductive organs of the female.

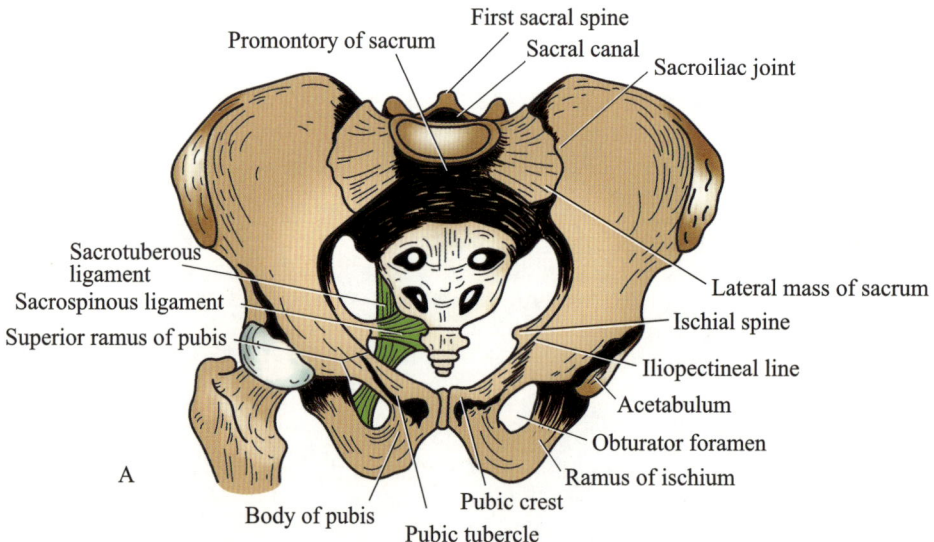

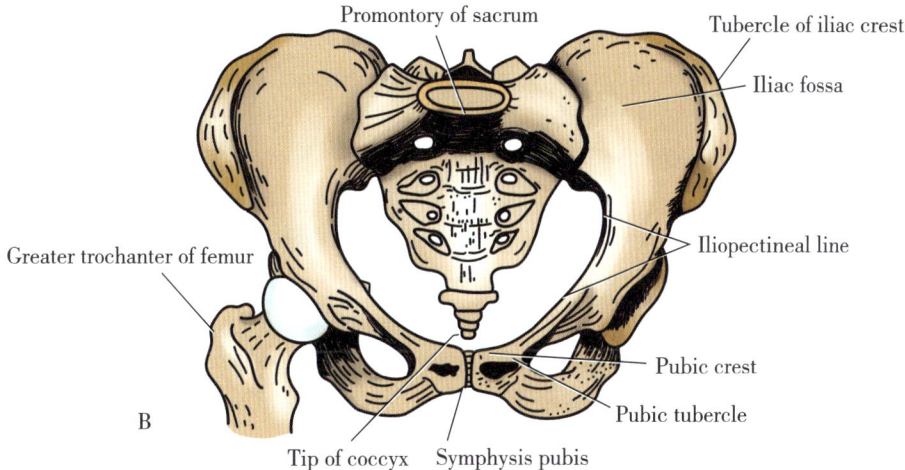

Figure 5-1 Anterior view of the male pelvis (A) and female pelvis (B)

As the formation of the bony pelvis, the two hip bones meet anteriorly at the pubic symphysis; posteriorly they articulate with the sacrum at the sacroiliac joints. The bony pelvis thus forms a ring that protects the pelvic contents.

The pelvis is divided into the greater pelvis (false pelvis), which lies above the pelvic brim (pelvic inlet), and the lesser pelvis, which lies between the pelvic inlet and pelvic outlet. The pelvic inlet lies at about 45° to the pelvic outlet (Figure 5-2).

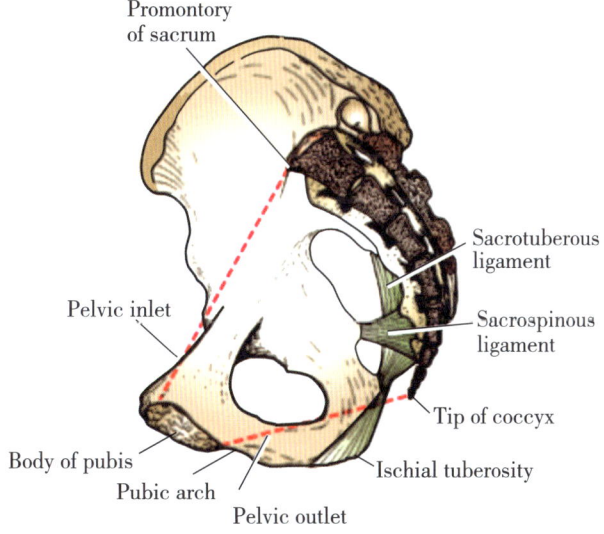

Figure 5-2 Right half of the pelvis

(1) Sacrum

It consists of the fused five sacral vertebrae. There are anterior and posterior sacral foramina for passage of the anterior and posterior rami of the sacral spinal nerves. The sacrum articulates with the hip bones via its articular surface of the sacroiliac joints.

(2) Hip bone

It is formed by the fusion of the ilium, the ischium, and the pubic bone shortly after puberty. The iliac fossa of ilium gives rise to the iliacus muscle. The ilium contributes to the formation of the acetabulum and the bony margin of the greater sciatic notch. The pubic bones articulate in the midline at the pubic symphysis. Each pubic bone has a superior and inferior ramus. The superior ramus forms the superior border of the obturator foramen. The inferior ramus unites the pubis with the ischial bone to form the ischiopubic ramus. The posterior border of the ischium contributes to the formation of the greater and lesser sciatic notches. The two notches are separated by the ischial spine. The sacrotuberous and sacrospinous ligaments transform the notches into the greater and lesser sciatic foramina.

(3) Male and female pelves

The male and female pelves may show a great deal of sexual dimorphism. The largest diameter of the pelvic inlet is the transverse diameter, while the largest diameter of the pelvic outlet is the anteroposterior diameter. As the foetal head enters the pelvic inlet, its maximum diameter lies across the pelvis, but as it descends through the birth canal, the head rotates through 90°, so that its maximum diameter lies anteroposteriorly at the pelvic outlet (Figure 5-3).

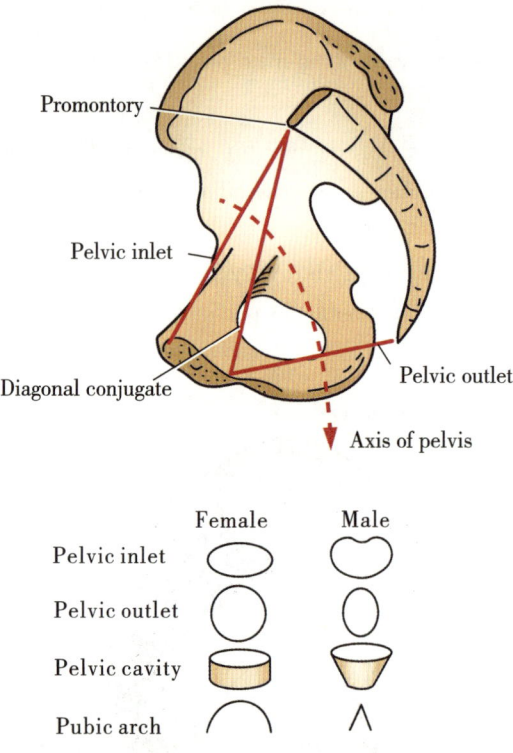

Figure 5-3　Pelvic inlet, pelvic outlet, diagonal conjugate, and axis of the pelvis

5.2　The pelvis

5.2.1　Pelvic wall and pelvic floor

The side wall of the pelvis is formed by the hip bone with the obturator internus muscle. The posterior wall is formed by the sacrum and the piriformis muscle as it passes into the greater sciatic foramen (Figure 5-4-Figure 5-6).

5.2.2 The pelvic floor

The pelvic floor is formed by the funnel-shaped pelvic diaphragm, which consists of the lavator ani and coccygeus muscles and the fascia covering the superior and inferior aspects of these muscles. The pelvic floor forms a gutter of muscle around the terminal parts of the rectum and the prostate and urethra in the male and the vagina and urethra in the female

The pelvic diaphragm, which consists of the levator ani and coccygeus muscles (Figure 5-7) and the fascia covering the superior and inferior aspects of these muscles, stretches between the pubis anteriorly and the coccyx posteriorly and from one lateral pelvic wall to the other.

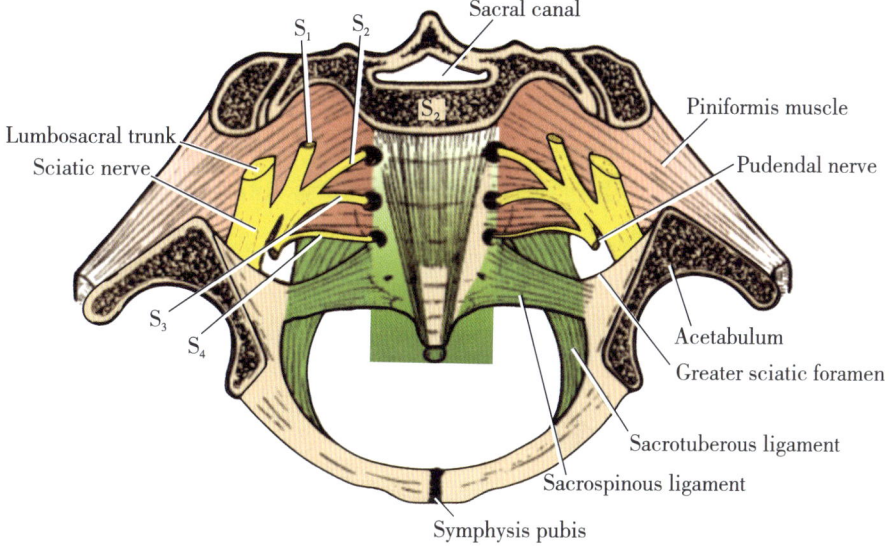

Figure 5-4 Posterior wall of the pelvis

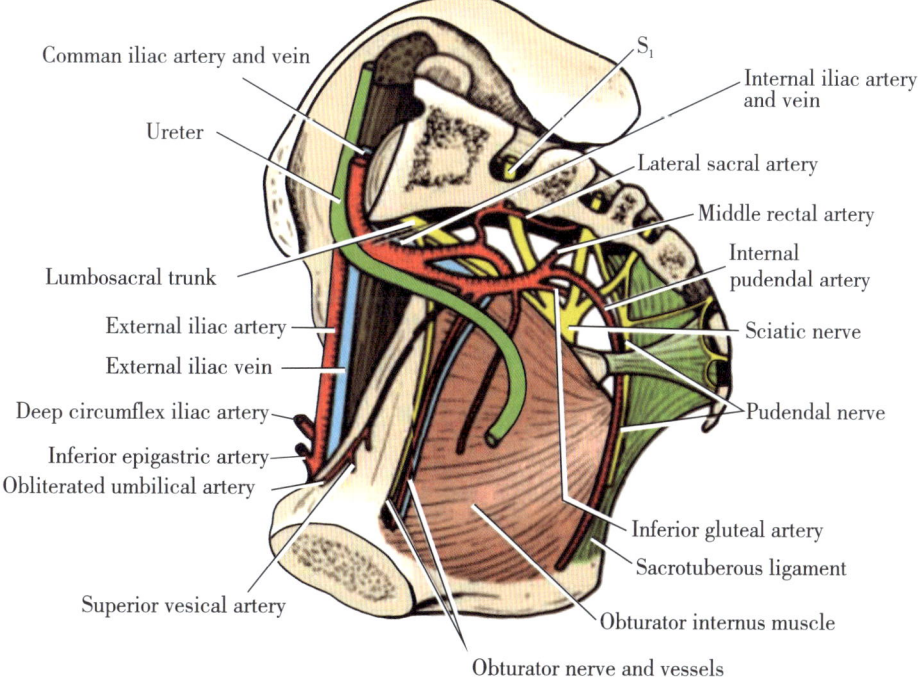

Figure 5-5 Lateral wall of the pelvis

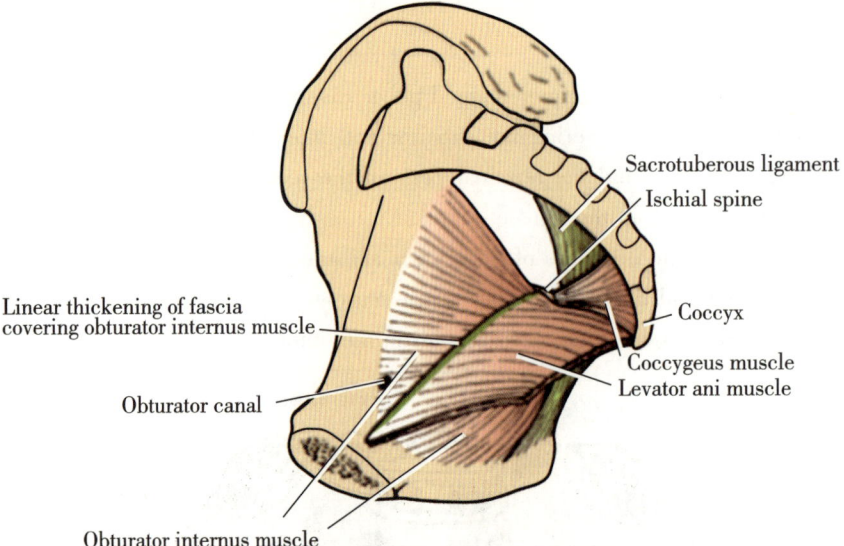

Figure 5-6 Inferior wall or floor of the pelvis

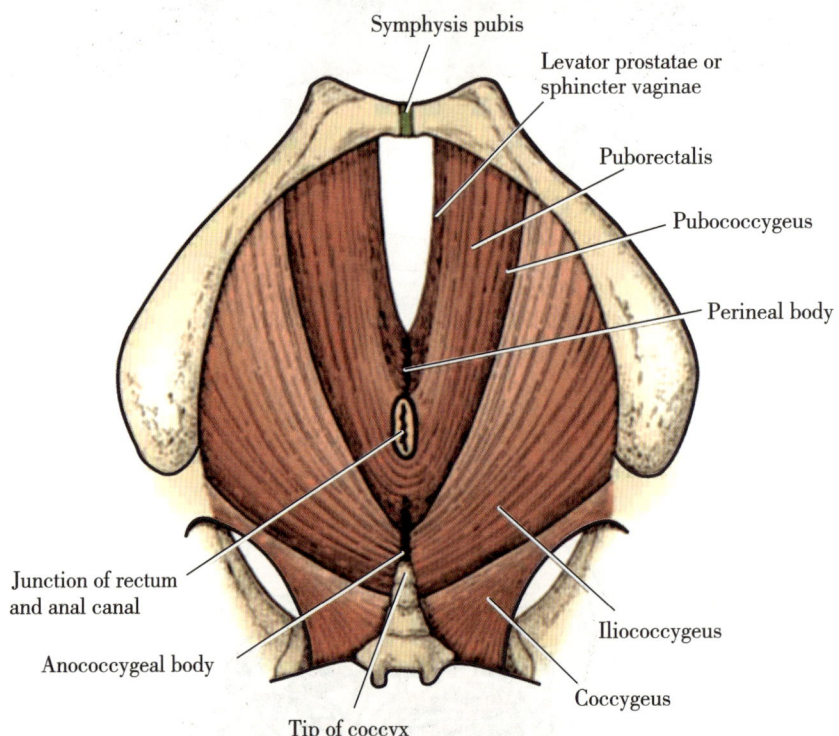

Figure 5-7 Levator ani muscle and coccygeus muscle seen on their inferior aspects

(Note that the levator ani is made up of several different muscle groups. The levator ani and coccygeus muscles with their fascial coverings form a continuous muscular floor to the pelvis, known as the pelvic diaphragm)

5.2.3 Pelvic fascia

Over the pelvic wall, the fascia is a strong membrane covering the obturator internus and piriformis muscles. Over the pelvic floor, the fascia consists of loose areolar tissue. The fascia condenses around the neurovascular bundles to 5 form ligaments and also gives rise to the puboprostatic and pubovesical ligaments in the male and female, respectively. The fascia varies in thickness over the pelvic viscera (Figure 5-8, Figure 5-9).

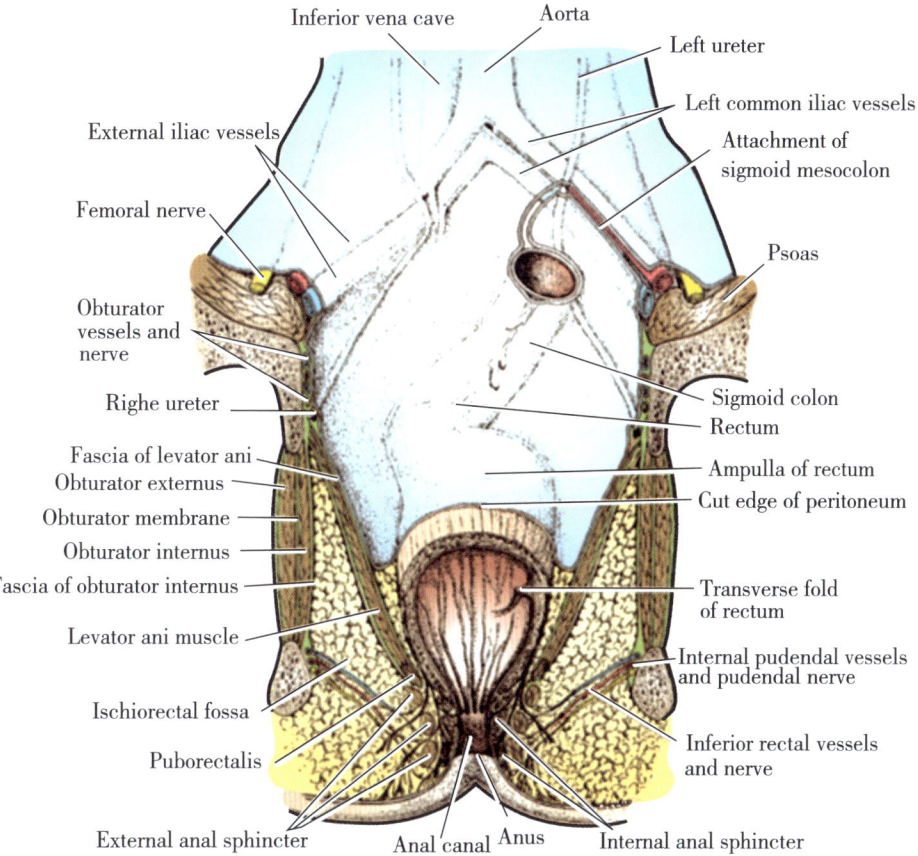

Figure 5-8 Coronal section through the pelvis

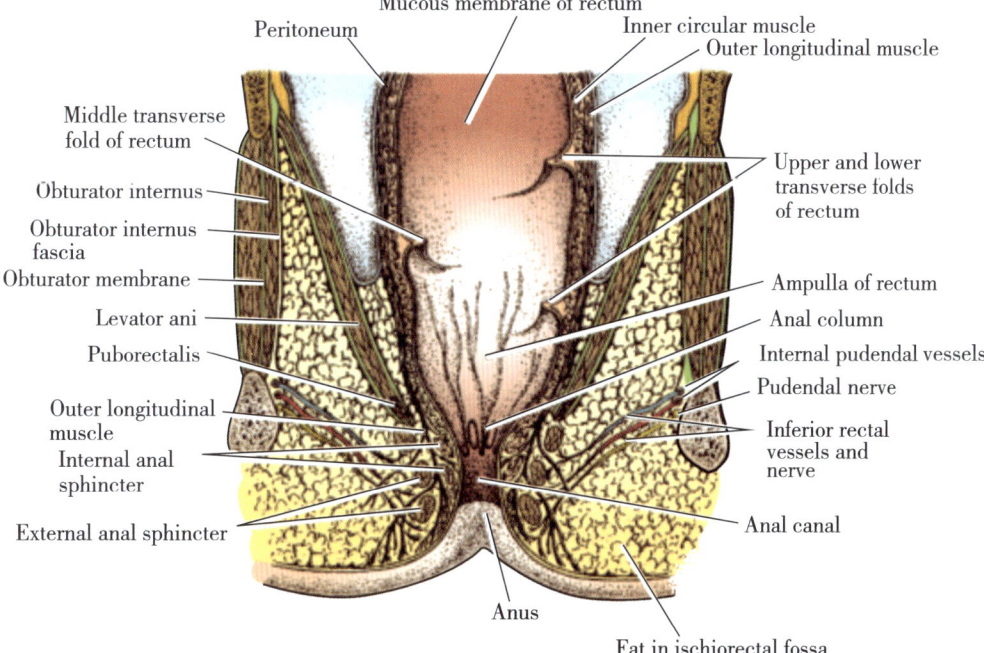

Figure 5-9 Coronal section through the pelvis showing the rectum and the pelvic floor

5.3 Pelvic organs

The organs of male and femal pelves are shown in Figure 5-10 and Figure 5-11.

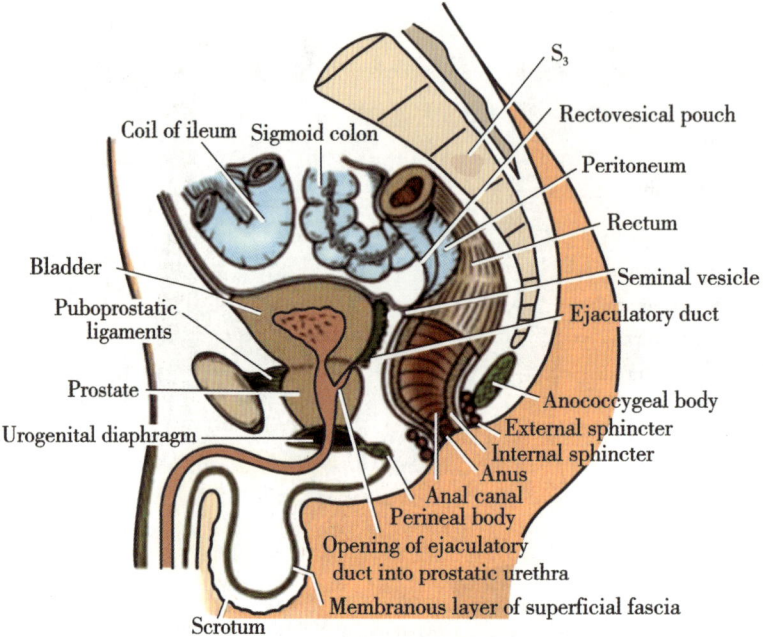

Figure 5-10 Sagittal section of the male pelvis

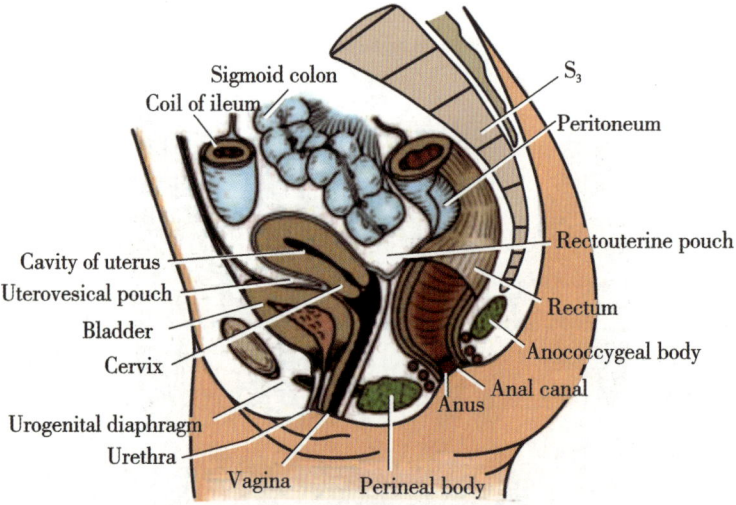

Figure 5-11 Sagittal section of the female pelvis

5.3.1 Rectum

The rectum commences as a continuation of the sigmoid colon at the level of the third piece of the sacrum. It ends at the anorectal junction by piercing 6 the pelvic floor at the border of the puborectalils muscle to become the anal canal(Frgure 5-12).

The rectum has three lateral curves and its lowest part dilates as the rectal ampulla. There are also three transverse folds containing both mucous membrane and circular muscle.

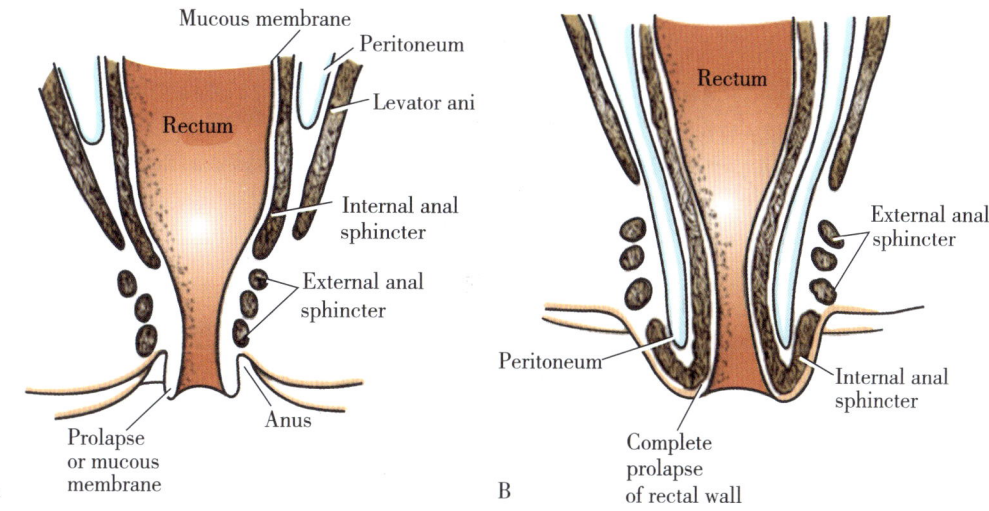

A. Incomplete rectal (mucosal) prolapse; B. Complete rectal prolapse.

Figure 5-12　Coronal section of the rectum and anal canal

The rectum has no mesentery. Peritoneum covers the upper third of the rectum at the front and sides, and the middle third of the rectum at the front. The lower third lies below the level of the peritoneum, and the latter is reflected onto the bladder or vagina to form the rectovesical or rectouterine pouch.

(1) Vessels of the rectum

Blood supply is from the superior, middle, and inferior rectal arteries. The superior rectal artery is a continuation of the inferior mesenteric artery. The rectal plexus of veins drains into the inferior mesenteric vein (portal system of veins). The rectal plexus is also drained by the middle and inferior rectal veins, which are systemic veins (Figure 5-13).

(2) Nerves of the rectum

The nerve supply of the rectum consists of:

1) Sympathetic—hypogastric plexus (Figure 5-14).

2) Parasympathetic—pelvic splanchnic nerves, which are motor to the rectal muscles.

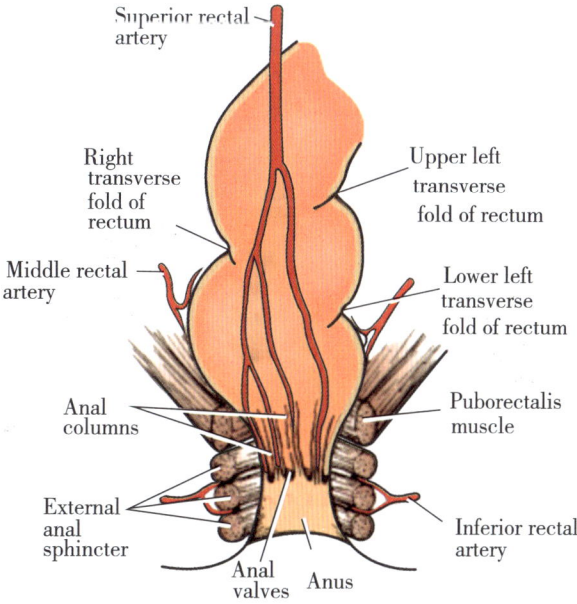

Figure 5-13　Blood supply to the rectum

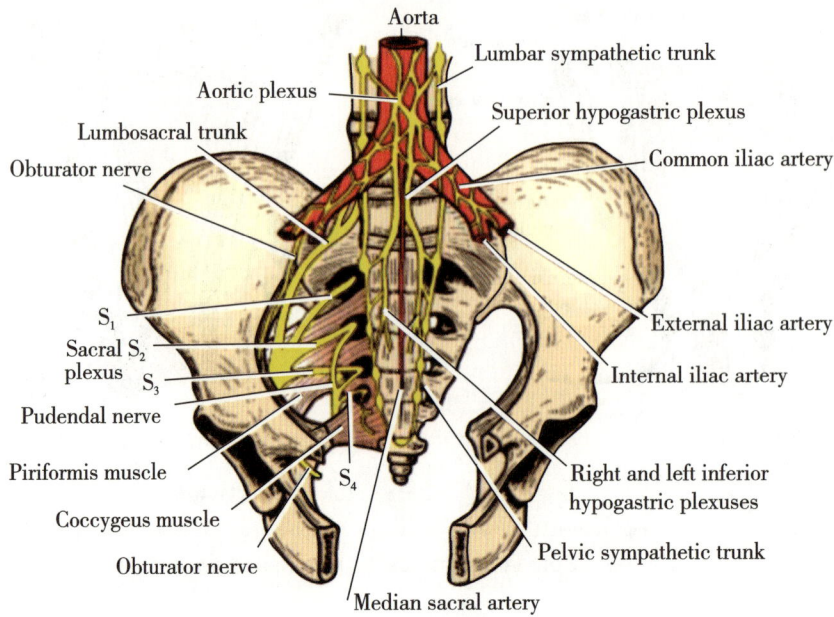

Figure 5–14 Posterior pelvic wall showing the sacral plexus, superior hypogastric plexus, and right and left inferior hypogastric plexuses.
(Pelvic parts of the sympathetic trunks are also shown)

5.3.2 Bladder

The anatomy of the bladder forms an extraperitoneal muscular urine reservoir that lies behind the pubic symphysis in the pelvis (Figure 5–15). The adult bladder is located in the anterior pelvis and is enveloped by extraperitoneal fat and connective tissue. It is separated from the pubic symphysis by an anterior prevesical space known as the retropubic space (of Retzius). The dome of the bladder is covered by peritoneum, and the bladder neck is fixed to neighboring structures by reflections of the pelvic fascia and by true ligaments of the pelvis. The undistended bladder is a pyramid-shaped organ. The apex points towards the pubic symphysis and the medial umbilical ligament is attached to it. The base is triangular, where the ductus deferens and the seminal vesicles are attached, and the ureter enters the bladder at its superolateral surface (Figure 5–16). In female, the base is firmly attached to the vaginal wall and the upper part of the cervix by connective tissue. Two inferolateral surfaces become continuous with each other at the retropubic space. The urethra leaves the bladder at its inferior angle.

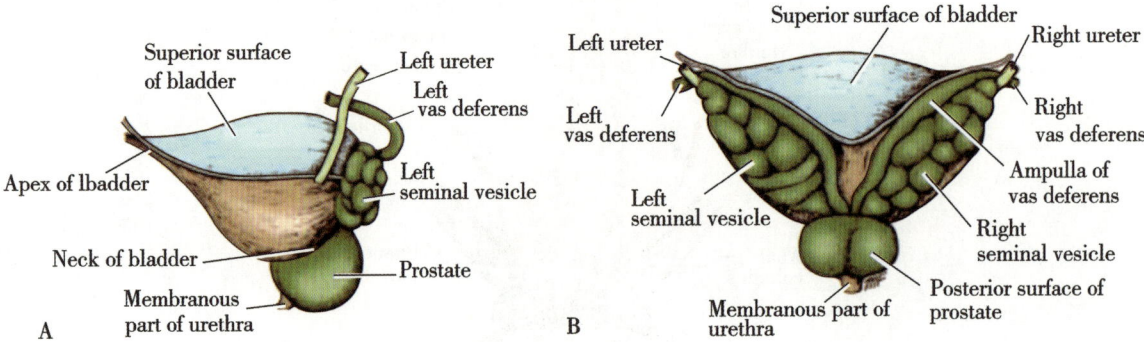

A. Lateral view of the bladder, prostate, and left seminal vesicle; B. Posterior view of the bladder, prostate, vasa deferentia, and seminal vesicles.

Figure 5–15 The bladder and prostate

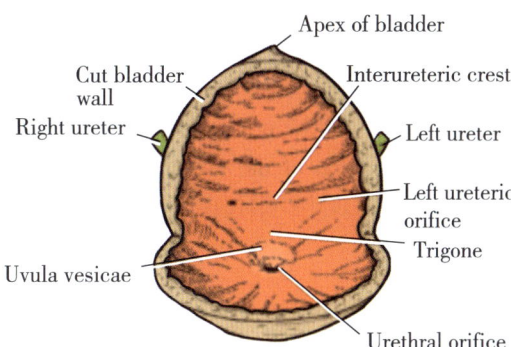

Figure 5-16　Interior of the bladder in the male as seen from in front

(1) Bladder neck

The bladder neck serves as an internal sphincter. At the bladder neck, the muscular bladder wall is more organized, and 3 relatively distinct layers become apparent. The inner longitudinal layer fuses with the inner longitudinal layer of the urethra. The middle circular layer is most prominent in the proximity of the bladder neck, and it fuses with the deep trigonal muscle. The outer longitudinal layer contributes some anterior fibers to what becomes the pubovesical muscles, terminating on the posterior 10 surface of the pubic bone. In males, the bladder neck is contiguous with the prostate, which is attached to the pubis by puboprostatic ligaments. In females, pubourethral ligaments support the bladder neck and urethra.

A normal bladder functions through a complex coordination of musculoskeletal, neurologic, and psychological functions that allow filling and emptying of the bladder contents. The prime effector of continence is the synergic relaxation of detrusor muscles and contraction of the bladder neck and pelvic floor muscles. The normal adult bladder accommodates 300–600 mL of urine; a central nervous system (CNS) response is usually triggered when the volume reaches 400 mL. However, urination can be prevented by cortical suppression of the peripheral nervous system or by voluntary contration of the external urethral sphincter.

(2) Trigone

The trigone is a triangular structure formed by the internal urethral opening and the orifices of the right and left ureter. The superior border of the trigone is a raised area called the interureteric ridge. Deep to the mucosa are 2 muscular layers. The superficial layer connects to longitudinal urethral musculature. The deep muscle fuses with detrusor and Waldeyer sheath, the fibromuscular covering of the intramural ureter. The intramural ureter enters the bladder wall obliquely. The muscle fibers are longitudinal in orientation at this point. This segment of the ureter is about 1.5 cm in length. Blood supply of the bladder is from the superior and inferior vesical arteries, with minor contribution from the obturator, uterine, inferior gluteal, and vaginal arteries. Veins form the vesicoprostatic plexus (vesicous plexus in female), which drain into the internal iliac veins.

(3) The nerve supply

1) Parasympathetic (motor)—pelvic splanchnic nerves 12.

2) Sympathetic—the superior hypogastric and pelvic plexuses.

5.3.3　The male urethra

The prostatic urethra has an elevated central region on its posterior wall, the urethral crest. The crest expands to form the seminal colliculus on which lies the prostatic utricle. The orifices of the ejaculatory duct open on either side of this. The membranous urethra lies between the apex of the prostate and the bulb of the penis. It is surrounded by the sphincter urethrae and the perneal membrane. The bulbourethral glands lie on either side of it. The spongy urethra passes through the bulb, corpus spongiosum, and glans of the penis. Immediately before the external urethral orifice, the urethra expands to form the navicular fossa.

The female urethra, being shorter than that of the male, is more prone to urinary tract infections by ascending organisms.

5.3.4 Prostate

A normal prostate gland is approximately 20 g in volume, 3 cm in length, 4 cm wide, and 2 cm in depth (Figure 5–17). As men get older, the prostate gland is variable in size secondary to benign prostatic hyperplasia.

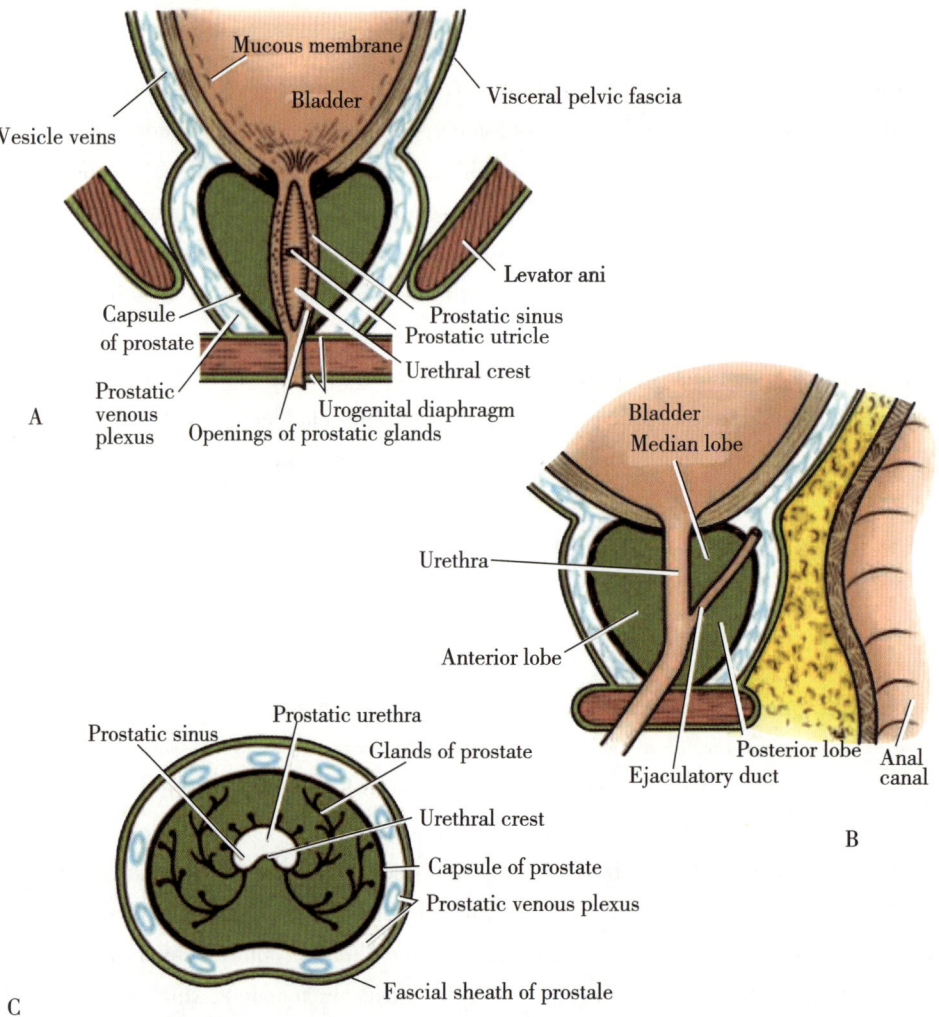

Figure 5-17 Prostate in coronal section (A), sagittal section (B), and horizontal section (C)
(In the coronal section, note the openings of the ejaculatory ducts on the margin of the prostatic utricle)

The gland is located posterior to the pubic symphysis, superior to the perineal membrane, inferior to the bladder, and anterior to the rectum. The base of the prostate is in continuity with the bladder and the prostate ends at the apex before becoming the striated external urethral sphincter. The sphincter is a vertically oriented tubular sheath that surrounds the membranous urethra and prostate.

(1) Prostate gland, posterior view

The prostate is enclosed by a capsule composed of collagen, elastin and large amounts of smooth muscle. The prostate is covered by 3 distinct layers of fascia on the anterior, lateral, and posterior aspects. The anterior and anterolateral fascia is in direct continuity of the true capsule; this is the location of the deep dorsal vein of the penis and its tributaries. Laterally, the fascia fuses with the levator fascia. The outer longitudinal fibers of the detrusor muscle fuse and blend with the fibromuscular tissue of the capsule. The posterior aspect is covered by the rectovesical fascia.

The rectovesical fascia is a connective tissue that is located between the anterior wall of the rectum and posterior aspect of the prostate. This fascial layer covers the prostate and seminal vesicles posteriorly and extends caudally to terminate as a fibrous plate just below the urethra at the level of the external urethral sphincter. This is described as a medial fibrous raphe which has a distal extension to the level of the central tendon of the perineum.

The gland is supported anteriorly by the puboprostatic ligaments and inferiorly by the external urethral sphincter and perineal membrane. The puboprostatic ligaments are actually pubovesical ligaments; however, with the growth of the prostate from puberty, these ligaments have the appearance of terminating into the prostate.

The prostate is surrounded by the puborectal portion of the levator ani. The seminal vesicles lie superior to the prostate under the base of the bladder and are approximately 6 cm in length. Each seminal vesicle joins its corresponding ductus deferens to form the ejaculatory duct before entering the prostate.

(2) Ductus (vas) deferens

The ductus (vas) deferens is the continuation of the epididymis; it is 30–45 cm long and conveys sperm to the ejaculatory ducts. The convoluted portion of the ductus deferens becomes straighter (diameter, 2–3 mm) as it travels posterior to the testis and medial to the epididymis. Subsequently, the ductus ascends on the posterior aspect of the spermatic cord until it reaches the deep inguinal ring, where it participates in the formation of the spermatic cord and loops over the inferior epigastric artery.

At this point, the ductus travels along the lateral pelvic wall, medial to the distal ureter, along the posterior wall of the bladder until it reaches the seminal vesicles dorsal to the prostate. Each ductus deferens has an artery usually derived from the superior vesical artery (artery to the ductus), with venous drainage to the pelvic venous plexus. Lymphatic drainage of the ductus deferens is to the external and internal iliac nodes and innervation is mainly sympathetic from the pelvic plexus.

(3) Ejaculatory ducts

The ejaculatory ducts are 2 cm in length and derived from the union of the seminal vesicle and the ampulla of the vas deferens. Each duct starts at the base of the prostate and terminates at the seminal colliculus (verumontanum). The vasculature, innervation, and lymphatics of the ejaculatory ducts are the same as for the ductus deferens.

(4) Seminal vesicle

The seminal vesicles are bilateral, lobulated glands. They are soft and approximately 5–7 cm long. The vesicles are blind pouches and are rounded on their most superior aspects and taper to their inferior aspects, where they constrict to ultimately form short ducts. They descend inferomedially while lying on the fundic portion of the posterior surface of the urinary bladder. The seminal vesicles are immediately inferior and lateral to the ampullary portions of the ductus deferentes. This bilateral arrangement most closely resembles the letter "V".

(5) Anterior aspect of the seminal vesicles, terminal parts of the deferent ducts, and the prostate

The ureters pass in between the superior, rounded aspects of the seminal vesicles and the superior portions of the ampullae of the ductus deferentes. The short ducts of the seminal vesicles join the lateral aspects of the ductus deferentes at an acute angle, creating the ejaculatory ducts at the base of the prostate gland.

The seminal vesicles lie below the inferior-most aspect of the peritoneum in the pelvic cavity. They are covered by endopelvic fascia, which is an abundant extraperitoneal connective tissue.

The seminal vesicles receive their arterial supply in a way that is similar to that of the prostate gland. The primary arterial supply is from the inferior vesical, internal pudendal, and middle rectal arteries. These 3 primary sources all arise from the anterior division of the internal iliac artery.

5.3.5　Uterus

The uterus is a dynamic female reproductive organ that is responsible for several reproductive functions, including menses, implantation, gestation, labor, and delivery. It is responsive to the hormonal milieu within the body, which allows adaptation to the different stages of a woman's reproductive life. The uterus adjusts to reflect changes in ovarian steroid production during the menstrual cycle and displays rapid growth and specialized contractile activity during pregnancy and childbirth. It can also remain in a relatively quiescent state during the prepubertal and postmenopausal years.

Uterus is a muscular organ that accommodates the developing embryo. Most of the wall is smooth muscle, the myometrium.

Uterus has three main parts: the fundus lies above the entrance of the fallopian tube; the body receives the fallopian tubes; the cavity of the uterus occupies the body; the cervical is the narrowest part of the uterus. It has a supravaginal part and a aginal part. The vaginal fornix surrounds the cervix, deepest posteriorly. The cervical anal is continuous with the uterine cavity at the internal os, and opens into the vagina the external os.

Uterus is a pear-shaped organ located in the female pelvis between the urinary bladder anteriorly and the rectum posteriorly (Figure 5-18, Figure 5-19). The average dimensions are approximately 8 cm long, 5 cm across, and 4 cm thick, with an average volume between 80 mL and 200 mL.

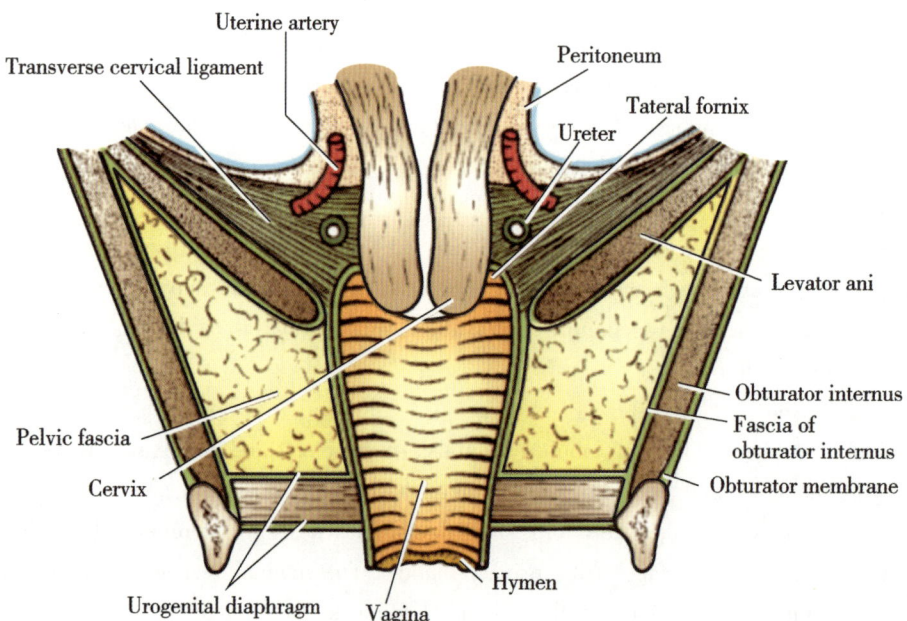

Figure 5-18　Coronal section of the pelvis showing relationship of the levators ani muscles and the transverse cervical ligaments to the uterus and vagina

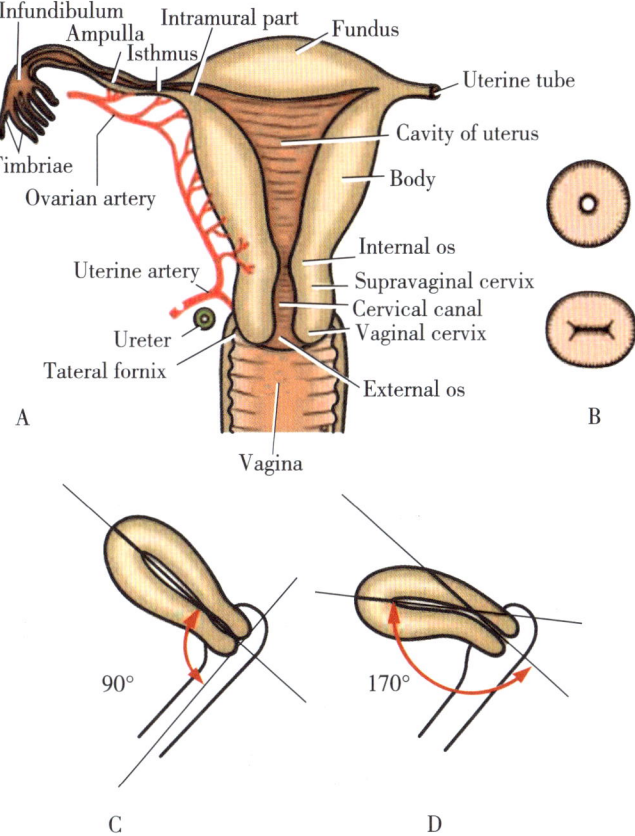

A. Different parts of the uterine tube and the uterus; B. External os of the cervix, (above) nulliparous, (below) parous; C. Anteverted position of the uterus; D. Anteverted and anteflexed position of the uterus.

Figure 5-19　Uterine and uterus

(1) Blood supply of the aterus

Blood is provided to the uterus by the ovarian and uterine arteries, the latter of which arise from the anterior divisions of the internal iliac artery. The uterine artery occasionally gives off the vaginal artery (although this is usually a separate branch of the internal iliac around), which supplies the upper vagina, and the arcuate arteries, which surround the uterus. It then further branches into the radial arteries, which penetrate the myometrium to provide blood to all layers, including the endometrium.

(2) Positions of the uterus

The uterine position can also be described based on the relative location of the fundus; that is, an anteflexed uterus, which is normal, is where the fundus tilts forward, and a retroflexed uterus is tilted backward.

5.3.6　Uterine tube

The uterine tubes, also known as oviducts or fallopian tubes, are the female structures that transport the ova from the ovary to the uterus each month. In the presence of sperm and fertilization, the uterine tubes transport the fertilized egg to the uterus for implantation.

The uterine tubes are uterine appendages located bilaterally at the superior portion of the uterine cavity. These tubes exit the uterus through an area referred to as the cornua, forming a connection between the endometrial and peritoneal cavities. Each uterine tube is approximately 10 cm in length and 1 cm in diameter and is situated within the mesosalpinx. The mesosalpinx is a fold in the broad ligament. The distal portion of the uterine tube ends in an orientation encircling the ovary. The primary function of the uterine tubes is to transport sperm toward the egg, which is released by the ovary, and to then allow passage of the fertilized egg back to the uterus for implantation. Figure 5-20 shows an ectopic pregnancy in the uterine tube.

A uterine tube contains 3 parts. The first segment, closest to the uterus, is called the isthmus. The second segment is the ampulla, which becomes more dilated in diameter and is the most common site for fertilization. The final segment, located farthest from the uterus, is the infundibulum. The infundibulum gives rise to the fimbriae, fingerlike projections that are responsible for picking up the egg released by the ovary.

The arterial supply to the uterine tubes is from branches of the uterine and ovarian arteries; these small vessels are located within the mesosalpinx.

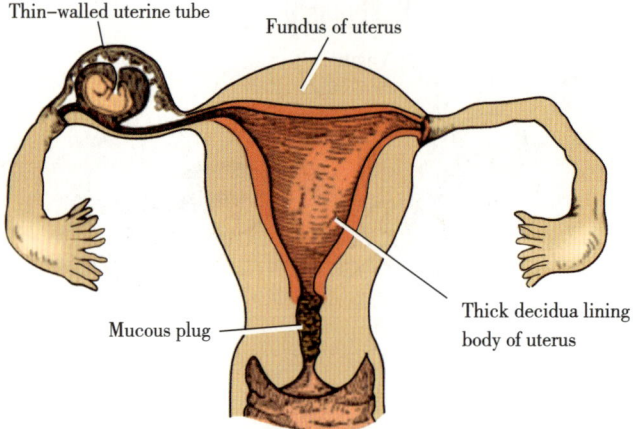

Figure 5 – 20 An ectopic pregnancy located where the ampulla of the uterine tube narrows down to join the isthmus

(Note the thin tubal wall compared to the thick decidua that lines the body of the uterus)

5.3.7 Ovary

The ovaries are the female pelvic reproductive organs that house the ova and are also responsible for the production of sex hormones. They are paired organs located on either side of the uterus within the broad ligament below the uterine (fallopian) tubes.

The ovary is within the ovarian fossa, a space that is bound by the external iliac vessels, obliterated umbilical artery, and the ureter. The ovaries are responsible for housing and releasing ova, or eggs, necessary for reproduction. At birth, a female has approximately (1-2) million eggs, but only 300 of these eggs will ever become mature and be released for the purpose of fertilization.

Anatomy of the ovaries is displayed in Figure 5-21.

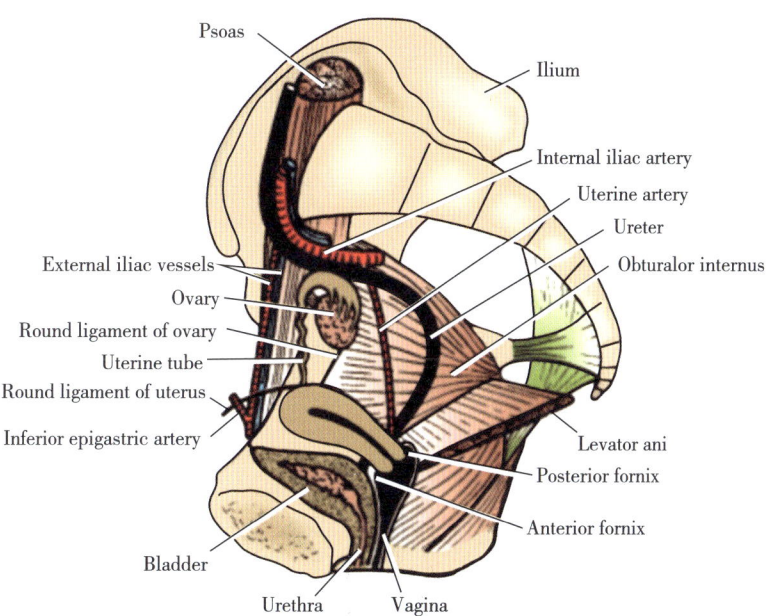

Figure 5-21 Right half of the pelvis showing the ovary, the uterine tube, and the vagina

(1) Ovaries, sagittal view

The ovaries are small, oval-shaped, and grayish in color, with an uneven surface. The actual size of an ovary depends on a woman's age and hormonal status; the ovaries, covered by a modified peritoneum, are approximately 3-5 cm in length during childbearing years and become much smaller and then atrophic once menopause occurs. A cross-section of the ovary reveals many cystic structures that vary in size. These structures represent ovarian follicles at different stages of development and degeneration.

(2) Ovarian ligament

Several paired ligaments support the ovaries. The ovarian ligament connects the uterus and ovary. The posterior portion of the broad ligament forms the mesovarium, which supports the ovary and houses its arterial and venous supply. The suspensory ligament of the ovary (infundibular pelvic ligament) attaches the ovary to the pelvic sidewall. This larger structure also contains the ovarian artery and vein, as well as nerve supply to the ovary.

(3) Blood supply, nerve supply, and lymph drainage

Blood supply to the ovary is via the ovarian artery; both the right and left arteries originate directly from the descending aorta. The ovarian artery and vein enter and exit the ovary at the hilum. The left ovarian vein drains into the left renal vein, and the right ovarian vein empties directly into the inferior vena cava.

Nerve supply to the ovaries runs with the vasculature via the suspensory ligament of the ovary, entering the ovary at the hilum. Supply is through the ovarian, hypogastric, and aortic plexuses.

Lymph drainage of the ovary is primarily to the lateral aortic nodes; however, the iliac nodes are also involved.

5.4 The perineum

The cavity of the pelvis is divided by the pelvic diaphragm into the main pelvic cavity above and the perineum below. When seen from below with the thighs abducted, the perineum is diamond-shaped and is bounded anteriorly by the symphysis pubis, posteriorly by the tip of the coccyx, and laterally by the ischial tuberosities. The lateral boundaries of perineum are the inferior rami of the pubes, the rami of ischia and the sacrotuberous ligaments. A line joining the anterior parts of the ischial tuberosities divides the perineum into a large posterior anal region(triangle) and a small anterior urogenital region(triangle)(Figure 5-22).

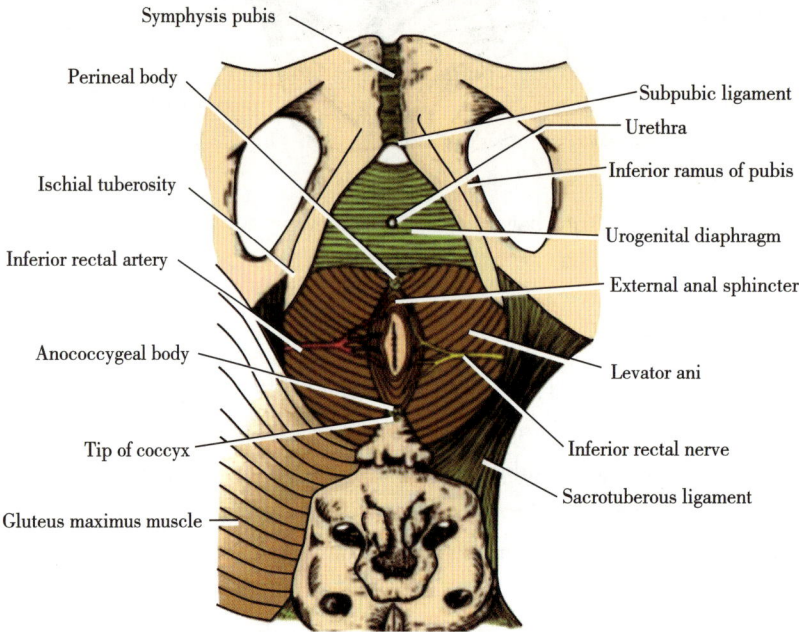

Figure 5-22　Anal triangle and urogenital triangle in male

5.4.1　Anal triangle

The anal triangle is bounded behind by the tip of the coccyx and on each side by the ischial tuberosity and the sacrotuberous ligament, overlapped by the border of the gluteus maximus muscle. The anus, or lower opening of the anal canal, lies in the midline, and on each side is the ischiorectal fossa. The skin around the anus is supplied by the inferior rectal (hemorrhoidal) nerve. The lymph vessels of the skin drain into the medial group of the superficial inguinal nodes.

5.4.1.1　Anal canal

(1) Location and description

The anal canal is about 4 cm long and passes downward and backward from the rectal ampulla to the anus. Except during defecation, its lateral walls are kept in apposition by the levatores ani muscles and the anal sphincters.

(2) Relations

Posteriorly: the anococcygeal body, which is a mass of fibrous tissue lying between the anal canal and the coccyx.

Laterally: the fat-filled ischiorectal fossae.

Anteriorly: in the male, the perineal body, the urogenital diaphragm, the membranous part of the urethra, and the bulb of the penis. In the female, the perineal body, the urogenital diaphragm, and the lower part of the vagina.

(3) Structure

1) The mucous membrane of the upper half of the anal canal is derived from hindgut entoderm. It has the following important anatomic features.

It is lined by columnar epithelium.

It is thrown into vertical folds called anal columns, which are joined together at their lower ends by small semilunar folds called anal valves (remains of proctodeal membrane).

The nerve supply is the same as that for the rectal mucosa and is derived from the autonomic hypogastric plexuses.

It is sensitive only to stretch.

The arterial supply is that of the hindgut–namely, the superior rectal artery, a branch of the inferior mesenteric artery. The venous drainage is mainly by the superior rectal vein, a tributary of the inferior mesenteric vein, and the portal vein.

The lymphatic drainage is mainly upward along the superior rectal artery to the pararectal nodes and then eventually to the inferior mesenteric nodes.

2) The mucous membrane of the lower half of the anal canal is derived from ectoderm of the proctodeum. It has the following important features.

It is lined by stratified squamous epithelium, which gradually merges at the anus with the perianal epidermis.

There are no anal columns.

The nerve supply is from the somatic inferior rectal nerve; it is thus sensitive to pain, temperature, touch, and pressure.

The arterial supply is the inferior rectal artery, a branch of the internal pudendal artery. The venous drainage is by the inferior rectal vein, a tributary of the internal pudendal vein, which drains into the internal iliac vein (Figure 5-23).

The lymph drainage is downward to the medial group of superficial inguinal nodes.

The pectinate line indicates the level where the upper half of the anal canal joins the lower half.

3) Muscle coat

As in the upper parts of the intestinal tract, it is divided into an outer longitudinal and an inner circular layer of smooth muscle.

4) Anal sphincters

The anal canal has an involuntary internal sphincter and a voluntary external sphincter.

The internal sphincter is formed from a thickening of the smooth muscle of the circular coat at the upper end of the anal canal. The internal sphincter is enclosed by a sheath of striped muscle that forms the voluntary external sphincter.

The external sphincter can be divided into three parts.

A subcutaneous part, which encircles the lower end of the anal canal and has no bony attachments.

A superficial part, which is attached to the coccyx behind and the perineal body in front.

A deep part, which encircles the upper end of the anal canal and has no bony attachments (Figure 5-24).

At the junction of the rectum and anal canal, the internal sphincter, the deep part of the external sphincter, and the puborectalis muscles form a distinct ring, called the anorectal ring, which can be felt on rectal examination (Figure 5-25).

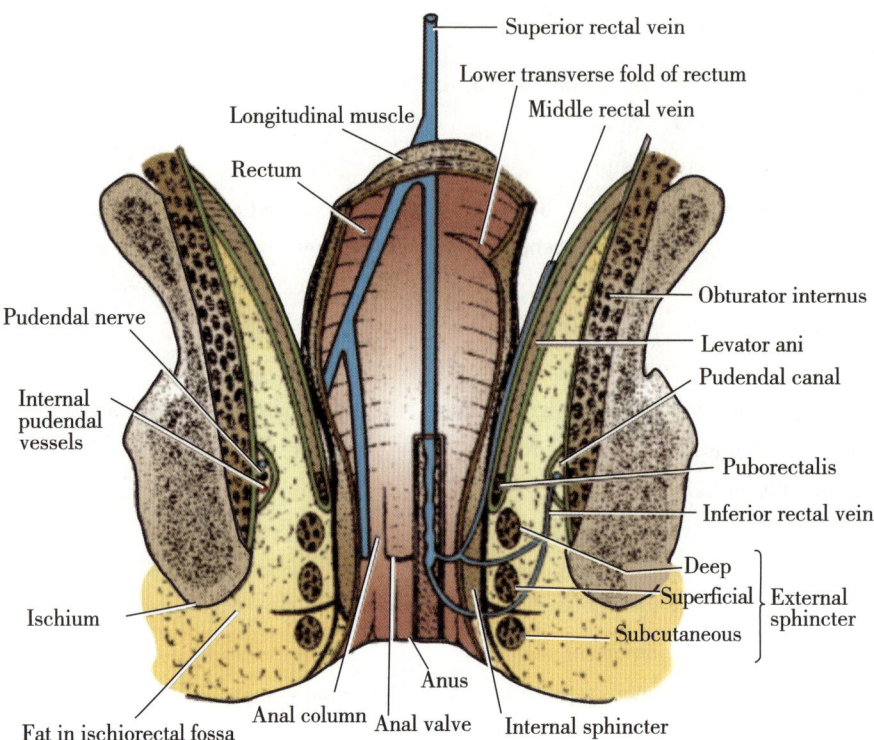

Figure 5-23 Coronal section of the pelvis and the perineum showing venous drainage of the anal canal

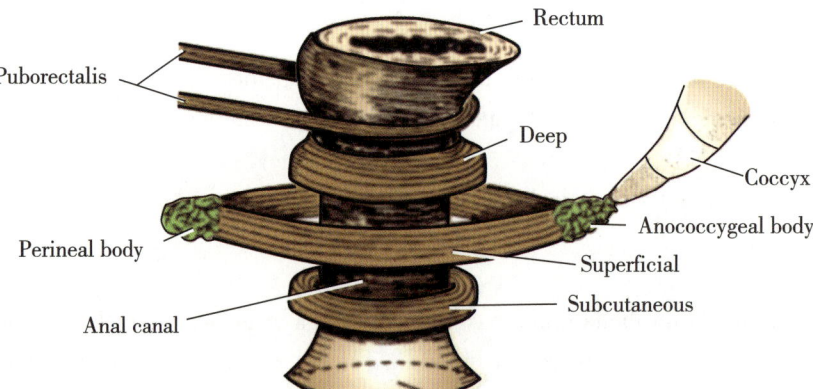

Figure 5-24 Arrangement of the muscle fibers of the puborectalis muscle and different parts of the external anal sphincter

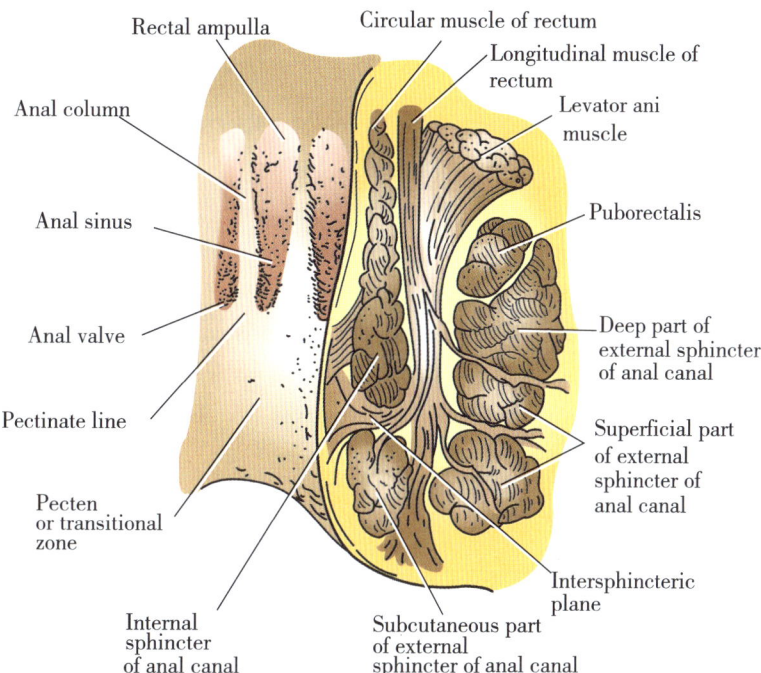

Figure 5-25　Coronal section of the anal canal showing the detailed anatomy of the mucous membrane and the arrangement of the internal and external anal sphincters

[Note that the terms "pectinate line" (the line at the level of the anal valves) and "pecten" (the transitional zone between the skin and the mucous membrane) are sometimes used by clinicians]

5.4.1.2　Ischiorectal fossa

The ischiorectal fossa (ischioanal fossa) is a wedge-shaped space located on each side of the anal canal. The base of the wedge is superficial and formed by the skin. The edge of the wedge is formed by the junction of the medial and lateral walls. The medial wall is formed by the sloping levator ani muscle and the anal canal. The lateral wall is formed by the lower part of the obturator internus muscle, covered with pelvic fascia.

(1) Contents of fossa

The ischiorectal fossa is filled with dense fat, which supports the anal canal and allows it to distend during defecation. The pudendal nerve and internal pudendal vessels are embedded in a fascial canal, the pudendal canal, on the lateral wall of the ischiorectal fossa, on the medial side of the ischial tuberosity. The inferior rectal vessels and nerve cross the fossa to reach the anal canal.

(2) Pudendal nerve

The pudendal nerve is a branch of the sacral plexus and leaves the main pelvic cavity through the greater sciatic foramen. After a brief course in the gluteal region of the lower limb, it enters the perineum through the lesser sciatic foramen. The nerve then passes forward in the pudendal canal and, by means of its branches, supplies the external anal sphincter and the muscles and skin of the perineum.

1) Inferior rectal nerve

This runs medially across the ischiorectal fossa and supplies the external anal sphincter, the mucous membrane of the lower half of the anal canal, and the perianal skin.

2) Dorsal nerve of the penis (or clitoris)

This is distributed to the penis (or clitoris).

3) Perineal nerve

This supplies the muscles in the urogenital triangle and the skin on the posterior surface of the scrotum (or labia majora).

(3) Internal pudendal artery

The internal pudendal artery is a branch of the internal iliac artery and passes from the pelvis through the greater sciatic foramen and enters the perineum through the lesser sciatic foramen.

Inferior rectal artery: this supplies the lower half of the anal canal.

Branches to the penis in the male and to the labia and clitoris in the female.

Internal pudendal vein: the internal pudendal vein receives tributaries that correspond to the branches of the internal pudendal artery.

5.4.2 Urogenital triangle

The urogenital triangle is bounded in front by the pubic arch and laterally by the ischial tuberosities.

5.4.2.1 Superficial fascia

The superficial fascia of the urogenital triangle can be divided into a fatty layer and a membranous layer.

The fatty layer (fascia of Camper) is continuous with the fat of the ischiorectal fossa and the superficial fascia of the thighs. In the scrotum, the fat is replaced by smooth muscle, the dartos muscle. The dartos muscle contracts in response to cold and reduces the surface area of the scrotal skin.

The membranous layer (Colles' fascia) is attached posteriorly to the posterior border of the urogenital diaphragm and laterally to the margins of the pubic arch; anteriorly it is continuous with the membranous layer of superficial fascia of the anterior abdominal wall (Scarpa's fascia). The fascia is continued over the penis (or clitoris) as a tubular sheath. In the scrotum (or labia majora), it forms a distinct layer.

5.4.2.2 Urogenital diaphragm

The urogenital diaphragm is a triangular musculofascial diaphragm situated in the anterior part of the perineum, filling in the gap of the pubic arch. It is formed by the sphincter urethrae and the deep transverse perineal muscles, which are enclosed between a superior and an inferior layer of fascia of the urogenital diaphragm. The inferior layer of fascia is often referred to as the perineal membrane.

Anteriorly, the two layers of fascia fuse, leaving a small gap beneath the symphysis pubis. Posteriorly, the two layers of fascia fuse with each other and with the membranous layer of the superficial fascia and the perineal body. Laterally, the layers of fascia are attached to the pubic arch. The closed space that is contained between the superficial and deep layers of fascia is known as the deep perineal pouch.

5.4.2.3 Contents of the male urogenital triangle

In the male, the triangle contains the penis and scrotum.

(1) Contents of the superficial perineal pouch in the male

The superficial perineal pounch contains the bulbospongiosus muscles, ischiocavernosus muscles, superficial transverse perineal muscles, perineal branch of the pudendal nerve, perineal body.

(2) Contents of the deep perineal pouch in the male

The deep perineal pouch contains the membranous part of the urethra, the sphincter urethrae, the bulbourethral glands, the deep transverse perineal muscles, the internal pudendal vessels and their branches, and the dorsal nerves of the penis.

5.4.2.4 Contents of the female urogenital triangle

In the female, the triangle contains the external genitalia and the orifices of the urethra and the vagina (Figure 5-26).

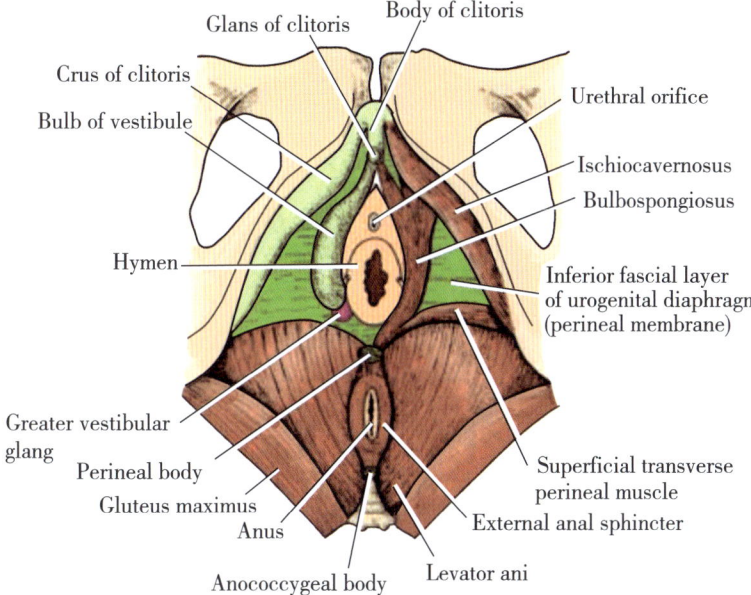

Figure 5-26 Root and body of the clitoris and the perineal muscles

(1) Contents of the superficial perineal pouch in the female

The superficial perineal pouch contains structures forming the root of the clitoris and the muscles that cover them, namely, the bulbospongiosus muscles and the ischiocavernosus muscles.

(2) Contents of the deep perineal pouch in the female

The deep perineal pouch contains part of the urethra; part of the vagina; the sphincter urethrae, which is pierced by the urethra and the vagina; the deep transverse perineal muscles; the internal pudendal vessels and their branches; and the dorsal nerves of the clitoris.

5.4.2.5 Anal canal

The anal canal is the most terminal part of the lower gastrointestinal (GI) tract/large intestine, which lies between the anal verge (anal orifice, anus) in the perineum below and the rectum above. Confusion and controversy exist regarding the anatomy of the anorectal region in anatomy and surgical texts. The description in this topic is from below upwards, as that is how this region is usually examined in clinical practice.

The pigmented, keratinized perianal skin of the buttocks (around the anal verge) has skin appendages (e.g., hair, sweat glands, sebaceous glands); compare this with the anal canal skin above the anal verge, which is also pigmented and keratinized but does not have skin appendages.

In anatomy texts, the rectum changes to the anal canal at the dentate line. For surgeons, however, the demarcation between the rectum above and the anal canal below is the anorectal ring. The following is the description of the surgical anal canal.

The anal canal is completely extraperitoneal. The length of the (surgical) anal canal is 3-5 cm, with two thirds of this being above the dentate line and one third below the dentate line (anatomical anal canal).

The epithelium of the (anatomical) anal canal (between the anal verge below and the dentate line above) is variously described as anal mucosa or anal skin. The author feels that it should be called anal skin (anoderm), as it looks like (pigmented) skin, is sensitive like skin, and is keratinized (but does not have skin appendages).

The dentate line (also called the pectinate line) is the site of fusion of the proctodeum below and the postallantoic gut above. It is a wavy demarcation formed by the anal valves (transverse folds of mucosa) at the inferior-most ends of the anal columns. Anal glands open above the anal valves into the anal crypts. The dentate line is not seen on inspection in clinical practice, but under anesthesia the anal canal descends down, and the dentate line can be seen on slight retraction of the anal canal skin.

From a surgical perspective, the anal canal just above the dentate line for 1-2 cm is called the transition zone. Beyond this transition zone, the (surgical) anal canal is lined with columnar epithelium. Anal columns (of Morgagni) are 5-10 longitudinal (vertical) mucosal folds in the upper part of the anal canal.

At the bottom of these columns are anal crypts, or sinuses, into which open the anal glands and anal papillae. Three of these columns (left lateral, right posterior, and rightanterior, at 3, 7, and 11 o'clock position in supine position) are prominent; they are called anal cushions and contain branches and tributaries of superior rectal (hemorrhoidal) artery and vein. When prominent, veins in these cushions form the internal hemorrhoids.

The anorectal ring is situated about 5 cm from anus. At the anorectal angle, the rectum turns backwards to continue as the anal canal.

Levator ani and coccygeus muscles form the pelvic diaphragm. Lateral to the anal canal are the ischioanal fossae (1 on either side), below the pelvic diaphragm. The anterior relations of the anal canal are, in males, the seminal vesicles, prostate, and urethra, and, in females, the cervix and vagina. In front of (anterior to) the anal canal is the rectovesical fascia (of Denonvilliers), and behind (posterior) is the presacral endopelvic fascia (of Waldeyer), under which lie a rich presacral plexus of veins. Posterior to the anal canal lie the tip of the coccyx and lower sacrum.

Blood supply and lymphatics: the anal canal above the dentate line is supplied by the terminal branches of the superior rectal (hemorrhoidal) artery, which is the terminal branch of the inferior mesenteric artery. The middle rectal artery (a branch of the internal iliac artery) and the inferior rectal artery (a branch of the internal pudendal artery) supply the lower anal canal.

Underneath the anal canal skin (below the dentate line) lies the external hemorrhoidal plexus of veins, which drains into systemic veins. Underneath the anal canal mucosa (above dentate line) lies the internal hemorrhoidal plexus of veins, which drains into the portal system of veins. The anorectum is, therefore, an important area of portosystemic venous connection (the other being the esophagogastric junction).

Lymphatics from the anal canal drain into the superficial inguinal group of lymph nodes.

5.4.2.6 Penis

The penile shaft is composed of 3 erectile columns, the 2 corpora cavernosa and the corpus spongiosum, as well as the columns' enveloping fascial layers, nerves, lymphatics, and blood vessels, all covered by skin. The 2 suspensory ligaments, composed of primarily elastic fibers, support the penis at its base.

The paired corpora cavernosa contain erectile tissue and are each surrounded by the tunica albuginea, a dense fibrous sheath of connective tissue with relatively few elastic fibers. The corpora cavernosa communicate freely through an incomplete midline septum. Proximally, at the base of the penis, the septum is more complete; ultimately, the corpora diverge, forming the crura, which attach to the ischiopubic rami.

The tunica albuginea consists of 2 layers: the outer longitudinal and the inner circular. The tunica albuginea becomes thicker ventrally where it forms a groove to accommodate the corpus spongiosum. The tunica albuginea of the corpus spongiosum is considerably thinner (< 0.5 mm) than that of the corpora cavernosa (approximately 2 mm). Along the inner aspect of the tunica albuginea, flattened columns or sinusoidal trabeculae composed of fibrous tissue and smooth muscle surround the endothelial-lined sinusoids (cavernous spaces). In addition, a row of structural trabeculae arises near the junction of the 3 corporal bodies and inserts in the walls of the corpora about the midplane of the circumference.

Structure of the tunica albuginea: the erectile tissue within the corpora contains arteries, nerves, muscle fibers, and venous sinuses lined with flat endothelial cells, and it fills the space of the corpora cavernosa. The cut surface of the corpora cavernosa looks like a sponge. There is a thin layer of areolar tissue that separates this tissue from the tunica albuginea.

Blood flow to the corpora cavernosa is via the paired deep arteries of the penis (cavernosal arteries), which run near the center of each corpora cavernosa.

Arterial supply of the penis: the single corpus spongiosum lies in the ventral groove between the 2 corpora cavernosa. The urethra passes through the corpus spongiosum. The corpus spongiosum possesses a much thinner and more elastic tunica albuginea to allow for distention of the corpus spongiosum for passage of the ejaculate through the urethra. The thinner tunica albuginea of the corpus spongiosum also allows the corpus to become less rigid during erection. Hence, the distal extension of the spongiosum, the glans penis, covers the tips of the corpora cavernosa to provide a cushioning effect. The urethral meatus is positioned just slightly on the ventral surface of the glans and is slitlike. The edge of the glans overhangs the shaft of the penis, forming a rim called the corona.

The three erectile bodies are surrounded by deep penile (Buck) fascia, the dartos fascia, and the penile skin. The deep penile fascia is a strong, deep, fascial layer that is immediately superficial to the tunica albuginea. It is continuous with the deep fascia of the muscles covering the crura and bulb of the penis, the ischiocavernosus and bulbospongiosus.

On the dorsal aspect of the corpora cavernosa, the deep dorsal vein and paired dorsal arteries and branches of the dorsal nerves are contained within the deep penile fascia. This fascia splits to surround the corpus spongiosum, and it extends into the perineum as the deep fascia of the ischiocavernosus and bulbospongiosus muscles.

The deep penile fascia encloses these muscles and each crus of the corpora cavernosa and the bulb of the corpus spongiosum, adhering these structures to the pubis, ischium, and the urogenital diaphragm.

The penile skin is continuous with that of the lower abdominal wall. Distally, the penile skin is confluent with the smooth, hairless skin covering the glans. At the corona, it is folded on itself to form the prepuce (foreskin), which overlies the glans. The subcutaneous connective tissue of the penis and scrotum has abundant smooth muscle and is called the dartos fascia, which continues into the perineum and fuses with the superficial perineal (Colle) fascia. In the penis, the dartos fascia is loosely attached to the skin and deep penile fascia and contains the superficial arteries, veins, and nerves of the penis.

5.4.2.7 Female external genitalia

The vulva, also known as the pudendum, is a term used to describe those external organs that may be visible in the perineal area (Figure 5-27, Figure 5-28). The vulva consists of the following organs: mons pubis, labia minora and majora, hymen, clitoris, vestibule, urethra, Skene glands, greater vestibular (Bartholin) glands, and vestibular bulbs.

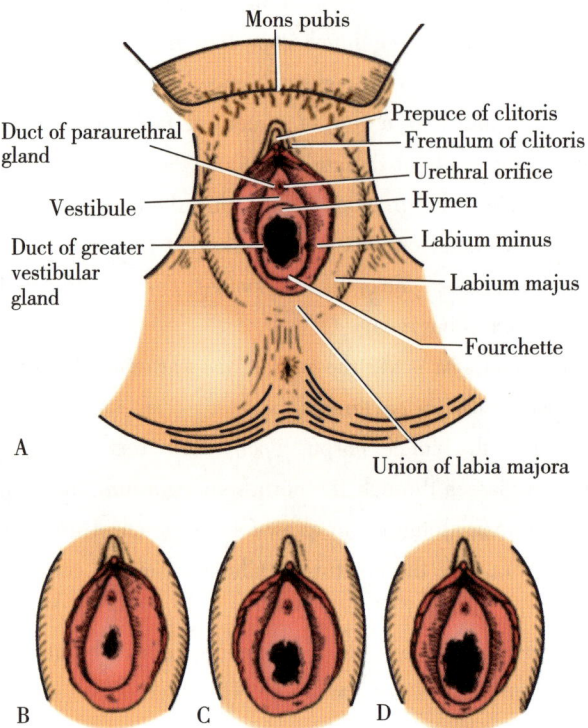

Figure 5-27 Vulva (A) and the different appearances of the hymen in a virgin (B), a woman who has had sexual intercourse (C), and a multiparous woman (D)

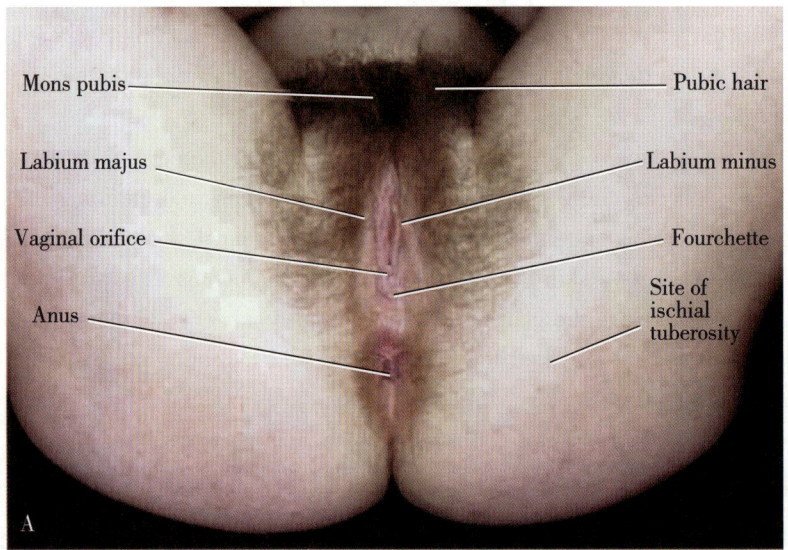

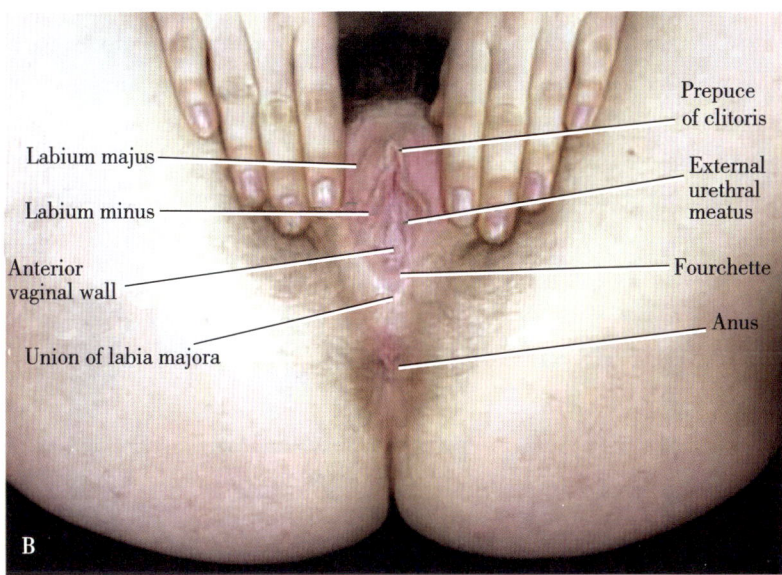

A. With labia together; B. With labia separated.

Figure 5-28　The perineum in a 25-year-old woman (inferior view)

The boundaries include the mons pubis anteriorly, the rectum posteriorly, and the genitocrural folds (thigh folds) laterally.

(1) Mons pubis

The mons pubis is the rounded portion of the vulva where sexual hair development occurs at the time of puberty. This area may be described as directly anterosuperior to the pubic symphysis.

(2) Labia

The labia majora are 2 large, longitudinal folds of adipose and fibrous tissue. They vary in size and distribution from female to female, and the size is dependent upon adipose content. They extend from the mons anteriorly to the perineal body posteriorly. The labia majora have hair follicles.

The labia minora, also known as nymphae, are 2 small cutaneous folds that are found between the labia majora and the introitus or vaginal vestibule. Anteriorly, the labia minora join to form the frenulum of the clitoris.

(3) Hymen

The hymen is a thin membrane found at the entrance to the vaginal orifice. Often, this membrane is perforated before the onset of menstruation, allowing flow of menses. The hymen varies greatly in shape.

(4) Clitoris

The clitoris is an erectile structure found beneath the anterior joining of the labia minora. Its width in an adult female is approximately 1 cm, with an average length of 1.5-2.0 cm. The clitoris is made up of 2 crura, which attach to the periosteum of the ischiopubic rami. It is a very sensitive structure, analogous to the male penis. It is innervated by the dorsal nerve of the clitoris, a terminal branch of the pudendal nerve.

(5) Vestibule and urethra

Between the clitoris and the vaginal introitus (opening) is a triangular area known as the vestibule, which extends to the posterior fourchette. The vestibule is where the urethral (urinary) meatus is found, approximately 1 cm anterior to the vaginal orifice, and it also gives rise to the opening of the Skene glands bilaterally. The urethra is composed of membranous connective tissue and links the urinary bladder to the vestibule externally. A female urethra ranges in length from 3.5 cm to 5.0 cm.

(6) Skene and Bartholin glands

The Skene glands secrete lubrication at the opening of the urethra. The greater vestibular (Bartholin) glands are also responsible for secreting lubrication to the vagina, with openings just outside the hymen, bilaterally, at the posterior aspect of the vagina. Each gland is small, similar in shape to a kidney bean.

(7) Vestibular bulbs

Finally, the vestibular bulbs are 2 masses of erectile tissue that lie deep to the bulbocavernosus muscles bilaterally.

5.5 Main contents of the pelvis and perineum

Pelvis	
Pelvic brim	
✓ This is the inlet of the true pelvis, i. e. , above the inlet is the greater/false pelvis, while below it is the lesser true pelvis ✓ It is oriented at an oblique plane, 50° – 60° to the horizontal	
Boundaries	
Anteriorly	✓ Upper margin of pubic symphysis
Posteriorly	✓ Sacral promontory
Either side	✓ Linea terminalis, which includes anterior margin of ala of sacrum, iliopectinal line, pectineal line, pubic tubercle and pubic crest
Shape	
✓ In males: heart-shaped, widest towards the back ✓ In female: transversely oval, widest further forward ✓ Indentation by the promontory is more marked in males than in females	
Relations	
At the sacral promontory	
✓ Medial plane—medial sacral artery ✓ Medially—hypogastric plexus ✓ Laterally—pelvic sympathetic and ganglia	
At the ala of the sacrum	
From medial to lateral are as follows: ✓ Lumbosacral trunk ✓ Iliolumbar artery ✓ Obturator nerve running towards obturator foramen ✓ On left side→ superior erior rectal artery	
At sacroiliac joint	
✓ Bifurcation of common iliac vessels into internal and external iliac vessels	

- ◊ Internal iliac vessels: cross pelvic brim to enter pelvis
- ◊ External iliac vessels: related along outer edge of pelvic brim
- ✓ Ureter passes into pelvic cavity lying on the bifurcation
  - ◊ On left side: medial limb of pelvic mesocolon

At iliopectineal line

- ✓ Ovary lies just below pelvic brim in front of ureter
- ✓ Psoas major
- ✓ External iliac, genitofemoral and gonadal vessels
  - ◊ In female: the uterine artery crosses the iliopectineal line to enter the broad ligament
  - ◊ More anteriorly, vas deferens (in male)
- ✓ Round ligament of uterus (in female)

At pectineal line

- ✓ Attached is:
  - ◊ Pectineal ligament laterally
  - ◊ Lacunar ligament medially
- ✓ Conjoint tendon deep to lacunar ligament
- ✓ Femoral ring is lateral to lacunar ligament
- ✓ Pubic branch of inferior epigastric artery crosses lateral margin of lacunar ligament

At pubic tubercle

- ✓ Attached is medial end of inguinal ligament
- ✓ In male: crossed by spermatic cord

At pubic crest

- ✓ Attached is the rectus abdominis
- ✓ Bladder is posterior

Pelvic diaphragm

- ✓ This includes the levator ani and coccygeus
- ✓ The pelvic diaphragm separates the pelvis from the perineum
- ✓ The muscle fibres slope backward and downwards to the midline making a gutter-shaped pelvic floor

Levator ani

This is composed of:

- ✓ Levator prostate in male/pubovaginalis in female
  - ◊ Sling around prostate/vagina and inserted into perineal body
- ✓ Puborectalis
  - ◊ Sling around junction of rectum and anal canal
- ✓ Pubococcygeus
  - ◊ Inserted into anococcygeal body and coccyx
- ✓ Iliococcygeus
  - ◊ Inserted into anococcygeal body and coccyx

Origin	✓ From the white line (thickening of pelvic fascia over obturator internus) ✓ Stretched from posterior surface of body of pubis to ischial spine
Insertion	✓ Surround prostate/vagina and inserted into perineal body ✓ Surround rectum ✓ Also inserted into anococcygeal body and tip of coccyx
Nerve supply	✓ Branch from S_4 ✓ Branch from pudental nerve

Coccygeus

Origin	✓ From ischial spine ✓ Sacrotuberous ligament
Insertion	✓ SV_5 ✓ Anococcygeal body and coccyx
Nerve supply	✓ Branches from S_4 and S_5

Actions of pelvic diaphragm

✓ Close posterior part of pelvic outlet
✓ Levator ani fix the perineal body and supports pelvic viscera
✓ Resist high intra-abdominal pressure and maintain continence of bladder and rectum
✓ Prevents prolapse of pelvic viscera
✓ Involved in the mechanics of labour

Relations of pelvic diaphragm

✓ Superior/pelvic surface covered with pelvic fascia, which separates it from bladder, prostate, rectum and peritoneum in male; bladder, vagina, rectum and peritoneum in female
✓ Inferior/perineal surface covered with anal fascia
✓ Anterior borders of the 2 muscles are superior by a triangular space for passage of
    ◊ Urethra (in male) or urethra and vagina (in female)
✓ Superiorly are 3 ligaments
    ◊ Pubocervical
    ◊ Cardinal
    ◊ Sacrocervical

Chinical notes: The muscles of the pelvic floor may be injured during parturition. This may lead to prolapse of the uterus and rectum

Superficial perineal pouch

Boundaries

Superiorly	✓ UG diaphragm
Inferiorly	✓ Membranous layer of superficial fascia

Laterally	✓ Attachment of membranous layer of superficial fascia and UG diaphragm to pubic arch
Posteriorly	✓ Fusion of upper and lower walls
Anteriorly	✓ Open

Contents in male

✓ Crura of the penis covered medially by the ischiocavernosus muscles
✓ Bulb of the penis containing proximal part of penile urethra covered by bulbospongiosus muscles
✓ Supficial transverse perinea muscles
✓ Perineal body—attached to centre of posterior margin of UG diaphragm provide attachment for
  ◊ External anal sphincter
  ◊ Bulbospongiosus
  ◊ Superficial transverse perinea
  ◊ Perineal branch of pudendal nerve

Muscles in male

	Ischiocavernosus	Bulbospongiosus	Superficial transverse perinei
Origin	✓ Ischial tuberosity	✓ Perineal body	✓ Ischial ramus
Insertion	✓ Fascia covering corpus cavernosum	✓ Fascia of bulb of penis ✓ Corpus spongiosum and cavernosum	✓ Perineal body
Nerve supply	✓ Perineal branch of pud nerve	✓ Perineal branch of pud nerve	✓ Perineal branch of pud nerve
Actions	✓ Assist erection of penis	✓ Compress urethra and assist in erection of penis	✓ Fix perineal body and help suppor pelvic viscera

Contents in female

✓ Crura of clitoris covered medially by ischiocavernosus muscles
✓ Bulbs of the vestibule covered by bulbospongiosus muscles
✓ Superficial transverse perineal muscles
✓ Perineal body
  ◊ Situated between vagina and anal canal
  ◊ Provide attachment for perineal muscles
  ◊ More important than in male because it indirectly supports weight of pelvic viscera especially uterus
✓ Perineal branch of pudendal nerve

Muscles in female

	Ischiocavernosus	Bulbospongiosus	Superficial transverse perinei
Origin	✓ Ischial tuberosity	✓ Perineal body	✓ Ischial ramus
Insertion	✓ Fascia covering corpus cavernosum	✓ Fascia covering corpora cavernosum of clitoris	✓ Perineal body

Nerve supply	✓ Perineal branch of pud nerve	✓ Perineal branch of pud nerve	✓ Perineal branch of pud nerve
Actions	✓ Assist erection of clitoris	✓ Sphincter of vagina ✓ Assist erection of clitoris	✓ Fix perineal body and help suppor pelvic viscera

Chinical notes

In males	In females
✓ During straddle – type accidents, urethra is damaged ✓ Urine leaks into superficial perineal pouch and inflammation causes swelling at level of ischial tuberosity	✓ Damage to perineal body, especially during parturition ✓ May result in permanent weakness of pelvic floor (and prolapse of uterus)

Deep perineal pouch

Boundaries

Superiorly	✓ Superior fascia of UG diaphragm
Inferiorly	✓ Inferior fascia of UG diaphragm (perineal membrane)
Laterally	✓ Both superior and inferior fascia attached to pubic arch
Anteriorly	✓ The 2 layers fuse
Posteriorly	✓ The 2 layers fuse ✓ Also fuse with membranous layer of superficial fascia and perineal body

Thus the deep perineal pouch is completely closed

Contents in male

✓ Sphincter urethrae muscle
✓ Deep transverse perinei muscles
✓ Membranous urethra
✓ Bulbo-urethral (Cowper's) glands
    ◊ 2 small glands
    ◊ Embedded in sphincter urethrae
    ◊ Its ducts pierce inferior fascia of UG diaphragm and enter penile urethra
✓ Inferior pudendal artery
✓ Artery to crura of penis
✓ Dorsal artery of penis
✓ Dorsal nerve of penis

Muscles in male

	Sphincter urethrae	Deep transverse perinea
Origin	✓ Pubic arch	✓ Ischial ramus
Insertion	✓ Surrounds urethra	✓ Perineal body
Nerve supply	✓ Perineal branch of pud nerve	✓ Perineal branch of pud nerve

Actions	✓ Voluntary sphincter of urethra	✓ Fixes perineal body

Contents in female		
✓ Sphincter urethrae muscle ✓ Deep transverse perinei muscles ✓ Part of vagina-pierce sphincter urethrae ✓ Membranous part of urethra-pierce sphincter urethrae ✓ Internal pudendal art-gives branches to the clitoris ✓ Dorsal nerve to clitoris		

Muscles in female		
✓ Sphincter urethrae—same as for male ✓ Deep transverse perinea—same as for male		

Clinical notes		
✓ Rupture of membranous part of urethra ✓ Urine escapes into deep perineal pouch		

Ischiorectal fossa

✓ It is a wedge-shaped space on each side of the anal canal

Boundaries	
Base	✓ Skin and fascia
Apex	✓ Meeting of medial and lateral walls
Medial wall	✓ Levator ani with anal fascia superiorly ✓ External anal sphincter with fascia inferiorly
Lateral wall	✓ Is vertical ✓ Obturator internal with fascia and obturator foramen ✓ Medial surface of ischial tuberosity below attachment of obturator fascia
Anteriorly	✓ Posterior border of perineal membrane and body of pubis
Posteriorly	✓ Gluteus maximus ✓ Sacrotuberous ligament

Recesses	
Anterior recess	✓ Proceeds forward above UG diaphragm till limited by anal fascia
Posterior recess	✓ Deep to sacrotuberous ligament
Horse-shoe recess	✓ Connects the 2 fossae behind to anal canal

Contents	
✓ Ischiorectal pad of fat ✓ Pudendal canal with its contents (pudendal nerve and internal pudendal vessels) ✓ Lies along lateral wall of fossa ✓ Inferior rectal nerves and vessels arch downward from lateral to medial	

- ✓ Perineal branch of S_4 nerve
- ✓ Posterior scrotal nerves and vessels
- ✓ Perforating cutaneous branches of S_2 and S_3 nerve

Chinical notes

- ✓ Allow distension of rectum and anal canal during passage of feces
- ✓ Common sites of absecesses
- ✓ Fat acts as support for rectum, thus disease causes prolapse of rectum
- ✓ Poorly vasculated→ infections are diff to clear with antibiotics
- ✓ Pudendal nerve may be blocked by anaesthetic during forceps delivery

Peritoneum in female pelvis

- ✓ Peritoneum descending over pelvic brim is separated from:
  - ◊ Part of posterior abdominal wall by rectum
  - ◊ Part of anterior abdominal wall by bladder
  - ◊ Pelvic floor by CT, nerves and vessels
- ✓ Posteriorly, peritoneum extends from right to left uninterrupted until at left sacro–iliac joint, it is confluent with base of sigmoid mesocolon
- ✓ The latter has an inverted V-shaped base with the ureter passing below its apex
- ✓ Below this, the peritoneum is related to the rectum in the following mamnner
  - ◊ Upper 1/3 of rectum→ covers anterior and lateral surfaces
  - ◊ Middle 1/3 of rectum→ covers anterior surface only
  - ◊ Lower 1/3 of rectum→ uncovered
- ✓ Para-rectal fossae formed on either side of rectum
- ✓ From middle 1/3 of retum, peritoneum is reflected onto posterior surface of upper part of vagina→ rectouterine pouch (of Douglas)
- ✓ The lateral edges of the pouch are marked by uterosacral (rectouterine) folds formed by uterosacral ligament
- ✓ From the vagina, the peritoneum continues over posterior surface of uterus→ over fundus → downward on anterior surface
- ✓ At level of anterior fornix of vagina, peritoneum is reflected onto posterior surface of bladder→ continues onto superior surface
- ✓ Note: lateral surfaces of bladder are not covered. On each side of superior surface is paravesical fossa whose lateral limit is marked by peritoneum covering round ligament of uterus. This reflection from uterus onto bladder→ uterovesical fossa
- ✓ The broad ligament is a fold of peritoneum raised by the fallopian tubes
- ✓ The anterior surface is continuous with the posterior at the superior free border which contains the fallopian tube
- ✓ It is divided into
  - ◊ Mesosalpinx
  - ◊ Mesometrium
  - ◊ Mesovarium
  - ◊ Infundibulopelvic ligament
- ✓ Inferiorly, the broad ligament spreads out to cover floor of pelvis
- ✓ The peritoneum stops at inner mucosal surface of ovarian fimbrae

- ✓ Thus, it presents 2 deficiencies (1 on each side) which allows communication with external environment
- ✓ The ovarian fossa is formed between elevation produced by the obliterated umbilical artery and the ureter posteriorly
- ✓ It lies on the lateral pelvic wall and has the ovary resting within its boundaries

Chinical notes

- ✓ Hysterosalpingography
  - ◊ Radioactive material is injected into uterus. If uterine tubes are patent, readioactivity will spill into peritoneal cavity via deficiencies in peritoneum
- ✓ Access to peritoneal cavity is via posterior wall of vagina and hence rectouterine pouch (of Douglas)
  - ◊ Insertion of scaples
  - ◊ Extraction of ova for in vitro fertilisation

Broad ligaments (of the uterus)

- ✓ These are 2 layered folds of peritoneum which suspend the uterus to the lateral pelvic wall
- ✓ It has anterior and posterior layers and a free upper border
- ✓ Superiorly the 2 layers are continuous over the uterine tube
- ✓ Inferiorly and laterally the 2 layers spread out to cover the pelvic floor and wall

Parts of the broad ligament

Mesosalpinx	✓ Between uterine tube and mesoovarian
Mesometrium	✓ Below ligament of the ovary
Mesovarium	✓ Reflection from posterior layer onto hilus of ovary ✓ Continuous with germinal epithelium of ovary
Infundibulopelvic ligament	✓ Covers infundibulum of uterine tube ✓ Continues to lateral pelvic wall

Contents of broad ligament

- ✓ Uterine tube in free upper border
- ✓ 2 ligaments
  - ◊ Round ligament of uterus
  - ◊ Ligament of ovary
- ✓ 2 vessels
  - ◊ Uterine artery
  - ◊ Ovarian artery
- ✓ 2 nerves
  - ◊ Uterovaginal plexus
  - ◊ Ovarian plexus
- ✓ 2 embryo remnants
  - ◊ Epoophoron
  - ◊ Paroophoron
- ✓ Lymphatics and LN

Rectum

- ✓ The rectum is about 12 cm long

Position and extent	
✓ Begins opposite SV_3 as continuation of sigmoid colon ✓ Passes downwards, following curve of sacrum and coccyx ✓ Ends at pelvic diaphragm 2.5 cm in front of tip of coccyx ✓ Pierces pelvic diaphragm to continue as anal canal	

Flexures		
	Flexures	Remarks
	3 lateral	✓ Uppermost and lowermost flexures directed to the right
	2 anteropost	✓ The first follows curvature of sacrum = sacral flexure ✓ The 2nd located at junction of rectum and anal canal = perineal flexure ✓ Perineal flexure is maintained by puborectalis sling

External apperance	

✓ The rectum can be distinguished by:
  ◊ Absence of mesentery and appendices epiploicae
  ◊ Absence of haustra
  ◊ Teniae coli to form longitudinal muscle coat	

Peritoneum	
Upper 1/3	✓ Peritoneum covers anterior and lateral surfaces
Middle 1/3	✓ Peritoneum covers anterior surface only
Lower 1/3	✓ Uncovered

Relations		

Anterior	In the male
	✓ Upper 2/3 (covered by peritoneum) is related to:
	  ◊ Sigmoid colon
	  ◊ Coils of ileum occupying rectovesical pouch
	✓ Lower 1/3 (devoid of peritoneum) is related to:
	  ◊ Posterior surface of bladder
	  ◊ Termination of vas deferens
	  ◊ Seminal vesicles
	  ◊ Prostate
		In the female
		✓ Upper 2/3 (covered by peritoneum) is related to:
		  ◊ Sigmoid colon
		  ◊ Coils of ileum occupying rectouterine pouch:
		✓ Lower 1/3 (devoid of peritoneum) is related to
		  ◊ Posteriorwall of vagina
		✓ Note: rectouterine pouch separates rectum from:
		  ◊ Lower part of uterus
		  ◊ Upper part of vagina

Posterior	✓ Sacrum ✓ Piriformis ✓ Levator ani and coccygeus ✓ Sacral plexus and symph trunks medial sacral vessels	
Lateral	✓ Lateral ligament of rectum ✓ In females, also uterosacral folds and ligament	

Blood supply	
Artery	Remarks
Superior rectal artery	✓ Supplies mucosa
Middle rectal artery	✓ Supplies muscular coat
Inferior rectal artery	✓ Anastomose with superior rectal artery
Medial sacral artery	✓ Supplies dilated lower part of rectum (ampulla)

Venous drainage

✓ Follow arteries
✓ However free anastomosis exist between the superior, middle and inferior rectal veins
  ↳ Porto-systemic anastomosis

Lymphatic drainage

✓ Into pararectal nodes
✓ Into inferior mesenteric nodes
✓ Into internal iliac nodes

Nerve supply

✓ Inferior hypogastric plexus
✓ Sympathetic nerve from L_1, L_2, parasympathetic nerve from S_2–S_4

Chinical notes

✓ Partial and complete prolapses of the rectum through the anus
✓ Varicosities of the rectal veins = hemorrhoids (piles)

Anal canal

The anal canal is about 4 cm long

Position and extent

✓ Begins at level of pelvic diaphragm as a continuation of the rectum
✓ Passes downwards and backwards from the perineal flexure of rectum (due to puborectalis sling)
✓ Opens at anal orifice in the perineum

Chinical notes: At the perineal flexure, the rectal angle prevents feces from entering the anal canal. The lumen of the anal canal is reduced to an anteropost slit when empty

Relations

		In the male	In the female
Anteriorly		✓ Perineal body ✓ UG diaphragm ✓ Membranous part of urethra ✓ Bulb of penis	✓ Perineal body ✓ UG diaphragm ✓ Lower part of vagina
Posteriorly		✓ Anoccoygeal body, which separates it from the coccyx	
Laterally		✓ Ischiorectal fossae containing fat, etc.	

Sphincters	
Internal anal sphincter	External anal sphincter

✓ Continuation of circular SM fibres of the rectum
✓ Encircles upper 3/4 of anal canal
✓ Involuntary
	✓ Composed of striated muscle
	✓ Voluntary
	✓ Consist of 3 parts
	  ◊ Deep part
	  ◊ Superficial part
	  ◊ Subcut part

The puborectalis part of levator ani blends with deep part of external anal sphincter to form a sling, cause rectum to join to anal canal at an angle	

Internal apperance	

Upper part of anal canal	✓ Derived from hindgut endoderm
	✓ Lined by columnar epithelium
	✓ Mucosa thrown into vertical folds called anal columns
	  ◊ Joined at their lower ends by
	  ◊ Small semilunar folds called anal valves
	✓ The upper part is separates from the lower part by the pectinate line (Hilton's white line)

Lower part of anal canal	✓ Derived from ectoderm ✓ No anal columns

Blood supply, venous drainage, lymphatic drainage and nerve supply		
	Upper part	Lower part
Blood supply	✓ Superior rectal artery (branch of inferior mes artery)	✓ Inferior rectal artery (branch of internal pudendal artery)
Venous drainage	✓ Superior rectal vein (into portal vein)	✓ Inferior rectal vein (pudendal vein)
Lymphatic drainage	✓ Inferior mesenteric nodes	✓ Superficial inguinal nodes
Nerve supply	✓ Autonomic nerve supply via inferior hypogastric plexus	✓ Somatic nerve supply via inferior rectal nerve (branch of pudendal nerve) and perineal branch of S_4

Chinical notes

✓ Hemorrhoids
  ◊ Internal (from superior rectal vein and tributaries)
  ◊ External (from inferior rectal vein and tributaries)
✓ Per rectal examination

Urinary bladder

✓ The bladder serves as a reservoir for urine
✓ It is the most anterior organ within the pelvic cavity and lies immediately behind the symphysis pubis, separated from it by the retropubic space

Parts and relations	
The empty bladder is pyramidal in shape	
Apex	✓ Directed towards pubic symphysis ✓ Continues upwards on anterior abdominal wall to umbilicus as the medial umbilical ligament
Superior surface	✓ Covered by peritoneum ✓ Related to 1 cm sigmoid colon ✓ Coils of ileum ✓ In females: also the uterus
Inferolat surface	✓ In front, related to 1 cm retropubic pad of fat ✓ Pubic bones ✓ More posteriorly, related to 1 cm obturator internal above ✓ Lev ani below ✓ Devoid of peritoneum
Posterior surface	✓ Triangular ✓ Covered by peritoneum only on upper part ✓ Superolat angles joined by the ureters ✓ Inferior angle gives rise to urethra ✓ In males: separated from rectum by 1 cm seminal vesicles ✓ Vas deferens ✓ Rectovesical suptum ✓ In females: posterior relation is the vagina
Neck	✓ In males: rest on base of prostate ✓ In females: rest on UG diaphragm

Peritoneum

Superior surface and upper part of posterior surface covered by peritoneum

Supports of bladder (fixation)

✓ Medial umbilical ligament
✓ Puboprostatic ligament in males
✓ Pubovesical ligament in females
✓ Lateral ligament of the bladder (rectovesicalis)

Inferior of bladder

✓ In an empty bladder, the greater part of mucosa shows irregular folds due to its loose attachment to the muscular coat
✓ The only smooth part is the trigone, which has the following boundaries
  ◊ Superiorly
    ◆ Interureteric ridge connecting ureteric openings
  ◊ On each side
    ◆ Line connecting each ureteric opening to internal urethral opening below

Blood supply
✓ From superior and inferior vesical artery
✓ Base is supplied by artery of ductus deferens in male, vaginal artery in female
Venous drainage
✓ Via vesical venous plexus
✓ Drains into iliac vein
Lymphatic drainage
✓ Mainly to external iliac nodes
✓ Base drains into internal iliac nodes
Nerve supply
✓ Vesical and prostatic plexuses
✓ Sympathetic fibres from $T_{10}-L_2$
✓ Parasympathetic from pelvic splanchnic nerve (S_2-S_4)
Chinical notes
✓ A full bladder may rise into the abdominal cavity
↳ May be ruptured by a blow to lower part of abdomen
✓ Rupture leads to leakage of urine into extraperitoneal space
✓ Bimanual palpation of the bladder

Prostate gland

✓ The prostate is shaped like an inverted pyramid, located in pelvis
✓ It is a fibromuscular and glandular organ that surrounds the prostatic urethra
✓ Dimensions: base = 4 cm×2 cm
✓ Height = 3 cm
✓ It lies between the neck of bladder (above) and UG diaphragm (below)
✓ It is an accessory gland in the male
Functions
✓ Production of a thin, milky fluid containing citric acid and acid phosphatase
✓ Added to semial fluid at ejaculation
Capsule
✓ Prostate is surrounded by fibrous capsule
✓ Outside capsule is a fibrous sheath (which is part of visceral layer of pelvic fascia)
✓ The fibrous sheath contains the prostatic venous plexus
Surfaces
✓ The prostate has a base, apex and 4 surfaces (anterior, posterior, and 2 lateral)
Lobes
It is completely divided into 5 lobes

Ant lobe	✓ Lies in front of urethra ✓ Devoid of glands
Medial lobe	✓ Wedge-shaped ✓ Lies between upper part of urethra and ejaculatory duct ✓ Related to trigone of bladder ✓ Rich is glands
Posterior lobe	✓ Behind urethra, below ejaculatory duct ✓ Contains glandular tissue
Left and right lateral lobes	✓ Lie on either side of urethra ✓ Separate by shallow vertical groove on posterior surface of prostate ✓ Rich in glands

Structures transversing prostate

✓ Prostatic urethra transverses it vertically
✓ Prostatic utricles is a blind sac directed upwards and backwards from urethral crest
✓ Ejaculatory ducts pass downwards and forwards and open into prostatic urethra on each side of prostatic utricle

Chinical notes: Prostatic glands open into prostatic sinus beside the urethral crest

Relations

Superiorly	✓ Neck of bladder
Inferiorly	✓ UG diaphragm
Anteriorly	✓ Pubic symphysis, separates by retropubic space containing fat ✓ Puboprostatic ligament connects fibrous sheath to posterior surface of pubic bones
Posteriorly	✓ Rectal ampulla, separates by rectovesical septum
Laterally	✓ Anterier fibres of levator ani

Blood supply

✓ Inferior vesical artery—branch of internal iliac artery
✓ Middle rectal artery—branch of anterior trunk of internal iliac artery
　◊ These form an outer subcapsular plexus and an inner periurethral plexus

Venous drainage

✓ The veins form the prostatic venous plexus around the prostate between the capsule and fibrous sheath
✓ Drain into internal iliac veins

Lymphatic drainage

✓ Mainly to internal iliac nodes and sacral nodes

Nerve supply

✓ Prostatic plexus of nerve
✓ Derived from lower part of inferior hypogastric plexus

Chinical notes

- ✓ Carcinoma of prostate
- ✓ Senile enlargement

Seminal vesicles

- ✓ These are 2 lobulated sacs lying on posterior surface of bladder
- ✓ Each is about 5 cm long and fusiform in shape
- ✓ They are directed upwards and laterally

Relations

Medially	✓ Terminal part of vas deferens
Posteriorly	✓ Rectum
Inferiorly	✓ Each seminal vesicle narrows and joins the vas deferens to form the ejaculatory ducts ✓ The 2 ducts run through the substance of the prostate to open into the prostatic urethra, lateral of opening of prostatic utricle

Functions of semincal vesicles

- ✓ Produce secretions which is added to seminal fluid
- ✓ Secretions contains substances which nourish the spermatozoa

Blood supply

- ✓ Artery of the ductus deferens

Venous drainage

- ✓ Into prostatic and vesical venous plexus

Lymphatic drainage

- ✓ External and internal iliac nodes

Nerve supply

- ✓ Inferior hypogastric and prostatic plexus
- ✓ Sympathetic supply from $T_{11}-L_1$
- ✓ Parasympathetic supply from S_2-S_4

Ovary

- ✓ The ovary is the germinal and endocrine gland of the female
- ✓ It is diamond-shaped
- ✓ Dimensions: 3 cm×2 cm×1 cm

Postion and orientation

- ✓ It is located in the ovarian fossa on lateral wall of pelvis
  - ◊ Behind the broad ligament, attached to back of broad ligament by mesovarium
- ✓ In nulliparous women: its long axis is vertcal
- ✓ In multiparous women: upper pole → lateral; lower pole → medial

Parts of ovary	
✓ Lateral and medial surfaces ✓ Upper (tubal) and lower (uterine) poles ✓ Anterior (mesovarian) and posterior (free) borders	
Relations	
Anteriorly	✓ Obliterated umbilical artery
Posteriorly	✓ Ureter ✓ Internal iliac artery ✓ The obturator nerve crosses floor of ovarian fossa
Posterolateral	✓ Rrimbrae of infundibulum of fallopian tube
Fixation	
Suspensory ligament	✓ Peritoneal fold running from its upper extremity to the iliac vessels ✓ Between attachment of mesovarium and lateral wall of pelvis ✓ Carries ovarian vessels, nerves, and lymphatics
Round ligament of ovary	✓ From upper end to lateral wall of uterus to medial margin of ovary ✓ Remains of upper part of gubenaculum (round ligament of uterus if remains of lower part)
Mesovarium	✓ Joins anterior border to posterior side of broad ligament ✓ Transmits vessels and nerves
Blood supply	
✓ Ovarian artery ◊ Branch of aorta at LV_1 level ◊ Sends branches to ovary and uterine tubes ◊ Anastomose with uterine artery	
Venous drainage	
✓ Pampiniform plexus→ ovarian vein →right side into a IVC, left side into left renal vein	
Nerve supply	
✓ Ovarian plexus (derived fromrenal, aortic and hypogastric plexuses) ◊ Accompany ovarian artery ◊ Contains sympathetic nerve ($T_{10,11}$), parasympathetic nerve (S_{2-4}) ✓ Thus pain is referred to inguinal and vulval regions	
Lymphatic drainage	
✓ Pre-aortic nodes ✓ Para-aortic nodes	
Chinical notes	
✓ Before puberty, ovary is smooth and grayish pink, after puberty, it is puckered and turns gray	

- ✓ When old, it may shrivel
  - ↧ Ovarian cysts
  - ↧ Ovarian carcinomas
  - ↧ Prolapse of ovaries into rectouterine pouch

Uterus

✓ The uterus is the child-bearing organ in the female

Shape and size

✓ Hollow, pear-shaped with thick muscular walls
✓ In young nulliparous women, it measures 8 cm long, 5 cm wide and 2 cm thick

Position (location)

✓ Between bladder and rectum
✓ Lower end forms an approx right angle with vagina→ angle of anteversion

Parts and relations

The uterus is subdivided into a fundus, body, isthmus and cervix

Fundus

✓ Convex
✓ Directed anteriorly and superiorly
✓ Related to coils of small intestine

Body

Vesical surface	✓ Lies on superior surface of bladder ✓ Covered with peritoneum which is reflected onto bladder forming uterovesical pouch
Intestinal surface	✓ Related to sigmoid colon and coils of small intestines ✓ Covered with peritoneum
Lateral margins	✓ Receives uterine tubes, uterine vessels by the side ✓ Related to broad ligament (mesometrium) ✓ Round ligament and ligament to ovary attached here

✓ Cavity of body is triangular in coronal section, but merely a cleft in sagittal section

Isthmus

✓ Constricted part of uterus—1 cm in length
✓ Cavity called internal os

Cervix

✓ Extends downwards and backwards from isthmus
✓ Pierces anterior wall of vagina
✓ Divided into supravaginal and vaginal parts
  - ↧ Supravaginal part

◆ Anteriorly: bladder
◆ Posteriorly: coils of small intestine
◆ Laterally: uterine artery and ureter embedded in parametrium
◊ Vaginal part
◆ Protudes into vagina→ forms vaginal fornix

✓ The cavity of the cervix, the cervical canal, is spindle-shaped and communicates with cavity of body through internal os, and with the vagina through the external os

Peritoneum

✓ From middle 1/3 of rectum, peritoneum reflected
  ◊ Onto posterior surface of upper part of vagina
  ◊ Rectouterine pouch (of Douglas)
✓ Continues over intestinal surface of uterus (body)
✓ Passes round fundus
✓ Continues down over vesical surface of body
✓ At level of fornix (anterior) of vagina→peritoneum reflected onto posterior surface of bladder

Blood supply

✓ Uterine artery—branch of internal iliac artery
✓ Ovarian artery (partly)—branch of aorta arising from LV_1 level

Venous drainage

✓ Venous plexus drains through uterine, ovarian and vaginal veins
✓ Into internal iliac vein

Lymphatic drainage

✓ Fundus into para-aortic nodes
✓ Body and cervix into internal and external iliac nodes

Chinical notes: a few lymph vessels also drain into superficial inguinal nodes

Nerve supply

✓ Uterovaginal portions of inferior hypogastric plexus
✓ Sympathetic supply from T_{12}, L_1
✓ Parasympathetic supply from S_2–S_4

Chinical notes: ①Uterine examination by bimanual palpation. ②Prolapse of uterus

Normal position of the uterus

Anteverted	Anteflexed
✓ Extends forward and upwards from upper end of vagina at approx right angle	✓ Body bent downwards at its junction with the isthmus

This position is generally maintained by

✓ Muscles
✓ Fibromuscular structures
✓ Fascial condensations (ligaments) and possibly

Regional Anatomy

- ✓ Peritoneal folds

The following are important supports

1. Levator ani muscle

- ✓ Anterior fibers (pubovaginalis) form a sling and supports the vagina indirectly supports the uterus
- ✓ Firbes are inserted into perineal body

Chinical notes: If levator ani is torn during childbirth, support of the vagina is lost and it tends to sink into the vestibule along with the uterus (prolapse)

2. Perineal body

- ✓ Situated between vagina and rectum
- ✓ Stabilized by numerous muscles, e.g., superficial transverse perinei and external anal sphincter
- ✓ Acts as anchor for levator ani → maintain integrity of pelvic floor

3. Urogenital diaphragm

- ✓ Some fibres are attached to the vagina → help support both vagina and uterus

4. Ligaments

- ✓ These are condensations of pelvic fascia on upper surface of levator ani muscles
- ✓ They are attached to cervix and vagina
- ✓ Support uterus and keep cervix in proper position

Cardinal ligament	✓ Connect lateral aspects of cervix and upper vagina to lateral pelvic wall
Pubocervical ligament	✓ Connect cervix to posterior surface of pubis
Sacrocervical ligament	✓ Connect cervix and upper end of vagina to lower end of sacrum ✓ Forms 2 ridges, 1 on either side of rectouterine pouch ✓ Helps maintain uterine axis
Round ligament of the uterus	✓ Remnant of lower 1/2 of the gubernaculums ✓ Connects lateral angle of uterus to labia majora via the inguinal canal

5. Uterine axis

- ✓ Anteverted position of uterus prevents it from sagging down the vagina
- ✓ This axis is maintained by the round ligament of uterus and sacrocervical ligament

The following are also possible supports

- ✓ Broad ligament
- ✓ Uterovesical fold of peritoneum
- ✓ Rectouterine fold of peritoneum

Chinical notes

- ✓ Tear of the perineum may cause a prolapse of the uterus
- ✓ Also due to hard labour or weakness in any of the supports
- ✓ Uterine (fallopian) tubes
- ✓ The uterine tubes convey ova, from ovary towards the uterus and sperm in the opposite direction
- ✓ Fertilisation usually occurs in the tube

Location	
✓ At upper free border of broad ligament (mesosalpinx)	

Extent and course	
✓ 10 cm long	
✓ Runs laterally from uterus to uterine end of ovary	
✓ Passes upwards on mesovarian border	
✓ Arches over tubal end	
✓ Terminates on free border and medial surface of ovary	
✓ Not joined to ovary → ova released into peritoneal cavity	

Parts	
Infundibulum	✓ Lateral expanded part with abdominal ostium (opening) surrounded by finger-like fimbrae ✓ One fimbra = ovarian fimbra attaches it to tubal pole of ovary ✓ Inner surface lined by ciliated columnar epithelium
Ampulla	✓ Medial continuation of infundibulum ✓ Thin walled and dilated ✓ Follows a tortuous course, arching over ovary
Isthmus	✓ Constricted part medial to ampulla ✓ Has thicker walls than ampulla
Intramural	✓ Lies within uterine wall ✓ Opens into uterus at superior angles of uterine cavity by a narrow uterine ostium

Blood supply
✓ Medial 2/3 → uterine artery (branch of internal iliac)
✓ Lateral 1/3 → ovarian artery (from abdominal aorta)

Venous drainage
✓ Veins drain into
◊ Pampiniform plexus of ovary
◊ Uterine veins

Lymphatic drainage
✓ Most drain into lateral aortic and pre-aortic nodes
✓ Some (around isthmus) follows round ligament of uterus into superficial inguinal nodes

Nerve supply	
Sympathetic	Parasympathetic
✓ T_{10}–L_2	✓ Mainly from pelvic splanchnic nerve (S_2–S_4)
✓ Via inferior hypogastric plexus	✓ Via inferior hypogastric plexus

Chinical notes
✓ Tubal pregnancy—common ectopic pregnancy
✓ Sterility caused by blockage of tube (due to inflammation)

✓ Female sterilization by tubectomy—ligated and excised

Vagina

✓ The vagina is the female copulatory organ
✓ It extends upward and backward from vulva to uterus and is situated behind to the bladder and urethra in front of recturn and anal canal
✓ It measures about 8 cm long and has anterior and posterior walls which are normally in apposition
✓ In the virgin, lower end of vagina is partially closed by hymen (mucous membrane)
✓ After rupture, a round elevation called carunculae hymenale is formed
✓ At upper end, anterior wall is pierced by the cervix, lumen there is circular and can be divided into 4 fornices, i. e., anterior, posterior, right lateral and left lateral
✓ The anterior fornix is shallowest while posterior fornix is deepest

Relations

Anteriorly	✓ Upper 1/2: base of bladder ✓ Lower 1/2: urethra
Posteriorly	✓ Upper 1/3: Douglas pouch + loops of ileum and sigmoid colon ✓ Middle 1/3: ampulla of rectum ✓ Lower 1/3: anal canal and perineal body
Laterally	✓ Upper 1/3: transverse cervical ligament in which are embedded the network of vaginal veins; ureter, which is crossed by uterine artery ✓ Middle 1/3: pubococcygeus (part of levator ani) ✓ Lower 1/3: pierces UG diaphragm; related to bulb of vestibule, bulbospongiosus, greater vestibular glands (of Bartholini)

Blood supply

✓ Mainly by vaginal branch of internal iliac artery
✓ Also by uterine, middle rectal and internal pudendal artery
✓ Anastomosis of these forms the vaginal azygos arteries
　◊ In the midline artery anteriorly and posteriorly

Venous drainage

✓ Rich venous plexus→ vaginal vein → internal iliac vein

Lymphatic drainage

✓ Upper 1/3→ external iliac nodes
✓ Middle 1/3→ internal iliac nodes
✓ Lower 1/3→ medial group of superficial inguinal nodes

Nerve supply

Lower 1/3	Upper 2/3
✓ Pain sensitive ✓ Supplied by 　◊ Inferior rectal nerve (from pudendal nerve) 　◊ Dorsal labial branches of perineal nerve	✓ Pain insensitive ✓ Supplied by 　◊ Sympathetic L_1, L_2 　◊ Parasympathetic S_2, S_3, S_4

Supports of vagina

- ✓ Upper: levator ani, transverse cervical, pubocervical and sacrocervical ligament
- ✓ Middle: UG diaphragm
- ✓ Lower: perineal body

Chinical notes

- ✓ Prolapse of vagina
- ✓ Vaginal lacerations
- ✓ Vaginitis
- ✓ Vaginal examinations

Ductus (vas) deferens

- ✓ The ductus deferens is 45 cm long
- ✓ It is a thick-walled muscular tube in the male
  - ◊ It conveys mature sperm from epididyrnis to ejaculatory duct and urethra

Origin

- ✓ Continuation of tail of epididymis
- ✓ Tortuous, but gradually straightens out

Course and relations

- ✓ Pass upwards medial to epididymis
- ✓ Asc through superficial inguinal ring with other structures in spermatic cord
- ✓ Passes though inguinal canal to reach deep inguinal ring
- ✓ Emerge from deep inguinal ring and pass around lateral margin of inferior epigastric artery→ enters abdominal cavity

In abdomen	In pelvis
✓ Turns medially (around lateral margin of inferior epigastric artery) ✓ Cross external iliac artery ✓ Runs posteriorly, medially and upward→ follows slant of body pelvis ✓ Reach pectineal line of pubis ✓ Crosses this and enters pelvis	✓ Continues backwards ✓ Follows curvature of lateral pelvic wall and covered medially by peritoneum ✓ Directed towards ischial spine ✓ Cross medial side of umbilical artery, obturator nerve and vessels (branches of internal iliac artery) and the ureter ✓ After crossing the ureter, turns medially and downwards to run in sacrogenital fold ✓ Reaches posterior aspect of bladder ✓ Runs downward and medially on medial side of seminal vesicles ✓ In this region, the ductus deferens is enlarged and dilated→ ampulla ✓ Near base of prostate, the caliber is small again ✓ Ductus deferens joined to duct of seminal vesicles → common ejaculatory duct

Blood supply

- ✓ Artery of ductus deferens (branch of inferior vesical artery)
- ✓ Inferior vesical and middle rectal arteries

Venous drainage

- ✓ Via prostatic and vesical plexuses → internal iliac veins

Lymphatic drainage

- ✓ Into external iliac nodes

Nerve supply

- ✓ Autonomic fibres from superior and inferior hypogastric plexuses

Chinical notes: Vasectomy = sterilization of the male → ligation of ductus deferens

Male urethra

- ✓ The male urethra is about 20 cm in length
- ✓ It begins at the neck of the bladder and extends through the prostate, pelvic diaphragm, sphincter urethrae, root and body of penis, to the tip of the glans—ends at external urethral orifice

Course and relations

- ✓ It is subdivided into 3 parts: prostatic, membranous, and spongy/penile

Prostatic part

- ✓ 3 cm long
- ✓ Extends from internal urethral orifice at apex of trigone of bladder
- ✓ Traverses the prostate—ends at sphincter urethrae muscle
- ✓ Most dilatable part of urethra
- ✓ When empty, anterior and posterior walls are in contact
- ✓ Anterior and lateral walls folded longitudinally

Urethral crest	✓ Medial ridge
Seminal colliculus	✓ Ovoid enlargement of the crest ✓ Located approx at junction of ✓ Middle and lower 1/3 of prostatic part
Opening of prostatic utricle	✓ At summit of colliculus
Prostatic sinus	✓ Groove on each side of crest ✓ Most prostatic ducts open into it ✓ Some open into side of urethral crest
Openings of ejaculatory ducts	✓ On each side of opening of prostatic utricle

Membranous part

- ✓ About 1 cm long
- ✓ Extends from apex of prostate
    - ◊ Passes through pelvic diaphragm and sphincter urethrae
    - ◊ Ends at bulb of penis
- ✓ Shortest, narrowest and least dilatable part of urethra
- ✓ Immediately below sphincter urethrae, its walls are thinner
    - ◊ Most liable to rupture during injury

Spongy part

- ✓ 10–16 cm long
- ✓ Extends from bulbs→ body → glans of penis → ends at external urethral orifice
- ✓ Lies in the corpus spongiosum
- ✓ Shows 2 dilatations
    - ◊ In the bulb—intra-bulbar fossa
    - ◊ In the glans—navicular fossa
- ✓ Openings for glands
    - ◊ Bulbo-urethral glands open into ventral wall
    - ◊ Urethral glands open throughout its length

Blood supply, venous drainage, lymphatic drainage, nerve supply

	Prostatic part	Membranous part	Spongy part
Blood supply	✓ Inferior vesicle and middle rectal artery	✓ Artery of bulb of penis	✓ Urethral artery ✓ Deep and dorsal artery of penis
Venous drainage	✓ Via prostatic plexus → internal pudendal vein → internal iliac vein		
Lymphatic drainage	✓ Internal iliac nodes ✓ Some to external iliac nodes	✓ Deep inguinal nodes ✓ Some to external iliac nodes	
Nerve supply	✓ Prostatic plexus	✓ Branches of pud nerve	

Chinical notes

- ✓ Rupture of urethra
    - ◊ At junction of prostatic and membranous parts → urine leaks into extraperitoneal space around bladder
    - ◊ Membranous part → urine leaks into superficial perineal space may spread into penis, scrotum and front of abdomen
- ✓ Examination: by passing a catheter through it

Pudendal nerve

Origin

- ✓ Branch of sacral plexus
- ✓ S_2, S_3, S_4 (ant rami)

Course

- ✓ Leaves pelvis via greater sciatic foramen, below piriformis
- ✓ Enters gluteal region
- ✓ Drosses back of ischial spine, where it is medial to internal pudendal artery
- ✓ Enters perineum through lesser sciatic foramen
- ✓ Enters pudendal canal in lateral wall of ischiorectal fossa

Branches	
Inferior rectal nerve	✓ Runs medially across ischiorectal fossa in company with corresponding vessels ✓ Supplies: external anal sphincter, mucous membrane of lower 1/2 of anal canal and perianal skin
Perineal nerve	✓ Supplies: muscles of UG triangle and skin on posterior surface of scrotum/labia majora
Dorsal nerve of penis/clitoris	✓ Distributed to penis/clitoris

Clinical notes
✓ Can be blocked either through vagina or from perineum; area supplied by pudendal nerve is anaesthetized ✓ The pudendal nerve is the principal nerver supply of the perineum

Lumbar plexus
✓ Formed in the psoas muscle ✓ From the anterior rami of L_1–L_4 nerve ✓ Anterior rami receive GRC from sympathetic trunk ✓ L_1 and L_2 give off WRC to the sympathetic trunk ✓ Branches emerge from the lateral and medial borders of the muscle and from its anterior surface

Branches
✓ Iliohypogastric ✓ Ilioinguinal ✓ Genitofemoral ✓ Lateral femoral cut nerve of thigh ✓ Femoral nerve ✓ Obturator nerve

Branches emerging from lateral border of psoas		
Branches	Course	Supply
Iliohypogastric nerve (L_1)	✓ Lateral and anterior abdominal wall	✓ Skin of lower part of anterior abdominal wall
Ilioinguinal nerve (L_1)	✓ Lateral and anterior abdominal wall ✓ Through inguinal canal	✓ Skin of groin and scrotum/labium majus
Lateral cut nerve of thigh (L_2 and L_3)	✓ Crosses iliac fossa in front of iliacus muscle ✓ Enters thigh behind lateral end of inguinal ligament	✓ Skin over lateral surface of thigh
Femoral nerve (L_2, L_3, L_4)	✓ Runs downward and lateral between psoas and iliacus muscles ✓ Enters thigh behind the inguinal ligament and lateral to femoral sheath	✓ Iliacus muscle in thigh

Branches emerging from the medial border of psoas at brim of pelvis	
Branches	Course
Obturator nerve (L_2, L_3, L_4)	✓ Crosses pelvic brim in front of SI joint ✓ Behind common iliac vessels ✓ Leaves the pelvis by passing through obturator canal (i.e., upper part of obturator foramen devoid of obturator membrane) into the thigh, splits into anterior and posterior division that pass through the canal to enter the adductor region of the thigh
4th lumbar root of lumbosacral trunk	✓ Formation of sacral plexus ✓ Desc anterior to ala of sacrum joins 1st sacral nerve

Genitofemoral branch (L_1, L_2) emerging on anterior surface of psoas		
Branches	Course	Supply
Genital branch	✓ Enters spermatic cord	✓ Cremaster muscle
Femoral branch		✓ Small area of skin of thigh

Wang Mingyan, Meng Buliang, Zhang Yanyu

Chapter 6

The Upper Limb

6.1 Introduction

6.1.1 Boundaries and divisions

The upper limb is a multijointed lever that is freely movable on the trunk at the shoulder joint. At the distal end of the upper limb is the important organ, the hand. Much of the importance of the hand depends on the pincer—like action of the thumb, which enables one to grasp objects between the thumb and index finger.

The upper limb is divided into the shoulder (junction of the trunk with the arm), arm, elbow, forearm, wrist, and hand.

The shoulder region includes the axilla, the scapular region and the deltoid region. The arm and the forearm can be divided into anterior and posterior regions. The hand can be divided into the palm, the dorsum and the fingers.

6.1.2 Surface anatomy

6.1.2.1 Shoulder region

(1) Acromion

As the summit of shoulder region, it forms a sharp bony edge at the lateral extremity of the scapilar spine, and lies 2.5 cm immediately above the smooth bulge of the deltoid.

(2) Coracoid process

It lies immediately below the clavicle at the junction of the middle and lateral thirds, and is covered by the anterior fibers of the deltoid.

(3) Anterior and posterior axillary folds

They are the musculocutaneous folds situated in front and behind the axilla respectively. The anterior axillary fold is formed mainly by the rounded lower border of the pectoralis major, wheras the posterior one is formed by the latissimus dorsi and intimately related to teres major.

6.1.2.2 Arm

(1) Medial and lateral biceps brachii furrow

It protrudes on the anterior surface of the arm. The shallow furrows indicate its medial and lateral borders. When the elbow is flexed against resistance, the muscle becomes still more obvious and its tendon of insertion can be held between the finger and thumb and traced down into the cubital fossa.

(2) Deltoid tuberosity

It lies at the lateral side of the middle third of the humerus. The deltoid is inserted into it. Posterior and below this tuberosity, there is a faint spiral groove, called the sulcus for radial nerve. The radial nerve and the deep brachial vessels pass through it.

6.1.2.3 Elbow

(1) Medial and lateral epicondyles

They are important in the diagnosis of elbow injury. The medial epicondyle of the humerus is a conspicuous landmake and is easily felt, particularly when the elbow is flexed; proximally it can be traced as it continues upwards as the medial supracondylar ridge. The ulnar nerve can be rolled from side to side posterior to the base of the epicondyle. The lateral epicondyle is not so prominent but its posterior surface is easily palpated and its lateral margin can be traced upwards into the lateral supracondylar ridge on deep pressure.

(2) Olecranon

It is a bony prominence at the back of the elbow. When the elbow is straightened out to its full extension, the olecranon and medial and lateral epicondyles of the humerus lie in the same horizontal plane; when the elbow is been to a right angle, they are at the angles of an isosceles triangle "the posterior cubital trangle". The relative position of them will be changed in the dislocation of elbow joint. When the elbow is flexed to a right angle, a lateral cubital trangle is formed by the lateral epicondyle, the head of radius and the olecranon. When the elbow is extended, a depression between the olecranon, the head of radius and the capitulum of humerus is called the posterior cubital fossa.

6.1.2.4 Wrist and hand

(1) Styloid process

On the back of the wrist, the distal end of the ulna forms a round prominence, corresponding to the head of ulna. The more inner and narrower projecting of the head of the ulna is the styloid process, which is about 1 cm proximal to the tip of the styloid process of the radius and on a more posterior plane. The styloid process of the radius bounds the snuff box proximally.

(2) Dorsal tubercle

It locates on the back of wist and posterior surface of the distal end of radius. it is landmark for inserting the Kuntscher's nail to perform the internal fixation of the fracture of radius.

(3) Wrist crease

There are three creases on the skin of the anterior carpal region. The proximal crease is at the level of the head (or the styloid process) of the ulna. The distal crease crosses the pisiform bone to the tip of the styloid process of the radius. The middle crease is not constant.

(4) Distal transverse crease

It begins at or near the cleft between the index and middle fingers, runs to the ulnae border of the palm, and corresponds to the $2^{nd}-5^{th}$ metacarpophalangeal joints.

(5) Radial longitudinal crease (thenar crease)

It partially encircles the thenar eminence.

6.2 The pectoral region and axillary region

6.2.1 Boundaries of the axillary cavity

The axillary is a pyramidal region. So it has an apex, a base and four walls (Figure 6-1).

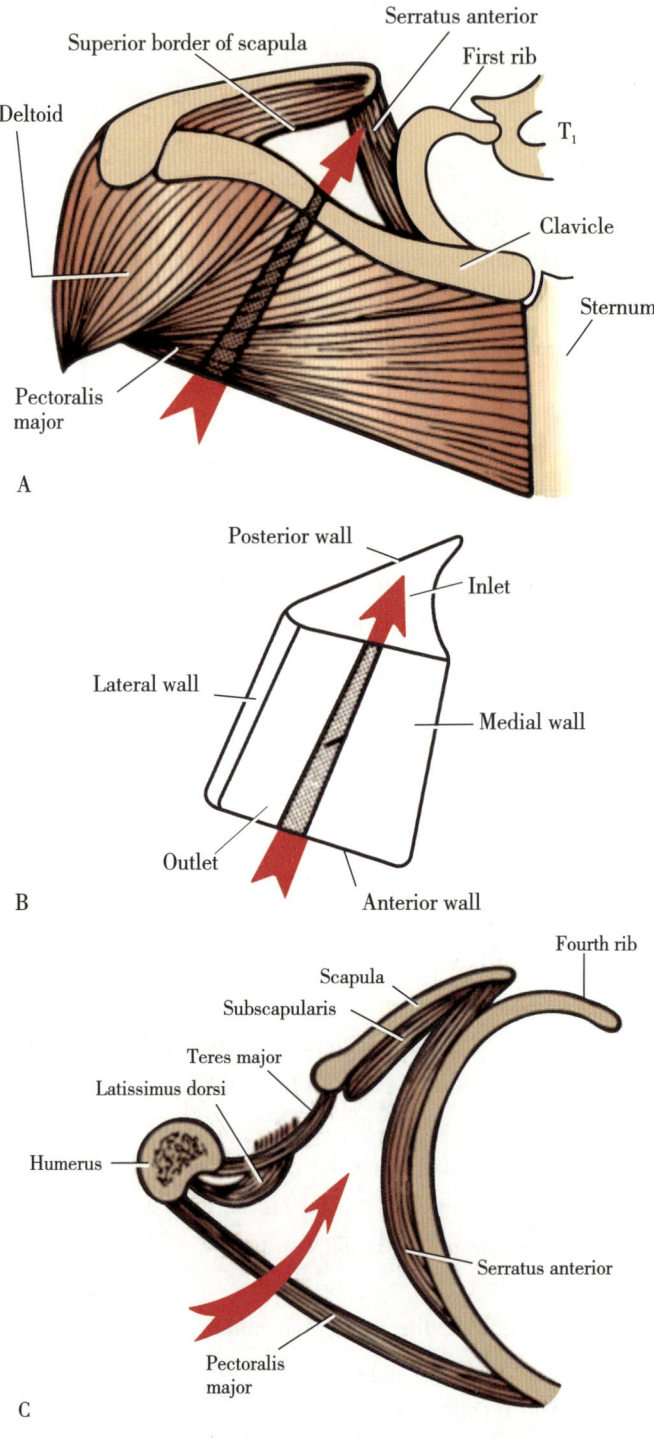

Figure 6-1   Inlet(A), walls(B), and outlet(C) of the right axilla

(1) The apex

The apex of the cavity is directed upwards to the root of the neck, and is formed by the first rib, the superior border of the scapula, the posterior surface of clavicle.

(2) The base

The base of the cavity is directed downwards, formed by the skin, the superficial fascia and the axillary fascia.

(3) The anterior wall

The anterior wall of the cavity is formed by the pectoralis major, the pectoralis minor and the clavipectoral fascia. The clavipectoral fascia is a strong fibrous sheet posterior to the pectoralis major and between the pectoralis minor and the clavicle, pierced by the cephalic vein, thoracoacromial vessels and lateral pectoral nerve.

(4) The posterior wall

The posterior wall is formed by the subscapularis, the teres major, the latissimus dorsi, the scapula.

In the posterior wall, there two important structures: the trangular space and the quadrangular space. The trangular space is the triangular space between the teres minor, the teres major, and the long head of the triceps brachii. It is pierced by the circumflex scapular vessels. The quadrangular space is the quadrangular space between the teres minor, the teres major, the long head of the brachii and the surgical neck of the humerus. It is pierced by the axillary nerve and the posterior humeral circumflex vessels.

(5) The medial wall

The medial wall is formed by first four ribs and their intercostal muscles, and the upper part of the serratus anterior.

(6) The lateral wall

The lateral wall is formed by the long head and the short head of the biceps brachii, the coracobrachialis, and the intertubercular sulcus of the humerus (Figure 6-2-Figure 6-4).

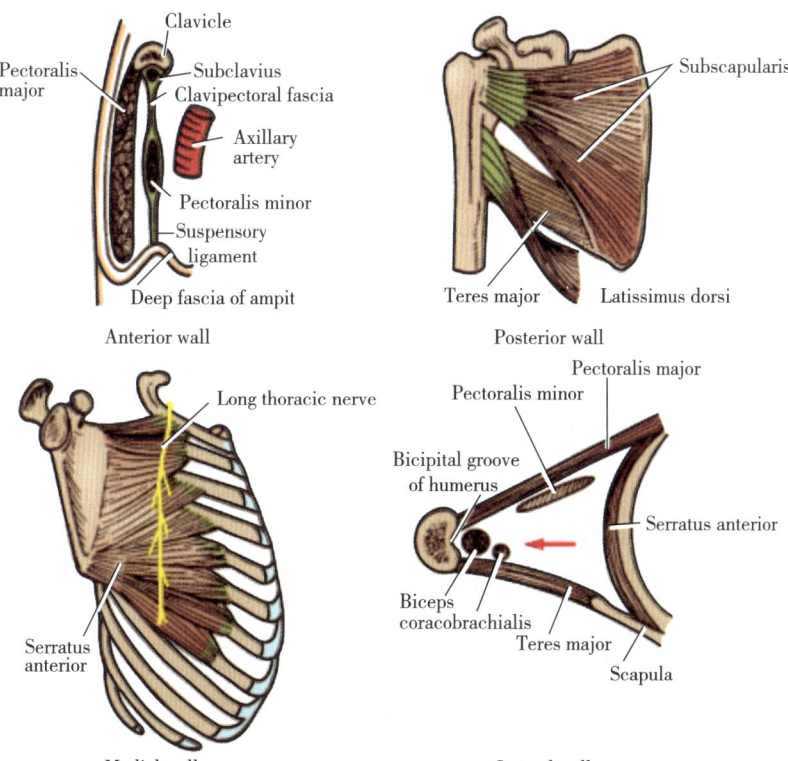

Figure 6-2 Structures that form the walls of the axilla

(The lateral wall is indicated by the arrow)

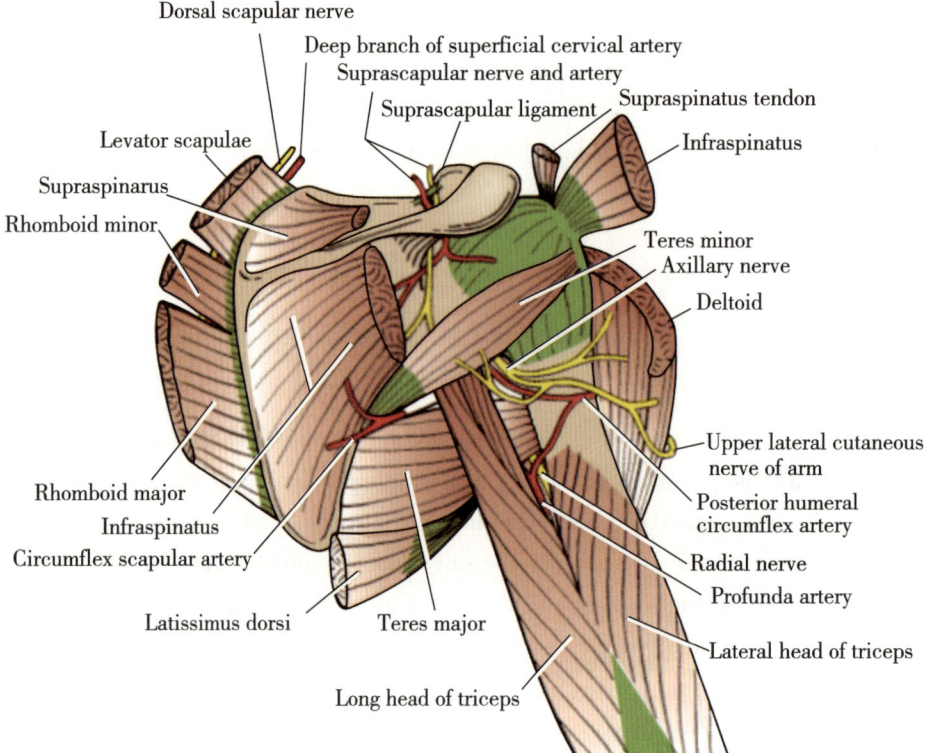

Figure 6–3 Muscles, nerves, and blood vessels of the scapular region
(Note the close relation of the axillary nerve to the shoulder joint)

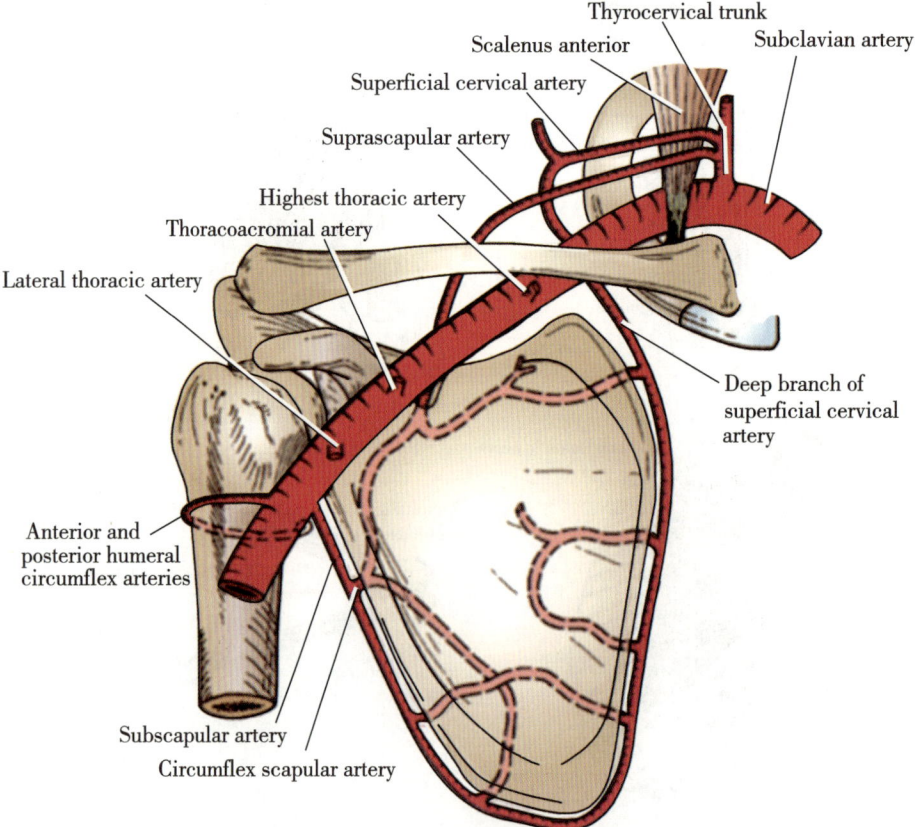

Figure 6–4 Arteries that take part in anastomosis around the shoulder joint

6.2.2 Contents of the axillary cavity

The main contents in the cavity include the axillary artery and its branches, the xillary vein and its tributaries, the brachial plexus and its branches, the axillary lymph nodes. And at same time, there are many fat and loose connective tissue in it (Figure 6-5-Figure 6-7).

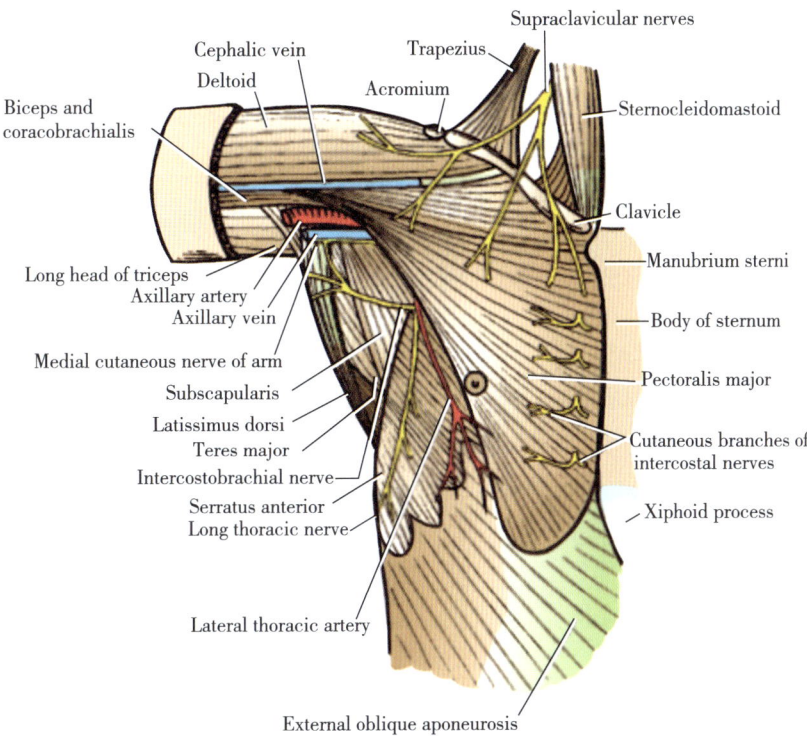

Figure 6-5 Pectoral region and axilla

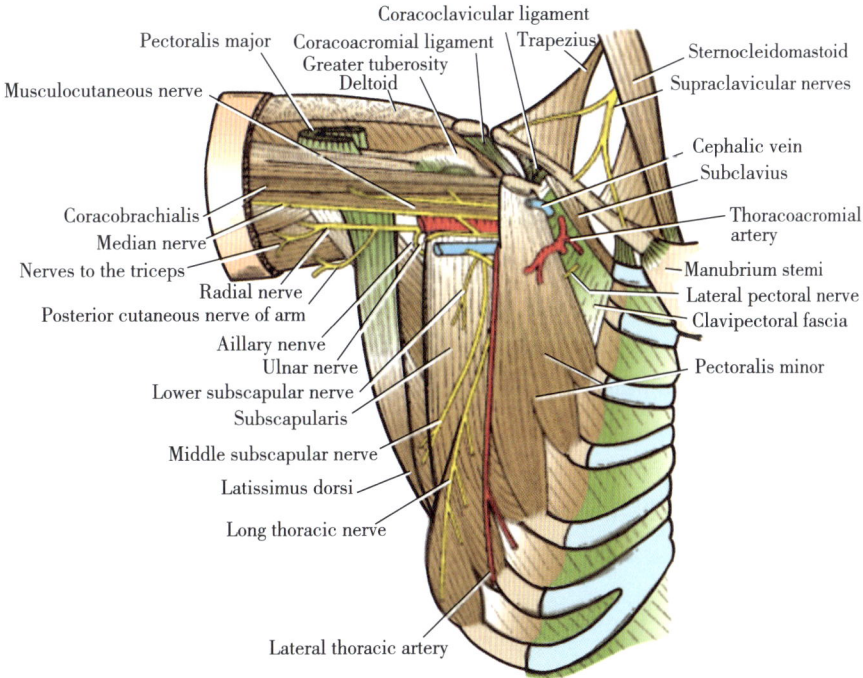

Figure 6-6 Pectoral region and axilla
(The pectoralis major muscle has been removed to display the underlying structures)

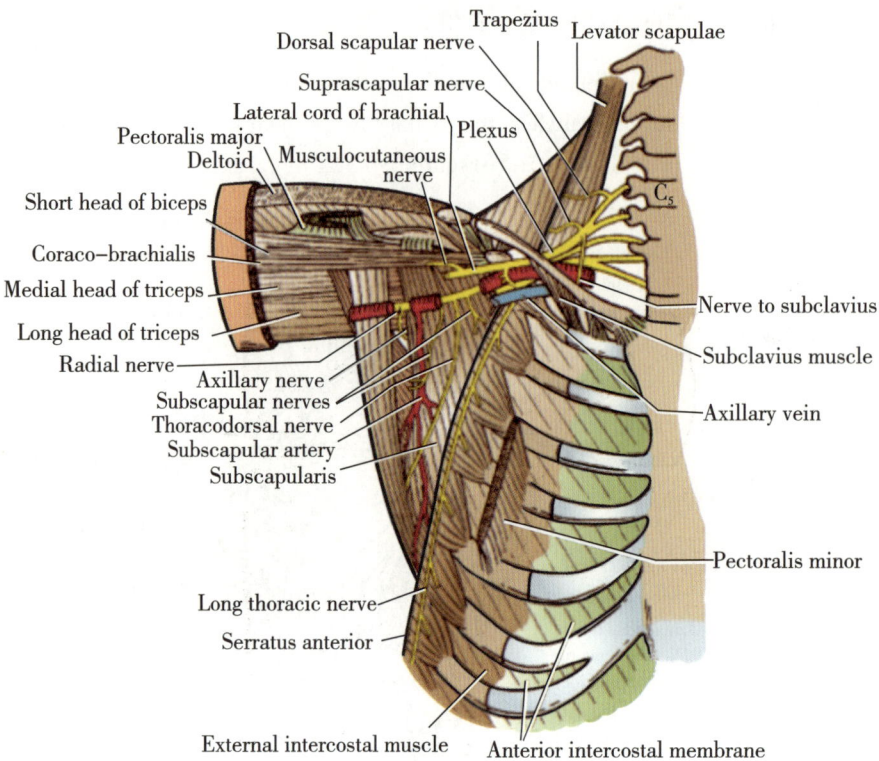

Figure 6-7 Pectoral region and axilla

(The pectoralis major and minor muscles and the clavipectoral fascia have been removed to display the underlying structures)

(1) The axillary artery

The axillary artery were divided into three parts by the pectoralis minor.

In the first part, there is only one branch, the superior thoracic artery, it upplies the anterior part of the first and the second intercostal spaces.

There are two branches coming from the trunk: the throracoacromial artery and the lateral thoracic artery. The throracoacromial artery pierces the clavipectoral fascia and divides into three branches immediately, one to the deltoid, one to the acromion, and the other goes to the pectorals. The lateral thoracic artery goes along the lower border of the pectoralis minor, mainly supplies the structures of the thoracic wall. In women, this artery is lager and gives the branch to breast.

There are three branches in the third part. The first is the subscapular artery. Usually this artery is the largest branch of the trunk. It has two branches: the circumflex scapular artery and the thoracodorsal artery. The circumflex artery pierces the triangular space to the back of the shoulder. The thoracodorsal artery goes to the latissimus dorsi. In the third part, there are two arteries go around humerus: the anterior humeral circumflex artery and the posterior humeral circumflex artery. The posterior humeral circumflex artery pierces the quadrangular space with the axillary nerve (Figure 6-8).

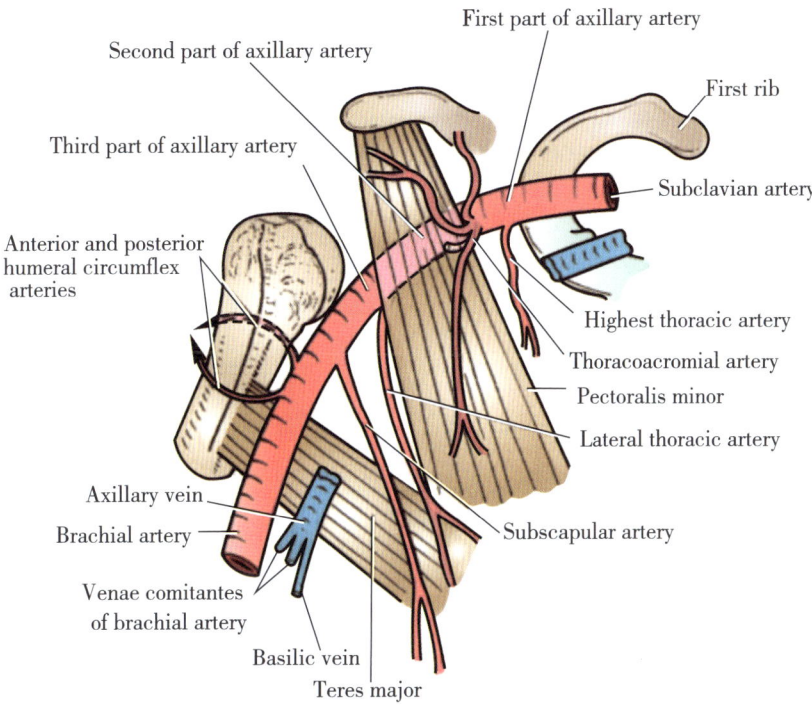

Figure 6-8 Parts of the axillary artery and its branches
(Note the formation of the axillary vein at the lower border of the teres major muscle)

(2) The main branches of the brachial plexus

There are many branches coming from the three cords of the brachial plexus, but the most important branches are the musculocutaneous nerve, the medial nerve, the ulnar nerve, the radial nerve and the axillary nerve.

The axillary sheath: the prevertebral layer of the deep cervical fascia extends from the neck and through the apex to the axillary cavity, in the cavity it encloses the axillary artery, the axillary vein and the brachial plexus, we call it axillary sheath (Figure 6-9-Figure 6-11).

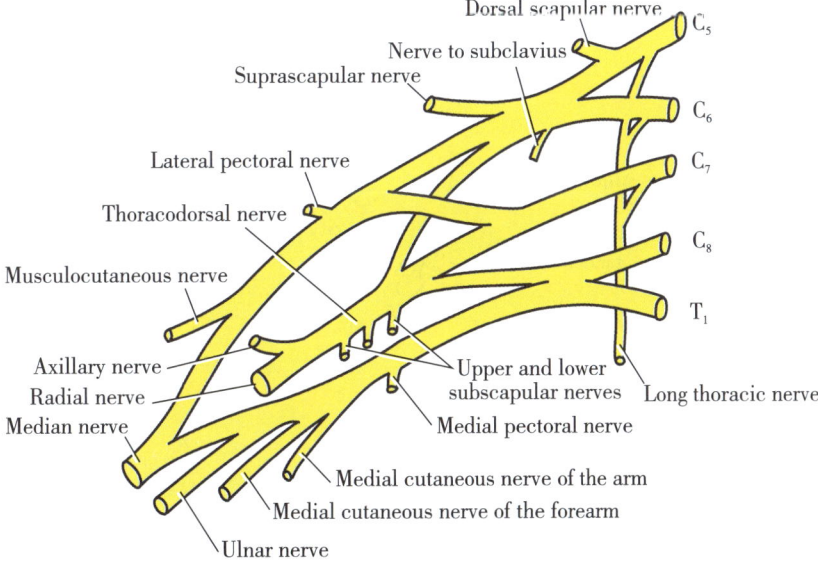

Figure 6-9 Roots, trunks, divisions, cords, and terminal branches of the brachial plexus

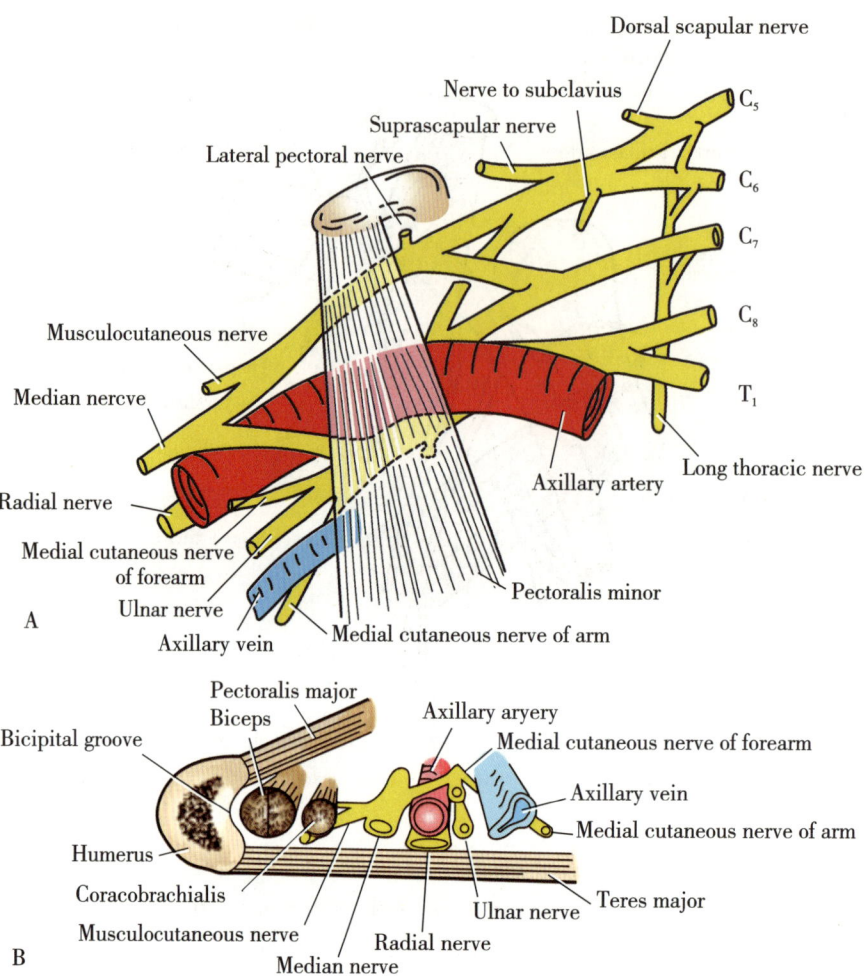

A. Relations of the brachial plexus and its branches to the axillary artery and vein; B. Section through the axilla at the level of the teres major muscle.

Figure 6-10　Brachial plexus and its branches

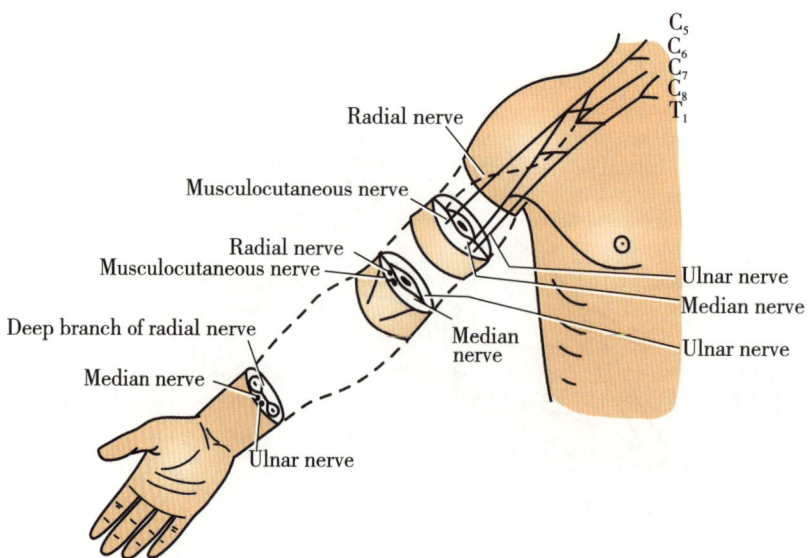

Figure 6-11　Distribution of the main branches of the brachial plexus to different fascial compartments of the arm and forearm

Because the fascia of the sheath comes from the prevertebral layer, so if there is a prevertebral abscess, the pus maybe spread to axilla through the axillary sheath. And when the surgical operation doing only on the lower part of the limb, we can inject the anesthetic into the axillary sheath to block the bracial plexus. But be careful not to damage the artery. So the operator should first touch the axillary according to its pulsation, and then insert the needle superior or inferior to the palpating index finger.

(3) The axillary lymph nodes

There are many lymph nodes in the axillary cavity and were divided into five groups. The nodes arrange along lower border of the pectoralis minor called the pectoral lymph nodes. The pectoral lymph nodes receive the vessels from the anterior and lateral thoracic wall, the central and lateral parts of the breast. The nodes arrange near the distal part of the axillary vein called the lateral lymph nodes and they receive the vessels from the upper limb. The nodes arrange near subscapular vessels called the subscapular lymph nodes and they receive the vessels from the scapular region and the back. The efferent vessels of these three group drain into the center group. The center group lies in the fat of the axillary cavity. And it's efferent vessels drain into the apical nodes. The apical nodes arrange near the upper part of the axillary cavity and receive the vessels from the center group and the upper part of the breast. And their efferent vessels form the subclavian trunk(Figure 6-12).

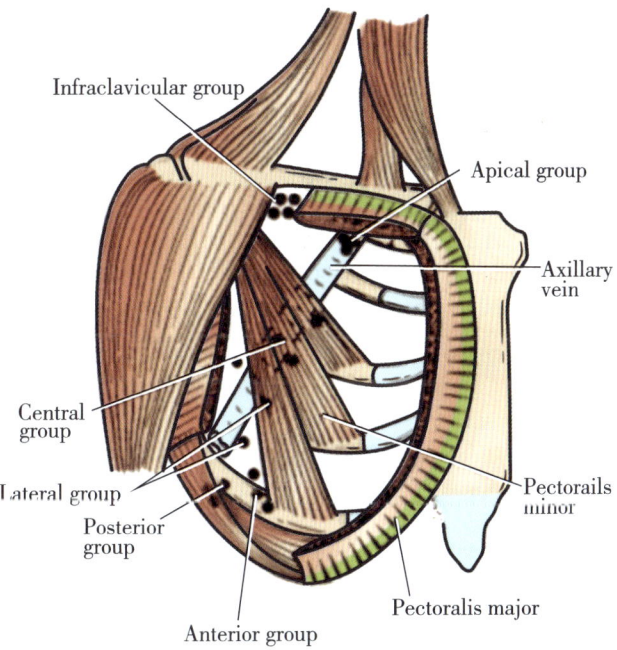

Figure 6-12   Different groups of lymph nodes in the axilla

(4) The lymphatic drainage of the breast

The cancer of breast is a common tumour happening in women, and it can spread through the lymphatic vessels. So studying the lymphatic drainage of the breast is very important.

Usually there are four pathways for lymphatic drainage(Figure 6-13).

1) The lymphatic vessels of the lateral and upper parts drain into the pectoral lymph nodes, this is the main lymphatic drainage of the breast, and usually is invaded early by the beast cancer.

2) The lymphatic vessels of the medial parts drain into the parasternal lymph nodes. These vessels can anastomose with the contralateral lymphatic vessels.

3) The lymphatic vessels of the inferomedial parts anastomose with the lymphatic vessels of the anterior

abdominal wall, the subdiaphragmatic and hepatic lymphatic vessels.

4) The deep lymphatic vessels of the breast pierce the pectoralis major and minor directly and axillary nodes receive more than 75% of lymph from the gland, and the remainder largely draining to parasternal nodes. So in the radical mastectomy, the pectoralis major and minor, the accessible lymph nodes must be removed thoroughly. When the operator working, he must be careful not to damage those important vessels and nerves going nearby. For example, when cutting the pectoralis major and minor, dealing with the clavipectoral dascia or removing the apical lymph nodes, he should protect the cephalic vein from damage. And when removing the pectoral lymph nodes, he should protect the long thoracic nerve; and when removing lateral and central lymph node, he should protect vessels and nerves in the axillary cavity especially the axillary vein; and when removing the subscapular lymph nodes, he should protect the thoracodorsal nerve.

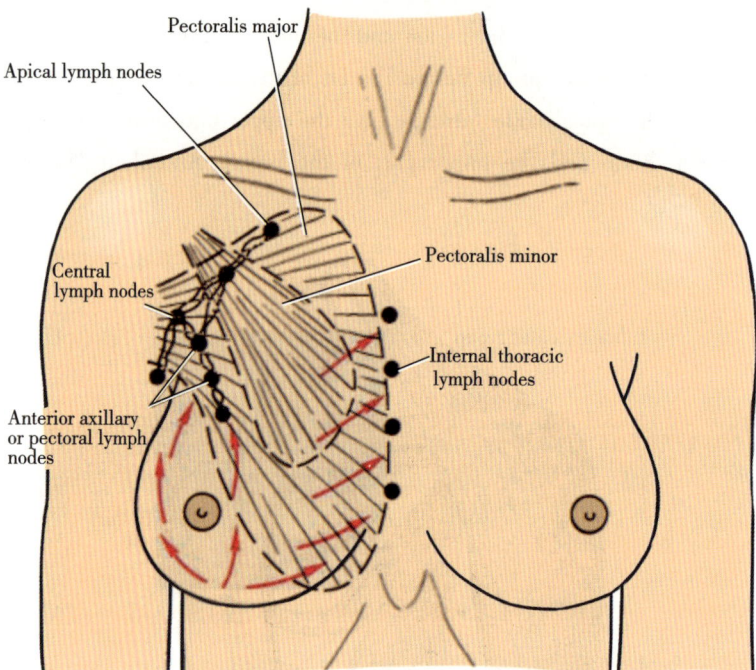

Figure 6-13 Lymph drainage of the breast

6.3 The anterior region of the arm, the elbow, the forearm, and the wrist

6.3.1 The superficial vein

There are two larger veins here. One is the cephalic vein, and the other is the basilic vein. The cephalic vein begins at the radial side of the dorsal venous rete of hand, and ascends to the elbow at the lateral side of the forearm, then goes into the cleft between the pectoralis major and deltoid, pierces the clavipectoral fascia and drains into the axillary vein(Figure 6-14).

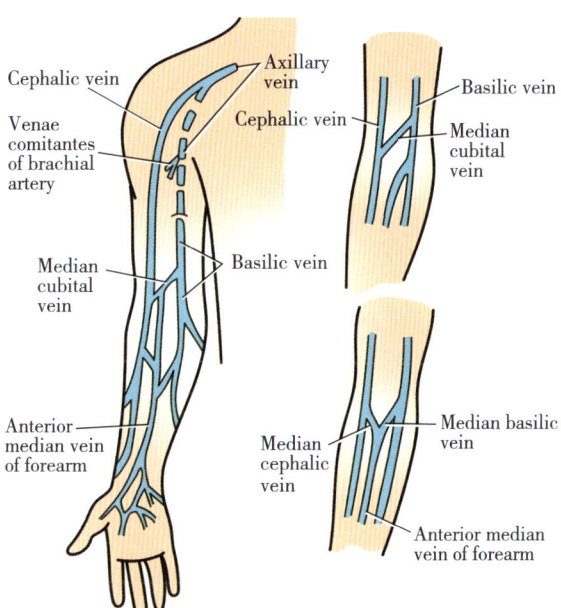

Figure 6-14 Superficial veins of the upper limb

(Note the common variations seen in the region of the elbow)

And the basilic vein begins at the unlar side of the dorsal venous rete of hand and ascends to the elbow at the medial side of the forearm, and then goes along the medial bicipital groove and pierces the deep fascia of the arm and drain into the axillary vein.

Some times there is a superficial vein connecting the cephalic vein and the basilic vein at the elbow. We call it the medial cubital vein. Usually it comes from the cephalic vein and drain into the basilic vein upward and medially. Vein punctures are often performed at upper limb with these superficial veins. Usually there is a large superficial vein at the anterior aspect of the elbow, sometimes maybe it is the medial cubital vein, and this superficial vein is connected with the deep vein, so we often make the vein punctures at the elbow.

The cutaneous innervation, the superficial lymphatics, the main arteries are showed in Figure 6-15-Figure 6-19.

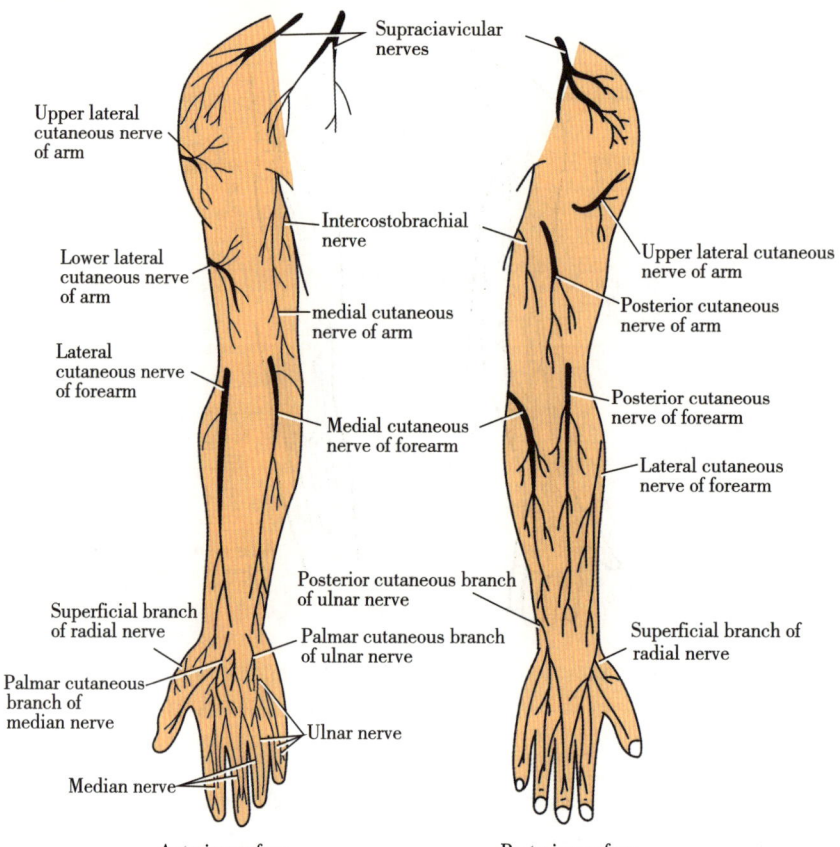

Figure 6–15 Cutaneous innervation of the upper limb

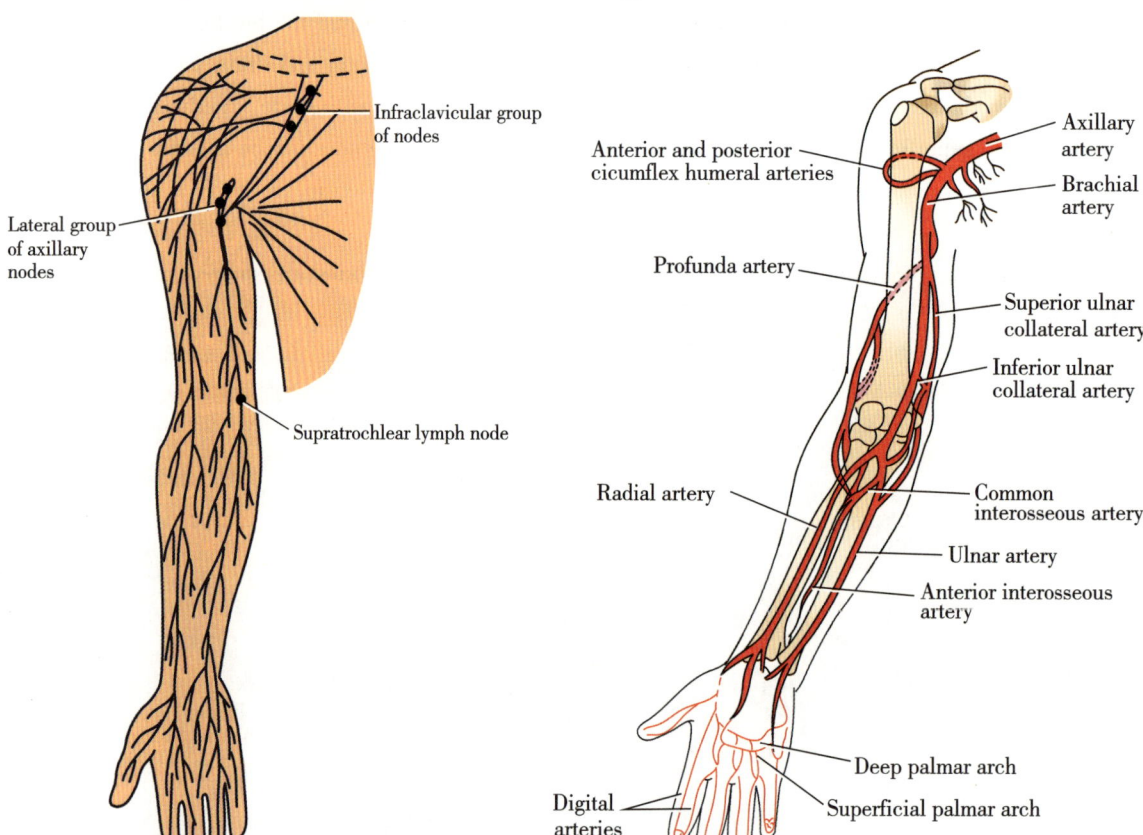

Figure 6–16 Superficial lymphatics of the upper limb
(Note the positions of the lymph nodes)

Figure 6–17 The main arteries of the upper limb

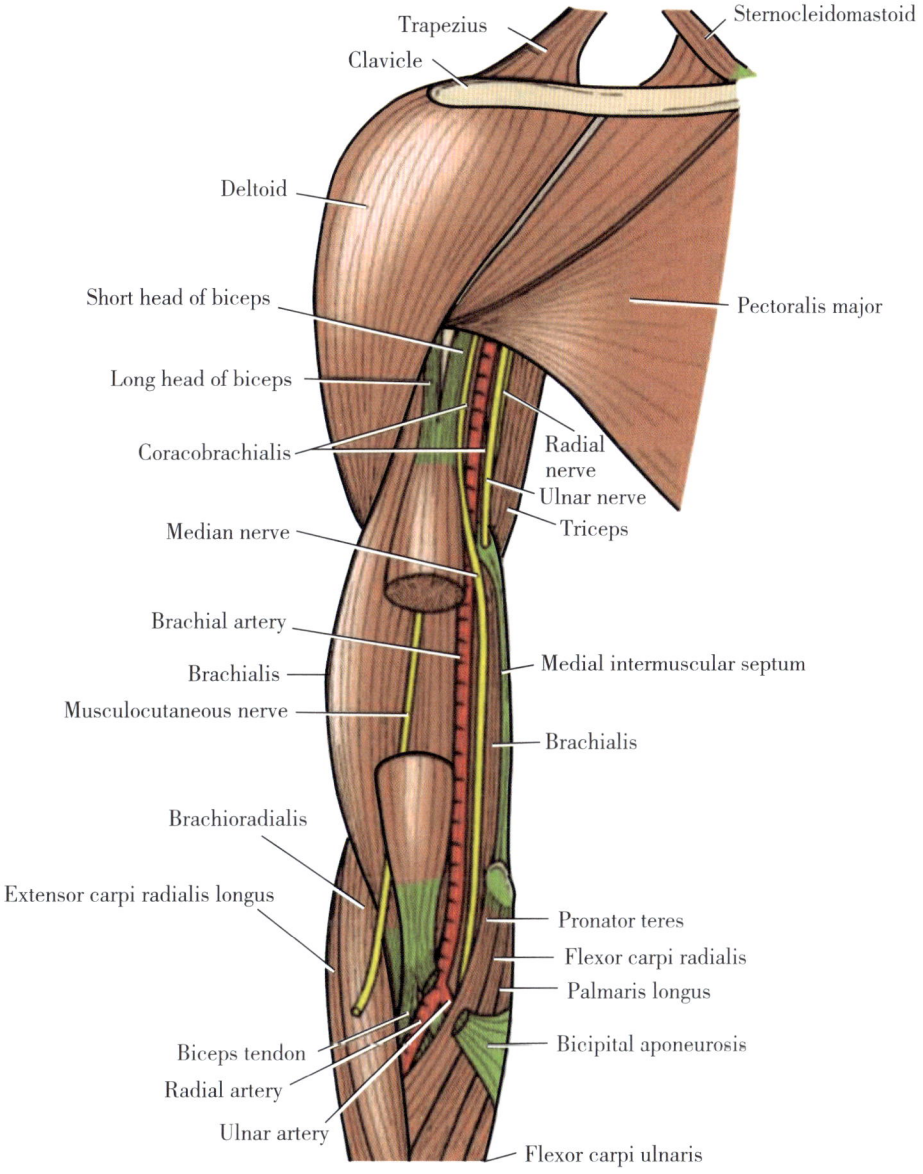

Figure 6-18 Anterior view of the upper arm
(The middle portion of the biceps brachii has been removed to show the musculocutaneous nerve lying in front of the brachialis)

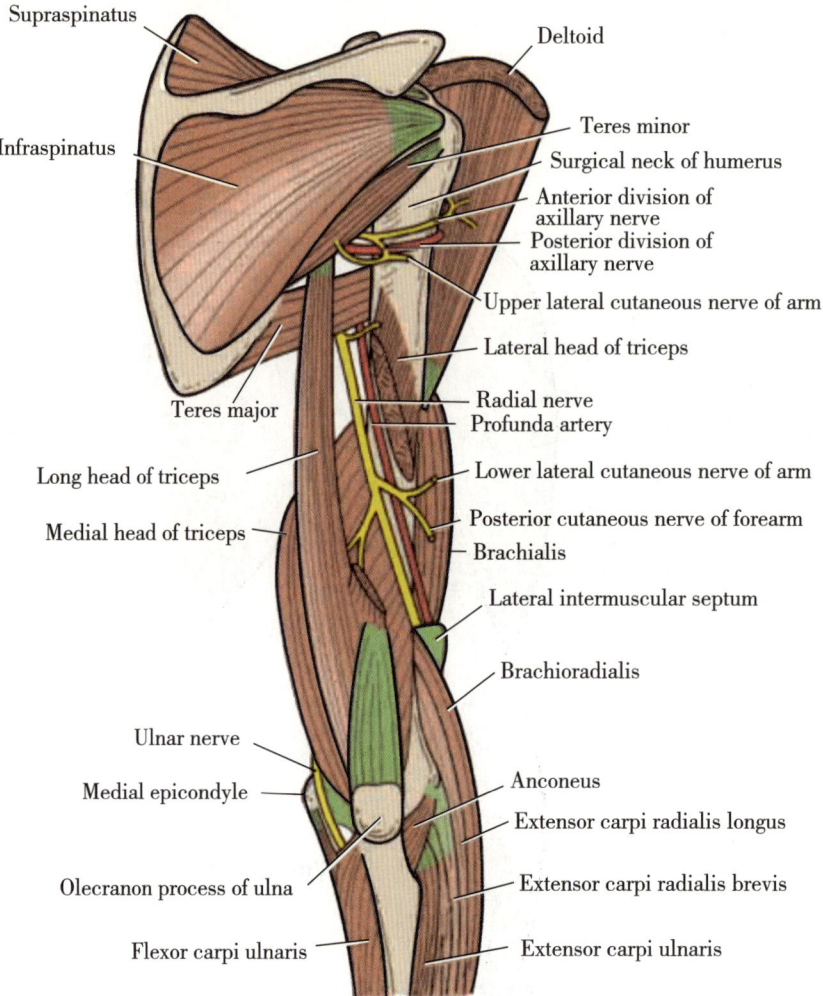

Figure 6-19   Posterior view of the upper arm
(The lateral head of the triceps has been divided to display the radial nerve and the profunda artery in the spiral groove of the humerus)

6.3.2 The cubital fossa

The cubital fossa is a triangular depression. If you remove the skin and the superficial fascia, you will find that all the content are deep to the aponeurosis of the biceps brachii and the deep fascia, so we can say the roof of the fossa is formed by the aponeurosis and the deep fascia. Then if you remove the deep fascia and cut off the apoeurosis, you can find the upper boundary is formed by an imaginary line connecting the two humeral epicondyles. The pronator teres is the inferomedial boundary and the brachioradialis is the inferolateral boundary. And the brachialis and supinator form the base of the fossa, and deep to all the content.

The contents in the cubital fossa arrange in a regular order. From the lateral side to the medial side, is the tendon of the biceps brachii, the terminal part of the brachil artery, and then the medial nerve. At the lower part of the fossa, the brachil artery divides into two branches: the radial artery and the ulnar artery (Figure 6-20).

The structures of forearm are showed in Figure 6-21-Figure 6-23.

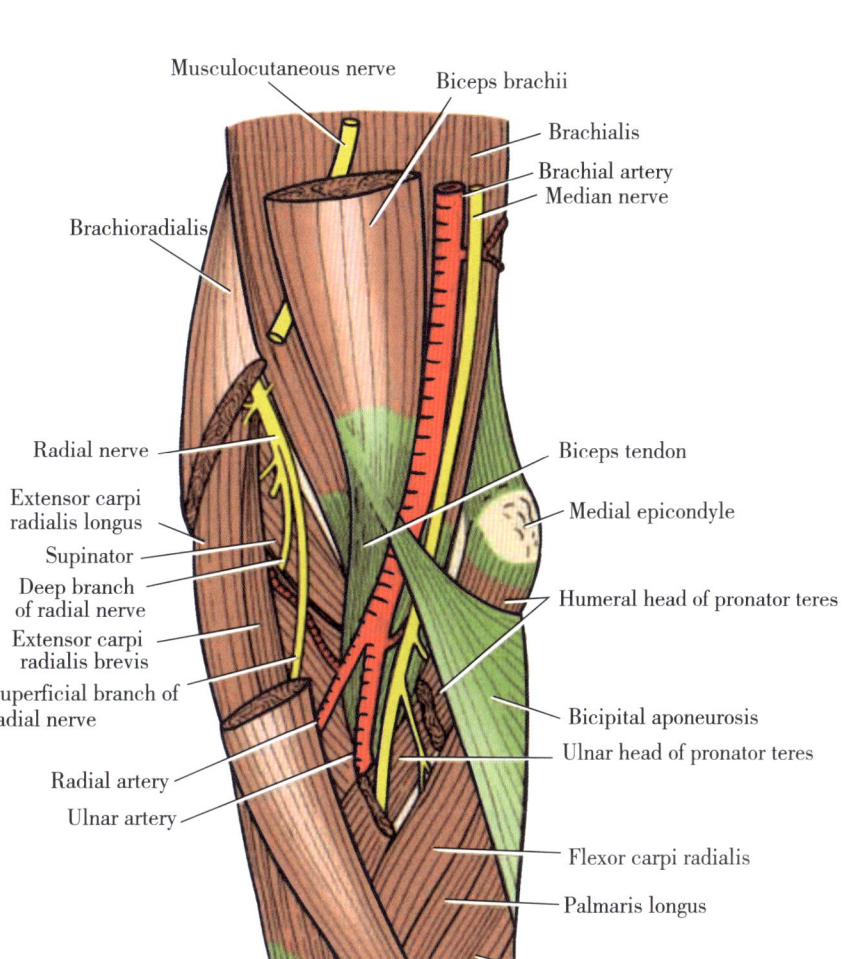

Figure 6–20   Right cubital fossa

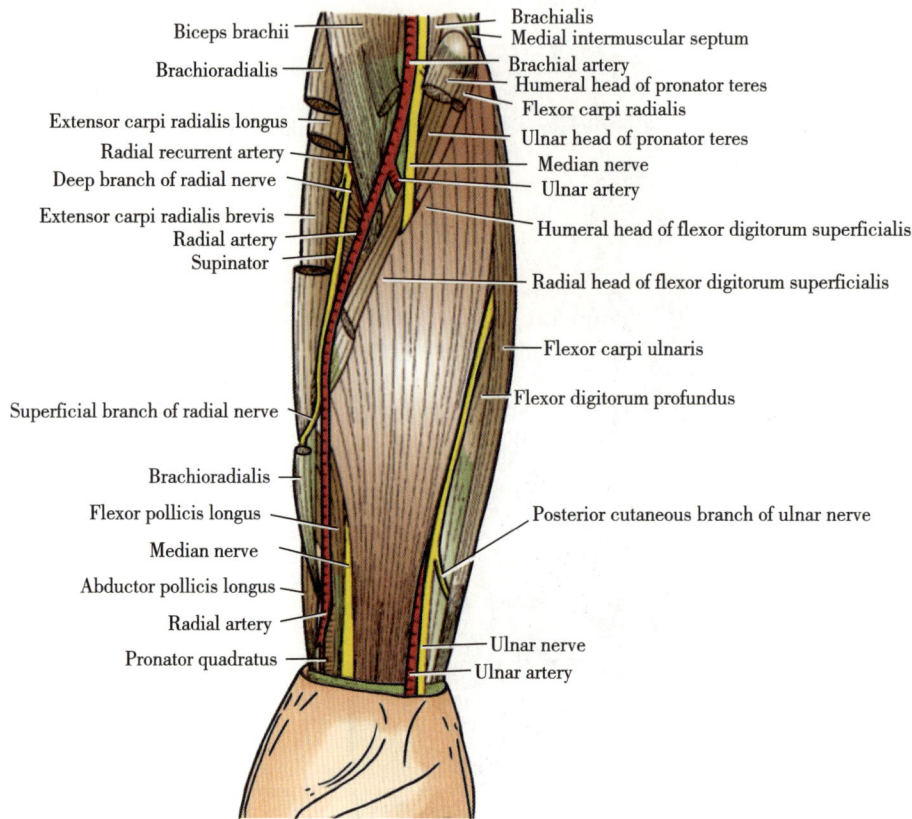

Figure 6-21　Anterior view of the forearm

(Most of the superficial muscles have been removed to display the flexor digitorum superficialis, medial nerve, superficial branch of the radial nerve, and radial artery. Note that the ulnar head of the pronator teres separates the medial nerve from the ulnar artery)

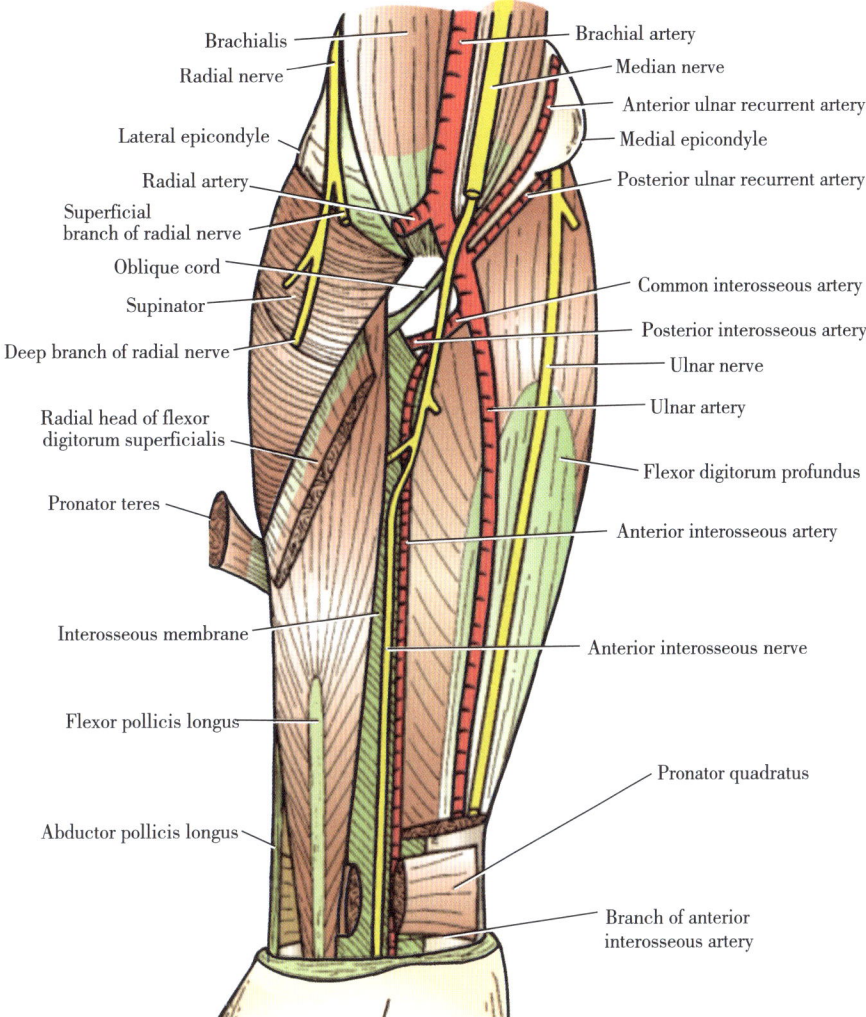

Figure 6-22 Anterior view of the forearm showing the deep structures

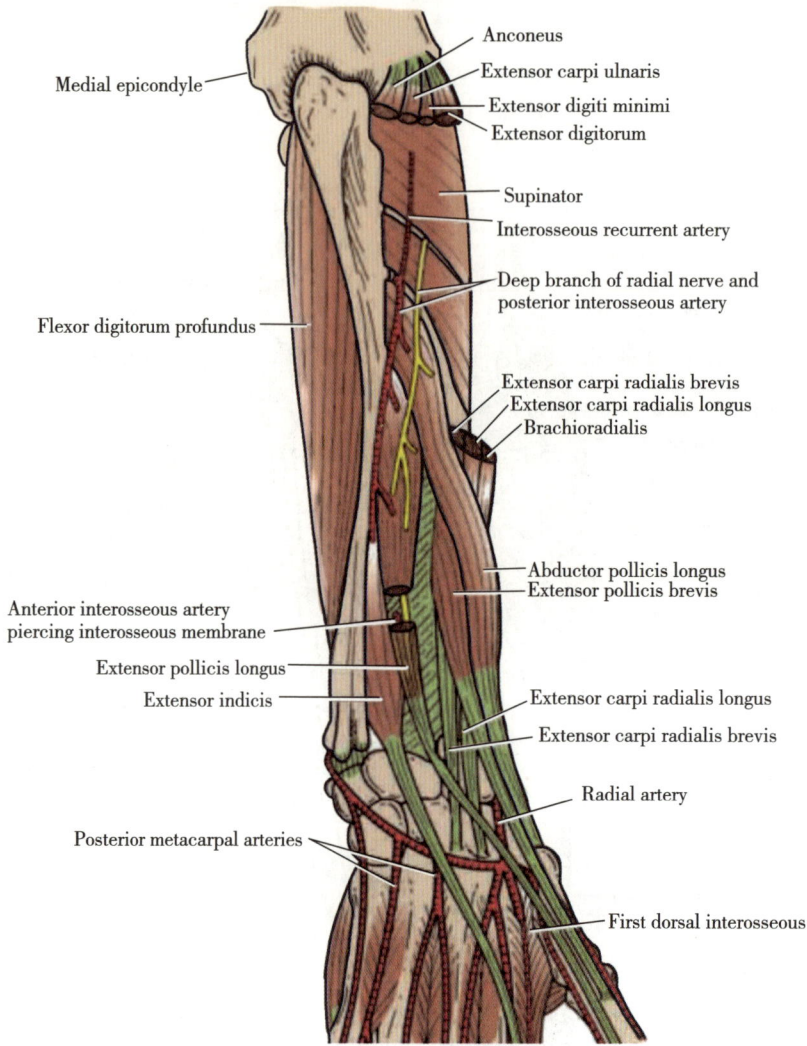

Figure 6-23 Posterior view of the forearm
(The superficial muscles have been removed to display the deep structures)

6.3.3 The carpal canal

First let's learn something about the deep fascia of the wrist. The deep fascia here includes two layers. The superficial layer of the deep fascia we call it the palmar carpal ligament. It is thickened by some transverse fibers. And the deep layer extends distally, we call it the flexor retinaculum. It is very thick. Both the ulnar end and the radial end of it is attached to some carpal bones. So there is a canal between the flexor retinaculum and the groove of the carpal bones, we call it the carpal canal. The medial nerve and nine tendons pass through the carpal canal to the palm. The nine tendons include the flexor digitorum superficialis, the tendons of the flexor digitorum profundus and the tendon of the pollicis longus. Because the flexor retinaculum is very thick, so it can protect the tendons and the medial nerve from some damage. But at the same time, any disease in the canal may injure the medial nerve. And the deep space of the forearm can communicates with the space of palm through the carpal canal. So the infection of the palm may extend to the forearm through this way.

The palm of the hand is showed in Figure 6-24–Figure 6-27.

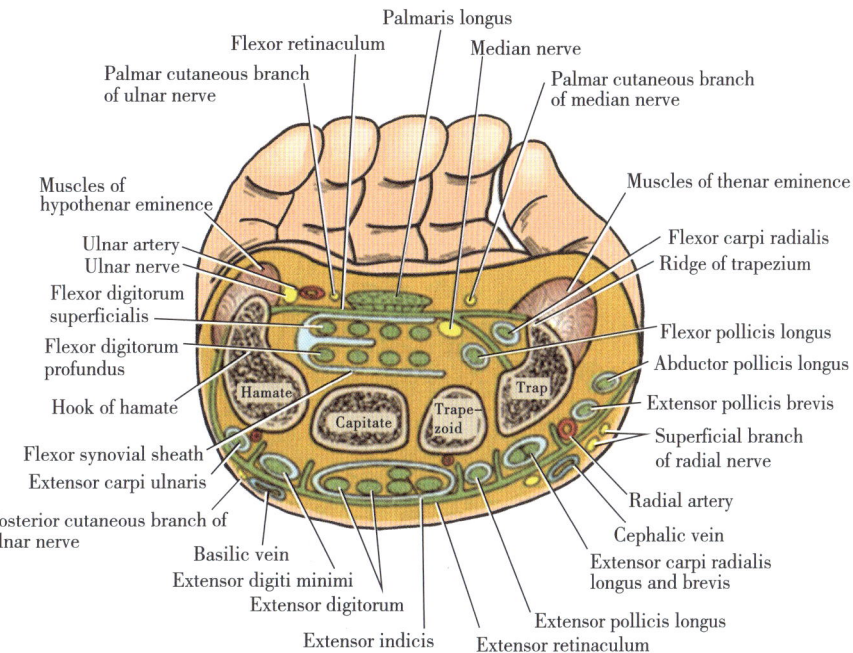

Figure 6-24　Cross section of the hand showing the relation of the tendons, nerves, and arteries to the flexor and extensor retinacula

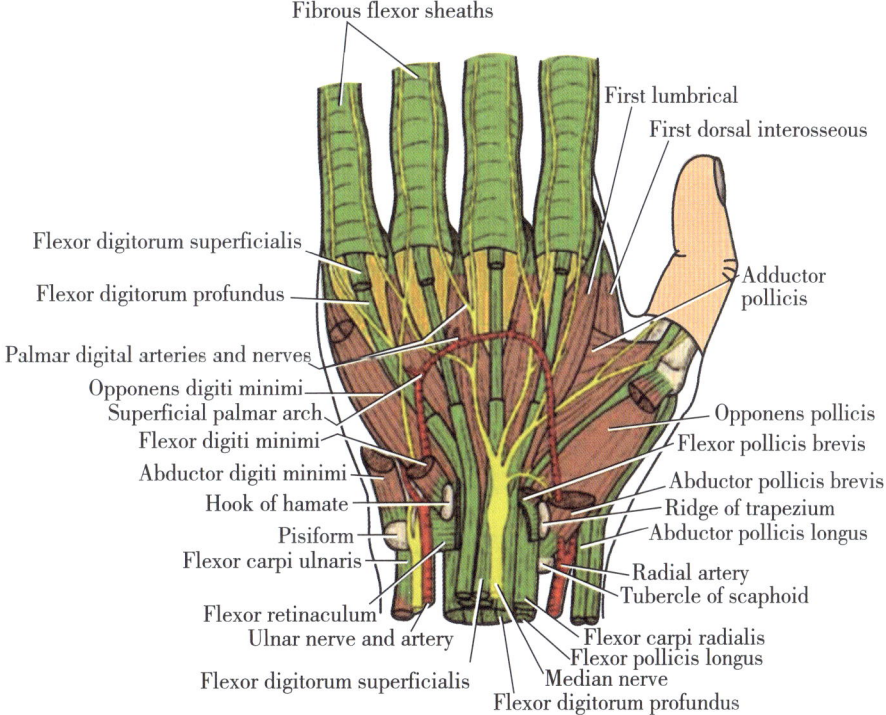

Figure 6-25　Anterior view of the palm of the hand

(The palmar aponeurosis and the greater part of the flexor retinaculum have been removed to display the superficial palmar arch, the medial nerve, and the long flexor tendons. Segments of the tendons of the flexor digitorum superficialis have been removed to show the underlying tendons of the flexor digitorum profundus)

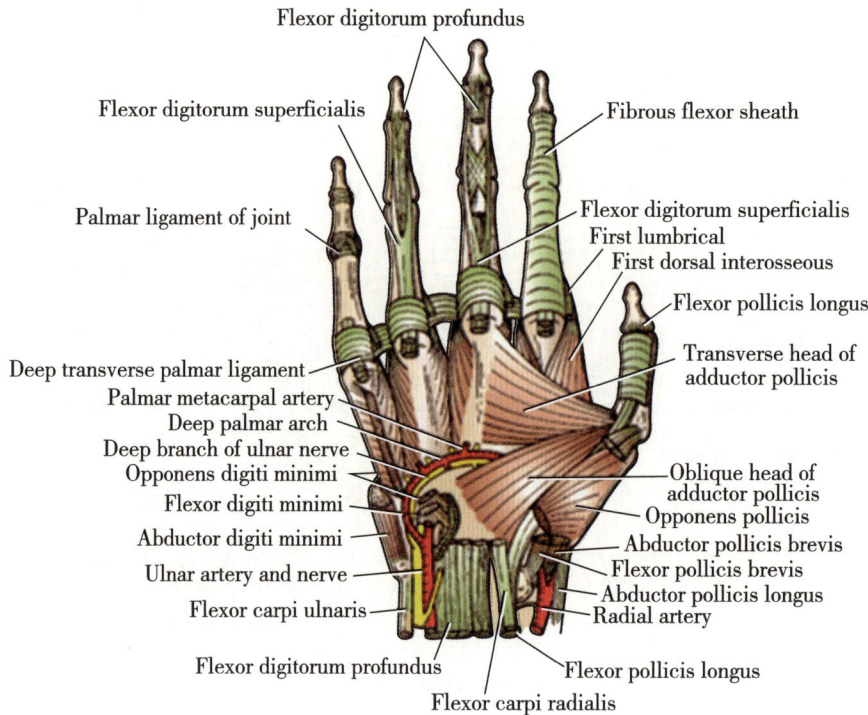

Figure 6-26 Anterior view of the palm of the hand
(The long flexor tendons have been removed from the palm, but their method of insertion into the fingers is shown)

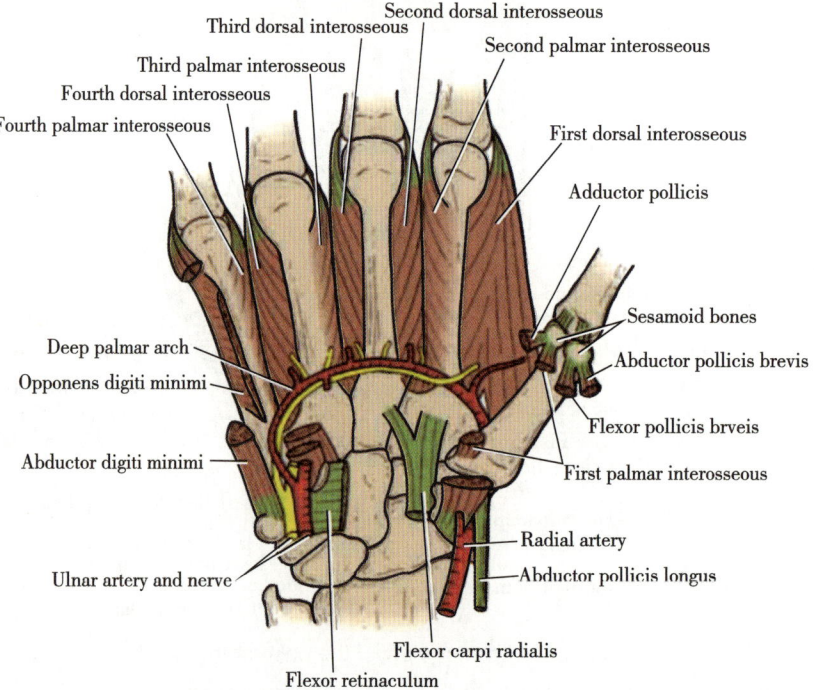

Figure 6-27 Anterior view of the palm of the hand showing the deep palmar arch and the deep terminal branch of the ulnar nerve

6.4 The posterior region of the arm, the elbow, the forearm, and the wrist

First, let's talk about the humeromuscular tunnel. It is located at the middle part on the back of the arm. And it extends downwards from the superomedial side to the inferolateral side. It is formed by the three heads of the triceps brachii and the sulcus for the radial nerve on the humerus. The radial nerve and deep brachial vessels pass through the humeromuscular tunnel. So if there is a fracture at the humeral shaft, the radial nerve may be injured. Over the cadaver to the prone position, abduct the upper limb and then make the incisions. Here we have two transverse incisions: one at the arm and the other at the wrist. Both of them continue with the anterior incisions. At the dorsum of hand, you should make a longitudinal incision in the midline and a curve incision along all the metacarpophalangeal joints.

Other structures of the posterior region of the arm, the elbow, the forearm, and the wrist are seen in the next section for details.

6.5 Main contents of the upper limb

6.5.1 Bones of upper limb

Clavicle
Description
✓ The clavicle, or collarbone, connects the upper limb to the trunk ✓ It is classed as a long bone, but is relatively short, attaching medially to the sternum, and laterally articulating with the acromion of the scapula ✓ It can be palpated along its length, and is visible under the skin in many people
Important landmarks
✓ The superior surface of the clavicle is subcutaneous ✓ The important landmarks can be seen on the inferior surface of the clavicle ✓ On the inferior surface near the lateral end of the clavicle, it possess the tubercle and ridge called conoid tubercle and trapezoid ridge ✓ The medial end of the clavicle is rounded and the lateral end is flattened

Superior view
Lateral — Acromial end
Medial — Sternal end

Inferior view
Lateral — Acromial end
Medial — Sternal end

Functions
✓ Fixes the limbs on the trunk ✓ Protects the vessels and nerves that lies below ✓ Transmits the weight of limbs to the trunk

Clinical importance
✓ The most common site of fracture is junction between medial 2/3 and lateral 1/3 ✓ The fracture occurs more commonly due to fall of outstretched hand ✓ After fracture, the lateral end of the clavicle is displaced inferiorly by the weight of the arm, and medially, by the pectoralis major. The medial end is pulled superiorly, by the sternocleidomastoid muscle. ✓ The suprascapular nerves (medial, intermedial and lateral) may be damaged by the upwards movement of the medial part of the fracture. These nerves innervate the lateral rotators of the upper limb at the shoulder—so damage results in unopposed medial rotation of the upper limb–the "waiters tip" position

Scapula

Description
✓ The scapula is also known as the shoulder blade. It articulates with the humerus at the glenohumeral joint, and with the clavicle at the acromioclavicular joint. In doing so, the scapula connects the upper limb to the trunk. It is a triangular, flat bone, which serves as a site for attachment for many muscles

Important landmarks
Costal surface
✓ It is also called anterior surface ✓ As the name costal surface indicates, this surface is related to ribcage ✓ The anterior or costal surface possess a concave depression on most of its surface called subscapularfossa, which provides an attachment to the muscle called subscapularis ✓ The "hook–like" projection originating from the superolateral aspect of costal surface is called corocoid process of scapula

Lateral surface

✓ The lateral surface of the scapula faces the humerus. It is the site of the glenohumeral joint, and of various muscle attachments
✓ Glenoid fossa—a shallow cavity, which articulates with the humerus to form the glenohumeral joint. The superior part of the lateral border is very important clinically, as it articulates with the humerus to make up the shoulder joint, or glenohumeral joint
✓ Supraglenoid tubercle—a roughening immediately superior to the glenoid fossa, this is the place of attachment of the long head of the biceps brachii
✓ Infraglenoid tubercle—a roughening immediately inferior to the glenoid fossa, this is the place of attachment of the long head of the triceps brachii

Posterior surface

✓ The posterior surface of the scapula faces outwards. It is a site of attachment for the majority of the rotator cuff muscles of the shoulder
✓ Spine—the most prominent feature of the posterior scapula. It runs transversely across the scapula, dividing the surface into two
✓ Infraspinous fossa—the area below the spine of the scapula, it displays a convex shape. The infraspinatus muscle originates from this area
✓ Supraspinous fossa—the area above the spine of the scapula, it is much smaller that the infraspinous fossa, and is more convex in shape. The supraspinatus muscle originates from this area
✓ Acromion—projection of the spine that arches over the glenohumeral joint and articulates with the clavicle

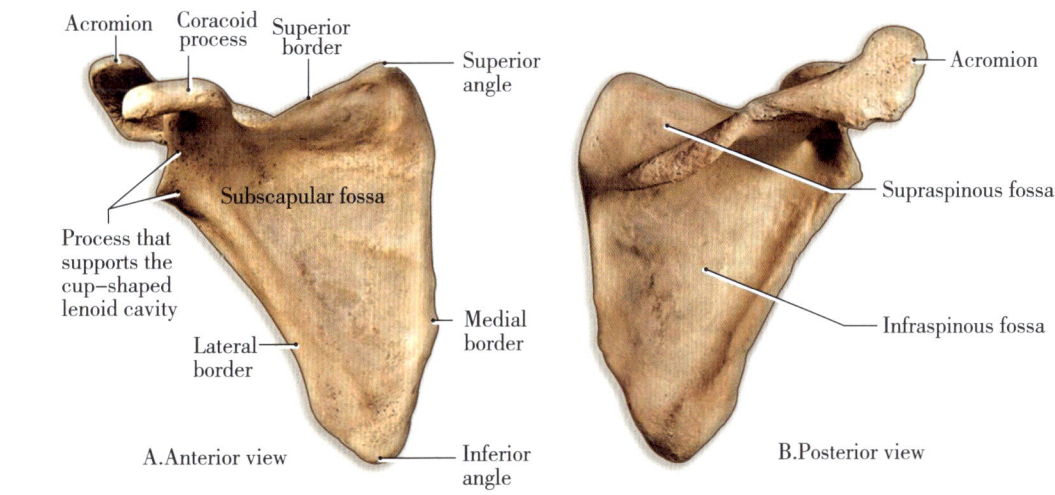

Clinical importance

Winging of scapula

✓ The serratus anterior muscle originating from the 2-8 ribs and inserted into the medial border of scapula supplied by long thoracic nerve (root value: C_5-C_7)
✓ The damage of the long thoracic nerve leads to the paralysis of the serratus anterior muscle which in turn causes the protrusion of scapula out of shoulder when pushing with the arm

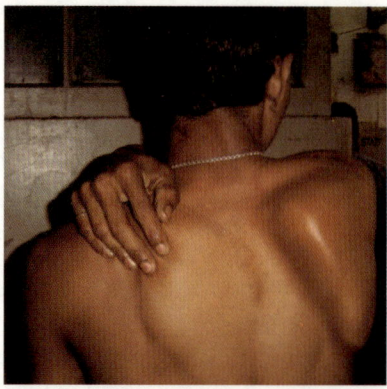

Humerus

Description

✓ The humerus is the bone that forms the upper arm, and joins it to the shoulder and forearm
✓ The proximal region articulates with the scapula and clavicle, forming part of the shoulder joint. Distally, the humerus articulates with the forearm bones (radius and ulna), to form the elbow joint
✓ The humerus acts as an attachment site for many muscles and ligaments, resulting in various raised roughening on the bony surface

Important landmarks

Upper part

✓ The upper part of the humerus articulates with the scapula to form the glenohumeral joint (shoulder joint)
✓ The important anatomical features of the proximal humerus are the head, anatomical neck, surgical neck, greater and lesser tubercles and intertubercular sulcus. A tubercle is a round nodule, and signifies an attachment site of a muscle or ligament
✓ The head of the humerus projects medially and superiorly to articulate with the glenoid cavity of the scapula.
The head is connected to the tubercles by the anatomical neck, which is short in width and nondescript.
✓ The greater tubercle is located laterally on the humerus. It has a anterior and posterior face. The greater tubercle serves as attachment site for 3 of the rotator cuff muscles (supraspinatus, infraspinatus and teres minor)
✓ The lesser tubercle is much smaller, and more medially located on the bone. It only has an anterior face. It is a place of attachment for the last rotator cuff muscle – subscapularis. Separating the two tubercles is a deep depression, called the intertubercular sulcus, or groove. The tendon of the long head of biceps brachii runs through this groove. The edges of the intertubercular sulcus are known as lips. Tendons of the pectoralis major, teres major and latissimus dorsi attach to the lips of the intertubecular sulcus
✓ The surgical neck runs from the tubercles to the shaft of the humerus

Shaft

✓ The shaft of the humerus contains some important bony landmarks such as the deltoid tuberosity and radial groove, and is the site of attachment for various muscles
✓ On the lateral side of the humeral shaft is a roughened surface where the deltoid muscle attaches. This is known is as the deltoid tuberosity

✓ The radial groove is shallow depression that runs diagonally down the posterior surface of the humerus, parallel to the deltoid tuberosity. The radial nerve and profunda brachii artery lie in this groove
✓ Other than the deltoid, the following muscles attach to the humerus:
  ◊ Anteriorly: corocobrachialis, deltoid, brachialis, brachioradialis
  ◊ Posterirly: medial and lateral heads of the triceps

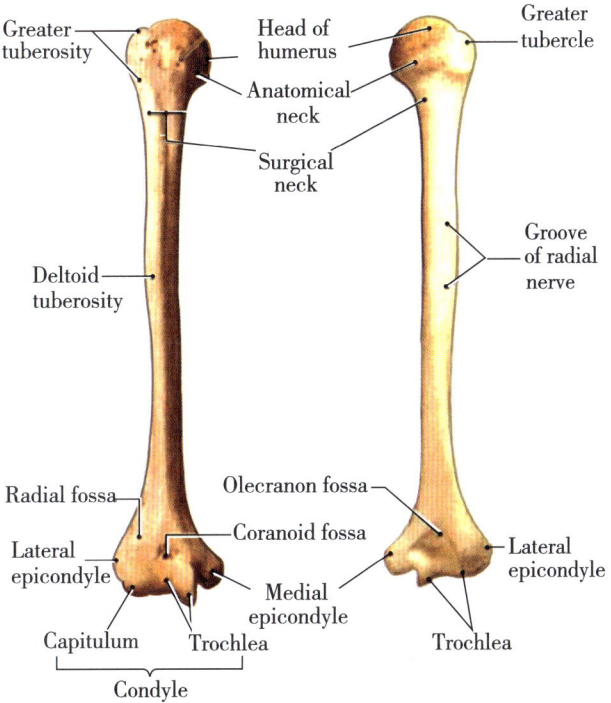

Lower part

✓ The lower part of the humerus articulates with the ulna and radius at the elbow joint. Here, the bone adopts a flattened, almost 2-D shape
✓ The lateral and medial borders of the humerus form medial and lateral supraepicondylar ridges. The lateral supraepidcondylar ridge is more roughened, as it is the site of attachment for many of the extensor muscles in the posterior forearm
✓ Immediately distal to the supraepicondylar ridges are the lateral and medial epicondyles–projections of bone. Both can be palpated at the elbow (the medial more so, as it is much larger). The ulnar nerve passes into the forearm along the posterior side of the medial epicondyle, and can also be palpated there
✓ The trochlea articulates with the ulna. It is located medially, and extends onto the posterior of the bone. Lateral to the trochlear is the capitulum, which articulates with the radius
✓ Also found on the distal portion of the humerus are three depressions, known as the coronoid, radial and olecranon fossae. They accommodate the forearm bones during movement at the elbow

Clinical importance

Surgical-neck fracture

✓ This is a frequent site of fracture (hence the name), this occurs by a direct blow to the area, or by falling on an outstretched hand

- ✓ It is important to consider the regional anatomy of this area to assess which vessels and nerves are a risk of damage. The key structures of concern is this scenario are the axillary nerve and posterior circumflex artery
- ✓ Damage to the axillary nerve will result in paralysis to the deltoid and teres minor muscles; the patient will not being able to abduct their arm
- ✓ The axillary nerve also innervates the skin over the lower deltoid (known as the regimental badge area), and so sensory innervation here could be lost

Mid-shaft fracture

- ✓ A mid-shaft fracture could easily damage the radial nerve and profunda brachii artery, as they are tightly bound in the radial groove
- ✓ The radial nerve innervates the extensors of the wrist. In the event of damage to this nerve, the extensors will be paralysed. This results in unopposed flexion of the wrist occurs, known as "wrist drop"
- ✓ There is also some sensory loss over the dorsal (posterior) surface of the hand, and the proximal ends of the lateral 3 and a half fingers dorsally

Fractures occurs at the lower part of humerus

- ✓ Supraepicondylar fractures and medial epicondyle fractures are common fracture types of the distal humerus. A supraepicondylar fracture occurs by falling on a flexed elbow. It is a transverse fracture, spanning between the two epicondyles
- ✓ Direct damage, or swelling can cause interference to the blood supply of the forearm from the brachial artery. The resulting ischaemia can cause Volkmann's ischaemic contracture-uncontrolled flexion of the hand, as flexors muscles become fibrotic and short. There also can be damage to the medial, ulnar or radial nerves
- ✓ A medial epicondyle fracture could damage the ulnar nerve, a deformity known as ulnar claw is the result. There will be a loss of sensation over the medial 1 and 1/2 fingers of the hand, on both the dorsal and palmar surfaces

Radius

Description

- ✓ The radius is a long bone in the forearm. It lies laterally and parallel to ulna, the second of the forearm bones.
- ✓ The radius pivots around the ulna to produce movement at the proximal and distal radio-ulnar joints

The radius articulates in four places

- ✓ Elbow joint—partly formed by an articulation between the head of the radius, and the capitulum of the humerus
- ✓ Proximal radioulnar joint—an articulation between the radial head, and the radial notch of the ulna
- ✓ Wrist joint—an articulation between the distal end of the radius and the carpal bones
- ✓ Distal radioulnar joint—an articulation between the ulnar notch and the head of the ulna

Important landmarks

Upper part of radius

- ✓ The proximal end of the radius articulates in both the elbow and proximal radioulnar joints

✓ Important bony landmarks include the head, neck and radial tuberosity
  ◊ Head of radius—a disk shaped structure, with a concave articulating surface. It is thicker medially, where it takes part in the proximal radioulnar joint
  ◊ Neck—a narrow area of bone, which lies between the radial head and radial tuberosity
  ◊ Radial tuberosity—a bony projection, which serves as the place of attachment of the biceps brachii muscle

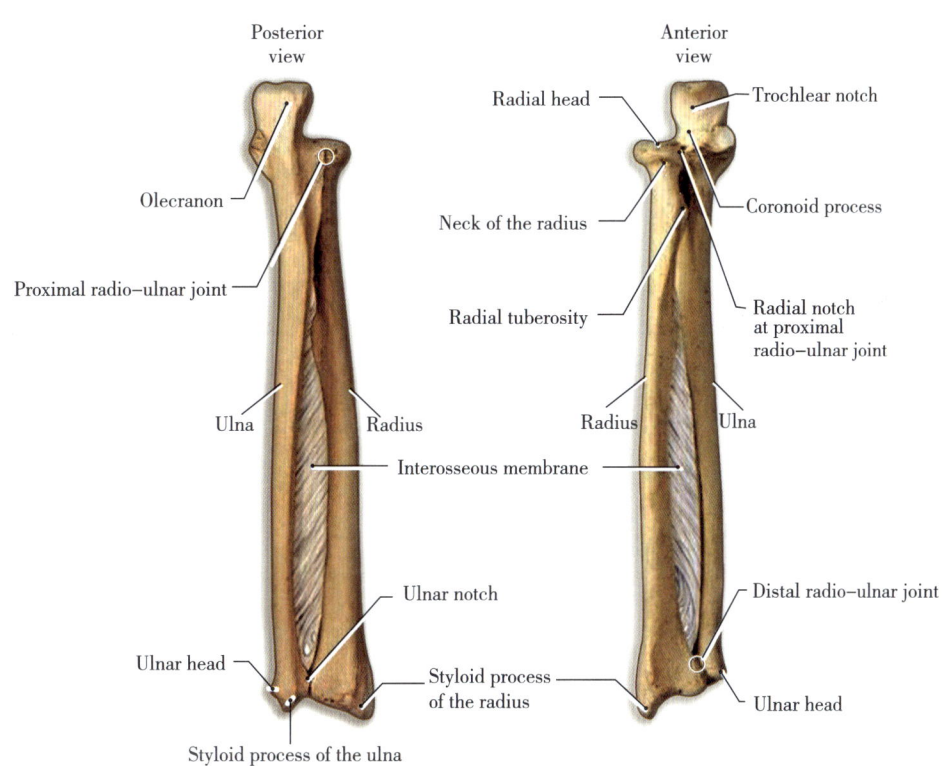

Shaft of radius

✓ The radial shaft expands in diameter as it moves distally. Much like the ulna, it is triangular in shape, with three borders and three surfaces

✓ In the middle of the lateral surface, there is a small roughening for the attachment of the pronator teres muscle

Distal region of radius

✓ In the distal region, the radial shaft expands to form a rectangular end. The lateral side projects distally as the styloid process. In the medial surface, there is a concavity, called the ulnar notch, which articulates with the head of ulna, forming the distal radioulnar joint

✓ The distal surface of the radius has two facets, for articulation with the scaphoid and lunate carpal bones. This makes up the wrist joint

Clinical importance

✓ The forearm is a common site for bone fractures. Here, we shall look at the common fracture types involving the radius

◊ Colles' fracture—the most common type of radial fracture. A fall onto an outstretched hand causing a fracture of the distal radius. The structures distal to the fracture (wrist and hand) are displaced posteriorly. It produces what is known as the "dinner fork deformity"

◊ Fractures of the radial head—this is characteristically due to falling on an outstretched hand. The radial head is forced into the capitulum of humerus, causing it to fracture

◊ Smith's fracture—a fracture caused by falling onto the back of the hand. It is the opposite of a Colles' fracture, as the distal fragment is now placed anteriorly

✓ The radius and the ulna are attached by the interosseous membrane. The force of a trauma to one bone can be transmitted to the other via this membrane. Thus, fractures of both the forearm bones are not uncommon. There are two classical fractures

◊ Monteggia's fracture—usually caused by a force from behind the ulna. The proximal shaft of ulna is fractured, and the head of the radius dislocates anteriorly at the elbow

◊ Galeazzi's fracture—a fracture to the distal radius, with the ulna head dislocating at the distal radio-ulnar joint

Ulna

Description

✓ The ulna is a long bone in the forearm. It lies medially and parallel to the radius, the second of the forearm bones. The ulna acts as the stablising bone, with the radius pivoting to produce movement

✓ Proximally, the ulna articulates with the humerus at the elbow joint. Distally, the ulna articulates with the radius, forming the distal radio-ulnar joint

Important landmarks

Upper part of ulna

✓ The upper portion of the ulna articulates with the trochlea of the humerus. To enable movement at the elbow joint, the ulna has a specialised structure, with bony prominences for muscle attachment

✓ Important landmarks of the proximal ulna are the olecranon, coronoid process, trochlear notch, radial notch and the tuberosity of ulna

◊ Olecranon—a large projection of bone that extends proximally, forming part of trochlear notch. It can be palpated as the "tip" of the elbow. The triceps brachii muscle attaches to its superior surface

◊ Coronoid process—this ridge of bone projects outwards in a anterior manner, forming part of the trochlear notch

◊ Trochlear notch—formed by the olecrannon and coronoid process. It is wrench shaped, and articulates with the trochlea of the humerus

◊ Radial notch—located on the lateral surface of the trochlear notch, this area articulates with the head of the radius

◊ Tuberosity of ulna—an roughening immediately distal of the coronoid process. It is where the brachialis muscle attaches

Shaft of ulna

✓ The ulnar shaft is triangular in shape, with three surfaces and three borders. It is moves distally, it decreases in width

The three surfaces
✓ Anterior—site of attachment for the pronator quadratus muscle distally ✓ Posterior—site of attachment for many muscles ✓ Medial—unremarkable
The three borders
✓ Posterior—palpable along the entire length of the forearm posteriorly ✓ Interosseous—site of attachment for the interosseous membrane, which spans the distance between the two forearm bones ✓ Anterior—unremarkable
Lower part of ulna
✓ The distal end of the ulna is much smaller in diameter that the proximal end. It is mostly unremarkable, terminating in a rounded head, with distal projection—the ulnar styloid process ✓ The head articulates with the ulnar notch of the radius to form the distal radio-ulnar joint
Clinical importance
✓ A fracture of the ulna alone (not involving the radius) usually occurs as a result of the ulna being hit by an object. The shaft is the most likely site of fracture. In this situation, the normal muscle tone will pull the proximal ulna posteriorly ✓ Less commonly, the olecrannon process can be fractured. This is caused by the patient falling on a flexed elbow. The triceps brachii can displace part of the fragment proximally ✓ The ulna and the radius are attached by the interosseous membrane. The force of a trauma to one bone can be transmitted to the other via this membrane. Thus, fractures of both the forearm bones are not uncommon
Hand
Description
✓ The bones of the hand provide support and flexibility to the soft tissues. They can be divided into three categories ◊ Carpal bones (most proximal)—a set of eight irregularly shaped bones. These are located in the wrist area ◊ Metacarpals—there are five metacarpals, each one related to a digit ◊ Phalanges (most distal)—the bones of the fingers. Each finger has three phalanges, except for the thumb, which has two important landmarks
Carpal bones
✓ The carpal bones are a group of eight, irregularly shaped bones. They are organised into two rows—proximal and distal ✓ In the proximal row, the bones are (lateral to medial) as follows: ◊ Scaphoid ◊ Lunate ◊ Triquetrum

- ◊ Pisiform—a sesamoid bone, formed within the tendon of the flexor carpi ulnaris
- ✓ In the distal row, the bones are (lateral to medial) as follows:
    - ◊ Trapesium
    - ◊ Trapezoid
    - ◊ Capitate
    - ◊ Hamate—has a projection on its palmar surface called the hook of hamate
- ✓ Proximally, the scaphoid and lunate articulate with the radius to form the wrist joint. In the distal row, all of the carpal bones articulate with the metacarpals

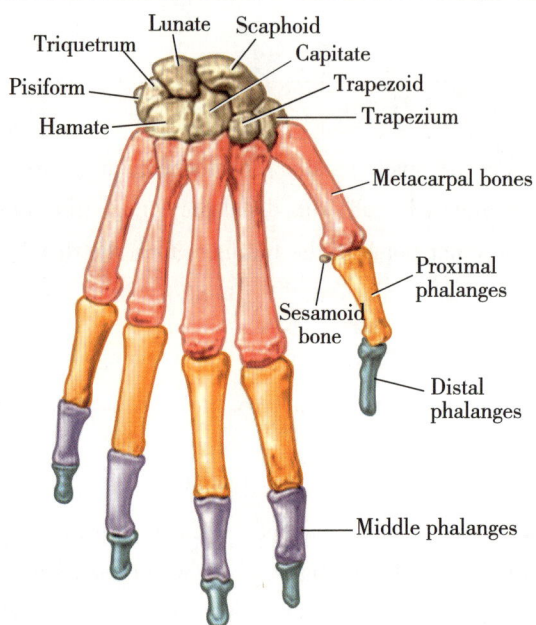

Metacarpal bones

- ✓ The metacarpal bones articulate proximally with the carpals, and distally with the proximal phalanges
- ✓ They are numbered, and each associated with a digit
    - ◊ Metacarpal I—Thumb
    - ◊ Metacarpal II—Index finger
    - ◊ Metacarpal III—Middle finger
    - ◊ Metacarpal IV—Ring finger
    - ◊ Metacarpal V—Little finger
- ✓ Each metacarpal consists of a base, shaft and a head. The medial and lateral surfaces of the metacarpals areconcave, allowing attachment of the interoessei muscles

Phalanges

- ✓ The phalanges are the bones of the fingers. The thumb has a proximal and distal phalanx, while the rest of the digits have proximal, middle and distal phalanges

Clinical importance

Carpals

- ✓ The two carpal bones that are most commonly fractured are the scaphoid and lunate. The most common mechanism of injury in both cases is falling on an outstretched hand

◊ The scaphoid is more commonly fractured. Characteristically there is pain and tenderness in the anatomical snuffbox. A fracture needs to be fixed quickly, as the off the blood supply to the proximal part of the bone can be cut off, causing it to undergo asvascular necrosis. Patients with an undiagnosed scaphoid fracture are very likely to develop wrist arthritis

◊ A lunate fracture occurs when falling on a outstretched hand causes hyperextension at the wrist. It is can be associated with some medial nerve damage

Metacarpals

✓ There are two common fractures of the metacarpals

◊ Boxer's fracture—a fracture of the 5th metacarpal neck. It is usually caused by a clenched fist striking a hard object. The distal part of the fracture is displaced posteriorly, producing shortening of the affected finger

◊ Bennett's fracture—a fracture of the 1st metacarpal base, extending into the carpometacarpal joint. It is caused by hyperabduction of the thumb

6.5.2 Deltoid and scapular region

Muscles of shoulder region						
Muscle	Origin	Insertion	Action	Innervation	Artery	Notes
Deltoid	Lateral one third of the clavicle, acromion, the lower lip of the crest of the spine of the scapula	Deltoid tuberosity of the humerus	Abducts arm; anterior fibers flex and medially rotate the arm; posterior fibers extend and laterally rotate the arm	Axillary nerve (C_5, C_6) from the posterior cord of the brachial plexus	Posterior circumflex humeral artery	The deltoid muscle is the principle abductor of the arm but due to poor mechanical advantage it can not initiate this action; it is assisted by the supraspinatus
Teres major	Dorsal surface of the inferior angle of the scapula	Crest of the lesser tubercle of the humerus	Adducts the arm, medially rotates the arm, assists in arm extension	Lower subscapular nerve (C_5, C_6) from the posterior cord of the brachial plexus	Circumflex scapular artery	Teres major inserts beside the tendon of latissimus dorsi, and assists latissimus in its actions
Triceps brachii	Long head: infraglenoid tubercle of the scapula. Lateral head: posterolateral humerus and lateral intermuscular septum. Medial head: posteromedial surface of the inferior 1/2 of the humerus	Olecranon process of the ulna	Extends the forearm; the long head extends and adducts arm	Radial nerve	Deep brachial (profunda brachii) artery	Long head of the triceps separates the triangular and quadrangular spaces (teres major, teres minor and the humerus are the other boundaries); all three heads of origin insert by a common tendon

Supraspinatus	Supraspinatous fossa	Greater tubercle of the humerus (highest facet)	Abducts the arm (initiates abduction)	Suprascapular nerve (C_5, C_6) from the superior trunk of the brachial plexus	Suprascapular artery	Supraspinatus initiates abduction of the arm, then the deltoid muscle completes the action; a member of the rotator cuff group
Infraspinatus	Infraspinatous fossa	Greater tubercle of the humerus (middle facet)	Laterally rotates the arm	Suprascapular nerve	Suprascapular artery	Infraspinatus, supraspinatus, teres minor and subscapularis are the rotator cuff muscles
Teres minor	Upper 2/3 of the lateral border of the scapula	Greater tubercle of the humerus (lowest facet)	Laterally rotates the arm	Axillary nerve (C_5, C_6) from the posterior cord of the brachial plexus	Circumflex scapular artery	Fixes the head of the humerus in the glenoid fossa during abduction and flexion of the arm; a member of the rotator cuff group
Subscapularis	Medial two thirds of the costal surface of the scapula (subscapular fossa)	Lesser tubercle of the humerus	Medially rotates the arm; assists extention of the arm	Upper and lower subscapular nerves (C_5, C_6)	Subscapular artery	Subscapularis, supraspinatus, infraspinatus, and teres minor are the rotator cuff muscles

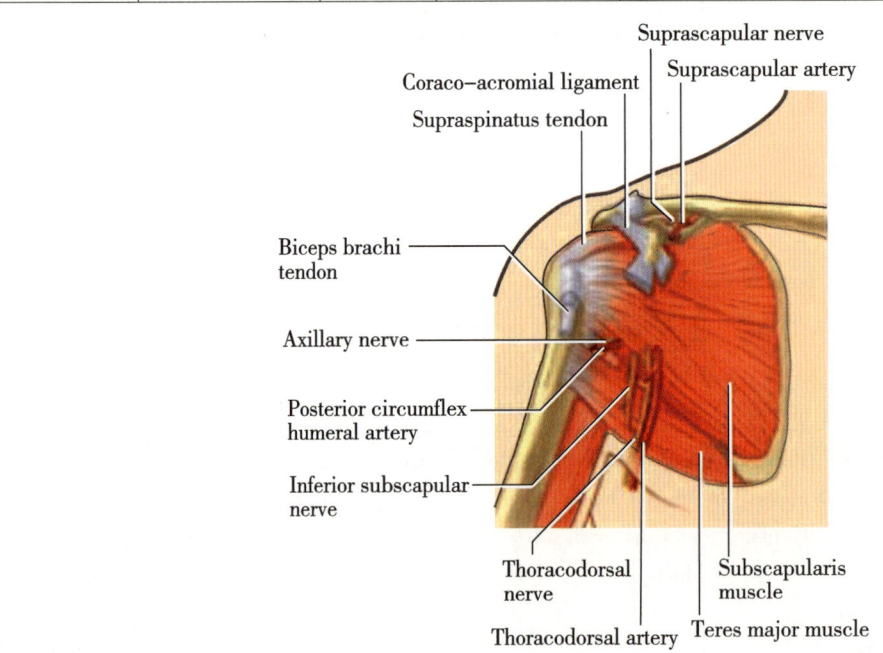

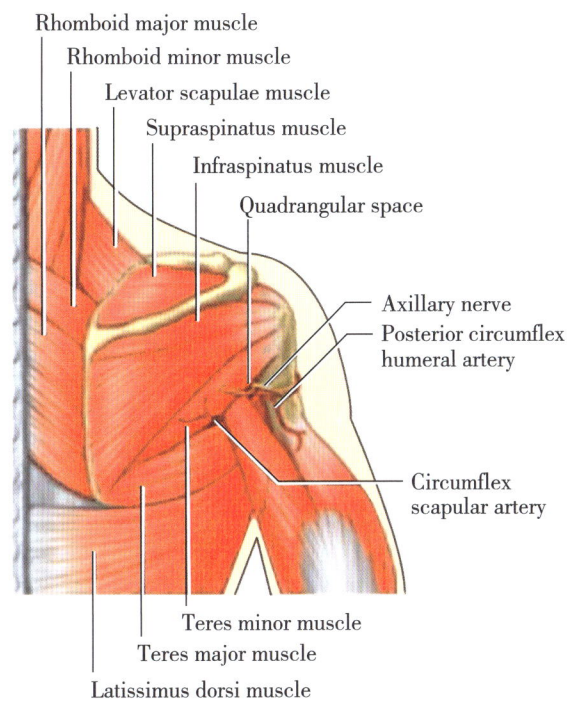

Blood supply of the shoulder

✓ Like the nerves in the shoulder, some of the arteries arise from the neck and some from the axillary region

✓ These vessels form an anastomotic system that establishes a potential alternative route for blood flow between the first part of the subclavian artery in the neck and the third part of the axillary artery before it enters the arm

✓ Circumscapular anastomosis—allows blood to reach the arm if the intervening arterial trunk becomes blocked

Subclavian artery—has four main branches before it becomes the axillary artery

✓ Vertebral artery

✓ Internal thoracic artery—descends posterior to the sternal end of the clavicle to supply the medial aspect of the thorax

✓ Thyrocervical trunk—has four main branches; two are important to the shoulder

◊ Inferior thyroid artery

◊ Ascending cervical artery

◊ Transverse cervical artery

◆ Passes through the trunks of the brachial plexus

◆ Superficial branch passes deep to the trapezius muscle following CN XI (spinal accessory nerve)

◆ Deep branch runs anterior to the rhomboid muscles and often joins with the dorsal scapular nerve

◆ Supplies the levator scapula and rhomboid muscles

◊ Suprascapular artery

• Passes posterior to the scapula above the suprascapular notch

• Supplies the supraspinatus and infraspinatus muscles

- ✓ Costocervical trunk—supplies deep cervical muscles and the first two intercostals spaces (deep cervical a and supreme intercostals artery)
- ✓ Dorsal scapular artery—if present, joins with the dorsal scapular nerve to supply the rhomboid muscles

Axillary artery—continuation of the subclavian artery

Starts at the lateral border of the 1st rib and runs to the inferior border of the teres major where it continues as the brachial artery. The axillary artery can be divided into 3 parts by the pectoralis minor muscle (proximal to, underneath, distal to) and has six branches

- ✓ First part of the axillary artery—runs from the lateral border of the first rib to the medial border of the pectoralis minor muscle and has one branch
  - ♦ Superior (supreme) thoracic artery—supplies muscles in the first two intercostals spaces and anastomoses with intercostals arteries
- ✓ Second part of the axillary artery—located behind the pectoralis minor muscle and has two branches
  - ♦ Thoracoacromial artery—short wide trunk that pierces the clavipectoral fascia and has four branches
    - ◆ Pectoral artery—pectoral muscles
    - ◆ Acromial artery—acromion process
    - ◆ Clavicular artery—clavicle and subclavius
    - ◆ Deltoid artery—deltoid muscle
  - ♦ Lateral thoracic artery—descends along the lateral border of the pectoralis minor muscle and supplies the pectoral muscles, the axillary lymph nodes and the breast
- ✓ Third part of the axillary artery—runs from the lateral border of the pectoralis minor muscle to the inferior border of the teres major muscle and has three branches
  - ♦ Subscapular artery—largest branch of the axillary artery that descends along the lateral border of the scapula and supplies the subscapularis, teres major, serratus anterior and latissimus dorsi muscles. It branches into the circumflex scapular and thoracodorsal arteries
  - ♦ Circumflex scapular artery—courses posteriorly around the lateral border of the scapula and passes between the teres major and subscapularis muscles. Passes through the triangular space to supply muscles of the dorsal surface of the scapula
  - ♦ Thoracodorsal artery—follows the lateral border of the scapula and supplies adjacent muscles, particularly the latissimus dorsi. Participates in the arterial anastomoses around the scapula
    - ◆ Anterior circumflex humeral artery—passes around the surgical neck of the humerus to anastomose with the posterior circumflex humeral artery. Supplies the coracobrachialis and biceps brachii muscles and the shoulder joint.
    - ◆ Posterior circumflex humeral artery—also passes around the surgical neck of the humerus and accompanies the axillary nerve posteriorly through the posterior wall of the axilla via the quadrangular space. Supplies the deltoid, teres major and minor, long head of the triceps as well as the shoulder joint

Chapter 6　The Upper Limb　365

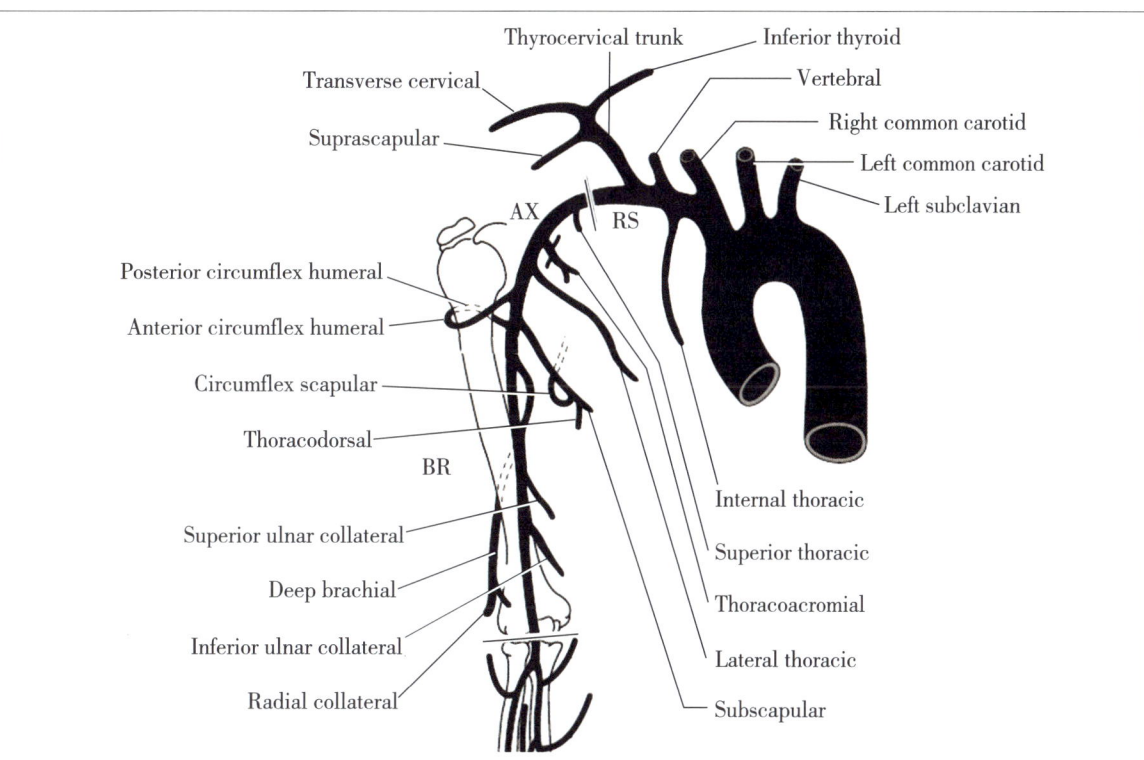

Joints of the shoulder

Acromioclavicular joint (AC joint)

✓ Type of joint—plane, synovial, articular capsule
✓ Movement—allows acromion to rotate on the clavicle during shoulder movements, especially flexion and abduction. Stabilizes movement during superior and inferior rotation of the scapula
✓ Ligaments
　◊ Acromioclavicular
　◊ Coracoclavicular
　　◆ Trapezoid (lateral)
　　◆ Conoid (medial)
　◊ Coracoacromial
✓ Blood supply
　◊ Suprascapular artery
　◊ Thoracoacromial artery—clavicular and acromial brances
✓ Nerve supply (pain and pprioception)
　◊ Supraclavicular nerve (cervical plexus)
　◊ Lateral pectoral nerve
　◊ Axillary nerve

Glenohumeral joint (GH joint)

✓ Type of joint—polyaxial synovial joint, "ball and socket"; fibrous capsule strengthened by ligaments and muscles; synovial membrane lines the fibrous capsule
✓ Glenoid fossa of the scapula—deepened by the glenoid labrum that is fibrocartilage
✓ Movements—flexion, extension, abduction, adduction, medial (internal) rotation, lateral (external) rotation

- ✓ Ligaments
  - ◊ Glenohumeral ligament—strengthens the joint anteriorly; fuses with the fibrous capsule
    - ◆ Superior
    - ◆ Middle
    - ◆ Inferior
  - ◊ Transverse humeral ligament—greater to lesser tubercles; forms canal for the tendon of the long head of the biceps; strengthens the joint anteriorly
  - ◊ Coracohumeral ligament—base of coracoid to greater tubercle of humerus
- ✓ Coracoacromial arch—provides extrinsic support superiorly; prevents superior displacement
  - ◊ Coracoid process
  - ◊ Acromion
  - ◊ Coracoacromial ligament
- ✓ Bursa—padlike sac or cavity found in the connective tissue; lined with synovial membrane; reduces friction between muscle/tendon and bone
  - ◊ Subacromial (deltoid)
  - ◊ Subscapular
- ✓ Blood supply
  - ◊ Anterior circumflex humeral artery
  - ◊ Posterior circumflex humeral artery
  - ◊ Suprascapular artery
- ✓ Nerve supply
  - ◊ Suprascapular nerve
  - ◊ Axillary nerve
  - ◊ Lateral pectoral nerve
- ✓ Joint stability
  - ◊ The shoulder joint is weakest inferiorly and usually dislocates inferiorly or downward—no tendon or ligament support
    - ◊ Superior—supraspinatus, coracoacromial arch
    - ◊ Posterior—infraspinatus, teres minor
    - ◊ Anterior—subscapularis, glenohumeral ligaments
    - ◊ Dislocations are described clinically by radiographs
      - ◆ Anterior—humeral head anterior to the infraglenoid tubercle and in front of the glenoid cavity
      - ◆ Posterior—humeral head posterior to the infraglenoid tubercle and lies in back of the glenoid cavity

Quadrangular space

- ✓ Borders
  - ◊ Upper—teres minor
  - ◊ Medial—long head of the triceps brachii
  - ◊ Lateral—shaft of the humerus
  - ◊ Lower—teres major
- ✓ Contents
  - ◊ Posterior circumflex humeral artery
  - ◊ Axillary nerve

Axillary nerve injuries

- ✓ Etiology
  - ↪ Fracture of the neck of the humerus
  - ↪ Dislocation of the glenohumeral joint
  - ↪ Entrapment in the quadrangular space
- ✓ Clinical findings
  - ↪ Loss of motor function of the deltoid and teres minor
  - ↪ Loss of sensory function to the skin over the lateral shoulder (superior lateral cutaneous nerve of the arm)

Triangular space

- ✓ Borders
  - ↪ Teres minor
  - ↪ Teres major
  - ↪ Long head of the triceps brachii
- ✓ Contents
  - ↪ Circumflex scapular artery

Blood supply of the scapula

Collateral circulation—anastomoses for blood supply to the scapula. These collateral pathways are important when the axillary or subclavian artery is ligated. Ligation of the axillary artery distal to the subscapular artery and proximal to the deep artery of the arm (profunda brachii) is dangerous as collateral circulation is inadequate

Arteries

- ✓ Suprascapular artery
- ✓ Circumflex scapular artery (subscapular artery)
- ✓ Transverse cervical artery/dorsal scapular artery
- ✓ Intercostal arteries

Dissections of scapular region

Surface anatomy of shoulder region

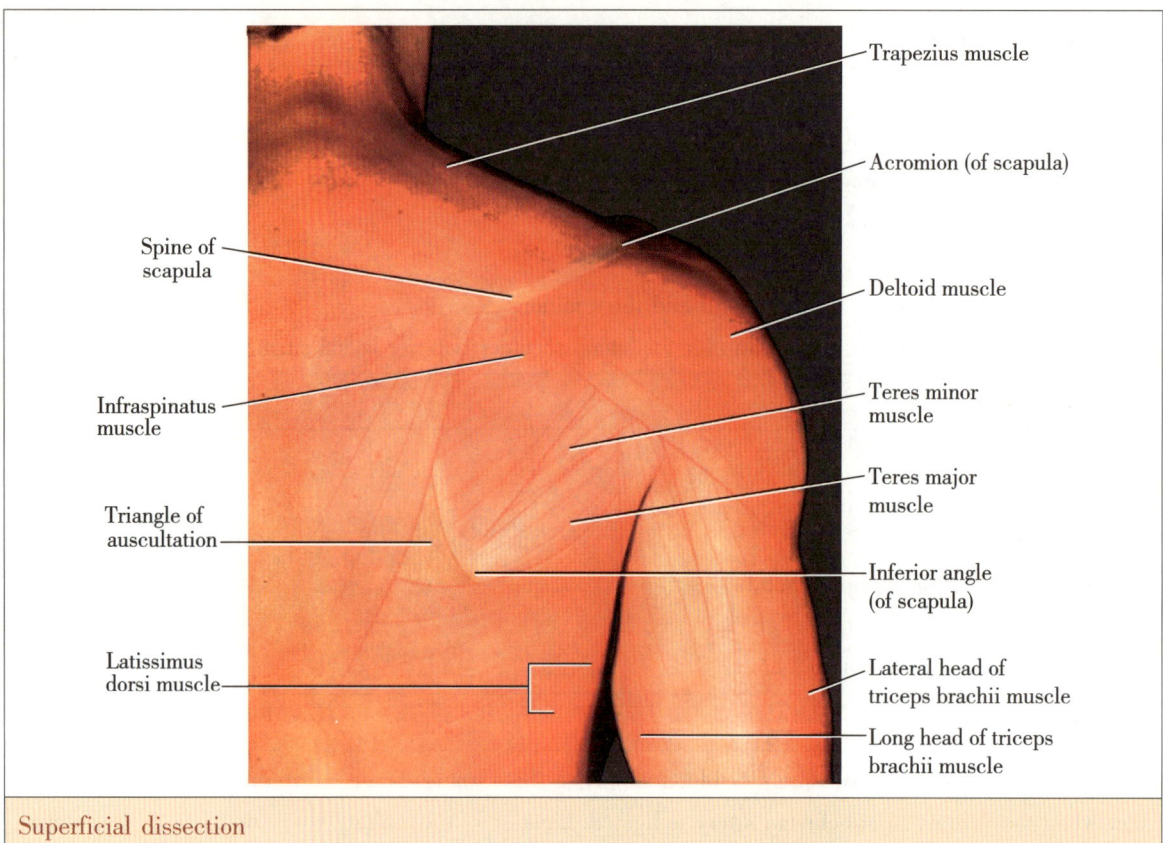

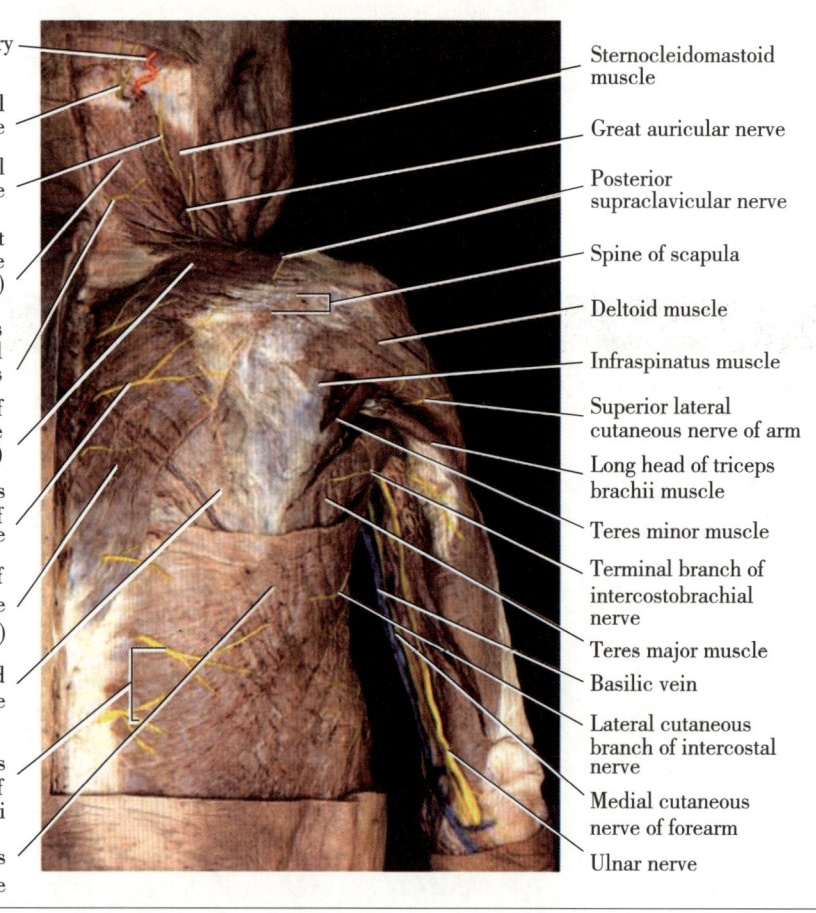

Superficial dissection

Intermediate dissection

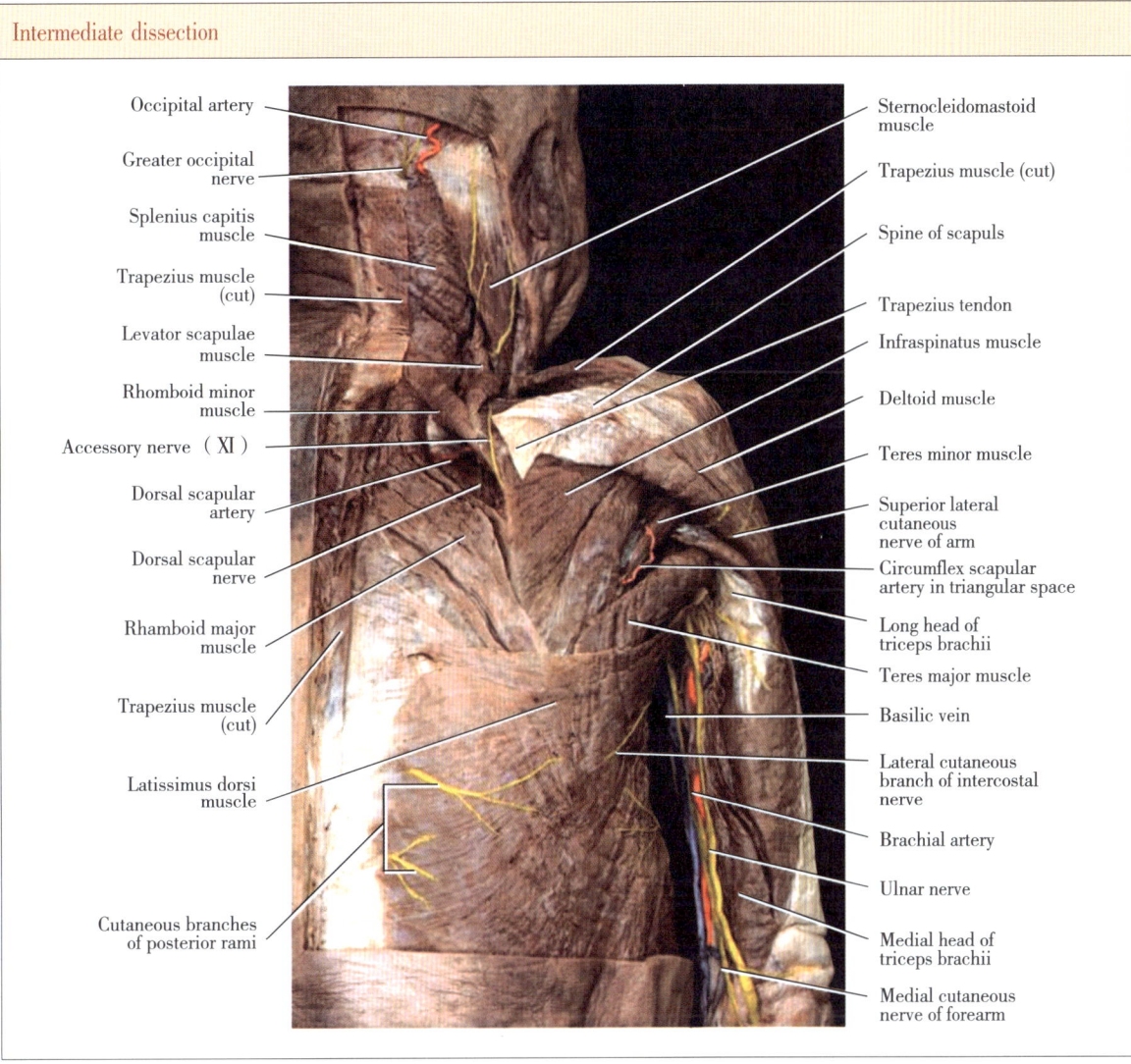

Deep dissection

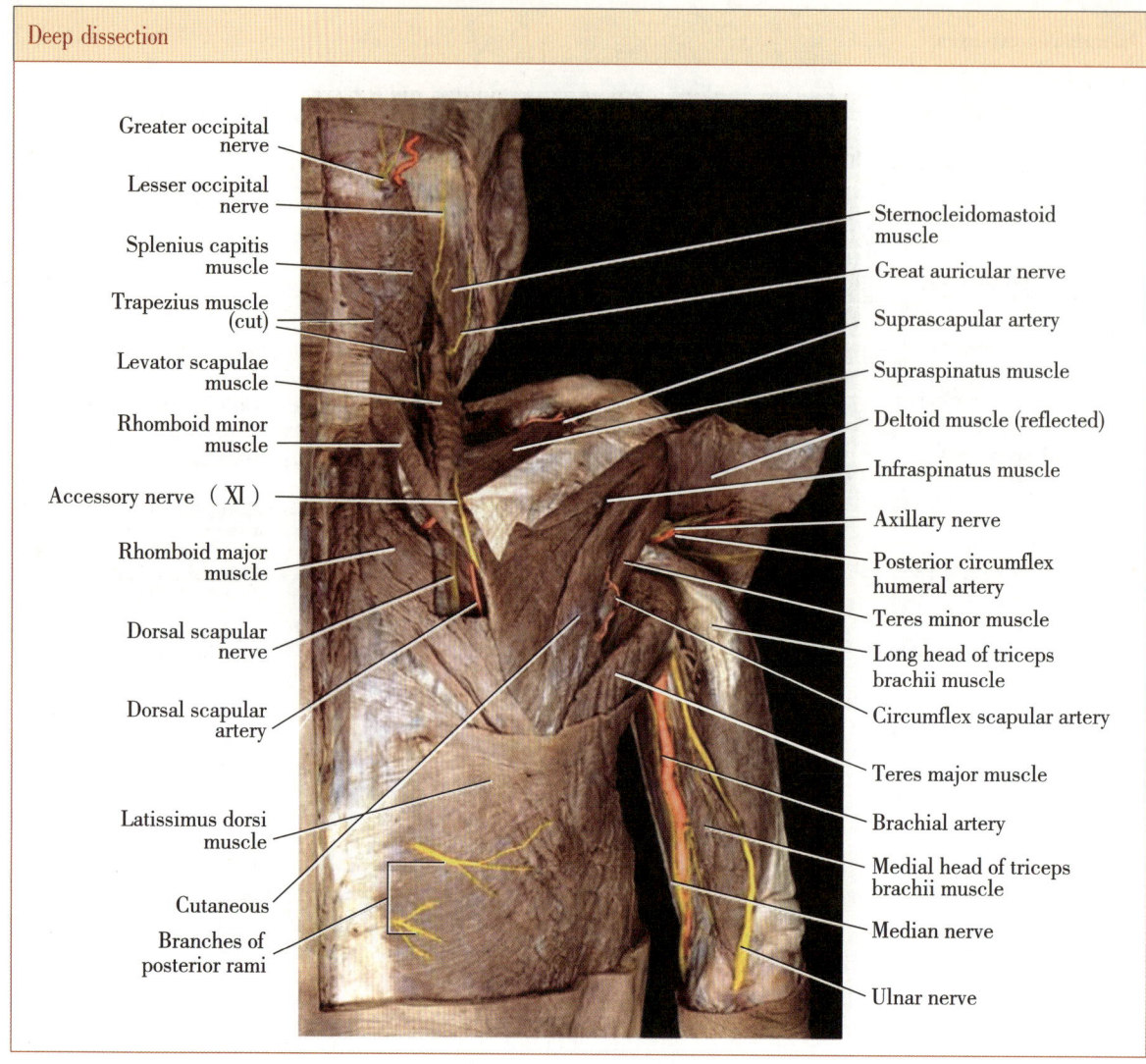

6.5.3 Arm and elbow

Overview

The arm

✓ Consists of the following

◊ 1 bone—humerus

◊ 2 muscle compartments

♦ Anterior compartment—innervated by the musculocutaneous nerve (C_5–C_6 to the motor components has some C_7 involved with the sensory component of the lateral cutaneous nerve of the forearm)

♦ Posterior compartment—innervated by the radial nerve (C_6–C_8)

◊ Blood supply—main blood supply is derived from branches of the deep artery of the arm (profunda brachii artery), with some contributions from the brachial artery

◊ Medial nerve

◊ Ulnar nerve

The elbow

✓ Consists of the following
  ◊ 3 bones—humerus, ulna, and radius
  ◊ Cubital fossa—a triangular region located on the volar surface of the elbow
  ◊ Common forearm flexor attachment—the medial epicondyle, where many of the forearm flexors attach (more detail later)
  ◊ Common forearm extensor attachment—the lateral epicondyle, where many of the forearm extensors attach (more detail later)
  ◊ The elbow's circulation is characterized by an extensive anastomosis (more detail later)
  ◊ Hilton's law—states that the nerves supplying a joint also supply the muscles moving the joint or the skin covering their attachments. Therefore, knowing muscles that cross the elbow provides information about the innervation of the joint and the skin of the region of the elbow (more detail later)

Surfaces—anterior and posterior

✓ Borders—medial and lateral
✓ Arm—1 bone, the humerus
✓ Forearm—2 bones, the radius and ulna
✓ Elbow—posterior aspect
✓ Cubital fossa—anterior aspect
✓ Forearm descriptions typically use the radial and ulnar border, since the forearm is so easily manipulated in space
✓ Carrying angle—the angle made by the intersection of the long axis of the arm and forearm. It is normally 10°–15° in men, and greater than 15° in women. The greater carrying angle in women is associated with the typically wider pelvis, that assists with moving the forearm away from the body when carrying heavy items

Muscle groups and fascia

✓ Muscle groups—arm
  ◊ Flexor compartment of the arm—anterior compartment
  ◊ Extensor compartment of the arm—posterior compartment
✓ Fascia
  ◊ Superficial fascia of the arm—brachial fascia, that consists of loose areolar tissue and variable amount of fat
  ◊ Deep fascia of the arm—brachial fascia, that consists of dense connective tissue, and two thickenings: ①lateral septa; ②medial septa. These two septa are boundaries that form the compartments of the arm

Dermatomes

✓ An area of skin supplied by one spinal root level, e.g., C_5
  ◊ Dermatomes overlap considerably which means that the loss of one spinal cord level (nerve root), usually does not result in the complete loss of sensation for that strip of skin. Typically, three adjacent spinal cord levels must be lost before a significant sensory deficit is apparent (but, loss of one level often results in some diminishment of sensation or an odd sensation in the affected dermatome)
  ◊ Dermatomes of the upper extremity: C_3, C_4, C_5, C_6, C_7, C_8, T_1

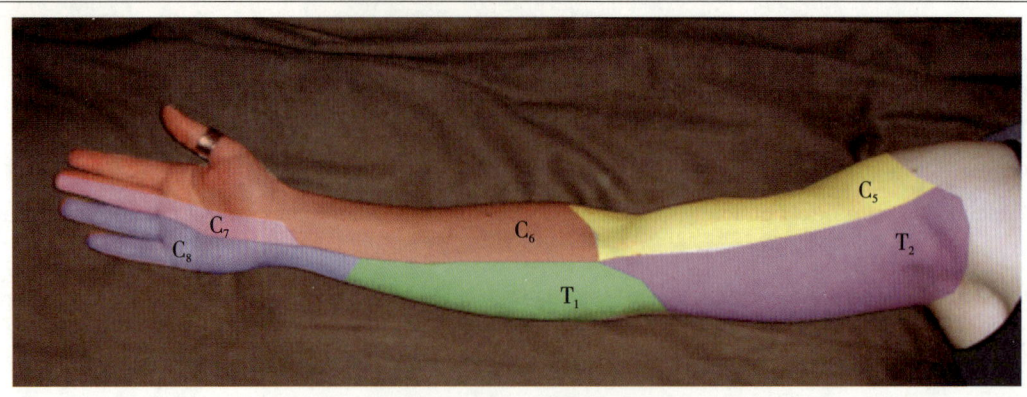

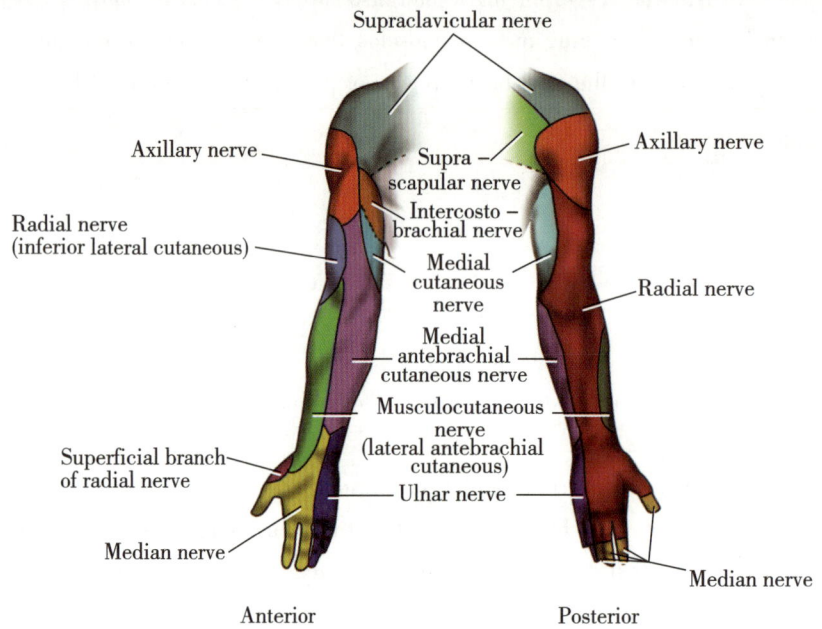

Peripheral nerve cutaneous innervation

✓ This is the region of skin innervated by a named peripheral nerve. Sensory deficits that are associated with the following peripheral nerves when injured occur within the upper extremity [thus not at the level of the nerve root exiting the foramina in the neck (between two adjacent vertebrae)], and typically have a different pattern than the dermatomes

✓ Peripheral cutaneous nerves of the upper extremity

♢ Supraclavicular nerve

♢ Axillary nerve—superior lateral cutaneous

♢ Radial nerve—three components: inferior lateral cutaneous, posterior cutaneous nerve of the forearm, and superficial radial nerve

♢ Medial cutaneous nerve of the arm (brachial cutaneous nerve) and medial cutaneous nerve of the forearm (antebrachial cutaneous nerve)—these both are direct branches from the medial cord of the brachial plexus

♢ Lateral cutaneous nerve of the forearm (lateral antebrachial cutaneous nerve)—the sensory component that is the continuation of the musculocutaneous nerve

◊ Medial nerve

◊ Ulnar nerve

Superficial veins

✓ Cephalic vein (found laterally in the forearm and arm, between the deltoid and pectoralis major)

◊ Pierces the clavipectoral fascia

◊ Empties into the axillary vein

✓ Basilic (found on the medial side of the arm)

◊ Ulnar side of forearm

◊ Pierces brachial fascia and ascends in anterior compartment of arm and empties into axillary vein

Muscles of the anterior compartment

✓ Coracobrachialis muscle

◊ Origin—tip of coracoid process

◊ Insertion—middle 1/3 of medial surface of humerus

◊ Action—flexion and adduction of the arm (affects the glenohumeral joint)

◊ Nerve—musculocutaneous (C_5–C_6)(C_7)

✓ Brachialis muscle

◊ Origin—distal 1/2 of anterior surface of the humerus

◊ Insertion—coronoid process and tuberosity of the ulna

◊ Action–forearm flexion (elbow)—most important flexor of the elbow, regardless of the position of the forearm ("workhorse" of the motion of elbow flexion)

◊ Nerve—musculocutaneous (C_5–C_6)(C_7)

✓ Biceps brachii muscle—as its name implies, it has two heads

◊ Origin

◆ Short head—tip of coracoid process of scapula

◆ Long head—supraglenoid tubercle of the scapula—from this point, the tendon passes through the glenohumeral joint, is surrounded by synovial membrane, and traverses the intertubercular groove (the position of the tendon is maintained in this groove by the transverse humeral ligament)

◊ Insertion—into the tuberosity of the radius and the fascia of the forearm via the bicipital aponeurosis

◊ Action—supinates foream and, when it is supinated, flexes the forearm (supinating a pronated forearm is the primary action of the biceps brachii)

◊ Nerve—musculocutaneous [C_5–C_6(C_7)]

◊ MSR—biceps reflex, C_5 primarily (C_5–C_6)

Muscles of the posterior compartment

✓ Triceps brachii muscle

◊ Origin

◆ Long head—infraglenoid tubercle of scapula

◆ Lateral head—posterior surface of humerus, superior to the radial groove

◆ Medial head—posterior surface of humerus, inferior to the radial groove. This is the true counterpart of the brachialis muscle, and it is active with all voluntary elbow extensions

◊ Insertion—proximal end of olecranon and fascia of the forearm

◊ Action—forearm extension (the elbow). The medial head is always active and the lateral and long heads provide additional power

◊ Nerve—radial (C_6–C_8)

◊ MSR—C_7 primarily (C_7–C_8)

✓ Anconeus muscle

◊ Origin—lateral epicondyle of the humerus

◊ Insertion—lateral side of the olecranon and superior part of the posterior surface of the ulna

◊ Action—forearm extension and stabilization of the joint

◊ Nerve—radial (C_7–T_1)

Muscle	Origin	Insertion	Action	Innervation	Artery	Notes
Anconeus	Lateral epicondyle of the humerus	Lateral side of the olecranon and the upper 1/4 of the ulna	Extends the forearm	Nerve to anconeus, from the radial nerve	Interosseous recurrent artery	None
Biceps brachii	Short head: tip of the coracoid process of the scapula. Long head: supraglenoid tubercle of the scapula	Tuberosity of the radius	Flexes the forearm, flexes arm (long head), supinates	Musculocutaneous nerve (C_5–C_6)	Brachial artery	A powerful supinator when the elbow is flexed; the bicipital aponeurosis, a membranous extension of the biceps brachii tendon, extends across the cubital fossa and protects the structures located there
Brachialis	Anterior surface of the lower one-half of the humerus and the associated intermuscular septa	Coronoid process of the ulna	Flexes the forearm	Musculocutaneous nerve (C_5–C_6)	Brachial artery, radial recurrent artery	A powerful flexor

Coracobra-chialis	Coracoid process of the scapula	Medial side of the humerus at mid-shaft	Flexes and adducts the arm	Musculocutaneous nerve (C_5–C_6)	Brachial artery	The musculocutaneous nerve usually passes through the coracobrachialis muscle to reach the other arm flexor muscles (biceps brachii and brachialis)
Triceps brachii	Long head: infraglenoid tubercle of the scapula. Lateral head: posterolateral humerus and lateral intermuscular septum. Medial head: posteromedial surface of the inferior 1/2 of the humerus	Olecranon process of the ulna	Extends the forearm; the long head extends and adducts arm	Radial nerve	Deep brachial (profunda brachii) artery	Long head of the triceps separates the triangular and quadrangular spaces (teres major, teres minor and the humerus are the other boundaries); all three heads of origin insert by a common tendon

Nerves of the anterior compartment of the arm

✓ Musculocutaneous nerve [C_5–C_6(C_7)] —the nerve of elbow flexion, forearm supination, and it provides the sensation for the lateral aspect of the forearm, once it emerges distally under the cover of the biceps brachii muscle (lateral cutaneous nerve of the forearm)

◊ Medial nerve (C_5–T_1)—Proximally, located anterolateral to brachial artery in the arm, but becomes medial to the brachial artery in the cubital fossa. Sends a branch to the pronator teres muscles (passes through the two heads of the pronator teres), and enters the flexor compartment of the wrist and hand. Provides sensation to the thumb, index, middle and 1/2 of the ring finger (palmar surface and tips of those fingers dorsally)

◊ Ulnar nerve [(C_7)C_8–T_1]—located posteromedial to the brachial artery in the arm. At a point approximately 1/2 way down the arm, the nerve pierces the medial intramuscular septum, then travels in the posterior compartment of the arm, passing behind (under) the medial epicondyle of the humerus (ulnar groove), into the forearm. This nerve will supply two muscles in the forearm and be the predominant nerve supply to the intrinsics in the hand. The ulnar nerve supplies sensation to both the palmar and dorsal surfaces of the little finger and the ulnar half of the ring finger

◊ Radial nerve (C_5–T_1)—in the proximal arm, the radial nerve is located posterior to the brachial artery. Below the teres major, the radial nerve enters the posterior compartment [along with the accompanying deep artery of the arm (profunda brachii artery)], then passes between the lateral and medial heads of the triceps (lies in the radial groove directly on the humerus). Ultimately, the radial nerve spirals around and pierces the lateral intramuscular septum to lie in the anterior compartment of the arm, just proximal to the elbow. In the region of the lateral epicondyle, the radial nerve divides into two branches that enter the forearm: ① superficial radial nerve (sensory only), that supplies sensation to the dorsum of the thumb, index, middle and 1/2 of the ring finger, except for the tips (supplied by the medial nerve); ② the deep radial nerve (posterior interosseous nerve after passing through the supinator), that innervates the extensors of the forearm

Chinical notes: Since the radial nerve lies directly on the humerus for a portion of its course, it is more vulnerable to injury with fractures of the humerus

Nerve	Source	Branches	Motor	Sensory	Notes
Musculocutaneous nerve	Lateral cord of the brachial plexus	Lateral antebrachial cutaneous nerve	Coracobrachialis muscle, biceps brachii muscle, brachialis muscle	Skin of the lateral side of the forearm	Musculocutaneous nerve usually passes through the coracobrachialis muscle
Radial nerve	Posterior cord of the brachial plexus	Posterior brachial cutaneous nerve, inferior lateral brachial cutaneous nerve, posterior antebrachial cutaneous nerve, superficial and deep branches	Muscles of the posterior arm: triceps brachii muscle, anconeus muscle. Muscles of the posterior forearm: brachioradialis, extensor carpi ulnaris muscle, extensor carpi radialis longus muscle, extensor carpi radialis brevis muscle, extensor digitorum muscle, extensor digiti minimi muscle, supinator muscle, abductor pollicis longus muscle, extensor pollicis longus muscle, extensor pollicis brevis muscle, extensor indicis muscle	Skin of the posterior arm, forearm and hand	All of the muscles on the posterior side of the arm and forearm are innervated by the radial nerve

The brachial artery

✓ It is the direct continuation of the axillary artery (name changes to the brachial as the artery passes the lower border of the teres major). During its course through the arm, the brachial artery lies on the coracobrachialis and brachialis muscles

✓ Terminates in the cubital fossa, dividing into the two major arteries of the forearm: the radial and ulnar arteries

✓ Major branch is the deep artery of the arm (profunda brachii artery) (that travels with the radial nerve). This is the chief source of blood supply to the arm, with branches to the humerus, branches contributing to the anastamoses of the shoulder and elbow. Named branches that stem off of the deep artery of the arm (profunda brachii artery) include:

◊ Radial collateral artery

◊ Middle collateral artery

◊ Superior ulnar collateral artery (arises in the middle of the arm and travels with the ulnar nerve)

◊ Inferior ulnar collateral artery (arises above the elbow, and provides an anastomosis with the posterior and anterior recurrent arteries (from the ulnar artery). This network assists with blood flow around the elbow

Artery	Source	Branches	Supply to	Notes
Anterior circumflex humeral	Axillary artery, 3rd part	Unnamed muscular branches	Deltoid muscle; arm muscles near the surgical neck of the humerus	Anterior circumflex humeral artery anastomoses with the posterior circumflex humeral artery
Posterior circumflex humeral	Axillary artery, 3rd part	Unnamed muscular branches	Deltoid muscle; arm muscles near the surgical neck of the humerus	Posterior circumflex humeral artery anastomoses with the anterior circumflex humeral artery; it passes through the quadrangular space with the axillary nerve
Brachial	Axillary artery (brachial artery is the continuation of the axillary artery distal to the teres major muscle)	Deep brachial artery, superior ulnar collateral artery, nutrient artery, inferior ulnar collateral artery; terminal branches are the radial artery and the ulnar artery	Arm, forearm and hand	Brachial artery normally terminates by branching within the cubital fossa, but high branching may occur

Brachial, deep	Brachial artery	Ascending branch; terminal branches are the middle collateral artery and radial collateral artery	Muscles and tissues of the posterior compartment of the arm	Deep brachial artery spirals around the shaft of the humerus in the radial groove where it is susceptible to injury in mid-shaft fractures
Collateral, inferior ulnar	Brachial artery	Unnamed muscular branches	Lower medial arm	Anastomoses with the anterior ulnar recurrent artery
Collateral, middle	Deep brachial artery	Unnamed muscular branches	Medial head of triceps, anconeus	Anastomoses with the interosseous recurrent artery
Collateral, radial	Deep brachial artery	Unnamed muscular branches	Lower lateral arm	Travels with the radial nerve; anastomoses with the radial recurrent artery
Collateral, superior ulnar	Brachial artery	Unnamed muscular branches	Medial arm muscles	Travels with the ulnar nerve; anastomoses with posterior ulnar recurrent artery

The brachial veins

✓ The brachial veins are deep veins (collect blood from deep tissue), paired, and they ascend one on each side of the brachial artery
✓ They are derived from the union of the radial and ulnar veins, returning blood from the forearm
✓ The brachial veins terminate proximally into the axillary vein

The cubital fossa

✓ The cubital fossa is a space in the anterior aspect of the elbow that contains all the major nerves and vessels, except for the ulnar artery (that does not pass through this space since it passes posterior to the medial epicondyle of the humerus)
✓ Boundaries
  ♦ Floor—brachialis muscle
  ♦ Roof—antebrachial fascia
  ♦ Medial boundary—pronator teres
  ♦ Lateral boundary—brachioradialis muscle
✓ Contents of the cubital fossa
  ♦ Biceps tendon
  ♦ Brachial artery (and beginning bifurcation of the ulnar and radial arteries)
  ♦ Medial nerve [that may give off a branch (anterior interosseous nerve), while still in the cubital fossa]
  ♦ Radial nerve (with both the superficial and deep components)
  ♦ Basilic and cephalic veins

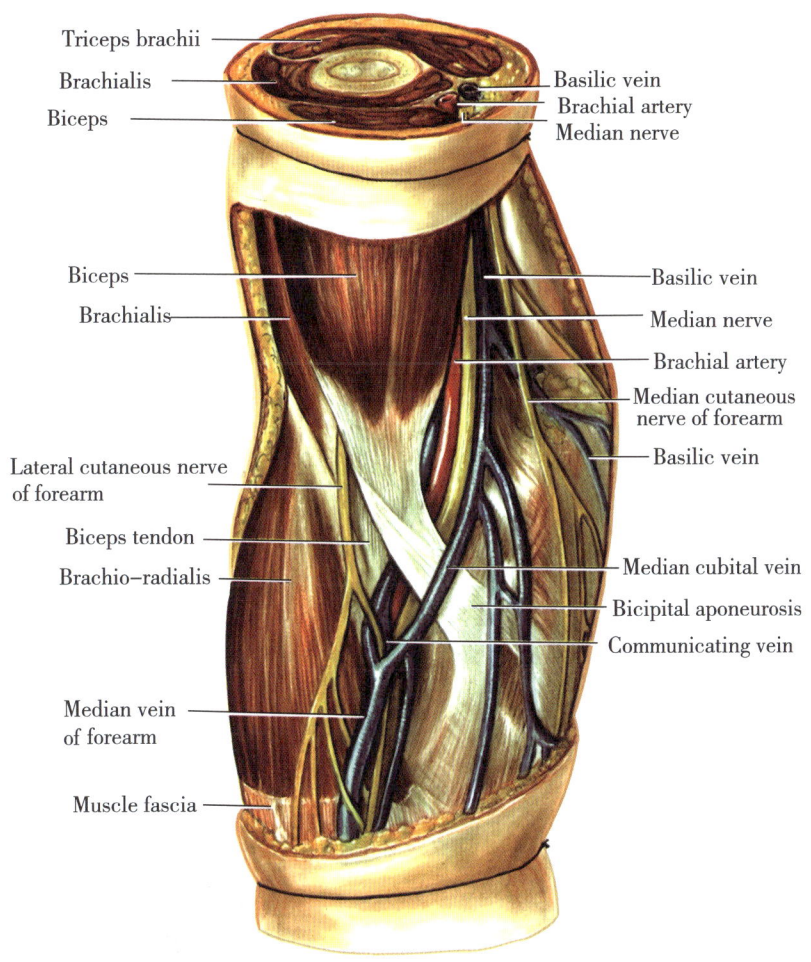

The elbow joint

✓ A compound synovial joint
✓ Has two bones: the radius and the ulna, both articulate with the humerus bone
✓ Characteristics of the elbow joint
  ▷ The joint cavity is continuous with that of the proximal radioulnar joint (thus, a single capsule)
  ▷ The joint between the humerus and the ulna is a uniaxial hinge joint, permitting only flexion and extension
✓ Elbow joint articular surfaces
  ▷ Proximally, the articular surfaces consist of the capitulum of the humerus and the trochlea of the humerus
  ▷ Distally, the articular surfaces consist of the head of the radius and the trochlear notch of the ulna
  ▷ In the anatomical position, the humeroradial joint is located laterally, and the humeroulnar joint is located medially
✓ Elbow joint—capsule, ligaments and bursae
  ▷ Articular capsule
    ◆ Thin, anteriorly and posteriorly
    ◆ Reinforced by collateral ligaments

◊ Ligaments—most of these are thickenings of the joint capsule and are difficult to visualize as discrete ligaments during dissection, particularly on the medial side of the joint
  ◆ Annular ligament (ring ligament)—passes from the radial notch around the head of the radius
  ◆ Ulnar collateral ligament—from the medial epicondyle to the olecranon process, to the coronoid process (often identified as having three parts: anterior, posterior, and oblique band)
  ◆ Radial collateral ligament—from the lateral epicondyle and blends with the annular ligament
◊ Bursae—subcutaneous olecranon bursae

Elbow joint movements

✓ Flexion—made possible by the following:
  ◊ Brachialis
  ◊ Biceps brachii
  ◊ Brachioradialis
  ◊ Wrist and hand flexors [and extensor (brachioradialis)], that cross the elbow joint (i.e., forearm flexors that insert into the common flexor tendon, and forearm extensors that insert into the common extensor tendon that pass anterior to the axis of the elbow joint)

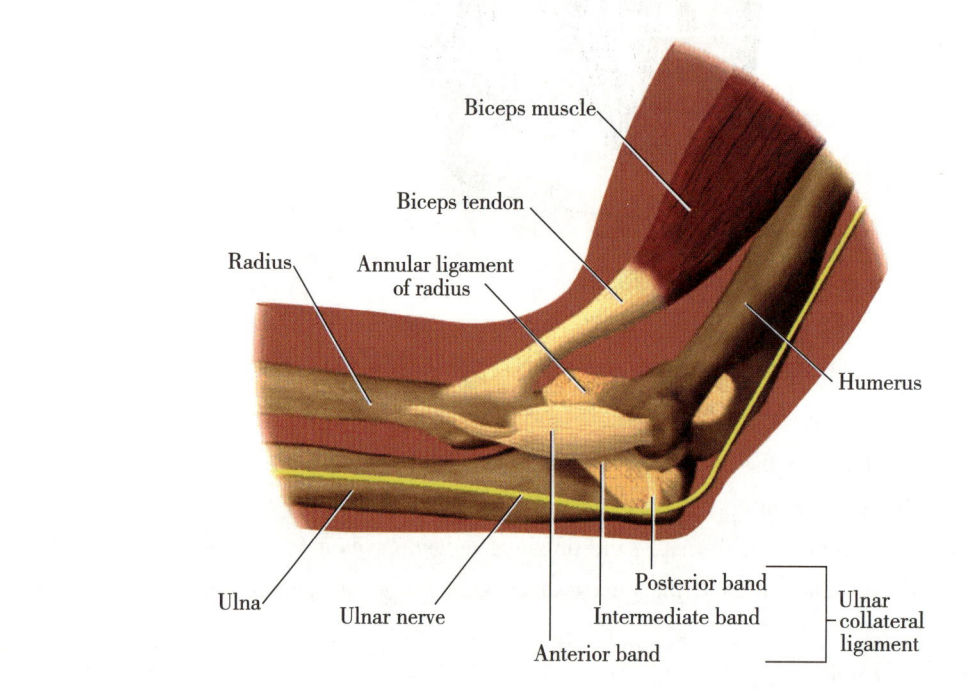

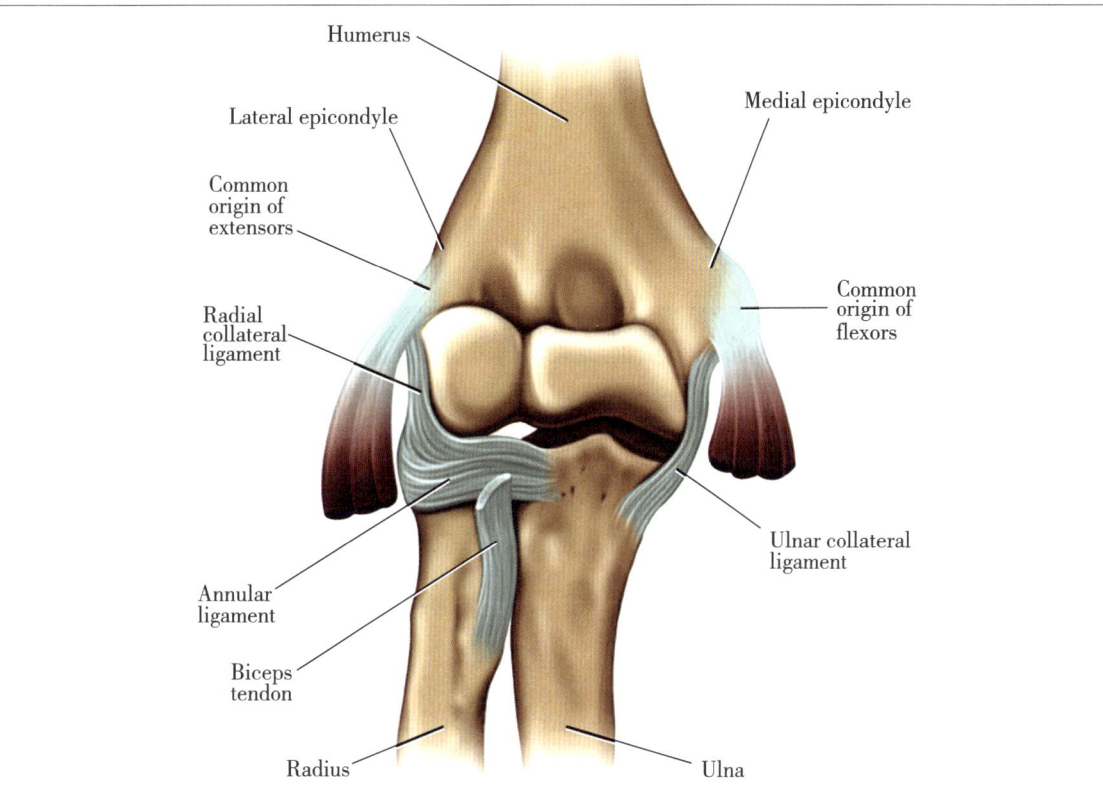

- ✓ Extension—made possible by the following:
  - ◊ Triceps brachii
  - ◊ Anconeus
  - ◊ Wrist and hand extensors (that insert into the common extensor tendon)

Elbow joint nerve supply

- ✓ Via Hilton's Law, four nerves supply the joint
  - ◊ Musculocutaneous nerve (anteriorly)
  - ◊ Medial nerve (anteriorly)
  - ◊ Radial nerve (posteriorly)
  - ◊ Ulnar nerve (posteriorly)

Elbow joint circulation

✓ Deep artery of the arm (profunda brachii artery) and its branches, the radial collateral artery and the middle collateral artery
✓ Brachial artery and its branches, the superior ulnar collateral artery and the inferior ulnar collateral artery
✓ Ulnar artery, with branches that pass back into the elbow via the anterior ulnar recurrent artery, the posterior ulnar recurrent artery, and the interosseous recurrent artery
✓ Radial artery, receives the radial recurrent artery
✓ Anastomoses and collateral circulation—rich anastomosis for the elbow joint

Chinical notes: Due the number of arteries and nerves in the region of the elbow joint, a serious injury to this joint can also result in a neurovascular injury

Other clinical correlations
✓ Elbow injury in children—subluxation of the radial head ✓ Dislocation of the elbow joint ✓ Elbow fractures

6.5.4 Forearm and hand

Anterior compartment of forearm and palmar aspect of hand		
Fasciae of anterior compartment		
Structure	Location/description	Notes
Fascia, antebrachial	Deep fascia which forms a tubular investment of the forearm muscles	Antebrachial fascia is attached to the radius via the lateral intermuscular septum; it is attached to the subcutaneous border of the ulna
Flexor retinaculum	A thickening of the deep fascia on the ventral surface of the wrist	Flexor retinaculum spans the ventral surfaces of the carpal bones (medially – scaphoid and trapezium; laterally – hamate and pisiform) to complete an osseofibrous tunnel for passage of the flexor tendons; tendons are surrounded by synovial tendon sheathes where they pass deep to retinacula
Palmar carpal ligament	A thickening of the antebrachial fascia on the ventral surface of the wrist	Palmar carpal ligament is a retinaculum that supports the tendons of the superficial flexor muscles; it is superficial and proximal to the flexor retinaculum of the wrist
Muscles/actions of anterior compartment		
✓ Ensheathed within antebrachial fascia		
Superficial flexor compartment		
✓ Common origin—medial epicondyle tendon		
Muscles lateral to medial		
Pronator teres muscle		
✓ Origin: 2 heads (common flexor tendon, coronoid process) ✓ Insertion: on middle shaft of radius ✓ Innervation: medial nerve passes between 2 heads and innervates this muscle ✓ Actions: pronator of forearm (speed and power); flexor of elbow joint		
Flexor carpi radialis muscle		
✓ Origin: common flexor tendon ✓ Passes through radial side of the transverse carpal ligament through a groove of the trapezium ✓ Insertion: base of 2nd, 3rd metacarpal ✓ Innervation: medial nerve ✓ Action: flexes carpals, abducts wrist ✓ Serves as a guide to radial artery—artery is lateral		

Palmaris longus muscle
✓ Origin: medial epicondyle if present, check this at the wrist on yourself ✓ Absent 13% of the time ✓ Insertion: palmar aponeurosis ✓ Innervation: medial nerve ✓ Action: literally helps you get a grip on things ✓ If tendon is present, the medial nerve is lateral to it
Flexor carpi ulnaris muscle
✓ Origin: medial epicondyle, medial border of ulna ✓ Insertion: pisiform, hamate, 5th metacarpal ✓ Innervation: ulnar nerve ✓ Action: flexes wrist, adducts wrist ✓ Compression neuropathy can occur between 2 heads of origin
Intermediate anterior compartment
Flexor digitorum superficialis muscle

✓ Origin
    ◊ Humeroulnar and radius connected by fibrous arch
    ◊ Common tendon of medial epicondyle of humerus
    ◊ Medial border of coronoid process of ulna
    ◊ Fibrous arch can cause a compression neuropathy
    ◊ Forms tendons 3 and 4 (superficial), 2 and 5 (deep)
    ◊ Passes distally through carpal tunnel
    ◊ Tendons split around deep flexor tendon at proximal phalanx
✓ Insertion: middle phalanx of digits
✓ Innervation: medial nerve
✓ Actions: flexes at the wrist, MP joint, PIP joint but not DIP joint

Deep anterior compartment (muscles lateral to medial)
Flexor pollicis longus
✓ Origin: anterior surface of radius and interosseus muscle ✓ Insertion: base of distal phalanx of pollex ✓ Innervation: anterior interosseus nerve (branch of medial nerve) ✓ Function: flexes MP joint, DIP of thumb
Flexor digitorum profundus
✓ Origin: arises from ulna, common aponeurosis with flexor carp ulnaris, interosseus membrane ✓ 4 discrete tendons, all lined in a row, pass through carpal tunnel at the wrist ✓ Insertion: distal phalanges 2-5

- ✓ Gives rise to 4 lumbrical muscles on radial side of tendons
- ✓ Dual innervation
    - ◊ 2 medial tendons—ulnar nerve
    - ◊ 2 lateral tendons—anterior interosseus branch of medial nerve
- ✓ Action
    - ◊ Flexes wrist, MP and 2 IP joints
    - ◊ Only flexor of DIP joint

Pronator quadratus muscle

- ✓ Name tells you its shape
- ✓ Origin: distal 1/4 of ulna, insertion—radius
- ✓ Function: initiates pronation of the forearm at the radioulnar joints and is the prime pronator
- ✓ Note: pronators are weaker than supinators (biceps, supinator muscle)
- ✓ Innervation: anterior interosseus nerve/medial nerve

Summary of the muscles in the anterior compartment

- ✓ All muscles are supplies by the medial and ulnar nerves except the brachioradialis
- ✓ Long flexors of the digits (FDS and FDP) also flex the metacarpophalangeal and wrist joints
- ✓ FDP flexes the digits in slow actions, but when speed and flexion against resistance are required, flexion of the digits is reinforced by the FDS
- ✓ When the wrist, metacarpophalangeal and interphalangeal joints are flexed, the flexor muscles are shortened; hence their actions are weakened

Muscle	Origin	Insertion	Action	Innervation	Artery	Notes
Flexor carpi radialis	Common flexor tendon from the medial epicondyle of the humerus	Base of the second and third metacarpals	Flexes the wrist, abducts the hand	Medial nerve	Ulnar artery	Functions synergistically with the extensor carpi radialis longus and brevis muscles to abduct hand
Flexor carpi ulnaris	Common flexor tendon and (ulnar head) from medial border of olecranon and upper 2/3 of the posterior border of the ulna	Pisiform, hook of hamate, and base of 5th metacarpal	Flexes wrist, adducts hand	Ulnar nerve	Ulnar artery	The ulnar nerve passes between the two heads of origin of the flexor carpi ulnaris muscle

Flexor digitorum profundus	Posterior border of the ulna, proximal 2/3 of medial border of ulna, interosseous membrane	Base of the distal phalanx of digits 2–5	Flexes the metacarpophalangeal, proximal interphalangeal and distal interphalangeal joints	Medial nerve (radial one-half); ulnar nerve (ulnar one-half)	Ulnar artery, anterior interosseous artery	Ulnar nerve innervates the portion of profundus that acts on digits 4 and 5 (the ulnar 2 digits)
Flexor digitorum superficialis	Humeroulnar head: common flexor tendon; radial head: middle 1/3 of radius	Shafts of the middle phalanges of digits 2–5	Flexes the metacarpophalangeal and proximal interphalangeal joints	Medial nerve	Ulnar artery	Medial nerve travels distally in the forearm on the deep surface of the flexor digitorum superficialis muscle
Flexor pollicis longus	Anterior surface of radius and interosseous membrane	Base of the distal phalanx of the thumb	Flexes the metacarpophalangeal and interphalangeal joints of the thumb	Medial nerve	Anterior interosseous artery	The tendon of flexor pollicis longus passes through the carpal tunnel with the other long digital flexor tendons and the medial nerve
Palmaris longus	Common flexor tendon, from the medial epicondyle of the humerus	Palmar aponeurosis	Flexes the wrist	Medial nerve	Ulnar artery	Palmaris longus is absent in about 13% of forearms; it may be present on one side only

Pronator quadratus	Medial side of the anterior surface of the distal 1/4 of the ulna	Anterior surface of the distal 1/4 of the radius	Pronates the forearm	Medial nerve via the anterior interosseous nerve	Anterior interosseous artery	Pronator quadratus is the deepest muscle in the distal forearm; it functions synergistically with pronator teres and has the same nerve supply
Pronator teres	Common flexor tendon and (deep or ulnar head) from medial side of coronoid process of the ulna	Midpoint of the lateral side of the shaft of the radius	Pronates the forearm	Medial nerve	Ulnar artery, anterior ulnar recurrent artery	Medial nerve passes between the two heads of origin of pronator teres

Neurovascular contributions

Ulnar nerve

✓ Deep (motor) branch of ulnar nerve.
✓ Common and proper digital branches of ulnar nerve.
✓ Dorsal cutaneous branch
✓ Sites at risk for injury and pathologies: when nerve passes posterior to the medial epicondyle of the humerus
  ▷ Injury here results in extensive motor and sensory loss to the hand
  ▷ Impaired adduction and when attempting to flex the wrist joint, the hand is drawn to the radial side by the FCR
  ▷ Clawhand injury: can't make a fist because of loss of flexion of 4th and 5th digits at the DIP joints
✓ Compression within the two heads of the flexor carpi ulnaris muscle
  ▷ Produces numbness and tingling of the medial part of the palm, 4th and 5th digits

Medial nerve

✓ Anterior interosseus nerve
✓ Palmar cutaneous nerve
✓ Recurrent (thenar, motor) branch of medial nerve
✓ Common and proper digital branches of medial nerve
✓ Sites at risk for injury
  ▷ Severed in elbow region
    ◆ Loss of flexion of the PIP joints of all digits

- ◆ Loss of flexion of the DIP joints of 2nd and 3rd digits due to loss of innervation to lumbrical muscles of these digits
  - ◊ Commonly injured proximal to flexor retinaculum (suicide attempts where wrists are slashed)
  - ◊ Compression near the elbow within the two heads of the pronator teres-pronator syndrome
    - ◆ Pain and tenderness in proximal aspect of anterior forearm

Radial artery and handout drawing

- ✓ Radial recurrents
- ✓ Deep (dorsal) palmar arterial arch
  - ◊ Princeps pollicis artery
  - ◊ Radialis indicis artery
  - ◊ Dorsal and palmar carpal arches
- ✓ Contribution to superficial palmar arterial arch
- ✓ Common place for measuring pulse rate
  - ◊ When the radial artery lies on the anterior surface of the distal end of the radius
  - ◊ Lateral to FCR muscle
  - ◊ Only covered by skin and fascia
  - ◊ If pulse can't be felt, try the other wrist due to an aberrant radial artery
  - ◊ Also can measure pulse in the anatomical snuffbox

Ulnar artery

Recurrent ulnar artery

- ✓ Common interosseus artery
  - ◊ Anterior and posterior interosseus arteries.
- ✓ Superficial palmar arch
  - ◊ Common and proper digital arteries
    - ◆ Contribution to deep palmar arterial arch
    - ◆ Palmar carpal arch

Palm of the hand

Functions of the hand

- ✓ With the hands the laborer supports a family, the parent loves and cares for a baby, the musician plays a sonata, the blind "read", and the deaf "talk"
- ✓ Pinching
- ✓ Precision handling
- ✓ Power gripping
- ✓ Free movements

Overview of volar (palmar) compartments and major components

- ✓ Thenar compartment
- ✓ Hypothenar compartment
- ✓ Interosseous/adductor compartment
- ✓ Central compartment and tendon sheaths from extrinsic flexors of the forearm

- ✓ Pulp space—located in the distal tip of each digit
- ✓ Arteries—ulnar artery and branches; radial artery and branches
- ✓ Nerves—ulnar nerve and branches; medial nerve and branches
- ✓ Two bony arches make possible the 3-dimensional features of the palm
  - ◊ The carpal arrangement and the angles of placement for the metacarpals make possible the intricate movements of the hand
  - ◊ Arches contribute to the hollowing of the palm
  - ◊ Arches assist with the ability to grip objects
  - ◊ Oblique palmar arch
    - ◆ Is visible when the hand is clenched or cupped
    - ◆ Is created by the relative mobility of the 4th and 5th metacarpals
    - ◆ Is used in either the power grip or the precision grip
  - ◊ Longitudinal palmar arch
    - ◆ Is created when the digits flex

Fascial considerations

Transverse carpal ligament or flexor retinaculum

- ✓ Converts the wrist region (carpal bones) into a C-shaped osseofibrous canal
- ✓ This connective tissue band is extremely tough and unyielding
- ✓ Any inflammation of the contents can create nerve problems—a problem known as carpal tunnel syndrome
- ✓ This spatial arrangement converts the carpel bones into a dorsally convex and ventrally concave carpal tunnel
- ✓ Carpal sulcus is deepened by these bony prominences on either side
- ✓ Radially: tubercles of the scaphoid and trapezium serve as lateral attachments
- ✓ Ulnarly: pisiform and hook of the hamate serve as medial attachments
- ✓ This anatomic arrangement defines a space for the transmission of long flexor tendons
- ✓ Superficially, the transverse carpal ligament, a band of fibrous connective tissue
  - ◊ Gives rise to the thenar and hypothenar musculature
  - ◊ Os crossed superficially by the ulnar nerve and artery and palmar branch of the medial nerve
  - ◊ Is crossed by the palmaris longus tendon (if present)
- ✓ Passing deep to the transverse carpal ligament (and within the carpal tunnel) are 9 long flexor tendons and 1 medial nerve (this is in the wrist not the palm)
  - ◊ Flexor digitorum superficialis (4 tendons)
  - ◊ Flexor digitorum profundus (4 tendons)
  - ◊ Flexor pollicis longus (1 tendon in the radial bursa)

Palmar aponeurosis

- ✓ Another dense thickening of connective tissue that is superficial and actually in the palm [It will require a very sharp scalpel blade (a new one) to eliminate of this tough layer]
- ✓ Proximally: this connective tissue is continuous with the flexor retinaculum. This layer receives the insertion of the palmaris longus

✓ Distally: 4 digital slips bifurcate and septa create definition around long flexor tendons. It extends attachments internally to the deep transverse metacarpal ligaments

Dupuytren's contracture is an unexplained contracture (shortening) of the collagen fibers in this aponeurosis. The fingers are drawn into permanent flexion and hence into a non-functional curled position. This fascial disease (nodules and thickened fibers) must be surgically excised so a patient can open up the palm of his/her hand

✓ Deep to and protected by the palmar aponeurosis, the roof of the central compartment of the palm is formed by the palmar aponeurosis
✓ Septa from the palmar aponeurosis dive deep and attach to the metacarpals. The lateral septum attaching to the 3rd metacarpal shaft, divides the central palm into 2 potential spaces/clefts where abscesses sometimes fester.
  ◊ Mid-palmar cleft (medial/ulnar side)—is sandwiched between the interosseous and central compartments
  ◊ Thenar cleft (lateral/radial side)—is sandwiched between the adductor and thenar compartments
✓ Palmaris brevis muscle
  ◊ It is a superficial muscle on the hypothenar side (ulnar side)
  ◊ It inserts into and wrinkles the proximal palmar skin
  ◊ It deepens the hollow of the hand when griping objects
  ◊ It is not within the hypothenar compartment but is superficial to it
  ◊ It is superficial to and thus somewhat protects the ulnar nerve and artery in the palm

Thenar and hypothenar compartments

Comparisons and contrasts

✓ Both compartments contain symmetrical muscle groups with identical functions
✓ All these muscles arise from either a carpal bone or the transverse carpal ligament
✓ Both compartments lie deep to the palmar aponeurosis
✓ There are only 2 noticeable differences between these two compartments of muscles
  ◊ The thenar muscular group is stronger and bulkier and innervated by motor branch of medial nerve
  ◊ The hypothenar muscular group is weaker and innervated by deep branch of the ulnar nerve
✓ All are considered intrinsic hand muscles
✓ The thumb is the most important digit
✓ 40% of hand function is dependent on the thumb
✓ The thumb allows for pinching/pickup movements
✓ If a thumb is amputated, it is either replanted with a great toe (thoe) or the ligaments and bones of the index finger are repositioned and the index finger is pollicized
✓ The tendon of insertion for the flexor pollicis brevis contains a sesamoid bone to allow for its unfettered movement over the interphalangeal joint

Interosseous/adductor compartments—functions, arrangements, innervations

✓ This group is innervated by the deep branch of ulnar nerve (all are intrinsic hand muscles)

Palmar interosseous muscles

✓ Unipennate muscles arising from palmar aspects of metacarpals—3 on each hand
✓ Insert into the dorsal extensor (hood) expansion
✓ Actions—PAD—adductors of digits—3rd digit is the central axis of the hand
  ◊ They flex MP joints, extend PIP and DIP joints along with the lumbrical muscles
  ◊ They are responsible for Z-movements (the opposite of claw hand)

Dorsal interosseous muscles

✓ Bipennate muscles arising from dorsal aspects of metacarpals—4 on each hand
✓ Insert into the extensor (hood) expansion
✓ Actions—DAB—abductors of digits—3rd digit serves as the central axis
  ◊ Flexes the MP joints, extends PIP and DIP joints along with lumbrical muscle
  ◊ Responsible for Z-movements (the opposite of claw hand)

Adductor pollicis muscles

✓ Oblique head of origin—base of 2nd and 3rd metacarpals
✓ Transverse head of origin—body of 3rd metacarpal
✓ Insertion—base of proximal phalanx of 1st digit
✓ Its tendon of insertion typically contains a sesamoid bone
✓ Action—take a guess about function
✓ A functional deficit in this muscle is tested by observing the ability of the patient to squeeze and retain a piece of paper between digit 1 and 2 when you gently try to tug it away
✓ Gamekeeper's thumb—a disruption to the adductor insertion and the ulnar collateral ligament on the ulnar side of the thumb

Central compartment (review)

Contents

✓ Flexor pollicis longus tendon
✓ An extrinsic hand muscle originating in the deep flexor forearm compartment
✓ Originates on the radius and interosseous membrane
✓ Inserts on the base of the distal phalanx of digit 1
✓ Its lubricating synovial sheath (known as the radial bursa) extends from the proximal border of the carpal tunnel to the distal phalanx of the 1st digit
✓ Flexor digitorum profundus tendons—4 in number

Extrinsic hand muscles

✓ Originate in the deep flexor forearm compartment
✓ Insert on the base of the distal phalanges of digits 2-5
✓ Their synovial sheaths are discontinuous and do not extend proximally into the palm
✓ A larger common bursa surrounding these tendons is found in the carpal region
✓ Individual bursae are present more distally in each digit and lubricate the tendon
✓ Are the only muscles that can flex the distal interphalangeal (DIP) joints

- ✓ Intrinsic hand muscles—4 lumbricals originate on these tendons
    - ◊ Lumbricals originate on the radial side of the FDP tendons
    - ◊ Insert into the dorsal extensor hood over digits 2–5
    - ◊ Flex the MP joints while extending PIP and DIP joints
    - ◊ Lumbrical mm for digits 2 and 3 are supplied by the medial nerve
    - ◊ These lumbricals are unipennate (arise from a single tendon)
    - ◊ Lumbrical mm for digits 4 and 5 are supplied by the ulnar nerve
    - ◊ These lumbricals are bipennate (arise from two adjacent tendons)
- ✓ Flexor digitorum superficialis tendons–4 in number
- ✓ Are considered extrinsic hand muscles
- ✓ Originate in the flexor forearm compartment
- ✓ Tendons are split by the FDP as it passes through on its way to insert into the base of distal phalanx
- ✓ FDS tendons insert on the middle phalanx for digits 2–5
- ✓ The FDS tendons are housed in the same synovial sheaths with the FDP tendons
- ✓ FDS flexes all joints that it crosses but has its greatest strength at the wrist joint

Introduction to the longitudinal aspects of the finger with its tendinous attachments

- ✓ Dorsal extension hood (expansion) and associated structures
- ✓ Boutonniere deformity—abnormality of a finger marked by the fixed flexion of the PIP joint and hyperextension of the DIP joint
- ✓ Mallet deformity or mallet finger—a permanently flexed terminal phalanx caused by injury to the extensor tendon

Synovial sheaths, pulleys, bursae, joint spaces

- ✓ Fibrous digital sheaths provide osseofibrous canals that closely bind the tendons to the phalanges—prevent "bowstringing" of the long flexor tendons
- ✓ The fibrous digital sheath functions as a series of pulleys
- ✓ They have named thickenings (important to hand surgeons) known as anular and cruciate ligaments
- ✓ Sheaths should permit unfettered movements of the tendons that glide through bursae that contain synovial fluid to lubricate and decrease friction
    - ◊ Tenosynovitis—a painful inflammation of these synovial pockets
    - ◊ Tenolysis—after injury the tendons can scar (become adherent) to the digital fibrous sheaths. This limits gliding movement. The result is a finger that becomes frozen. Surgery is required to cut loose the scar tissue to restore movement. If not corrected early after injury, the joint capsules and ligaments become too stiff to ever allow for finger flexion
- ✓ Nourishment to the tendons is supplied through tiny blood vessels that are conducted to the tendons from their deep surface by fragile connective tissue bridges known as vincula longa and vincula brevia
- ✓ The ulnar bursa is the synovial sheath surrounding the long tendons to the 5th digit
- ✓ This bursa extends from the distal fingertip to the proximal border of the carpal tunnel
- ✓ In the region of the central compartment (palm), it also encloses the proximal portions of the flexor digitorum superficialis and flexor digitorum profundus
- ✓ Parona's space—this is located in the distal forearm proximal to the carpal tunnel

- ✓ If an infection spreads proximally from a puncture wound on the tip of either digit 1 or 5, it may accumulate for a time in Parona's space and then advanced distally to the tip of the opposite digit. This results in a swollen hand and is known as a horseshoe abscess.
- ✓ Other types of inflammation—arthritis: destruction of the cartilage with swelling
- ✓ Osteoarthritis—wear and tear inflammatory processes: swelling of IP joints
- ✓ Rheumatoid arthritis—results in ulnar deviation typically at the MP joints

Blood supply to the hand—anastomoses rule

- ✓ When performing surgery on the hand, a tourniquet is applied at the arm region to ensure that blood flow is completely stopped. Otherwise this is one region where applying direct pressure over one artery (either the radial or ulnar arteries) will typically stop blood loss for a few secondly only

Superficial palmar (arterial) arch

- ✓ Located immediately deep to the palmar aponeurosis
- ✓ To approximate its location, extend your thumb and draw an imaginary line from the distal edge of the thumb across the center of the palm
- ✓ Is mainly a continuation of the ulnar artery although it may be completed on the lateral side by a superficial branch of the radial artery
- ✓ Gives rise to the common palmar digital arteries that branch into the proper digital arteries

Deep palmar (arterial) arch

- ✓ Located 1 cm proximal to the superficial palmar arch
- ✓ Is mainly a continuation of the deep branch of the radial artery although it may be completed from the medial side by a deep branch of the ulnar artery
- ✓ Lies deep to the central compartment but superficial to the interosseous compartment
- ✓ Branches
  - ◊ 3 palmar metacarpal arteries that anastomose with common palmar digital arteries
  - ◊ Perforating arteries that anastomose with dorsal metacarpal arteries
  - ◊ Nutrient arteries to metacarpal bones

Ulnar artery (medial aspect)

- ✓ Ulnar artery passes superficial to the transverse carpal ligament (flexor retinaculum)
- ✓ Obviously it is at risk of injury from glass shards or other sharp objects at this point
- ✓ It divides into a deep ulnar artery that dives through the hypothenar compartment
- ✓ The remaining ulnar artery continues as the superficial palmar arch
- ✓ More distally the superficial continuation of the ulnar artery (superficial palmar arterial arch) is protected by passing deep to the palmar aponeurosis
- ✓ The superficial palmar arch gives off common digital arteries
- ✓ The common digital arteries divide into proper digital arteries
- ✓ Proper digital arteries are frequently repaired during finger replantation surgery
- ✓ Deep ulnar artery dives into the hypothenar compartment
- ✓ It contributes to the deep palmar arch
- ✓ The deep palmar arch gives off palmar metacarpal arteries

Radial artery contributions (lateral aspect)

✓ The radial artery may send a small ventral contribution to the superficial (distal) palmar arch
✓ The radial artery passes dorsal to the palm in the anatomical snuffbox
✓ The deep radial artery typically gives off the princeps pollicis artery to the thumb
✓ The radial artery gives off the radialis indicis artery to the lateral side of the 2nd digit
✓ The deep radial artery is usually the main contributor to the deep (proximal) palmar arch
✓ The deep palmar arch gives off palmar metacarpal arteries
✓ The deep palmar arch anatomoses with the common digital arteries

Miscellaneous clinical considerations

Allen test—a test for perfusion in the hand. Without and adequate arterial supply, the hand will die so arterial supply is checked before surgery or to test when perfusion may have been compromised. An Allen's test is conducted by compressing both the ulnar and radial arteries, having the patient make a fist and then open the fist repeatedly several times while still compressing both arteries. Then one artery is released such as the radial artery. If the radial arterial contributions are not compromised, then the hand should flush from the radial side first to the ulnar side. This test is repeated but the ulcer artery. is then released. The hand should flush first on the ulnar side and become normal in color in 1–2 seconds. Such a test might be done before and after introduction of an arterial catheter into the radial artery. One must never allow arterial flow to the hand to be compromised for many minutes

✓ Arteriogram—dye is introduced to check for the patency of both arteries
✓ Pulp space—the distal volar tips of the fingers receive a rich infilling of capillaries from the paired digital arteries. If a finger tip is severed in children, it can typically be salvaged by pinning through bone it to stabilize the DIP joint and simply suturing the severed tip into place. Capillary networks will be quickly reestablished and the fingertip saved

Nerves for the volar aspect of the hand

Medial nerve

✓ Palmar cutaneous nerve—branches off proximal to the carpal tunnel
✓ Recurrent (thenar, motor) branch of the medial nerve
✓ Supplies motor innervations and proprioception to lumbricals 1 and 2
✓ Tinel's sign—an indication of irritability of a nerve. If during a physical exam the doctor percusses over a damaged nerve and an unpleasant distal tingling sensation is noted, then this is a positive sign that indicates nerve damage. This simple diagnostic tool is often used to determine whether patients are being honest about their symptoms. If a patient truly has carpal tunnel syndrome, a tapping over the medial nerve at the wrist will produce this unpleasant sensation

Ulnar nerve

✓ It gives off superficial dorsal and palmar cutaneous branches proximal to the wrist
✓ Ulnar nerve at the wrist passes superficial to the transverse carpal ligament
✓ Ulnar nerve passes deep to the palmar aponeurosis
✓ Deep (motor) branch of ulnar nerve innervates the hypothenar muscles
✓ Deep (motor) branch of the ulnar nerve passes through Guyon's canal

- ✓ The canal is a fibrosseous arch (pisi-hamate ligament) stretching between the pisiform and hook of the hamate
- ✓ The deep ulnar nerve is at risk of compression in this narrow passage
- ✓ Deep ulnar nerve supplies the interosseous/adductor compartment
- ✓ Deep ulnar nerve supplies sensation to the metacarpal bones and proprioception to the joints
- ✓ The continuation of the ulnar nerve remains superficial
- ✓ It supplies cutaneous sensation to the volar surface of digit 5 and medial portions of digit 4
- ✓ It also supplies sensation for the skin over the dorsal middle and distal phalanx and nail bed
- ✓ It supplies motor branches to lumbricals 3 and 4
- ✓ Begin to consider sites where the ulnar nerve would be at greatest risk of damage

Miscellaneous considerations/important clinical considerations

- ✓ Sensory nerve testing is performed by measuring 2-point tactile discrimination
- ✓ Motor nerve testing is accomplished using electromyography (EMG)
- ✓ Autonomic (sympathetic) nerve contributions
  - ◊ All nerves contain these components
  - ◊ Sweating palms (sudomotor) and constriction of blood vessels (vasoconstriction)
  - ◊ Raynaud's syndrome has an unexplained cause (etiology) but it involves over-stimulation of the sympathetic nervous system—resulting in painfully cold hands due to the excessive constriction of the blood vessels

Segmental (dermatome) innervations of the hand region versus cutaneous nerve patterns

- ✓ Segmental patterns exist because there are 31 pairs or segments of spinal cord that give rise to motor nerves to muscles at each level and receive sensory input at each spinal level
- ✓ Certain nerves migrate outward to the hand during limb bud development (e.g., C_5-T_1). Nerves from several spinal levels often group together as they travel down the highway to the limb (similar to how you flock together when you go out to lunch). These grouped nerves are very visible to surgeons and became named (e.g., the palmar branch of the medial nerve or the deep branch of the ulnar nerve)
- ✓ No matter how much these nerves appear to be a solid group, each individual spinal cord level retains its unique identity. It knows which spinal segment it belongs to (e.g., C_5, C_6, C_7, C_8, T_1)
- ✓ Each spinal cord segment (level) has certain muscles that it moves (a myotome innervation pattern) and certain areas of skin that it receives sensory input from (a dermatome innervation). This is what is meant by a segmental innervation pattern

Summary—the hand is more than the sum of its parts

- ✓ It serves as a manipulative tool
- ✓ It serves as a sensory organ sending messages to the central computer (the brain)
- ✓ Its loss is devastating. Hand specialists in plastic surgery, orthopedic surgery and physical therapy work together with the cooperative patient to maximize function

Posterior compartment of arm and dorsum of hand

- ✓ Posterior compartment is one of two compartments in the forearm (posterior and anterior)—the interosseous membrane that connects the radius and the ulna separates these

✓ Muscles in the posterior compartment can be grouped into two layers: superficial [with three subdivisions (lateral, intermediate, and medial) and a total of six muscles] and deep (with a total of five muscles)

　♢ The muscles in the superficial layer all have, at least in part, a common origin from the lateral epicondyle or lateral epicondylar ridge

　♢ Apart from the supinator (the most proximal deep muscle), the other four muscles of the deep layer have their origins distal to the lateral epicondyle

　♢ There are no intrinsic muscles on the dorsum of the hand—all finger function is the responsibility of muscles that originated in the forearm and extend into the hand. This is a positive design feature, since the operation and range of movement of the wrist and a digit requires that the bellies and tendons of the muscles be long

✓ All the muscles of the posterior compartment (extensor region of the forearm), are innervated by the radial nerve or its terminal extension (posterior interosseous nerve). The posterior compartment begins proximally at the elbow joint and ends distally at the wrist

✓ The radial nerve splits into:

　♢ Superficial radial nerve (purely sensory), supplying the dorsum of the thumb, index, middle and one-half of the ring finger, except for the tips (supplied by the medial nerve)

　♢ Posterior interosseous nerve (motor), supplying all of the muscles of the posterior compartment except for the lateral superficial group (that receives their innervations from the common radial nerve prior to its branching)

✓ All muscles of the forearm are enclosed by the fascia of the forearm (antebrachial fascia)

✓ Moving into the forearm, the extensors are held in place by an extensor retinaculum (thickening of deep fascia), that houses these long tendons in six compartments (more detail later)

✓ Finger function into extension is made possible by the long tendons that distally create extensor expansions (dorsal hoods), that when working with the lumbricals and interossei (palmar and dorsal), permit controlled motion at the MCP, PIP, and DIP joints

Superficial layer of forearm extensors—3 groups in this layer
Common point for all muscles in this layer—common extensor tendon originates from the lateral epicondyle and supracondylar ridge of the humerus
Lateral group: this group has 3 muscles, brachioradialis, extensor carpi radialis longus, and extensor carpi radialis brevis
Brachioradialis
✓ Origin: upper 2/3 of the lateral epicondylar ridge and adjacent intermuscular septum ✓ Insertion: base of the styloid process of the radius (does not cross the radiocarpal joint) ✓ Action: an elbow flexor; it has no action in the hands or digits ✓ Nerve: radial nerve (C_5–C_7)
Extensor carpi radialis longus
✓ Origin: lower $1/3^{rd}$ of lateral epicondylar ridge and adjacent intermuscular septum ✓ Insertion: dorsum of the second metacarpal bone of the hand

- ✓ Action: extension and abduction of the hand at the wrist
- ✓ Nerve: radial nerve supplies this muscle just before it subdivides into its deep and superficial parts (C_6–C_7)

Extensor carpi radialis brevis

- ✓ Origin: lateral epicondyle of the humerus
- ✓ Insertion: dorsum of the base of the 3rd metacarpal bone
- ✓ Action: extension and abduction of the hand at the wrist
- ✓ Nerve: deep radial nerve innervates this muscle just prior to its entry into the supinator muscle (C_7–C_8)
- ✓ Other facts associated with the lateral group of forearm extensors:
- ✓ Note that the radial nerve provides the motor supply to these muscles before it splits into the superficial and deep portions of the radial nerve—this is an important fact that can be used when determining the level of injury of the radial nerve
- ✓ In their passage under the extensor retinaculum, the tendons of the extensor carpi radialis longus and brevis tendons are enclosed in a single synovial sheath

Intermediate group: this group has 2 muscles, extensor digitorum, and extensor digiti minimi

Extensor digitorum (communis)

- ✓ Origin: common extensor tendon on the lateral epicondyle of the humerus
- ✓ Insertion: extensor expansion hood of the phalanges
- ✓ Action: extends the wrist, MCP and IP joints
- ✓ Nerve: posterior interosseous nerve (changes its name as it emerges from the supinator) (C_7–C_8)

Extensor digiti minimi (quinti)

- ✓ Origin: common extensor tendon on the lateral epicondyle of the humerus
- ✓ Insertion: tendon joins the ulnar side of the tendon of the extensor digitorum to the 5th digit and helps to form the extensor expansion over the fifth digit
- ✓ Action: provides independent extensor action for this digit
- ✓ Nerve: posterior interosseous nerve (C_7–C_8)

Medial group: this group consists of only one muscle, the extensor carpi ulnaris

Extensor carpi ulnaris

- ✓ Origin: lateral epicondyle and middle of the posterior border of the ulna
- ✓ Insertion: ulnar side of the base of the fifth metacarpal bone
- ✓ Action: adduction or ulnar deviation of the wrist. It is a weak extensor of the wrist
- ✓ Nerve: posterior interosseous branch of the radial (C_7–C_8)

Deep layer of forearm extensor muscles: 5 muscles in this group

- ✓ Common feature of all muscles in this group is that they are all innervated by the deep branch of the radial nerve or its continuation, the posterior interosseous nerve (although different root levels)

Supinator

- Origin: lateral epicondyle of the humerus, supinator crest and fossa of the ulna
- Insertion: fibers are arranged in two planes, between which the deep branch of the radial nerve lies; winds around the posterior and lateral neck of the radius to insert along the shaft of the radius
- Action: assists biceps brachii in supination of the forearm
- Nerve: deep branch of the radial nerve (C_5–C_6)
- *Clinical notes*: ①The supinator muscle is located in the upper $1/3^{rd}$ of the forearm, but it is completely hidden by superficial muscles. ②After the point where the deep radial nerve passes out of the supinator muscle, it is designated as the posterior interosseous nerve. In addition to innervating muscles of the posterior aspect of the forearm, it provides supply to the carpals and the digit joints

Abductor pollicis longus

- Origin: middle 1/3 of the posterior surface of the radius, lateral part of the posterior surface of the ulna below the anconeus
- Insertion: crosses the tendons of the extensor carpi radialis longus and brevis and inserts on the radial side of the base of the metacarpal bone of the thumb
- Action: abducts the thumb in concert with the abductor pollicis brevis (intrinsic thumb muscle)
- Nerve: posterior interosseous branch of the radial nerve (C_7–C_8)

Extensor pollicis brevis

- Origin: posterior surface of the ulna and the adjacent interosseous membrane
- Insertion: tendon passes obliquely across the tendons of both the radial extensors of the wrist and along the ulnar side of the first metacarpal bone to terminate on the base of the distal phalanx of the thumb
- Action: extends the MCP joint of the thumb
- Nerve: posterior interosseous branch of the radial nerve (C_7–C_8)

Extensor pollicis longus

- Origin: posterior surface of the ulna and adjacent interosseous membrane
- Insertion: tendon passes obliquely across the tendons of both the radial extensors of the wrist and along the ulnar side of the first metacarpal bone to terminate on the base of the distal phalanx of the thumb
- Action: extends the distal phalanx of the thumb
- Nerve: posterior interosseous branch of the radial nerve (C_7–C_8)
- *Clinical notes*: The tendon of this muscle passes around the dorsal radial tubercle and is at risk of damage by a superficial laceration

Extensor indicis

- Origin: posterior surface of the ulna and adjacent interosseous membrane
- Insertion: extensor expansion of the index finger
- Action: adds independent extensor power to the MCP joint of the finger
- Nerve: deep radial nerve (C_7–C_8)

Forearm serial cross sections

- Upper 1/3 of the forearm

- ✓ Middle 1/3 of the forearm
- ✓ Distal 1/3 of the forearm

Additional points associated with the superficial and deep (posterior interosseous) branches of the radial nerve

- ✓ Sensation to a portion of the dorsal forearm and dorsum of the hand is supplied by derivatives of the radial nerve
  - ◊ The posterior cutaneous nerve of the forearm is a direct branch off of the radial nerve, arising in the proximal 1/3 to middle 1/2 of the arm
  - ◊ The superficial branch of the radial nerve arises in the region of the lateral elbow, travels under cover of the brachioradialis, crosses the tendon of the EPL, and supplies the dorsal aspect of the thumb, index, middle and 1/2 of the ring finger (except the tips, that are supplied by the medial nerve)
- ✓ Arises from a common radial nerve in the anterior compartment
- ✓ Gains entrance into the posterior compartment by running lateral to the radius, moving between the supinator, dividing that muscle into two heads
- ✓ Innervates all muscles within the posterior compartment, except the lateral superficial group (receive their innervations from the common radial nerve prior to its branching)
- ✓ While injury to the common radial nerve produces "wrist drop", injury to the deep radial nerve results only in weakened extension of the wrist and a loss of the extension at the MCP joint

Arterial supply to the posterior compartment

The posterior interosseous branch of the ulnar artery and the anterior interosseous artery (distally)

- ✓ The posterior interosseous branch of the ulnar artery arises from the common interosseous branch of the ulnar artery in the anterior compartment
  - ◊ It gains entrance to the posterior compartment by passing between the radius and the ulna at the superior margin of the interosseous membrane, then emerges from under the inferior border of the supinator, where it joins and travels with the deep radial nerve
  - ◊ It gives rise to the interosseous recurrent artery, which is part of the collateral circulation around the elbow
- ✓ The anterior interosseous artery penetrates the interosseous membrane in the distal $1/3^{rd}$ of the forearm and supplies the region distal to that point, since the posterior interosseous branch of the ulnar artery is exhausted by that point

Dorsum of the hand

Extensor retinaculum

- ✓ Thickening of the deep fascia over the dorsal aspect of the distal forearm (does not overlie the carpal bones)
  - ◊ Extends from the radius to the styloid process of the ulna to the pisiform and triquetral bones
- ✓ The extensor retinaculum forms 6 compartments containing the long tendons of the extensor group of muscles—the compartments are:
  - ◊ Compartment 1—tendons of the extensor pollicis brevis and abductor pollicis longus
  - ◊ Compartment 2—tendons of the extensor carpi radialis brevis and extensor carpi radialis longus

◊ Compartment 3—single tendon of the extensor pollicis longus

◊ Compartment 4—tendons of the extensor digitorum and extensor indicis

◊ Compartment 5—single tendon of the extensor digiti minimi

◊ Compartment 6—single tendon of the extensor carpi ulnaris

✓ Key points associated with the compartments

◊ To avoid friction, each compartment is provided with a synovial sheath or tendinous bursa, which extends above and below the retinaculum

◊ Infections of these synovial sheaths are rare

◊ As it passes deep to the retinaculum, extensor pollicis longus is passing medial to the dorsal tubercle of the radius, using it as a pulley; distally it turns to the thumb, thus creating the "anatomical snuff box"

◆ Dorsal portion of the radial artery and the scaphoid are palpable in the snuff box

Oblique intertendinous connections

✓ Three oblique bands unite the 4 flattened tendons of the extensor digitorum on the dorsum of the hand, proximal to the knuckles

✓ The presence of these intertendinous connections restricts independent extension of the fingers, especially the ring finger

Extensor expansions (dorsal hoods)

✓ On the distal ends of the metacarpals and on the digits, the extensor tendons become flattened, widening and becoming reinforced by transversely-oriented fibers as they do so

◊ Forms a visor-like hood covering the dorsum and sides of each metacarpal head and proximal phalanx, called an extensor expansion or dorsal hood

◊ Via the transversely-oriented fibers, each hood is anchored on each side to the palmar ligament; thus the extensor tendon is retained in the midline of the digit

✓ On the proximal phalanx, the expansion divides into a medial band, which passes to the base of the middle phalanx, and into 2 lateral bands, which pass to the base of the distal phalanx

◊ The tendon of extensor digitorum pulls mostly via the medial band

✓ Each lateral band is joined by half an interosseous muscle tendon (the other half passes directly to the base of the proximal phalanx)

✓ The lateral band on the radial side is joined by the entire tendon of the lumbrical muscle

◊ In attaching to the lateral bands, the tendons of the interossei and lumbricals pass ventral to the point of rotation of the metacarpophalangeal joint; after their attachment, the lateral bands pass dorsal to the points of rotation of the proximal and distal interphalangeal joints.

◊ Thus, when acting independent of the long extensor, the interossei and lumbricals act in concert to produce flexion at the MP joint and extension at the two IP joints

◊ In ulnar paralysis, the extensor digitorum is unopposed at the MP joint, and the long flexors innervated by the medial nerve are unopposed at the PIP and DIP joints, thus the clawhand results

◊ When the MP joints are extended by the long flexor tendon, the palmar and dorsal interossei may be selectively activated to produce adduction and abduction, respectively, at the MP joints via their direct attachment to the bases of the proximal phalanges, the movements are ineffective in ulnar paralysis

Nail and nailbed

Superficial venous and lymph drainage of the upper extremity

√ Superficial veins of the forearm are the: cephalic, basilic, and medial antebrachial veins
√ Lymph from the wrist and forearm drains into the cubital lymph nodes, eventually making its way to the axillary lymph nodes

Clinical correlates

Elbow tendinitis

√ Painful condition that may follow repetitive use of the superficial extensor muscles of the forearm
√ Repeated forceful flexion and extension of the wrist strain the attachment of the common tendon, producing inflammation of the periosteum of the lateral epicondyle
√ Pain is felt over the lateral epicondyle and radiates down the posterior surface of the forearm

Mallet finger

√ DIP joint is suddenly being forced into extreme flexion
√ Avulse the attachment of a long extensor tendon from the base of the distal phalanx
√ Patient cannot extend the DIP joint

Fracture of the scaphoid

√ Most frequently fractured carpal bone
√ Localized tenderness in the anatomical snuff box
√ May lead to avascular necrosis

Synovial cyst of the wrist

√ Nontender cystic swelling ("ganglion") on the dorsum of the wrist
√ Cystic swellings are close to and often communicate with the synovial sheaths
√ Attachment of the extensor carpi radialis brevis tendon into base of the 3rd metacarpal is a common site
√ Flexion of the wrist makes the cyst enlarge and it may be painful

Radial tunnel syndrome

√ Thought to be caused by entrapment of the posterior interosseous nerve at the arcade of Frohse (radial tunnel)—symptoms mimic those of resistant tennis elbow syndrome
√ Several studies have shown needle EMG abnormalities in the extensor digitorum in patients with resistant tennis elbow
√ Forceful supination appears to increase the electrophysiological findings, when present

√ While clinical (and some electrophysiological) findings suggest the presence of this syndrome, there is as yet no solid evidence to state that refractory tennis elbow is due to entrapment of the posterior interosseous nerve

Radial nerve injury

√ With a humeral fracture, the radial nerve (and thus the extensors of the forearm and hand) is at high risk, due to its proximity to the bone

Xian Dehai

Chapter 7

The Lower Limb

7.1 Introduction

The primary function of the lower limbs is to support the weight of the body and to provide a stable foundation in standing, walking, and running; they have become specialized for locomotion.

Because the two hip bones articulate posteriorly with the trunk at the strong sacroiliac joints and anteriorly with each other at the symphysis pubis, the lower limbs are very stable and can bear the weight of the body.

7.1.1 Boundary and division

The lower limb connects to the trunk. It is bounded anteriorly by the inguinal groove that connected with abdomen, and posteriorly by iliac crest that connected with the waist and sacrum.

The lower limb is divided into four parts: buttock (hip), thigh, leg and foot. The term "leg" refers only to the portion of the lower limb between the knee and ankle, not to the entire lower limb. The surface anatomy of the lower limb can be studied on a living subject or the cadaver. Place the cadaver in the supine position and palpate the following structures: medial malleolus, lateral malleolus, medial femoral epicondyle, lateral femoral epicondyle, patella, pubic tubercle, anterior superior iliac spine, and iliac crest. The top of the iliac crests marks the level of the fourth lumbar vertebral body (L_4), above or below which lumbar puncture may be performed.

7.1.2 Suface anatomy

(1) The gluteal region and thigh

The iliac crest can be felt through the skin along its entire length, it ends anteriorly as the anterior superior iliac spine and posteriorly as the posterior superior iliac spine. The tubercle of iliac crest is a prominence felt on the outer surface of the iliac crest about 5 cm behind the anterior superior iliac spine. The spine of the fourth lumbar vertebra lies on the line connecting the highest points of the two sides of the iliac crest. The ischial tuberosity can be easily palpated medially in the lower part of the gluteal region as the hip joint is flexed, it forms the posterior aspect of the body of ischium. The greater trochanter can be felt laterally in the middle part of the gluteal region and is about 10 cm behind the iliac tubercle. The symphysis pubis is the cartilaginous joint that lies in the midline between the rami of the pubic bones, it can be palpated in this region. The pubic crest forms the upper border of the superior ranus of the pubis and ends laterally as the pubic tubercle. Lateral to the pubic tubercle, a resilent band can be felt in the inguinal groove, it is the inguinal ligament which lies between the anterior surface of the thigh and abdomen.

(2) The knee

In front of the knee joint, the patalla forms a prominent landmark. When the quadriceps femoris is relaxed, this bone is freely mobile from side to side. The strong parellar ligament stretches inferiorly from the patella to the tibial tuberosity. At the lateral and medial sides of the patella, the lateral and medial condyles of the femur and the tibia can be palpated. Each condyle of the femur has a flattened conical projection, the epicondyle of the femur. Above the medial epicondyle, the adductor tubercle for the attachment of the tendon of a adductor magnus is readily palpable. On the lateral side, the tendon of biceps femoris can be felt when the knee is bent, and the tendons of semitendinosus and semimembranosus are on the medial side. The tendon of the biceps femoris inserts into the head of the fibula.

(3) The leg

The shaft of the tibia is subcutaneous and readily felt from the tibial tuberosity to the anterior margin of the medial malleolus. The fibular head which can be felt as a knob of bone lies the lateral side of the knee. The neck of the fibula is a slender part below the head. The below part of the fibula can be palpated obviously on the lateral side of the leg.

(4) The foot

The medial malleolus and lateral malleous are the important landmarks, which are the projections of the lower end of the tibia and the fibula respectively. The teno calcaneus is on the posterior of the ankle, and the calcaneal tuberosity lies below it. The tuberosity of the navicular bone and the fifth matatarsal bone are palpated on the middle part of the medial side and the lateral side of the foot.

7.2 The front and medial aspects of the thigh

7.2.1 Skin of the thigh

7.2.1.1 Cutaneous nerves

The lateral cutaneous nerve of the thigh, a branch of the lumbar plexus ($L_2 - L_3$), enters the thigh behind the lateral end of the inguinal ligament. Having divided into anterior and posterior branches, it supplies the skin of the lateral aspect of the thigh and knee. It also supplies the skin of the lower lateral quadrant of the buttock.

The femoral branch of the genitofemoral nerve, a branch of the lumbar plexus ($L_1 - L_2$), enters the thigh behind the middle of the inguinal ligament and supplies a small area of skin. The genital branch supplies the cremaster muscle.

The ilioinguinal nerve, a branch of the lumbar plexus (L_1), enters the thigh through the superficial inguinal ring. It is distributed to the skin of the root of the penis and adjacent part of the scrotum (or root of the clitoris and adjacent part of the labium majus in the female) and to a small skin area below the medial part of the inguinal ligament.

The medial cutaneous nerve of the thigh, a branch of the femoral nerve, supplies the medial aspect of the thigh and joins the patellar plexus.

The intermediate cutaneous nerve of the thigh, a branch of the femoral nerve, divides into two branches that supply the anterior aspect of the thigh and joins the patellar plexus.

Branches from the anterior division of the obturator nerve supply a variable area of skin on the medial aspect of the thigh.

The patellar plexus lies in front of the knee and is formed from the terminal branches of the lateral, intermediate, and medial cutaneous nerves of the thigh and the infrapatellar branch of the saphenous nerve (Figure 7-1).

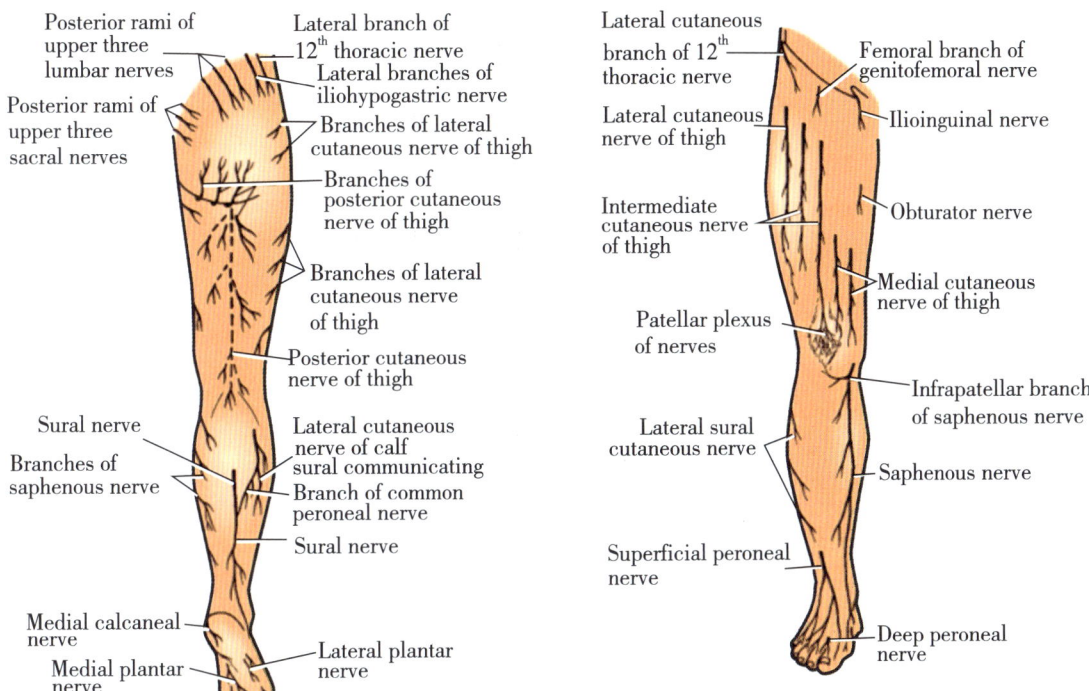

Figure 7-1　Cutaneous nerves of the posterior and anterior surface of the right lower limb

7.2.1.2　Superficial Veins

The superficial veins of the leg are the great and small saphenous veins and their tributaries (Figure 7-2). They are of great clinical importance.

The great saphenous vein drains the medial end of the dorsal venous arch of the foot and passes upward directly in front of the medial malleolus. It then ascends in company with the saphenous nerve in the superficial fascia over the medial side of the leg. The vein passes behind the knee and curves forward around the medial side of the thigh. It passes through the lower part of the saphenous opening in the deep fascia and joins the femoral vein about 4 cm below and lateral to the pubic tubercle.

The great saphenous vein possesses numerous valves and is connected to the small saphenous vein by one or two branches that pass behind the knee. Several perforating veins connect the great saphenous vein with the deep veins along the medial side of the calf.

At the saphenous opening in the deep fascia, the great saphenous vein usually receives three tributaries that are variable in size and arrangement: the superficial circumflex iliac vein, the superficial epigastric vein, and the superficial external pudendal vein (Figure 7-3). These veins correspond with the three branches of the femoral artery found in this region.

An additional vein, known as the accessory vein, usually joins the main vein about the middle of the thigh or higher up at the saphenous opening.

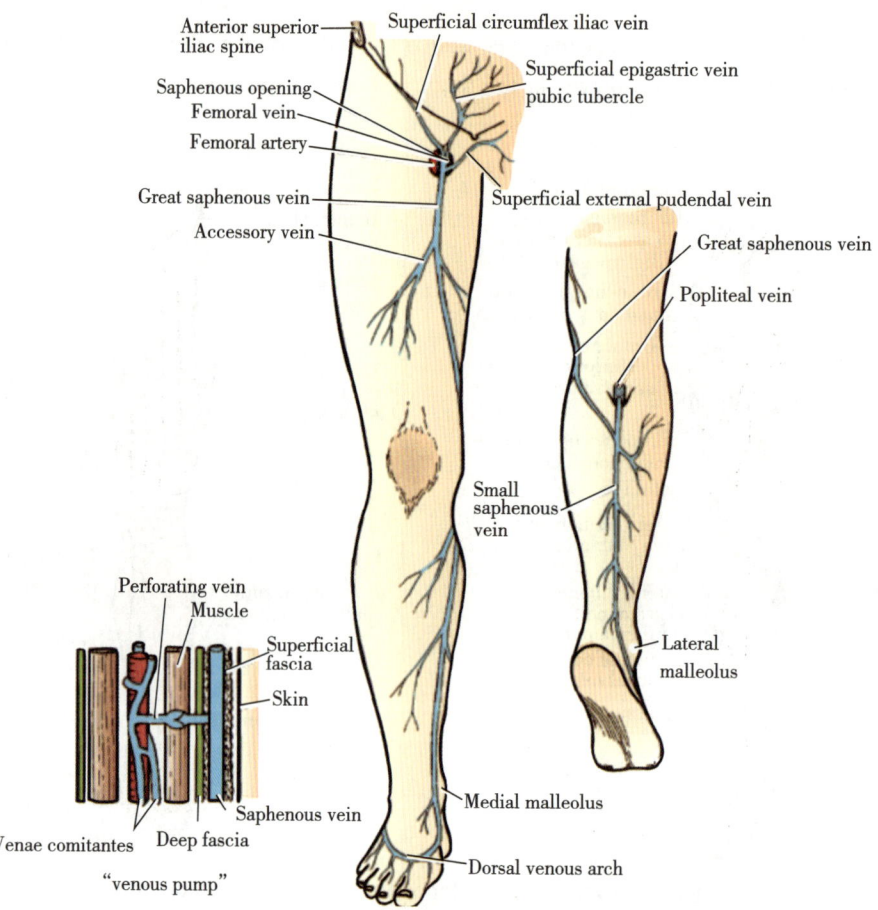

Figure 7-2 Superficial veins of the right lower limb

(Note the importance of the valved perforating veins in the "venous pump")

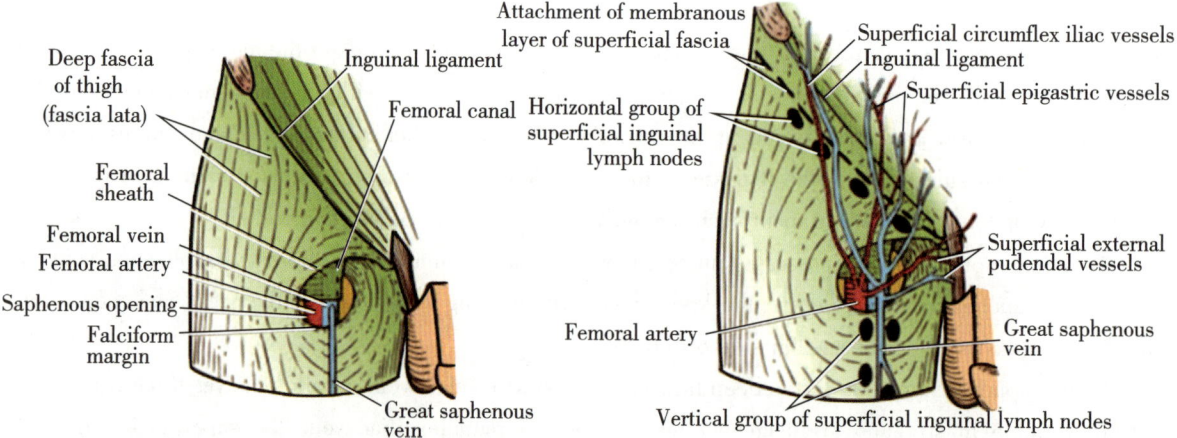

Figure 7-3 Superficial veins, arteries, and lymph nodes over the right femoral triangle

(Note the saphenous opening in the deep fascia and its relationship to the femoral sheath. Note also the line of attachment of the membranous layer of superficial fascia to the deep fascia, about a fingerbreadth below the inguinal ligament)

7.2.1.3 Inguinal lymph nodes

The inguinal lymph nodes are divided into superficial and deep groups (Figure 7-4).

(1) Superficial inguinal lymph nodes

The superficial nodes lie in the superficial fascia below the inguinal ligament and can be divided into a horizontal and a vertical group.

The horizontal group lies just below and parallel to the inguinal ligament. The medial members of the group receive superficial lymph vessels from the anterior abdominal wall below the level of the umbilicus and from the perineum. The lymph vessels from the urethra, the external genitalia of both sexes (but not the testes), and the lower half of the anal canal are drained by this route. The lateral members of the group receive superficial lymph vessels from the back below the level of the iliac crests.

The vertical group lies along the terminal part of the great saphenous vein and receives most of the superficial lymph vessels of the lower limb.

The efferent lymph vessels from the superficial inguinal nodes pass through the saphenous opening in the deep fascia and join the deep inguinal nodes.

(2) Deep inguinal lymph nodes

The deep nodes are located beneath the deep fascia and lie along the medial side of the femoral vein, the efferent vessels from these nodes enter the abdomen by passing through the femoral canal to lymph nodes along the external iliac artery.

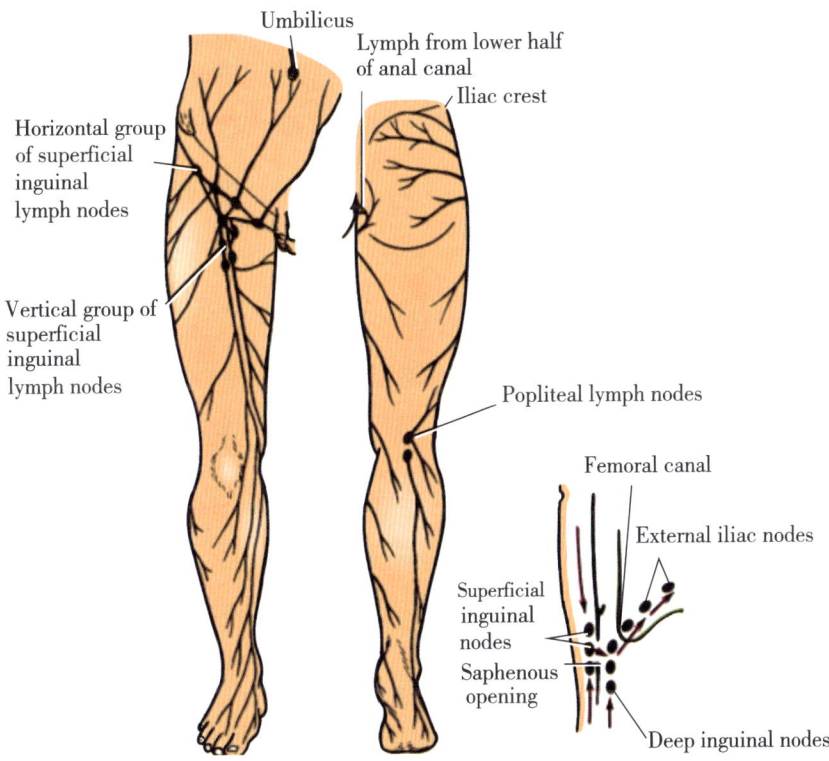

Figure 7-4 Lymph drainage for the superficial tissues of the right lower limb and the abdominal walls below the level of the umbilicus

(Note the arrangement of the superficial and deep inguinal lymph nodes and their relationship to the saphenous opening in the deep fascia. Note also that all lymph from these nodes ultimately drains into the external iliac nodes via the femoral canal)

7.2.2　Superficial fascia of the thigh

The membranous layer of the superficial fascia of the anterior abdominal wall extends into the thigh and is attached to the deep fascia (fascia lata) about a fingerbreadth below the inguinal ligament. The fatty layer of the superficial fascia on the anterior abdominal wall extends into the thigh and continues down over the lower limb without interruption.

7.2.3 Deep fascia of the thigh (fascia lata)

The deep fascia encloses the thigh like a trouser leg and at its upper end is attached to the pelvis and the inguinal ligament. On its lateral aspect, it is thickened to form the iliotibial tract, which is attached above to the iliac tubercle and below to the lateral condyle of the tibia. The iliotibial tract receives the insertion of the tensor fasciae latae and the greater part of the gluteus maximus muscle. In the gluteal region, the deep fascia forms sheaths, which enclose the tensor fasciae latae and the gluteus maximus muscles.

The saphenous opening is a gap in the deep fascia in the front of the thigh just below the inguinal ligament. It transmits the great saphenous vein, some small branches of the femoral artery, and lymph vessels. The saphenous opening is situated about 4 cm below and lateral to the pubic tubercle. The falciform margin is the lower lateral border of the opening, which lies anterior to the femoral vessels. The border of the opening then curves upward and medially, and then laterally behind the femoral vessels, to be attached to the pectineal line of the superior ramus of the pubis.

The saphenous opening is filled with loose connective tissue called the cribriform fascia.

7.2.4 Fascial compartments of the thigh

Three fascial septa pass from the inner aspect of the deep fascial sheath of the thigh to the linea aspera of the femur. By this means, the thigh is divided into three compartments, each having muscles, nerves, and arteries. The compartments are anterior, medial, and posterior in position.

The contents of the anterior fascial compartment of the thigh are as follows.

Muscles: sartorius, iliopsoas, pectineus, and quadriceps femoris.

Blood supply: femoral artery.

Nerve supply: femoral nerve.

Note the following: action of quadriceps femoris muscle (quadriceps mechanism).

The quadriceps femoris muscle, consisting of the rectus femoris, the vastus intermedius, the vastus lateralis, and the vastus medialis, is inserted into the patella and via the ligamentum patellae, is attached to the tibial tuberosity. Together, they provide a powerful extensor of the knee joint. Some of the tendinous fibers of the vastus lateralis and vastus medialis form bands, or retinacula, which join the capsule of the knee joint and strengthen it. The lowest muscle fibers of the vastus medialis are almost horizontal and prevent the patella from being pulled laterally during contraction of the quadriceps muscle. The tone of the quadriceps muscle greatly strengthens the knee joint.

The rectus femoris muscle also flexes the hip joint.

7.2.5 Femoral triangle

The femoral triangle is a triangular depressed area situated in the upper part of the medial aspect of the thigh just below the inguinal ligament. Its boundaries are as follows.

Superiorly: the inguinal ligament.

Laterally: the medial border of the sartorius.

Medially: the medial border of the adductor longus.

Its floor is gutter shaped, from lateral to medial formed by the iliopsoas, the pectineus and the adductor longus. Its roof is formed by the skin and fasciae of the thigh.

The femoral triangle contains the terminal part of the femoral nerve and its branches, the femoral artery and its branches, the femoral vein and its tributaries, the adductor canal and the deep inguinal lymph nodes (Figure 7-5).

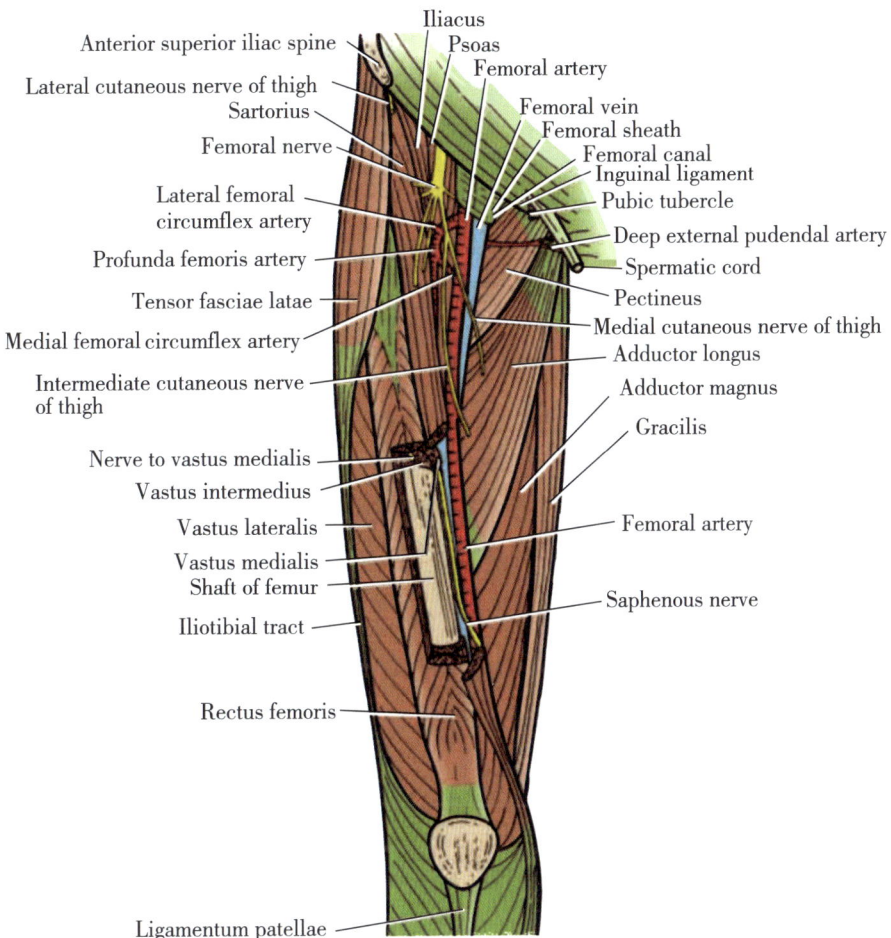

Figure 7-5 Femoral triangle and adductor (subsartorial) canal in the right lower limb

7.2.6 Adductor (subsartorial) canal

The adductor canal is an intermuscular cleft situated on the medial aspect of the middle third of the thigh beneath the sartorius muscle. It commences above at the apex of the femoral triangle and ends below at the opening in the adductor magnus. In cross section, it is triangular, having an anteromedial wall, a posterior wall and a lateral wall. The anteromedial wall is formed by the sartorius and fascia. The posterior wall is formed by the adductor longus and magnus. The lateral wall is formed by the vastus medialis.

The adductor canal contains the terminal part of the femoral artery, the femoral vein, the deep lymph vessels, the saphenous nerve, the nerve to the vastus medialis and the terminal part of the obturator nerve (Figure 7-6).

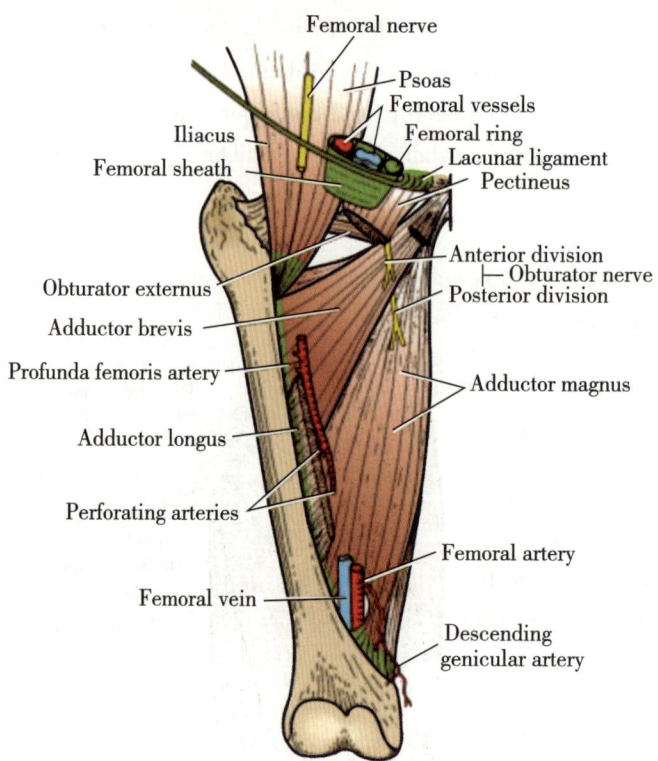

Figure 7-6 Relationship between the obturator nerve and the adductor muscles in the right lower limb

7.2.7 Femoral sheath

The femoral sheath is a downward protrusion into the thigh of the fascial envelope lining the abdominal walls. Its anterior wall is continuous above with the fascia transversalis, and its posterior wall with the fascia iliaca. The sheath surrounds the femoral vessels and lymphatics for about 2.5 cm below the inguinal ligament. The femoral artery, as it enters the thigh beneath the inguinal ligament, occupies the lateral compartment of the sheath. The femoral vein, as it leaves the thigh, lies on its medial side and is separated from it by a fibrous septum and occupies the intermediate compartment. The lymph vessels, as they leave the thigh, are separated from the vein by a fibrous septum and occupy the most medial compartment (Figure 7-7).

The femoral canal is a small medial compartment for the lymph vessels. It is about 1.3 cm long, and its upper opening is called the femoral ring. The femoral septum, which is a condensation of extraperitoneal tissue, closes the ring. The femoral canal contains fatty connective tissue, all the efferent lymph vessels from the deep inguinal lymph nodes, and one of the deep inguinal lymph nodes.

The femoral sheath is adherent to the walls of the blood vessels and inferiorly blends with the tunica adventitia of these vessels. The part of the femoral sheath that forms the medially located femoral canal is not adherent to the walls of the small lymph vessels; it is this site that forms a potentially weak area in the abdomen. A protrusion of peritoneum could be forced down the femoral canal, pushing the femoral septum before it. Such a condition is known as a femoral hernia and is described below.

The femoral ring has the following important relations: anteriorly, the inguinal ligament; posteriorly, the pectineal ligament; medially, the lacunar ligament, and laterally, the femoral vein.

The lower end of the canal is normally closed by the adherence of its medial wall to the tunica adventitia of the femoral vein. It lies close to the saphenous opening in the deep fascia of the thigh.

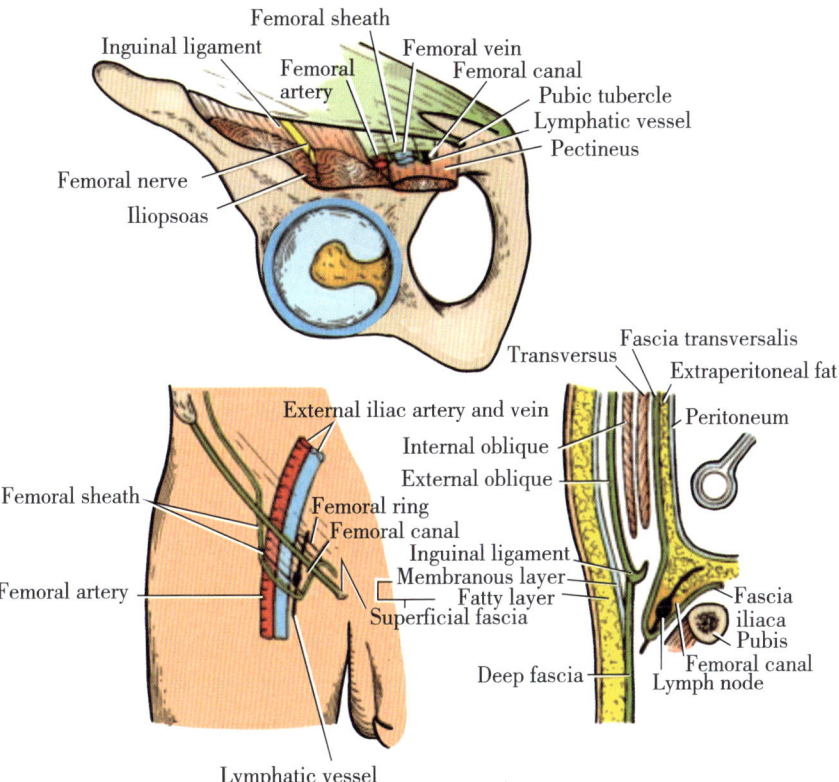

Figure 7-7　Right femoral sheath and its contents

7.2.8　Contents of the anterior fascial compartment of the thigh

7.2.8.1　Femoral artery

　　The femoral artery enters the thigh from behind the inguinal ligament, as a continuation of the external iliac artery. Here, it lies midway between the anterior superior iliac spine and the symphysis pubis.

　　The femoral artery is the main arterial supply to the lower limb. It descends almost vertically toward the adductor tubercle of the femur and ends at the opening in the adductor magnus muscle by entering the popliteal space as the popliteal artery.

　　Branches of femoral artery are as follows (Figure 7-8).

　　(1) The superficial circumflex iliac artery is a small branch that runs up to the region of the anterior superior iliac spine.

　　(2) The superficial epigastric artery is a small branch that crosses the inguinal ligament and runs to the region of the umbilicus.

　　(3) The superficial external pudendal artery is a small branch that runs medially to supply the skin of the scrotum (or labium majus).

　　(4) The deep external pudendal artery runs medially and supplies the skin of the scrotum (or labium majus).

　　(5) The profunda femoris artery is a large and important branch that arises from the lateral side of the femoral artery about 4 cm below the inguinal ligament. It passes medially behind the femoral vessels and enters the medial fascial compartment of the thigh. It ends by becoming the fourth perforating artery. At its origin, it gives off the medial and lateral femoral ircumflex arteries, and during its course it gives off three perforating arteries.

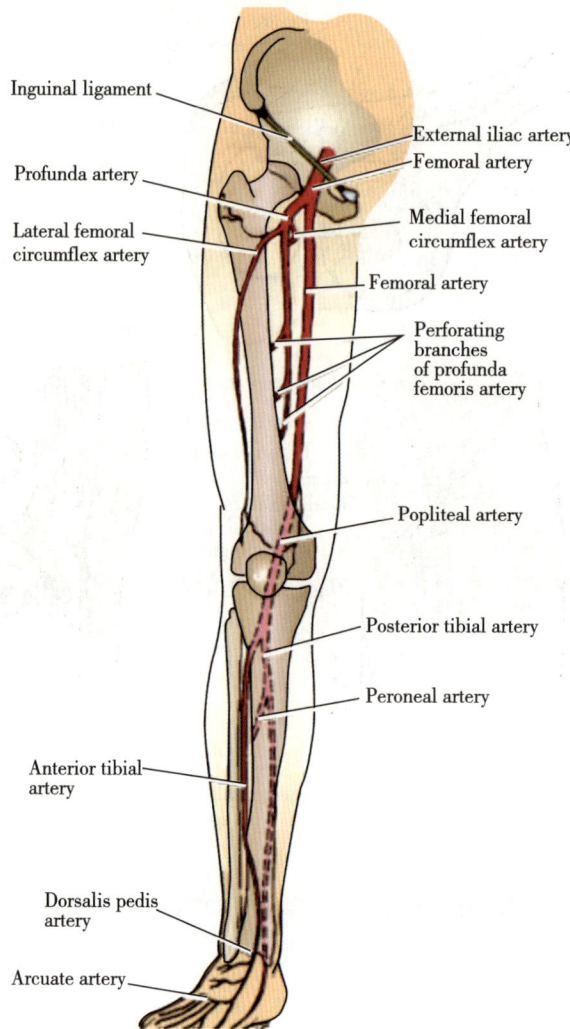

Figure 7-8 Major arteries of the lower limb

(6) The descending genicular artery is a small branch that arises from the femoral artery near its termination. It assists in supplying the knee joint.

7.2.8.2 Femoral vein

The femoral vein enters the thigh by passing through the opening in the adductor magnus as a continuation of the popliteal vein. It ascends through the thigh, lying at first on the lateral side of the artery, then posterior to it, and finally on its medial side.

It leaves the thigh in the intermediate compartment of the femoral sheath and passes behind the inguinal ligament to become the external iliac vein.

The tributaries of the femoral vein are the great saphenous vein and veins that correspond to the branches of the femoral artery. The superficial circumflex iliac vein, the superficial epigastric vein and the external pudendal veins drain into the great saphenous vein.

7.2.8.3 Lymph nodes of the anterior fascial compartment of the thigh

The deep inguinal lymph nodes are variable in number, but there are commonly three. They lie along the medial side of the terminal part of the femoral vein, and the most superior is usually located in the femoral canal. They receive all the lymph from the superficial inguinal nodes via lymph vessels that pass through the cribriform fascia of the saphenous opening. They also receive lymph from the deep structures of the lower limb that have ascended in lymph vessels alongside the arteries, some having passed through the popliteal nodes. The efferent lymph vessels from the deep inguinal nodes ascend into the abdominal cavity through the femoral canal and drain into the external iliac nodes.

7.2.8.4 Nerve supply of the anterior fascial compartment of the thigh

(1) Femoral nerve

The femoral nerve is the largest branch of the lumbar plexus (L_2, L_3, and L_4). It emerges from the lateral border of the psoas muscle within the abdomen and passes downward in the interval between the psoas and iliacus. It lies behind the fascia iliaca and enters the thigh lateral to the femoral artery and the femoral sheath, behind the inguinal ligament. About 4 cm below the inguinal ligament, it terminates by dividing into anterior and posterior divisions. The femoral nerve supplies all the muscles of the anterior compartment of the thigh. Note that the femoral nerve does not enter the thigh within the femoral sheath.

(2) Branches

1) Anterior division

The anterior division gives off two cutaneous and two muscular branches. The cutaneous branches are the medial cutaneous nerve of the thigh and the intermediate cutaneous nerves that supply the skin of the medial and anterior surfaces of the thigh, respectively. The muscular branches supply the sartorius and the pectineus.

2) Posterior division

The posterior division gives off the cutaneous branch and the saphenous nerve. The muscular branches to the quadriceps muscle. The saphenous nerve runs downward and medially and crosses the femoral artery from its lateral to its medial side. It emerges on the medial side of the knee between the tendons of the sartorius and gracilis, then it runs down the medial side of the leg in company with the great saphenous vein. It passes in front of the medial malleolus and along the medial border of the foot, where it terminates in the region of the ball of the big toe.

The muscular branch of the rectus femoris also supplies the hip joint; the branches to the three vasti muscles also supply the knee joint.

7.2.9 Contents of the medial fascial compartment of the thigh

Muscles: gracilis, adductor longus, adductor brevis, adductor magnus, and obturator externus.

Blood supply: profunda femoris artery and obturator artery.

Nerve supply: obturator nerve.

7.2.9.1 Muscles of the medial fascial compartment of the thigh

Note the adductor magnus is a large, triangular muscle consisting of adductor and hamstring portions. The adductor hiatus is a gap in the attachment of this muscle to the femur, which permits the femoral vessels to pass from the adductor canal downward into the popliteal space.

7.2.9.2 Blood supply of the medial fascial compartment of the thigh

(1) Profunda femoris artery

The profunda femoris artery is a large artery that arises from the lateral side of the femoral artery in the femoral triangle, about 4 cm below the inguinal ligament. It descends in the interval between the adductor longus and adductor brevis and then lies on the adductor magnus, where it ends as the fourth perforating artery.

Branches of profunda femoris artery are as follows.

1) Medial femoral circumflex artery

This passes backward between the muscles that form the floor of the femoral triangle and gives off muscular branches in the medial fascial compartment of the thigh. It takes part in the formation of the cruciate anastomosis.

2) Lateral femoral circumflex artery

This passes laterally between the terminal branches of the femoral nerve. It breaks up into branches that supply the muscles of the region and takes part in the formation of the cruciate anastomosis.

3) Four perforating arteries

Three of these arise as branches of the profunda femoris artery; the fourth perforating artery is the terminal part of the profunda artery. The perforating arteries run backward, piercing the various muscle layers as they go. They supply the muscles and terminate by anastomosing with one another and with the inferior gluteal artery and the circumflex femoral arteries above and the muscular branches of the popliteal artery below.

(2) Profunda femoris vein

The profunda femoris vein receives tributaries that correspond to the branches of the artery. It drains into the femoral vein.

(3) Obturator artery

The obturator artery is a branch of the internal iliac artery. It passes forward on the lateral wall of the pelvis and accompanies the obturator nerve through the obturator canal (i.e., the upper part of the obturator foramen). On entering the medial fascial compartment of the thigh, it divides into medial and lateral branches, which pass around the margin of the outer surface of the obturator membrane. It gives off muscular branches and an articular branch to the hip joint.

(4) Obturator vein

The obturator vein receives tributaries that correspond to the branches of the artery. It drains into the internal iliac vein.

7.2.9.3 Nerve supply of the medial fascial compartment of the thigh

(1) Obturator nerve

The obturator nerve arises from the lumbar plexus (L_2–L_4) and emerges on the medial border of the psoas muscle within the abdomen. It runs forward on the lateral wall of the pelvis to reach the upper part of the obturator foramen, where it divides into anterior and posterior divisions.

(2) Branches

1) The anterior division passes downward in front of the obturator externus and the adductor brevis and behind the pectineus and adductor longus. It gives muscular branches to the gracilis, adductor brevis, and adductor longus, and occasionally to the pectineus. It gives articular branches to the hip joint and terminates as a small nerve that supplies the femoral artery. It contributes a variable branch to the subsartorial plexus and supplies the skin on the medial side of the thigh.

2) The posterior division pierces the obturator externus and passes downward behind the adductor brevis and in front of the adductor magnus. It terminates by descending through the opening in the adductor magnus to supply the knee joint. It gives muscular branches to the obturator externus, to the adductor part of the adductor magnus, and occasionally to the adductor brevis.

7.3 The gluteal region, the back of the thigh and the popliteal fossa

7.3.1 The gluteal region

The gluteal region, or buttock, is bounded superiorly by the iliac crest and inferiorly by the fold of the buttock. The region is largely made up of the gluteal muscles and a thick layer of superficial fascia(Figure 7-9, Figure 7-10).

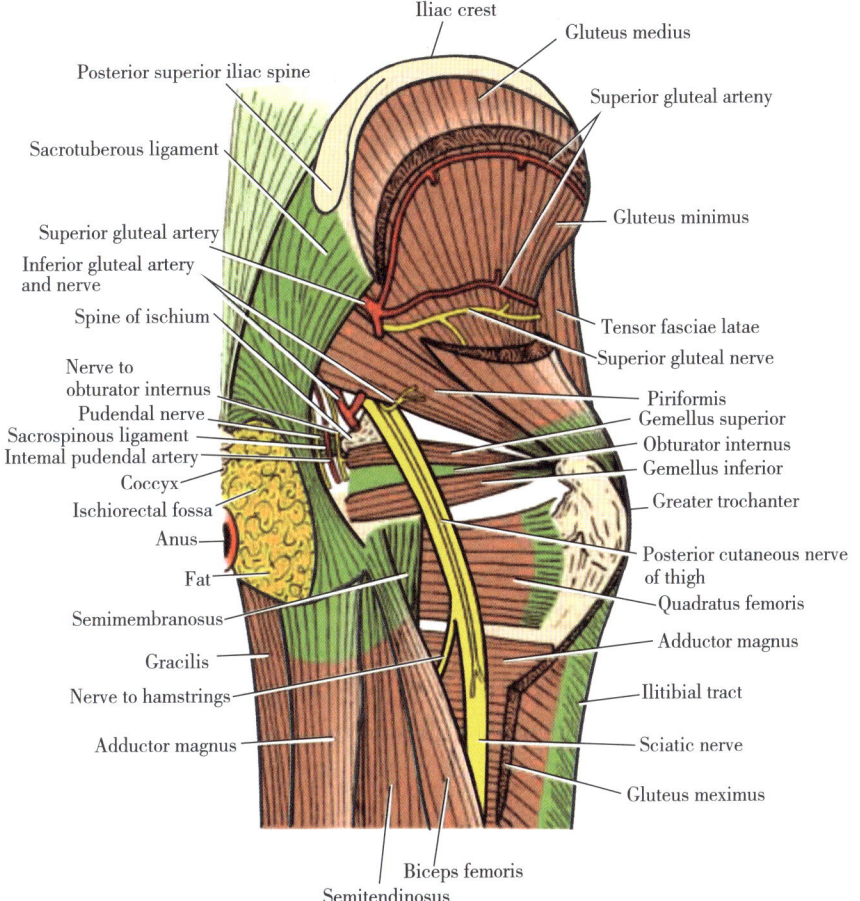

Figure 7-9 Structures in the right gluteal region

(The greater part of the gluteus maximus and part of the gluteus medius have been removed)

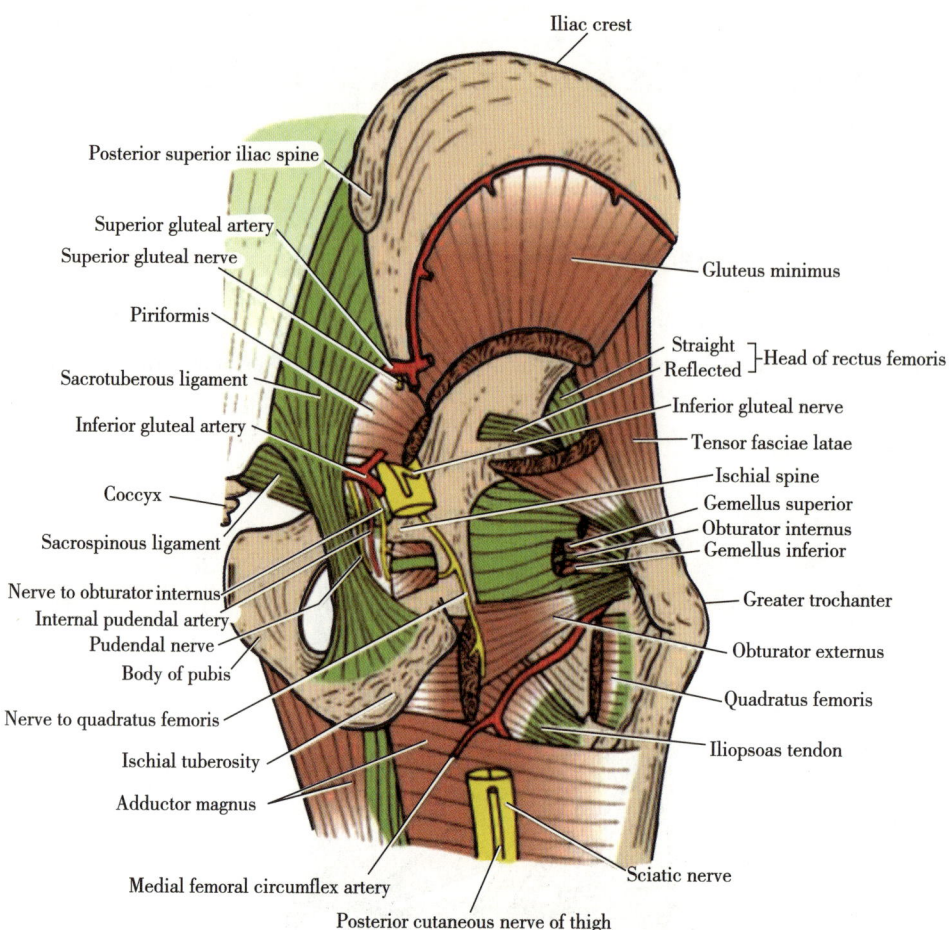

Figure 7-10 Deep structures in the right gluteal region
(The gluteus maximus and the gluteus medius muscles have been completely removed)

7.3.1.1 The skin of the buttock

The cutaneous nerves are derived from posterior and anterior rami of spinal nerves, as follows.

(1) The upper medial quadrant is supplied by the posterior rami of the upper three lumbar nerves and the upper three sacral nerves.

(2) The upper lateral quadrant is supplied by the lateral branches of the iliohypogastric (L_1) and 12th thoracic nerves (anterior rami).

(3) The lower medial quadrant is supplied by branches from the posterior cutaneous nerve of the thigh (S_1-S_3, anterior rami).

The skin over the coccyx in the floor of the cleft between the buttocks is supplied by small branches of the lower sacral and coccygeal nerves.

The lymph vessels drain into the lateral group of the superficial inguinal nodes.

7.3.1.2 Fascia of the buttock

The superficial fascia is thick, especially in women, and is impregnated with large quantities of fat. It contributes to the prominence of the buttock.

The deep fascia is continuous below with the deep fascia (fascia lata) of the thigh. In the gluteal region, it splits to enclose the gluteus maximus muscle. Above the gluteus maximus, it continues as a single layer that covers the outer surface of the gluteus medius and is attached to the iliac crest. On the lateral surface of the thigh, the fascia is thickened to form a strong, wide band, the iliotibial tract. This is attached above to the tubercle of the iliac crest and below to the lateral condyle of the tibia. The iliotibial tract forms a sheath for the tensor fasciae latae muscle and receives the greater part of the insertion of the gluteus maximus.

7.3.1.3 Muscles of the gluteal region

The muscles of the gluteal region include the gluteus maximus, the gluteus medius, the gluteus minimus, the tensor fasciae latae, the piriformis, the obturator internus, the superior and inferior gemelli, and the quadratus femoris.

Note the following:

(1) The gluteus maximus is the largest muscle in the body. It lies superficial in the gluteal region and is largely responsible for the prominence of the buttock.

(2) The tensor fasciae latae runs downward and backward to its insertion in the iliotibial tract and thus assists the gluteus maximus muscle in maintaining the knee in the extended position.

(3) The piriformis lies partly within the pelvis at its origin. It emerges through the greater sciatic foramen to enter the gluteal region. Its position serves to separate the superior gluteal vessels and nerves from the inferior gluteal vessels and nerves.

(4) The obturator internus is a fan-shaped muscle that lies within the pelvis at its origin. It emerges through the lesser sciatic foramen to enter the gluteal region. The tendon is joined by the superior and inferior gemelli and is inserted into the greater trochanter of the femur.

(5) Three bursae are usually associated with the gluteus maximus: between the tendon of insertion and the greater trochanter, between the tendon of insertion and the vastus lateralis, and overlying the ischial tuberosity.

7.3.1.4 Nerves of the gluteal region

(1) Sciatic nerve

The sciatic nerve, a branch of the sacral plexus (L_4-L_5; S_1-S_3), emerges from the pelvis through the lower part of the greater sciatic foramen. It is the largest nerve in the body and consists of the tibial and common peroneal nerves bound together with fascia. The nerve appears below the piriformis and curves downward and laterally, lying successively on the root of the ischial spine, the superior gemellus, the obturator internus, the inferior gemellus, and the quadratus femoris to reach the back of the adductor magnus. It is related posteriorly to the posterior cutaneous nerve of the thigh and the gluteus maximus. It leaves the buttock region by passing deep to the long head of the biceps femoris to enter the back of the thigh.

Occasionally, the common peroneal nerve leaves the sciatic nerve high in the pelvis and appears in the gluteal region by passing above or through the piriformis muscle.

The sciatic nerve usually gives no branches in the gluteal region.

(2) Posterior cutaneous nerve of the thigh

The posterior cutaneous nerve of the thigh, a branch of the sacral plexus, enters the gluteal region through the lower part of the greater sciatic foramen below the piriformis muscle. It passes downward on the posterior surface of the sciatic nerve and runs down the back of the thigh beneath the deep fascia. In the popliteal fossa, it supplies the skin.

Branches are as follows.

1) Gluteal branches to the skin over the lower medial quadrant of the buttock.

2) Perineal branch to the skin of the back of the scrotum or labium majus.

3) Cutaneous branches to the back of the thigh and the upper part of the leg.

(3) Superior gluteal nerve

The superior gluteal nerve, a branch of the sacral plexus, leaves the pelvis through the upper part of the greater sciatic foramen above the piriformis. It runs forward between the gluteus medius and minimus, supplies both, and ends by supplying the tensor fasciae latae.

(4) Inferior gluteal nerve

The inferior gluteal nerve, a branch of the sacral plexus, leaves the pelvis through the lower part of the greater sciatic foramen below the piriformis. It supplies the gluteus maximus muscle.

(5) Nerve to the quadratus femoris

A branch of the sacral plexus, the nerve to the quadratus femoris leaves the pelvis through the lower part of the greater sciatic foramen. It ends by supplying the quadratus femoris and the inferior gemellus.

(6) Pudendal nerve and the nerve to the obturator internus

Branches of the sacral plexus, the pudendal nerve, and nerve to the obturator internus leave the pelvis through the lower part of the greater sciatic foramen, below the piriformis. They cross the ischial spine with the internal pudendal artery and immediately re-enter the pelvis through the lesser sciatic foramen; they then lie in the ischiorectal fossa. The pudendal nerve supplies structures in the perineum. The nerve to the obturator internus supplies the obturator internus muscle on its pelvic surface.

7.3.1.5 Arteries of the gluteal region

(1) Superior gluteal artery

The superior gluteal artery is a branch from the internal iliac artery and enters the gluteal region through the upper part of the greater sciatic foramen above the piriformis. It divides into branches that are distributed throughout the gluteal region.

(2) Inferior gluteal artery

The inferior gluteal artery is a branch of the internal iliac artery and enters the gluteal region through the lower part of the greater sciatic foramen, below the piriformis. It divides into numerous branches that are distributed throughout the gluteal region.

(3) The trochanteric anastomosis

The trochanteric anastomosis provides the main blood supply to the head of the femur. The nutrient arteries pass along the femoral neck beneath the capsule. The following arteries take part in the anastomosis: the superior gluteal artery, the inferior gluteal artery, the medial femoral circumflex artery, and the lateral femoral circumflex artery.

(4) The cruciate anastomosis

The cruciate anastomosis is situated at the level of the lesser trochanter of the femur and, together with the trochanteric anastomosis, provides a connection between the internal iliac and the femoral arteries. The following arteries take part in the anastomosis: the inferior gluteal artery, the medial femoral circumflex artery, the lateral femoral circumflex artery, and the first perforating artery, a branch of the profunda artery.

7.3.2 The back of the thigh

Figure 7-11 and Figure 7-12 show the structures in the posterior aspect of the right thing.

Chapter 7 The Lower Limb 417

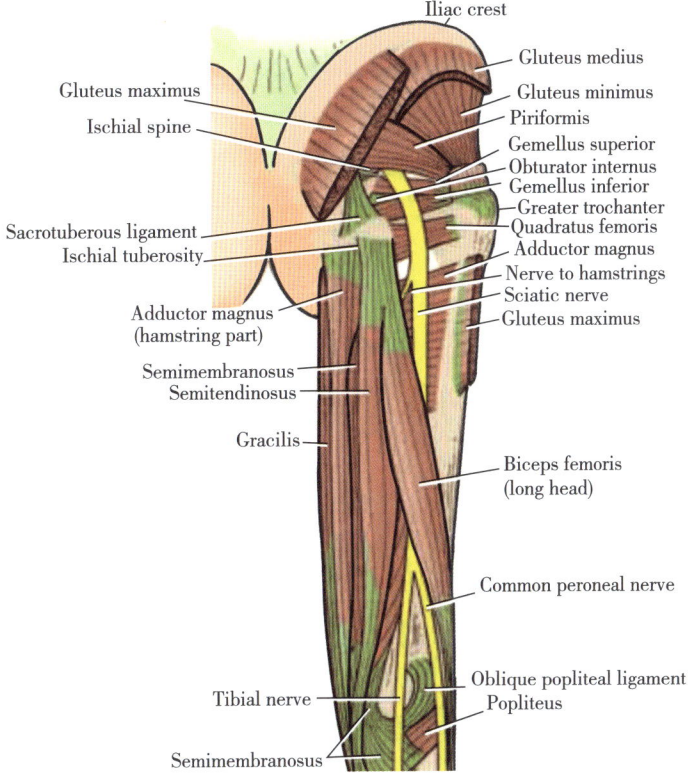

Figure 7-11 Structures in the posterior aspect of the right thigh

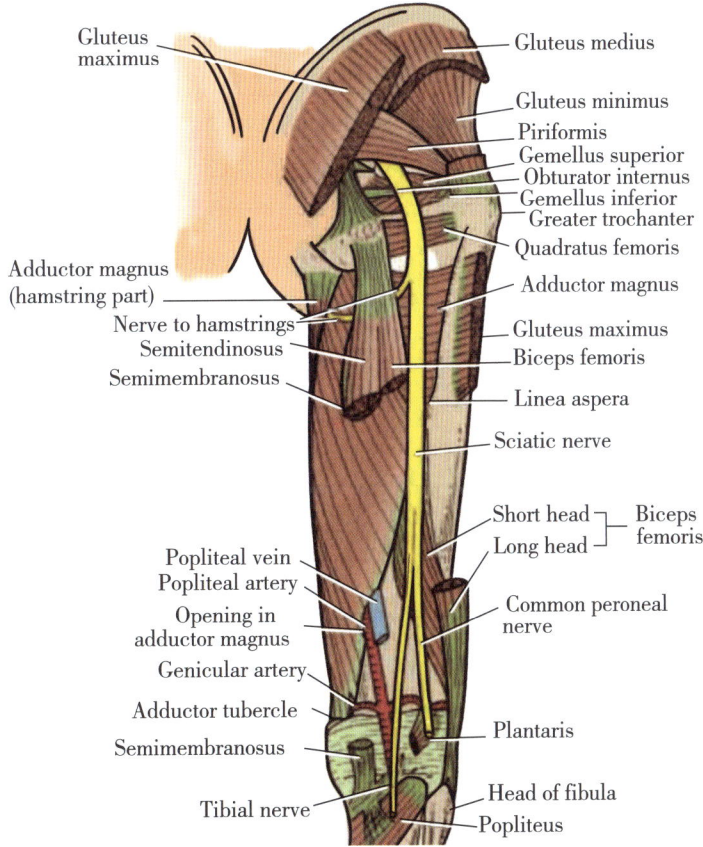

Figure 7-12 Deep structures in the posterior aspect of the right thigh

7.3.2.1 Cutaneous nerves

The posterior cutaneous nerve of the thigh, a branch of the sacral plexus, leaves the gluteal region by emerging from beneath the lower border of the gluteus maximus muscle. It descends on the back of the thigh, and in the popliteal fossa it pierces the deep fascia and supplies the skin. It gives off numerous branches to the skin on the back of the thigh and the upper part of the leg.

7.3.2.2 Superficial veins

Many small veins curve around the medial and lateral aspects of the thigh and ultimately drain into the great saphenous vein. Superficial veins from the lower part of the back of the thigh join the small saphenous vein in the popliteal fossa.

7.3.2.3 Lymph vessels

Lymph from the skin and superficial fascia on the back of the thigh drains upward and forward into the vertical group of superficial inguinal lymph node.

7.3.2.4 Contents of the posterior fascial compartment of the thigh

(1) Muscles: biceps femoris, semitendinosus, semimembranosus, and a small part of the adductor magnus (hamstring muscles).

(2) Blood supply: branches of the profunda femoris artery.

(3) Nerve supply: sciatic nerve.

Note the following:

(1) The biceps femoris muscle receives its nerve supply from the sciatic nerve, the long head from the tibial portion, and the short head from the common peroneal portion.

(2) The hamstring part of the adductor magnus muscle receives its nerve supply from the tibial portion of the sciatic nerve and the adductor part from the obturator nerve.

(3) The semimembranosus insertion sends a fibrous expansion upward and laterally, which reinforces the capsule on the back of the knee joint; the expansion is called the oblique popliteal ligament.

7.3.2.5 Blood supply of the posterior compartment of the thigh

The four perforating branches of the profunda femoris artery provide a rich blood supply to this compartment. The profunda femoris vein drains the greater part of the blood from the compartment.

7.3.2.6 Nerve supply of the posterior compartment of the thigh

(1) Sciatic nerve

The sciatic nerve, a branch of the sacral plexus ($L_4 - L_5$; $S_1 - S_3$), leaves the gluteal region as it descends in the midline of the thigh. It is overlapped posteriorly by the adjacent margins of the biceps femoris and semimembranosus muscles. It lies on the posterior aspect of the adductor magnus muscle. In the lower third of the thigh, it ends by dividing into the tibial and common peroneal nerves. Occasionally, the sciatic nerve divides into its two terminal parts at a higher level—in the upper part of the thigh, the gluteal region, or even inside the pelvis.

(2) Branches

1) The tibial nerve, a terminal branch of the sciatic nerve, enters the popliteal fossa.

2) The common peroneal nerve, a terminal branch of the sciatic nerve, enters the popliteal fossa on the lateral side of the tibial nerve.

3) Muscular branches to the long head of the biceps femoris, the semitendinosus, the semimembranosus, and the hamstring part of the adductor magnus. These branches arise from the tibial component of the sciatic

nerve and run medially to supply the muscles.

7.3.3 Popliteal fossa

The popliteal fossa is a diamond-shaped intermuscular space situated at the back of the knee. The fossa is most prominent when the knee joint is flexed. It contains the popliteal vessels, the small saphenous vein, the common peroneal and tibial nerves, the posterior cutaneous nerve of the thigh, the genicular branch of the obturator nerve, connective tissue, and lymph nodes (Figure 7-13, Figure 7-14).

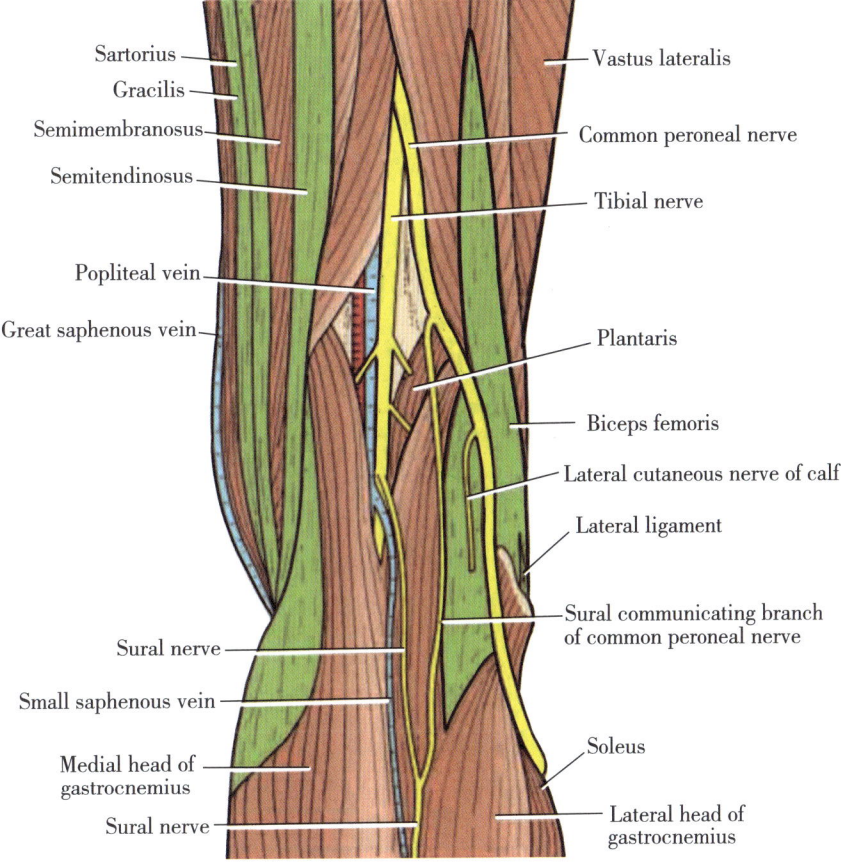

Figure 7-13　Boundaries and contents of the right popliteal fossa

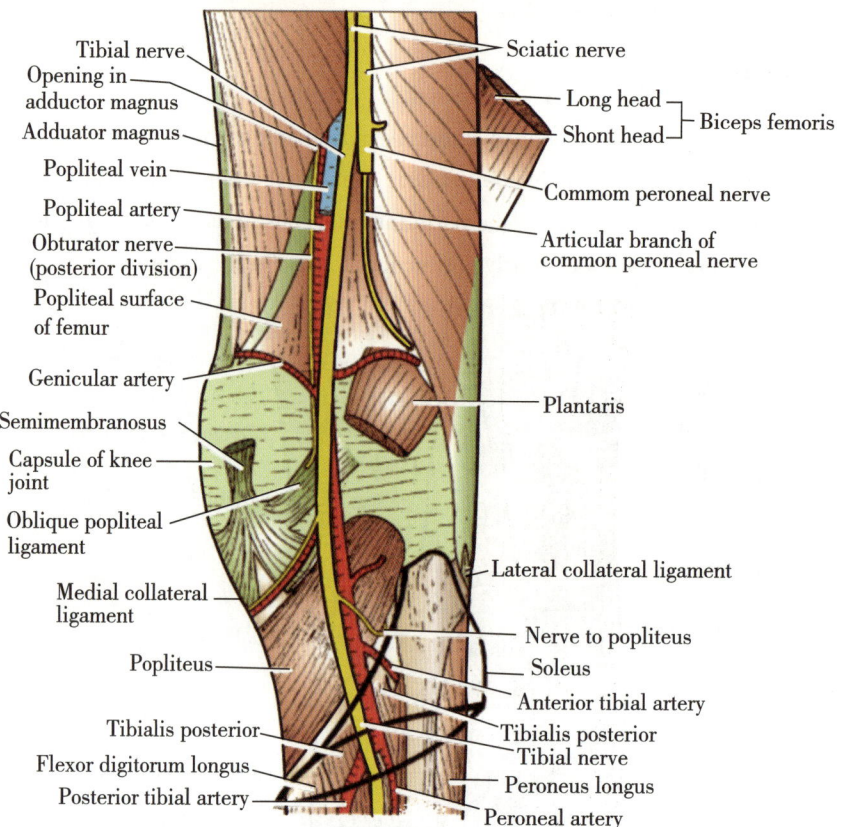

Figure 7-14 Deep structures in the right popliteal fossa
(The proximal end of the soleus muscle is shown in outline only)

7.3.3.1 Boundaries

Laterally: the biceps femoris above and the lateral head of the gastrocnemius and plantaris below.

Medially: the semimembranosus and semitendinosus above and the medial head of the gastrocnemius below.

The anterior wall or floor of the fossa is formed by the popliteal surface of the femur, the posterior ligament of the knee joint, and the popliteus muscle.

The roof is formed by skin, superficial fascia, and the deep fascia of the thigh.

7.3.3.2 Popliteal artery

The popliteal artery is deeply placed and enters the popliteal fossa through the opening in the adductor magnus, as a continuation of the femoral artery. It ends at the level of the lower border of the popliteus by dividing into anterior and posterior tibial arteries.

Anteriorly: the popliteal surface of the femur, the knee joint, and the popliteus muscle.

Posteriorly: the popliteal vein and the tibial nerve, fascia, and skin.

Branches: the popliteal artery has muscular branches and articular branches to the knee.

7.3.3.3 Popliteal vein

The popliteal vein is formed by the junction of the venae comitantes of the anterior and posterior tibial arteries at the lower border of the popliteus muscle on the medial side of the popliteal artery. As it ascends through the fossa, it crosses behind the popliteal artery so that it comes to lie on its lateral side. It passes through the opening in the adductor magnus to become the femoral vein.

The tributaries of the popliteal vein are as follows.

(1) Veins that correspond to branches given off by the popliteal artery.

(2) Small saphenous vein, which perforates the deep fascia and passes between the two heads of the gastrocnemius muscle to end in the popliteal vein.

7.3.3.4 Arterial anastomosis around the knee joint

To compensate for the narrowing of the popliteal artery, which occurs during extreme flexion of the knee, around the knee joint is a profuse anastomosis of small branches of the femoral artery with muscular and articular branches of the popliteal artery and with branches of the anterior and posterior tibial arteries.

7.3.3.5 Popliteal lymph nodes

About six lymph nodes are embedded in the fatty connective tissue of the popliteal fossa. They receive superficial lymph vessels from the lateral side of the foot and leg; these accompany the small saphenous vein into the popliteal fossa. They also receive lymph from the knee joint and from deep lymph vessels accompanying the anterior and posterior tibial arteries.

7.3.3.6 Tibial nerve

The tibial nerve is the larger terminal branch of the sciatic nerve, it arises in the lower third of the thigh. It runs downward through the popliteal fossa, lying first on the lateral side of the popliteal artery, then posterior to it, and finally medial to it. The popliteal vein lies between the nerve and the artery throughout its course. The nerve enters the posterior compartment of the leg by passing beneath the soleus muscle.

Branches are as follows.

(1) Cutaneous: the sural nerve descends between the two heads of the gastrocnemius muscle and is usually joined by the sural communicating branch of the common peroneal nerve. Numerous small branches arise from the sural nerve to supply the skin of the calf and the back of the leg. The sural nerve accompanies the small saphenous vein behind the lateral malleolus and is distributed to the skin along the lateral border of the foot and the lateral side of the little toe.

(2) Muscular branches supply both heads of the gastrocnemius and the plantaris, soleus, and popliteus.

(3) Articular branches supply the knee joint.

7.3.3.7 Common peroneal nerve

The common peroneal nerve is the smaller terminal branch of the sciatic nerve, it nerve arises in the lower third of the thigh. It runs downward through the popliteal fossa, closely following the medial border of the biceps muscle. It leaves the fossa by crossing superficially the lateral head of the gastrocnemius muscle. It then passes behind the head of the fibula, winds laterally around the neck of the bone, pierces the peroneus longus muscle, and divides into two terminal branches: the superficial peroneal nerve and the deep peroneal nerve. As the nerve lies on the lateral aspect of the neck of the fibula, it is subcutaneous and can easily be rolled against the bone.

7.3.3.8 Posterior cutaneous nerve of the thigh

The posterior cutaneous nerve of the thigh through the gluteal region and the back of the thigh terminates by supplying the skin over the popliteal fossa.

7.3.3.9 Obturator nerve

It leaves the subsartorial canal with the femoral artery by passing through the opening in the adductor magnus. The nerve terminates by supplying the knee joint.

7.3.3.10 Fascial compartments of the leg

The deep fascia surrounds the leg and is continuous above with the deep fascia of the thigh. Below the tibial condyles, it is attached to the periosteum on the anterior and medialborders of the tibia. Two intermuscular septa pass from its deep aspect to be attached to the fibula. These, together with the interosseous membrane, divide the leg into three compartments (anterior, lateral, and posterior), each having its own muscles, blood supply, and nerve supply.

7.3.3.11 Interosseous membrane

The interosseous membrane binds the tibia and fibula together and provides attachment for neighboring muscles.

7.3.3.12 Retinacula of the ankle

The retinacula are thickenings of the deep fascia that keep the long tendons around the ankle joint in position and act as pulleys.

7.3.3.13 Superior extensor retinaculum

The superior extensor retinaculum is attached to the distal ends of the anterior borders of the fibula and the tibia.

7.3.3.14 Inferior extensor retinaculum

The inferior extensor retinaculum is a Y-shaped band located in front of the ankle joint. Fibrous bands separate the tendons into compartments, each of which is lined by a synovial sheath.

7.3.3.15 Flexor retinaculum

The flexor retinaculum extends from the medial malleolus downward and backward to be attached to the medial surface of the calcaneum. It binds the tendons of the deep muscles of the back of the leg to the back of the medial malleolus as they pass forward to enter the sole. The tendons lie in compartments, each of which is lined by a synovial sheath.

7.3.3.16 Superior peroneal retinaculum

The superior peroneal retinaculum connects the lateral malleolus to the lateral surface of the calcaneum. It binds the tendons of the peroneus longus and brevis to the back of the lateral malleolus. The tendons are provided with a common synovial sheath.

7.3.3.17 Inferior peroneal retinaculum

The inferior peroneal retinaculum binds the tendons of the peroneus longus and brevis muscles to the lateral side of the calcaneum. The tendons each possess a synovial sheath, which is continuous above with the common sheath.

7.4 The anterior and lateral region of the leg

7.4.1 The front of the leg

7.4.1.1 Cutaneous nerves

The lateral cutaneous nerve of the calf, a branch of the common peroneal nerve, supplies the skin on the upper part of the lateral surface of the leg.

The superficial peroneal nerve, a branch of the common peroneal nerve, supplies the skin of the lower part of the anterolateral surface of the leg. The saphenous nerve, a branch of the femoral nerve, supplies the skin on the anteromedial surface of the leg.

7.4.1.2 Superficial veins

Numerous small veins curve around the medial aspect of the leg and ultimately drain into the great saphenous vein.

7.4.1.3 Lymph vessels

The greater part of the lymph from the skin and superficial fascia on the front of the leg drains upward and medially in vessels that follow the great saphenous vein, to end in the vertical group of superficial inguinal lymph nodes. A small amount of lymph from the upper lateral part of the front of the leg may pass via vessels that accompany the small saphenous vein and drain into the popliteal nodes.

7.4.1.4 Contents of the anterior fascial compartment of the leg (Figure 7-15, Figure 7-16)

Muscles: the tibialis anterior, extensor digitorum longus, peroneus tertius, and extensor hallucis longus.

Blood supply: anterior tibial artery.

Nerve supply: deep peroneal nerve.

(1) Muscles of the anterior fascial compartment of the leg

Note the following:

1) Extension, or dorsiflexion of the ankle, is the movement of the foot away from the ground.

2) The peroneus tertius muscle extends the foot at the ankle joint along with the other muscles in this compartment and is supplied by the deep peroneal nerve. The muscle also everts the foot at the subtalar and transverse tarsal joints along with the peroneus longus and brevis muscles but receives no innervation from the superficial peroneal nerve.

3) The extensor digitorum longus tendons on the dorsal surface of each toe become incorporated into a fascial expansion called the extensor expansion. The central part of the expansion is inserted into the base of the middle phalanx, and the two lateral parts converge to be inserted into the base of the distal phalanx.

(2) Artery of the anterior fascial compartment of the leg

1) Anterior tibial artery

The anterior tibial artery is the smaller of the terminal branches of the popliteal artery. It arises at the level of the lower border of the popliteus muscle and passes forward into the anterior compartment of the leg through an opening in the upper part of the interosseous membrane. It descends on the anterior surface of the interosseous membrane, accompanied by the deep peroneal nerve. In the upper part of its course, it lies deep beneath the muscles of the compartment. In the lower part of its course, it lies superficial in front of the lower end of the tibia. Having passed behind the superior extensor retinaculum, it has the tendon of the extensor hallucis longus on its medial side and the deep peroneal nerve and the tendons of extensor digitorum longus on its lateral side. It is here that its pulsations can easily be felt in the living subject. In front of the ankle joint, the artery becomes the dorsalis pedis artery.

2) Branches

- Muscular branches to neighboring muscles.
- Anastomotic branches that anastomose with branches of other arteries around the knee and ankle joints
- Venae comitantes of the anterior tibial artery join those of the posterior tibial artery in the popliteal fossa to form the popliteal vein.

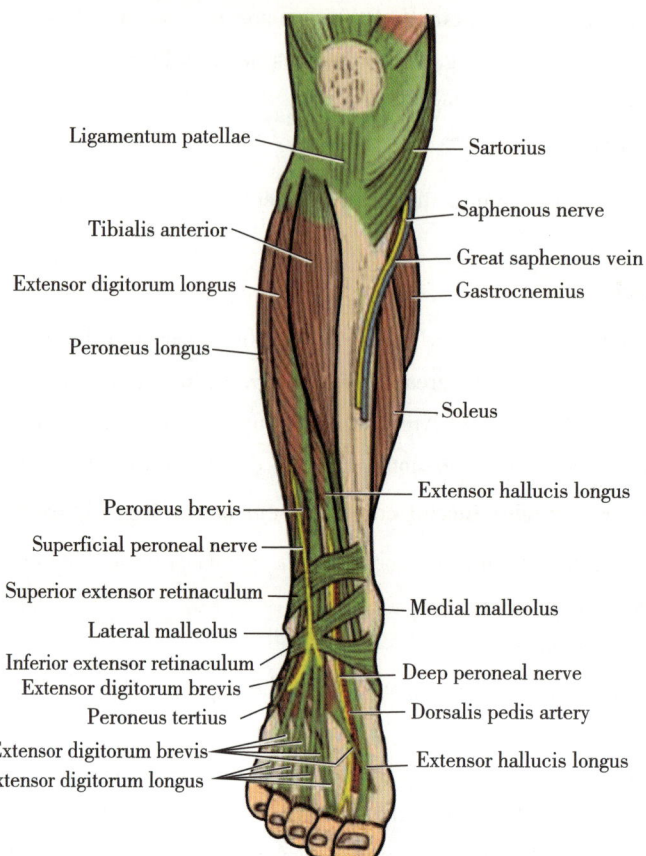

Figure 7–15   Structures in the anterior and lateral aspects of the right leg and the dorsum of the foot

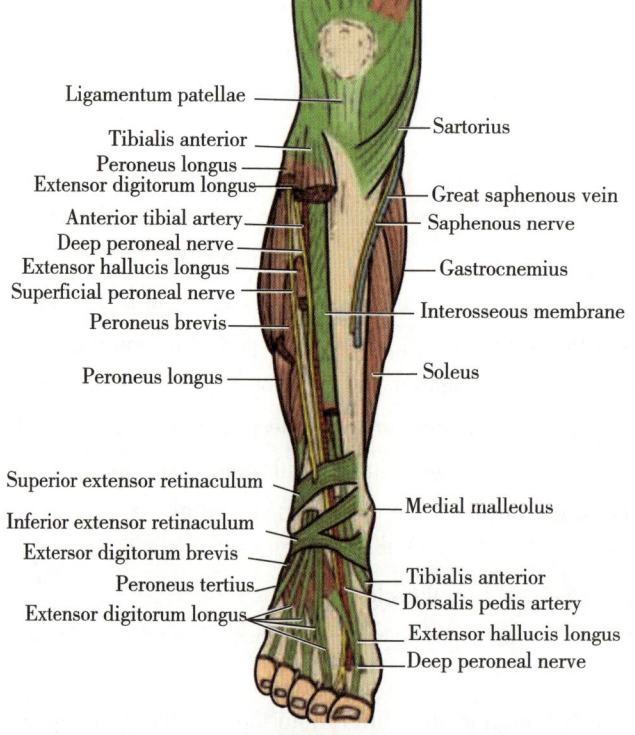

Figure 7–16   Deep structures in the anterior and lateral aspects of the right leg and the dorsum of the foot

(3) Nerve supply of the anterior fascial compartment of the leg

1) Deep peroneal nerve

The deep peroneal nerve is one of the terminal branches of the common peroneal nerve. It arises in the substance of the peroneus longus on the lateral side of the neck of the fibula. The nerve enters the anterior compartment by piercing the anterior fascial septum. It then descends deep to the extensor digitorum longus muscle, first lying lateral, then anterior, and finally lateral to the anterior tibial artery.

2) Branches

- Muscular branches to the tibialis anterior, the extensor digitorum longus, the peroneus tertius, and the extensor hallucis longus.
- Articular branch to the ankle joint.

7.4.1.5 Contents of the lateral fascial compartment of the leg

Muscles: peroneus longus and peroneus brevis.

Blood supply: branches from the peroneal artery.

Nerve supply: superficial peroneal nerve.

(1) Muscles of the lateral fascial compartment of the leg

Note the following: both the peroneus longus and brevis muscles flex the foot at the ankle joint and evert the foot at the subtalar and transverse tarsal joints. They also play an important role in holding up the lateral longitudinal arch in the foot. In addition, the peroneus longus tendon serves as a tie to the transverse arch of the foot.

(2) Artery of the lateral fascial compartment of the leg

Numerous branches from the peroneal artery, which lies in the posterior compartment of the leg, pierce the posterior fascial septum, and supply the peroneal muscles.

(3) Nerve of the lateral fascial compartment of the leg

1) Superficial peroneal nerve

The superficial peroneal nerve is one of the terminal branches of the common peroneal nerve. It arises in the substance of the peroneus longus muscle on the lateral side of the neck of the fibula. It descends between the peroneus longus and brevis, and in the lower part of the leg it becomes cutaneous.

2) Branches

- Muscular branches to the peroneus longus and brevis.
- Cutaneous: medial and lateral branches are distributed to the skin on the lower part of the front of the leg and the dorsum of the foot. In addition, branches supply the dorsal surfaces of the skin of all the toes, except the adjacent sides of the first and second toes and the lateral side of the little toe.

7.4.2 The back of the leg

7.4.2.1 Cutaneous nerves

The posterior cutaneous nerve of the thigh descends on the back of the thigh. In the popliteal fossa, it supplies the skin over the popliteal fossa and the upper part of the back of the leg.

The lateral cutaneous nerve of the calf, a branch of the common peroneal nerve, supplies the skin on the upper part of the posterolateral surface of the leg.

The sural nerve, a branch of the tibial nerve, supplies the skin on the lower part of the posterolateral surface of the leg.

The saphenous nerve, a branch of the femoral nerve, gives off branches that supply the skin on the posteromedial surface of the leg.

7.4.2.2 Superficial veins

The small saphenous vein arises from the lateral part of the dorsal venous arch of the foot. It ascends behind the lateral malleolus in company with the sural nerve. It follows the lateral border of the tendo calcaneus and then runs up the middle of the back of the leg. The vein pierces the deep fascia and passes between the two heads of the gastrocnemius muscle in the lower part of the popliteal fossa; it ends in the popliteal vein. The small saphenous vein has numerous valves along its course.

Tributaries are as follows.

(1) Numerous small veins from the back of the leg.

(2) Communicating veins with the deep veins of the foot.

(3) Important anastomotic branches that run upward and medially and join the great saphenous vein.

The mode of termination of the small saphenous vein is subject to variation: it may join the popliteal vein; it may join the great saphenous vein; or it may split in two, one division joining the popliteal and the other joining the great saphenous vein.

7.4.2.3 Lymph vessels

Lymph vessels from the skin and superficial fascia on the back of the leg drain upward and either pass forward around the medial side of the leg to end in the vertical group of superficial inguinal nodes or drain into the popliteal nodes.

7.4.2.4 Contents of the posterior fascial compartment of the leg (Figure 7-17, Figure 7-18)

The deep transverse fascia of the leg is a septum that divides the muscles of the posterior compartment into superficial and deep groups.

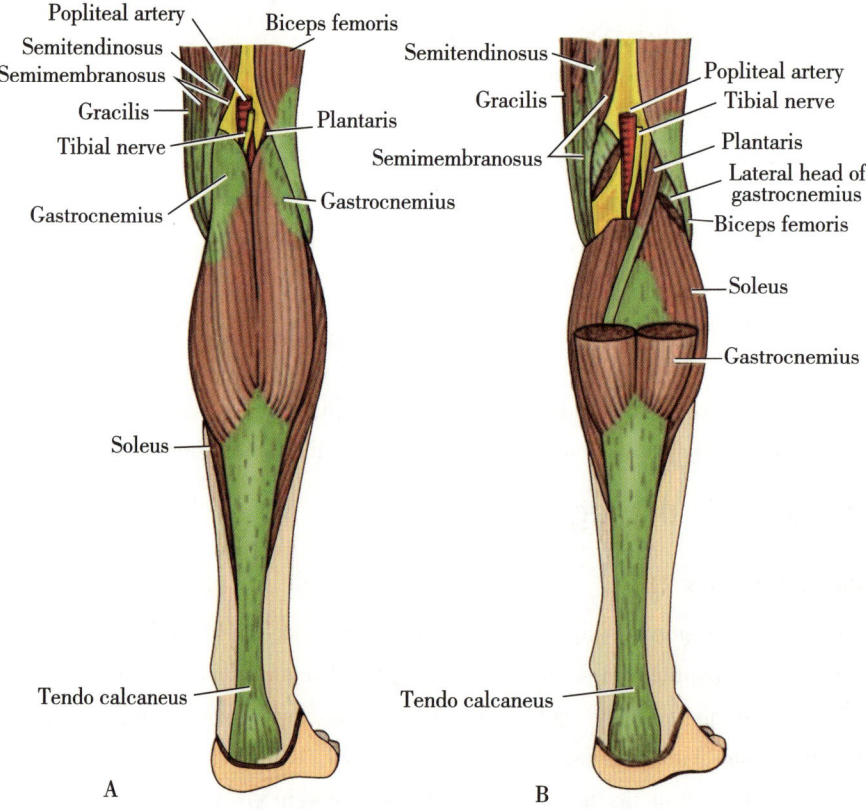

Figure 7-17　Structures in the posterior aspect of the right leg

(In B, part of the gastrocnemius has been removed)

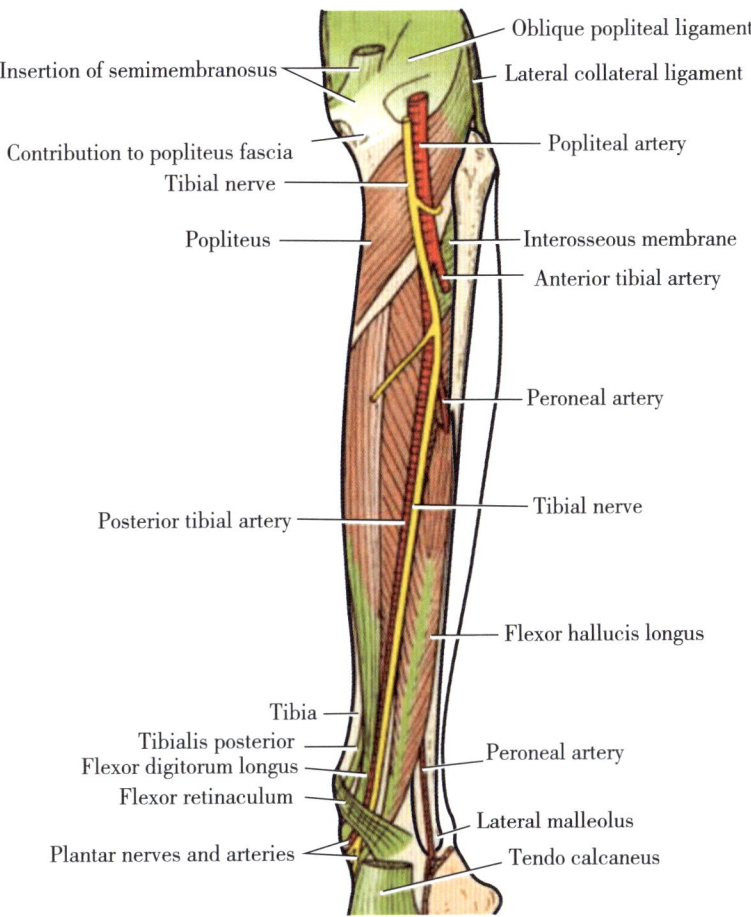

Figure 7-18 Deep structures in the posterior aspect of the right leg

Superficial group of muscles: gastrocnemius, plantaris, and soleus.

Deep group of muscles: popliteus, flexor digitorum longus, flexor hallucis longus, and tibialis posterior.

Blood supply: posterior tibial artery.

Nerve supply: tibial nerve.

(1) Muscles of the posterior fascial compartment of the leg: superficial group

Note the following: together, the soleus, gastrocnemius, and plantaris act as powerful plantar flexors of the ankle joint. They provide the main forward propulsive force in walking and running by using the foot as a lever and raising the heel off the ground.

(2) Muscles of the posterior fascial compartment of the leg: deep group

Note the following:

1) The popliteus muscle arises inside the capsule of the knee joint and is inserted into the upper part of the posterior surface of the tibia. The tendon separates the lateral ligament of the knee joint from the lateral meniscus so that the meniscus is not tethered to the ligament and is freer to move and adapt to the surfaces of the condyle of the femur and the tibia.

2) The popliteus muscle is responsible for "unlocking" the knee joint.

(3) Artery of the posterior fascial compartment of the leg

1) Posterior tibial artery

The posterior tibial artery is one of the terminal branches of the popliteal artery. It begins at the level of the lower border of the popliteus muscle and passes downward deep to the gastrocnemius and soleus and the deep transverse fascia of the leg. It lies on the posterior surface of the tibialis posterior muscle above and on the posterior surface of the tibia below. In the lower part of the leg, the artery is covered only by skin and fascia. The artery passes behind the medial malleolus deep to the flexor retinaculum and terminates by dividing into medial and lateral plantar arteries.

2) Branches

- Peroneal artery, which is a large artery that arises close to the origin of the posterior tibial artery. It descends behind the fibula, either within the substance of the flexor hallucis longus muscle or posterior to it. The peroneal artery gives off numerous muscular branches and a nutrient artery to the fibula and ends by taking part in the anastomosis around the ankle joint. A perforating branch pierces the interosseous membrane to reach the lower part of the front of the leg.
- Muscular branches are distributed to muscles in the posterior compartment of the leg.
- Nutrient artery to the tibia.
- Anastomotic branches, which join other arteries around the ankle joint.
- Medial and lateral plantar arteries.

Venae comitantes of the posterior tibial artery join those of the anterior tibial artery in the popliteal fossa to form the popliteal vein.

(4) Nerve of the posterior fascial compartment of the leg

1) Tibial nerve

The tibial nerve is the larger terminal branch of the sciatic nerve in the lower third of the back of the thigh. It descends through the popliteal fossa and passes deep to the gastrocnemius and soleus muscles. It lies on the posterior surface of the tibialis posterior and, lower down the leg, on the posterior surface of the tibia. The nerve accompanies the posterior tibial artery and lies at first on its medial side, then crosses posterior to it, and finally lies on its lateral side. The nerve, with the artery, passes behind the medial malleolus, between the tendons of the flexor digitorum longus and the flexor hallucis longus. It is covered here by the flexor retinaculum and divides into the medial and lateral plantar nerves.

2) Branches in the leg (below the popliteal fossa)

- Muscular branches to the soleus, flexor digitorum longus, flexor hallucis longus, and tibialis posterior.
- Cutaneous: the medial calcaneal branch supplies the skin over the medial surface of the heel.
- Articular branch to the ankle joint.
- Medial and lateral plantar nerves.

7.5 The region of the ankle and foot

7.5.1 The region of the ankle

Before learning the anatomy of the foot, it is essential that a student have a sound knowledge of the arrangement of the tendons, arteries, and nerves in the region of the ankle joint. From the clinical standpoint, the ankle is a common site for fractures, sprains, and dislocations.

7.5.1.1 Anterior aspect of the ankle

(1) Structures that pass anterior to the extensor retinacula from medial to lateral (Figure 7-19)

1) Saphenous nerve and great saphenous vein (in front of the medial malleolus).

2) Superficial peroneal nerve (medial and lateral branches).

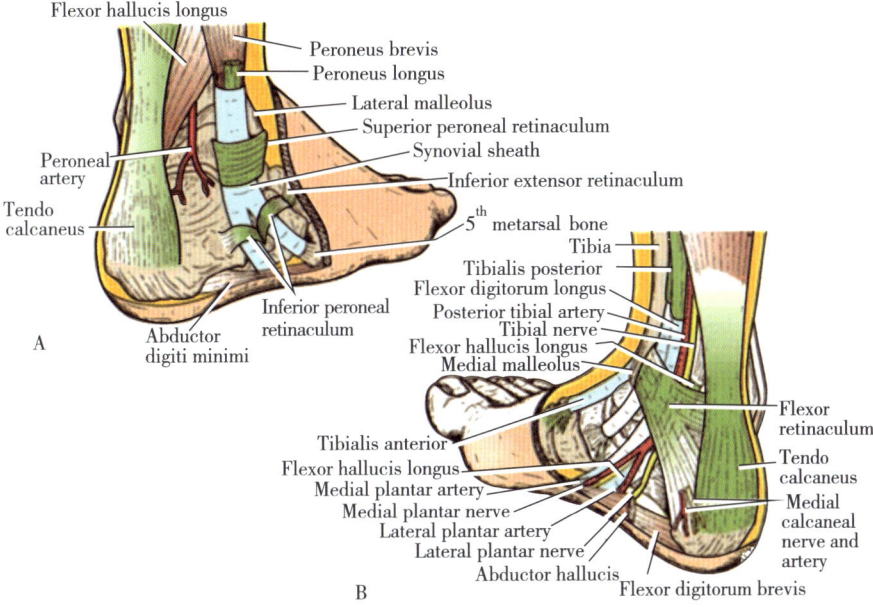

Figure 7-19 Structures passing behind the lateral malleolus (A) and the medial malleolus (B)

(Synovial sheaths of the tendons are shown in blue. Note the positions of the retinacula)

(2) Structures that pass beneath or through the extensor retinacula from medial to lateral

1) Tibialis anterior tendon.
2) Extensor hallucis longus tendon.
3) Anterior tibial artery with venae comitantes.
4) Deep peroneal nerve.
5) Extensor digitorum longus tendons.
6) Peroneus tertius.

As each of the above tendons passes beneath or through the extensor retinacula, it is surrounded by a synovial sheath.

The tendons of extensor digitorum longus and the peroneus tertius share a common synovial sheath.

(3) Structures that pass in front of the medial malleolus

1) Great saphenous vein.
2) Saphenous nerve.

7.5.1.2 Posterior aspect of the ankle

(1) Structures that pass behind the medial malleolus beneath the flexor retinaculum from medial to lateral

1) Tibialis posterior tendon.
2) Flexor digitorum longus.
3) Posterior tibial artery with venae comitantes.
4) Tibial nerve.
5) Flexor hallucis longus.

As each of these tendons passes beneath the flexor retinaculum, it is surrounded by a synovial sheath.

(2) Structures that pass behind the lateral malleolus superficial to the superior peroneal retinaculum

1) The sural nerve.

2) Small saphenous vein.

(3) Structures that pass behind the lateral malleolus beneath the superior peroneal retinaculum

The peroneus longus and brevis tendons share a common synovial sheath. Lower down, beneath the inferior peroneal retinaculum, they have separate sheaths.

(4) Structures that lie directly behind the ankle

The fat and the large tendo calcaneus lie behind the ankle.

7.5.2 The foot

The foot supports the body weight and provides leverage for walking and running. It is unique in that it is constructed in the form of arches, which enable it to adapt its shape to uneven surfaces. It also serves as a resilient spring to absorb shocks, such as in jumping.

7.5.2.1 The sole of the foot

(1) Skin

The skin of the sole of the foot is thick and hairless. It is firmly bound down to the underlying deep fascia by numerous fibrous bands. The skin shows a few flexure creases at the sites of skin movement. Sweat glands are present in large numbers.

The sensory nerve supply to the skin of the sole of the foot is derived from the medial calcaneal branch of the tibial nerve, which innervates the medial side of the heel; branches from the medial plantar nerve, which innervate the medial two thirds of the sole; and branches from the lateral plantar nerve, which innervate the lateral third of the sole.

(2) Deep fascia

The plantar aponeurosis is a triangular thickening of the deep fascia that protects the underlying nerves, blood vessels, and muscles. Its apex is attached to the medial and lateral tubercles of the calcaneum (Figure 7-20). The base of the aponeurosis divides into five slips that pass into the toes.

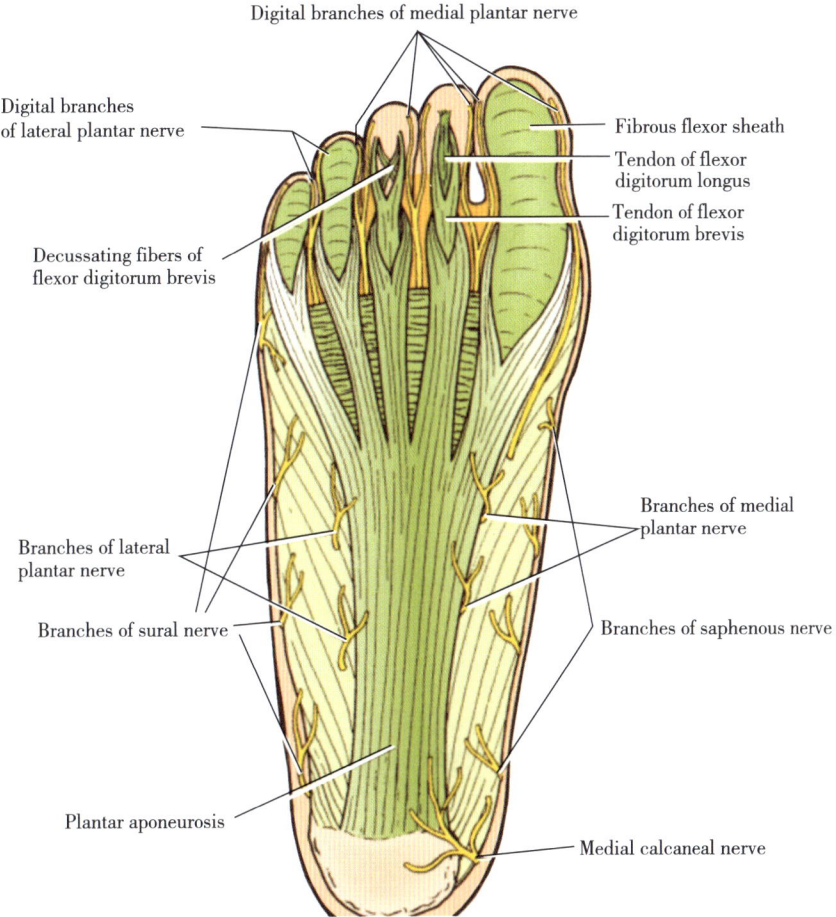

Figure 7-20 Plantar aponeurosis and cutaneous nerves of the sole of the right foot

(3) Muscles of the sole of the foot

The muscles of the sole are conveniently described in four layers from the inferior layer superiorly.

1) First layer: abductor hallucis, flexor digitorum brevis, abductor digiti minimi (Figure 7-21).

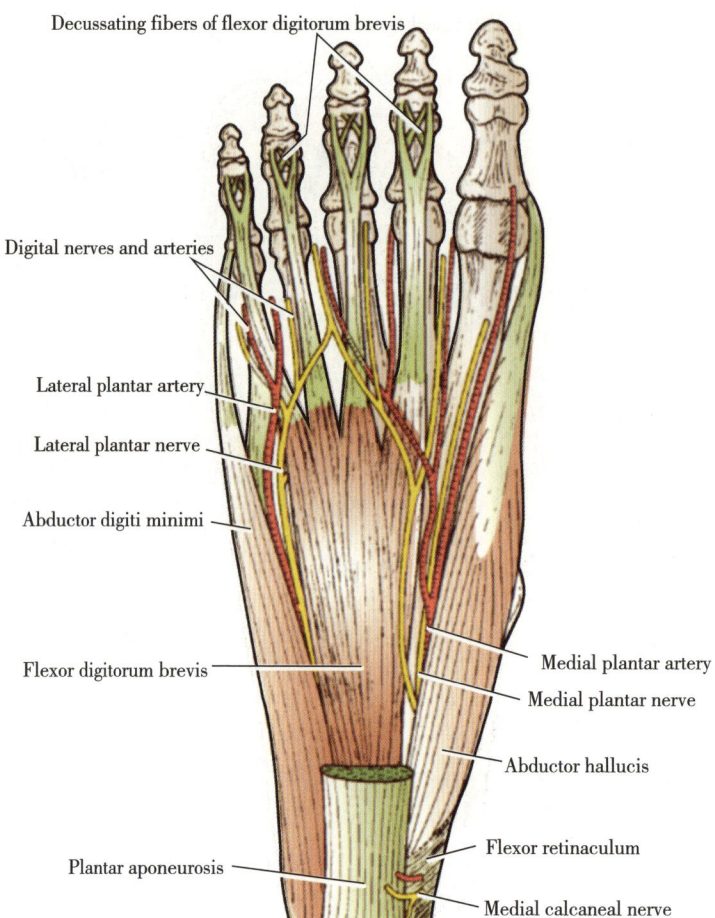

Figure 7-21　First layer of the plantar muscles of the right foot
(Medial and lateral plantar arteries and nerves are also shown)

2) Second layer: quadratus plantae, lumbricals, flexor digitorum longus tendon, flexor hallucis longus tendon (Figure 7-22).

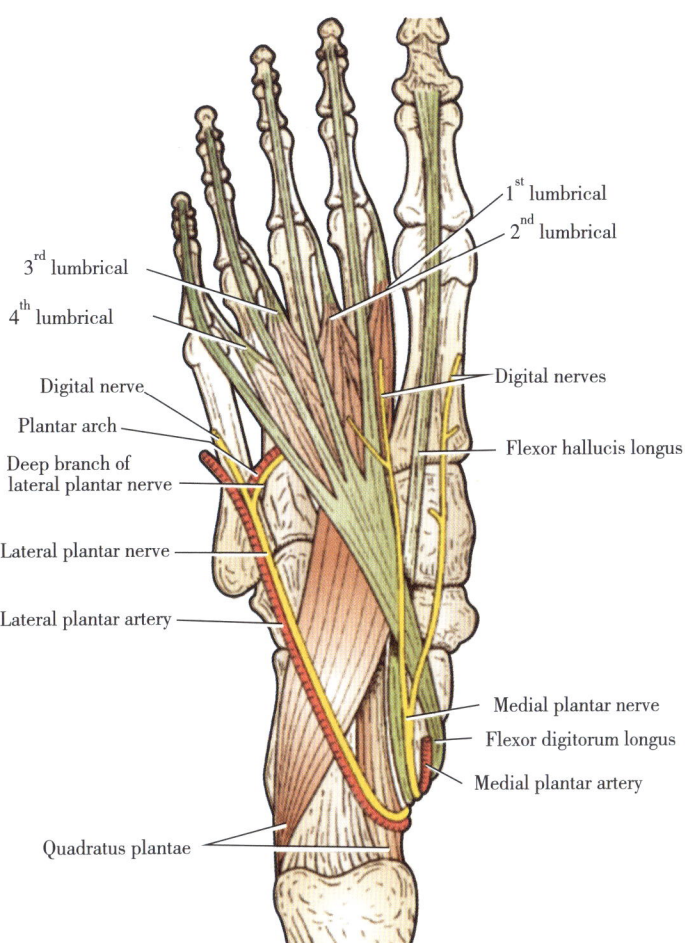

Figure 7-22 Second layer of the plantar muscles of the right foot

(Medial and lateral plantar arteries and nerves are also shown)

3) Third layer: flexor hallucis brevis, adductor hallucis, flexor digiti minimi brevis (Figure 7-23).

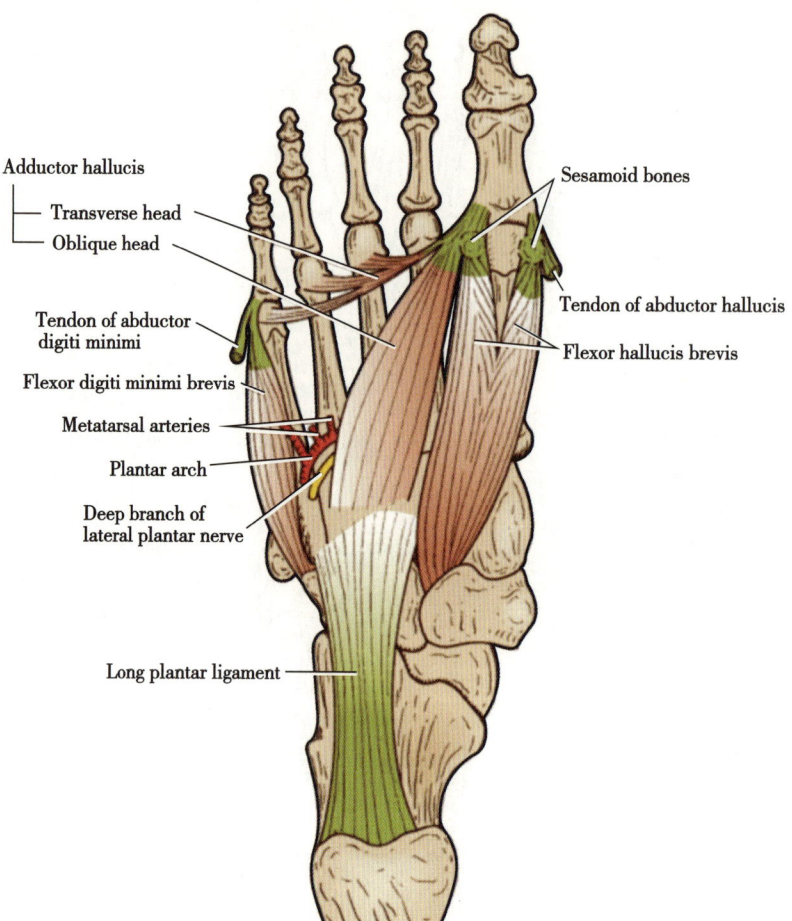

Figure 7-23　Third layer of the plantar muscles of the right foot

(The deep branch of the lateral plantar nerve and the plantar arterial arch are also shown)

4) Fourth layer: interossei, peroneus longus tendon, tibialis posterior tendon (Figure 7-24).

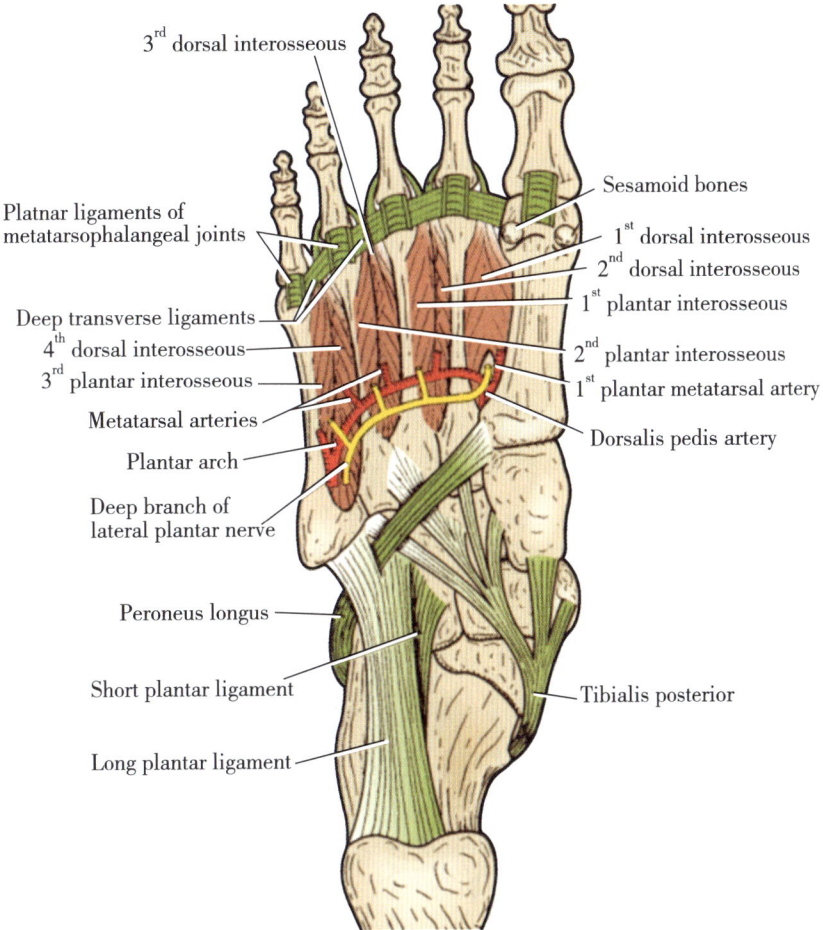

Figure 7-24 Fourth layer of the plantar muscles of the right foot
(The deep branch of the lateral plantar nerve and the plantar arterial arch are also shown. Note the deep transverse ligaments)

(4) Long tendons of the sole of the foot

1) Flexor digitorum longus tendon

The flexor digitorum longus tendon enters the sole by passing behind the medial malleolus beneath the flexor retinaculum. It passes forward across the medial surface of the sustentaculum tali and then crosses the tendon of flexor hallucis longus, from which it receives a strong slip. It is here that it receives on its lateral border the insertion of the quadratus plantae muscle. The tendon now divides into its four tendons of insertion, which pass forward, giving origin to the lumbrical muscles. The tendons then enter the fibrous sheaths of the lateral four toes. Each tendon perforates the corresponding tendon of flexor digitorum brevis and passes on to be inserted into the base of the distal phalanx. It should be noted that the method of insertion is similar to that found for the flexor digitorum profundus in the hand.

2) Flexor hallucis longus tendon

The flexor hallucis longus tendon enters the sole by passing behind the medial malleolus beneath the flexor retinaculum. It runs forward below the sustentaculum tali and crosses deep to the flexor digitorum longus tendon, to which it gives a strong slip. It then enters the fibrous sheath of the big toe and is inserted into the base of the distal phalanx.

3) Fibrous flexor sheaths

The inferior surface of each toe, from the head of the metatarsal bone to the base of the distal phalanx, is provided with a strong fibrous sheath, which is attached to the sides of the phalanges arrangement is similar to that found in the fingers. The fibrous sheath, together with the inferior surfaces of the phalanges and the interphalangeal joints, forms a blind tunnel in which lie the flexor tendons of the toe.

4) Synovial flexor sheaths (Figure 7-25)

The tendons of the flexor hallucis longus and the flexor digitorum longus are surrounded by synovial sheaths.

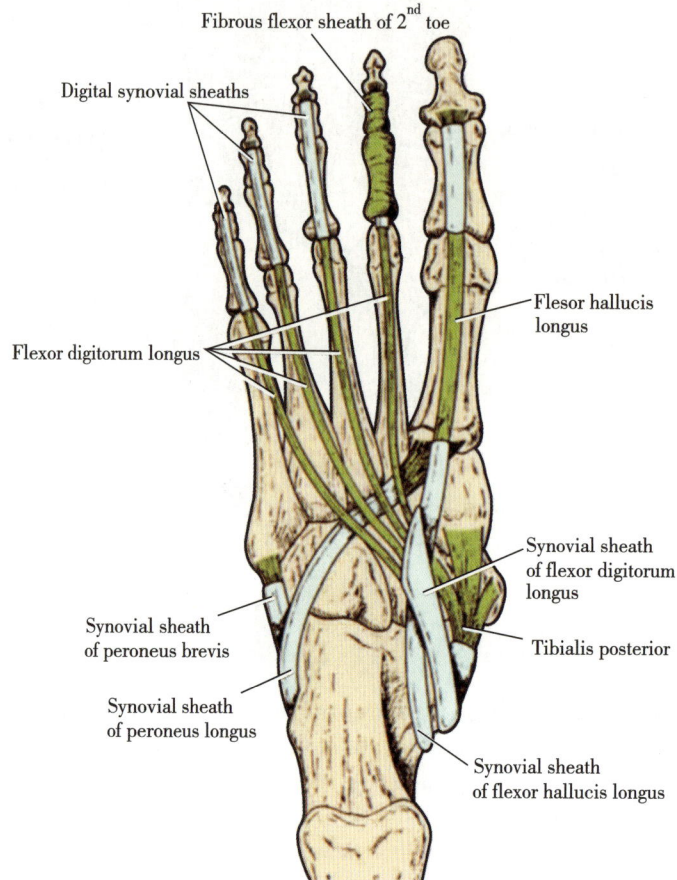

Figure 7-25 Synovial sheaths of the tendons seen on the sole of the right foot

5) Peroneus longus tendon

The peroneus longus tendon enters the foot from behind the lateral malleolus and runs obliquely across the sole to be inserted into the base of the first metatarsal bone and the adjacent part of the medial cuneiform.

The tendon grooves the inferior surface of the cuboid where it is held in position by the long plantar ligament and is surrounded by a synovial sheath.

6) Tibialis posterior tendon

The tibialis posterior tendon enters the foot from behind the medial malleolus. It passes beneath the flexor retinaculum and runs downward and forward above the sustentaculum tali to be inserted mainly into the tuberosity of the navicular. Small tendinous slips pass to the cuboid and the cuneiforms and to the bases of the second, third, and fourth metatarsals. The tendon is surrounded by a synovial sheath.

(5) Arteries of the sole of the foot

1) Medial plantar artery

The medial plantar artery is the smaller of the terminal branches of the posterior tibial artery. It arises beneath the flexor retinaculum and passes forward deep to the abductor hallucis muscle. It ends by supplying the medial side of the big toe. During its course, it gives off numerous muscular, cutaneous, and articular branches.

2) Lateral plantar artery

The lateral plantar artery is the larger of the terminal branches of the posterior tibial artery. It arises beneath the flexor retinaculum and passes forward deep to the abductor hallucis and the flexor digitorum brevis. On reaching the base of the 5th metatarsal bone, the artery curves medially to form the plantar arch and at the proximal end of the first intermetatarsal space joins the dorsalis pedis artery. During its course, it gives off numerous muscular, cutaneous, and articular branches. The plantar arch gives off plantar digital arteries to the toes.

3) Dorsalis pedis artery (the dorsal artery of the foot)

When entering the sole between the two heads of the first dorsal interosseous muscle, the dorsalis pedis artery immediately joins the lateral plantar artery.

4) Branches

The first plantar metatarsal artery, which supplies the cleft between the big and second toes.

(6) Veins of the sole of the foot

Medial and lateral plantar veins accompany the corresponding arteries, and they unite behind the medial malleolus to form the posterior tibial venae comitantes.

(7) Nerves of the sole of the foot

1) Medial plantar nerve

The medial plantar nerve is a terminal branch of the tibial nerve. It arises beneath the flexor retinaculum and runs forward deep to the abductor hallucis, with the medial plantar artery. It comes to lie in the interval between the abductor hallucis and the flexor digitorum brevis.

Branches are as follows.

• Muscular branches to the abductor hallucis, the flexor digitorum brevis, the flexor hallucis brevis, and the first lumbrical muscle.

• Cutaneous branches: plantar digital nerves run to the sides of the medial three and a half toes. The nerves extend onto the dorsum and supply the nail beds and the tips of the toes.

2) Lateral plantar nerve

The lateral plantar nerve is a terminal branch of the tibial nerve. It arises beneath the flexor retinaculum and runs forward deep to the abductor hallucis and the flexor digitorum brevis, in company with the lateral plantar artery. On reaching the base of the fifth metatarsal bone, it divides into superficial and deep branches.

Branches are as follows.

• From the main trunk to the quadratus plantae and abductor digiti minimi; cutaneous branches to the skin of the lateral part of the sole.

• From the superficial terminal branch to the flexor digiti minimi and the interosseous muscles of the fourth intermetatarsal space. Plantar digital branches pass to the sides of the lateral one and a half toes. The nerves extend onto the dorsum and supply the nail beds and tips of the toes.

• From the deep terminal branch. This branch curves medially with the lateral plantar artery and supplies the adductor hallucis; the second, third, and fourth lumbricals; and all the interossei, except those in the fourth intermetatarsal space.

7.5.2.2 The dorsum of the foot (Figure 7-26)

(1) Skin

The skin on the dorsum of the foot is thin, hairy, and freely mobile on the underlying tendons and bones.

The sensory nerve supply to the skin on the dorsum of the foot is derived from the superficial peroneal nerve, assisted by the deep peroneal, saphenous, and sural nerves.

The superficial peroneal nerve emerges from between the peroneus brevis and the extensor digitorum longus muscle in the lower part of the leg. It now divides into medial and lateral cutaneous branches that supply the skin on the dorsum of the foot; the medial side of the big toe; and the adjacent sides of the second, third, fourth, and fifth toes.

The deep peroneal nerve supplies the skin of the adjacent sides of the big and second toes.

The saphenous nerve passes onto the dorsum of the foot in front of the medial malleolus. It supplies the skin along the medial side of the foot as far forward as the head of the first metatarsal bone.

The sural nerve enters the foot behind the lateral malleolus and supplies the skin along the lateral margin of the foot and the lateral side of the little toe.

The nail beds and the skin covering the dorsal surfaces of the terminal phalanges are supplied by the medial and lateral plantar nerves.

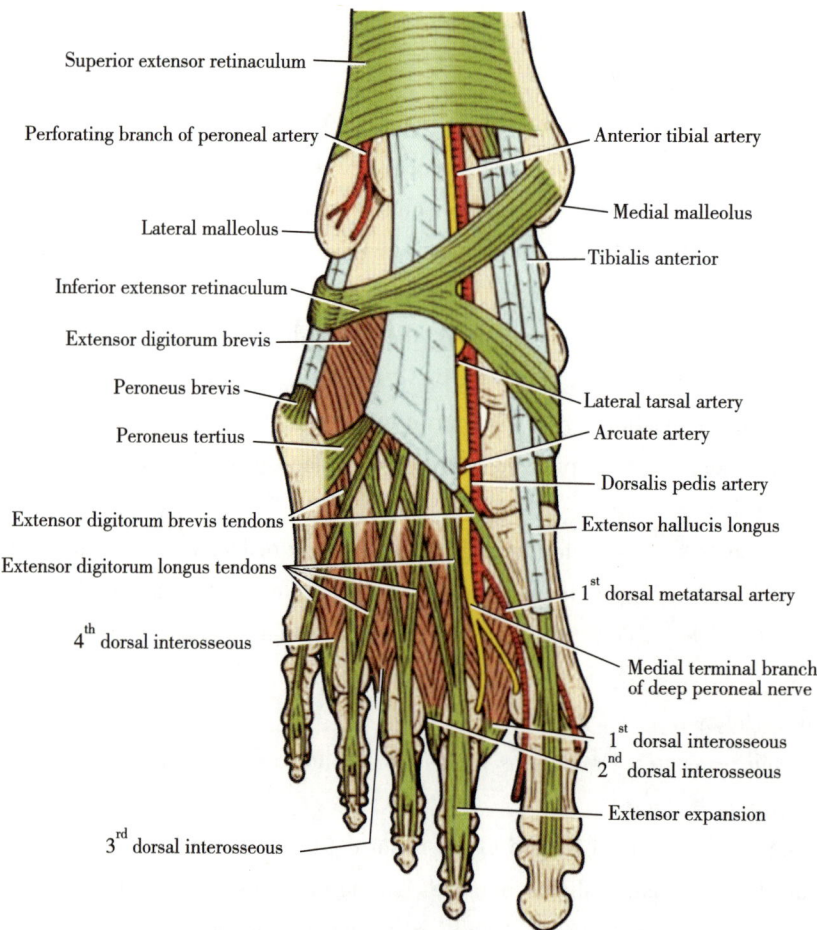

Figure 7-26 Structures in the dorsal aspect of the right foot

(2) Dorsal venous arch (or network)

The dorsal venous arch lies in the subcutaneous tissue over the heads of the metatarsal bones and drains on the medial side into the great saphenous vein and on the lateral side into the small saphenous vein. The great saphenous vein leaves the dorsum of the foot by ascending into the leg in front of the medial malleolus. The small saphenous vein ascends into the leg behind the lateral malleolus.

The greater part of the blood from the whole foot drains into the arch via digital veins and communicating veins from the sole, which pass through the interosseous spaces.

(3) Muscles of the dorsum of the foot

1) Extensor digitorum brevis

2) The insertion of the long extensor tendons

The tendon of extensor digitorum longus passes beneath the superior extensor retinaculum and through the inferior extensor retinaculum, in company with the peroneus tertius muscle. The tendon divides into four, which fan out over the dorsum of the foot and pass to the lateral four toes. Opposite the metatarsophalangeal joints of the second, third, and fourth toes, each tendon is joined on its lateral side by a tendon of extensor digitorum brevis.

On the dorsal surface of each toe, the extensor tendon joins the fascial expansion called the extensor expansion. Near the proximal interphalangeal joint, the extensor expansion splits into three parts: a central part, which is inserted into the base of the middle phalanx, and two lateral parts, which converge to be inserted into the base of the distal phalanx.

The dorsal expansion, as in the fingers, receives the tendons of insertion of the interosseous and lumbrical muscles.

(4) Arteries of the dorsum of the foot

1) Dorsalis pedis artery (the dorsal artery of the foot)

The dorsalis pedis artery begins in front of the ankle joint as a continuation of the anterior tibial artery. It terminates by passing downward into the sole between the two heads of the first dorsal interosseous muscle, where it joins the lateral plantar artery and completes the plantar arch. It is superficial in position and is crossed by the inferior extensor retinaculum and the first tendon of extensor digitorum brevis. On its lateral side lie the terminal part of the deep peroneal nerve and the extensor digitorum longus tendons. On the medial side lies the tendon of extensor hallucis longus. Its pulsations can easily be felt.

2) Branches

• Lateral tarsal artery, which crosses the dorsum of the foot just below the ankle joint.

• Arcuate artery, which runs laterally under the extensor tendons opposite the bases of the metatarsal bones. It gives off metatarsal branches to the toes.

• First dorsal metatarsal artery, which supplies both sides of the big toe.

(5) Nerve supply of the dorsum of the foot—deep peroneal nerve

The deep peroneal nerve enters the dorsum of the foot by passing deep to the extensor retinacula on the lateral side of the dorsalis pedis artery. It divides into terminal, medial, and lateral branches. The medial branch supplies the skin of the adjacent sides of the big and second toes. The lateral branch supplies the extensor digitorum brevis muscle. Both terminal branches give articular branches to the joints of the foot.

7.6 Main contents of lower limb

7.6.1 Anterior and medial compartments of thigh

Fascia of the lower limb
Deep fascia of the lower limb—especially strong (non-yielding) in the lower limb and invests limb like an elastic stocking
✓ Composed of fascia lata (deep fascia of the thigh), which is continuous with the crural fascia distally (discussed later), the other component of the deep fascia of the lower limb ◊ Attaches superiorly to inguinal ligament, pubic arch, body of pubis, and pubic tubercle as well as Scarpa's fascia (the membranous layer of subcutaneous tissue) of the lower abdominal wall ◊ Attaches laterally and posteriorly to the iliac crest ◊ Attaches posteriorly to the sacrum, the sacrotuberous ligament, and the ischial tuberosity ◊ Attaches distally to the exposed parts of bones around the knee ◊ Fascia lata encloses large thigh muscles and it is substantial, especially laterally where it is thickened and strengthened by additional longitudinal fibers to form the iliotibial tract, the conjoint aponeurosis of the tensor fasciae latae and gluteus maximus muscles
Clinical correlation: The iliotibial tract can be utilized as a donor site when making/repairing ligaments or repair of hernias
✓ Forms the dense layer of connective tissue (CT) between the subcutaneous tissue and the underlying muscles ✓ Separates muscles from one another and invest them (by forming fibrous fascial intermuscular septa)—three exist in the thigh (lateral, medial, and posterior) that arise from the deep aspect of the fascia lata to attach to the linea aspera of the femur ✓ Form the walls that separate the thigh muscles into three separate compartments (anterior, posterior, and medial), each containing a main function group of muscles, all of which are innervated by the same nerve ◊ Anterior compartment—composed of muscles that flex the hip and/or extend the leg at the knee. These muscles are located laterally to the sartorius muscle and include the pectineus muscle. Innervated by the femoral nerve (composed of ventral rami L_2–L_4) ◊ Posterior compartment—composed of muscles that extend the thigh at the hip and/or flex the leg at the knee. Innervated by the sciatic nerve (composed of ventral rami L_4–S_3) ◊ Medial compartment—composed of muscles that adduct the thigh at hip. Innervated by the obturator nerve (ventral rami L_2–L_4) ◊ Why is there no lateral compartment? Why are there no abductor muscles located laterally in the thigh? ◆ Attach to the posterior aspect of the linea aspera of the femur, so the femur is in the anterior compartment

◆ Lateral intermuscular septum is strong (as opposed to the medial and posterior which are relatively weak), and it extends from the iliotibial tract to the lateral lip of the linea aspera and lateral supracondylar line of the femur

▷ Unyielding nature prevents bulging of the muscles during contraction allowing the muscular contraction to be more efficient in pumping blood back to the heart

Saphenous opening of the fascia lata—a deficiency in the deep fascia lata inferior to the medial part of the inguinal ligament, approximately 4 cm inferolateral to the pubic tubercle

√ Through this opening pass the great saphenous vein, superficial epigastric vein, external pudendal vein, superficial circumflex iliac vein, accessory lateral saphenous vein, numeral efferent lymphatic vessels from the superficial inguinal lymph nodes, and arteries which accompany some of the veins

√ Ill-defined due to the presence of superficial inguinal lymph nodes, the lymph vessels, the veins, and loose connective tissue in the area. However, the long axis is vertical (about 3.75 cm in length)

√ Medial margin is smooth, but its superior, lateral, and inferior margins form a sharp, crescentic edge, the falciform margin. This sickle-shaped margin is joined at its medial margin by fibrofatty tissue called the cribiform fascia (sieve-like fascia derived from the thin, membranous subcutaneous tissue that spreads over and covers/fills the saphenous opening)

Superficial (subcutaneous) fascia of the lower limb

√ Consists of fat and connective tissue fibers that blend superficially with the dermis with no distinct plane of cleavage

√ Continuous with the superficial fascia of the anterolateral abdominal wall and buttock

√ Provides a pathway for superficial veins, lymphatic vessels, and cutaneous nerves

Endoabdominal (extraperitoneal) fascia also exists within the thigh. It is lining the subinguinal space, a passageway deep (posterior) to the inguinal ligament and anterior to the anterior brim of the pelvis

Divided into two compartments (lacunae) by iliopectineal arch (ligaments)

√ Muscular lacunae—lateral passageway for iliopsoas muscle and femoral nerve

√ Vascular lacunae—medial passageway for femoral vessels and femoral canal that tapers into a funnel-shaped fascial tube, the femoral sheath, a funnel-like downward prolongation of endoabdominal (extraperitoneal) fascia deep to the inguinal ligament into the thigh

▷ Particularly, a downward projection iliopsoas fascia (dorsally)

▷ A downward prolongation of transversalis fascia (ventrally)

▷ Narrow, inferior end of this funnel-shaped sheath fuses with the adventitia of the contained structures about two inches below the inguinal ligament

▷ Divided internally into three compartments by septa (also derived from extraperitoneal fascia of the abdomen)

◆ Lateral compartment—contains the femoral artery

◆ Intermediate compartment—contains the femoral vein

♦ Medial compartment (the femoral canal)—contains fatty connective tissue, a few lymphatic vessels, and sometimes a deep inguinal lymph nodes. The femoral canal lies between the compartment for the femoral vein and the lacunar ligament. The canal communicates superiorly with the extraperitoneal abdominal fascial space by an opening, the femoral ring. The canal is limited inferiorly by the blending of its medial wall with the adventitia of the femoral vein. During exercise, the femoral vein enlarges considerably and is accommodated by the canal medially. Femoral hernias (usually fatty) may protrude through the canal into the femoral triangle

Venous drainage of the lower limb

Superficial veins of lower limb—reside in the subcutaneous fascia and contain valves

Great saphenous vein—located medially and formed by the union of the dorsal vein of the great toe and the dorsal venous arch of the foot; longest vein in body

✓ Contains 10-12 valves (cup-like flaps of endothelium); more numerous in leg than in thigh; found inferior to the perforating veins; enables blood to overcome force of gravity on its way to the heart; subject to varicosities

✓ Has many important anatomical relationships: ascends anterior to the medial malleolus, passes posterior to the medial condyle of the femur (one hand-width posterior to the medial border of the patella) where it is accompanied by the saphenous nerve, traverse the saphenous opening in fascia lata, and empties into the femoral vein

✓ Anastomoses freely with the small saphenous vein

✓ Receives the superficial circumflex iliac, superficial epigastric, and external pudendal veins near its termination

Small (lesser) saphenous vein—located laterally and formed by the union of the dorsal vein of the small (little) toe with the dorsal venous arch

✓ Has many important anatomical relationships: ascends posterior to the lateral malleolus as a continuation of the lateral marginal vein, passes along the lateral border of the calcaneal tendon, inclines to the midline of the fibula and penetrates the deep fascia, ascends between the heads of the gastrocnemius muscle (accompanied by the medial sural nerve in this region), and pierces the deep fascia to empty into the popliteal vein in the popliteal fossa

✓ Diameter stays relatively same throughout length due to perforating veins

Perforating (communicating) veins—penetrate the deep fascia at an oblique angle, so that when muscles contract and pressure increases inside the deep fascia, blood is returned to the heart (musculovenous pump). Valves are present, which only allow the blood to have one pattern of drainage (to travel from superficial veins to deep veins via the perforating veins)

Clinical correlation: Varicose veins form when valves that usually prevent bloodflow from the deep veins through the perforating veins to the superficial veins are incompetent. As a result, the superficial veins become tortuous, elongated, and dilated. Varicose veins are common in the posteromedial parts of the lower limb

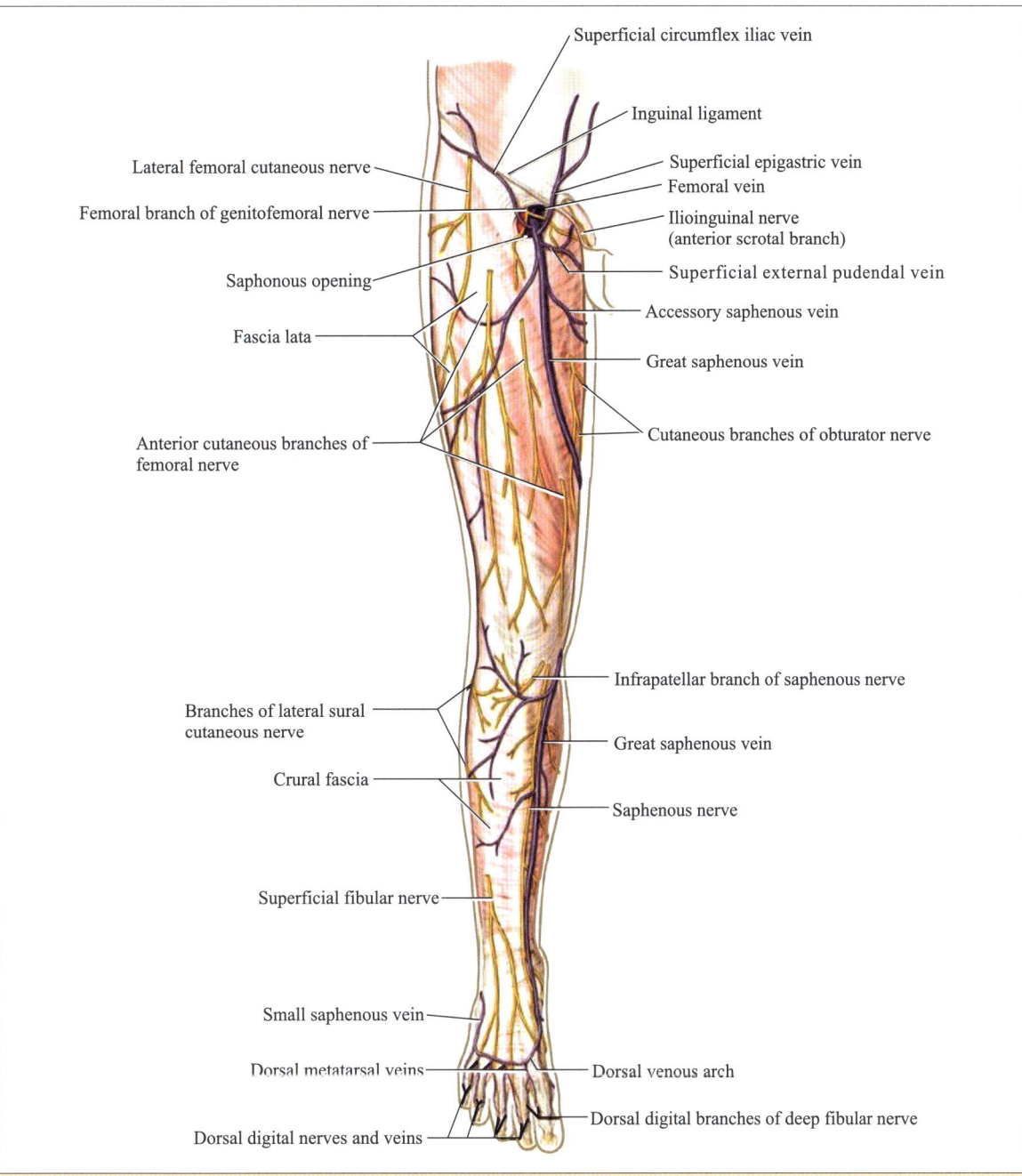

Deep veins of the lower limb—located beneath (deep to) the deep fascia within the same vascular sheath as the artery, whose pulsations also help to compress and move blood in the veins

These veins accompany all the major arteries and their branches. Instead of occurring as a single vein in the limbs (as often illustrated and discussed), the deep veins usually occur as paired, frequently interconnecting veins that flank the artery they accompany

Lymphatic drainage of the lower limb—has superficial and deep lymphatic vessels

✓ Superficial lymphatic vessels accompany the saphenous (great and small) veins and their tributaries. These lymphatic vessels accompanying the great saphenous vein end in the superficial inguinal lymph nodes. Most lymph from these 12–20 nodes passes directly to the external iliac lymph nodes (located along the external iliac veins); however, lymph may also pass to the deep inguinal lymph nodes

✓ Deep lymphatic vessels accompany the deep veins and enter the popliteal lymph nodes. From there, the deep lymphatic vessels ascend to the deep inguinal lymph nodes, which are connected to the external iliac lymph nodes and common iliac nodes. Lymph then proceeds to the lumbar nodes, which drain to the cisterna chili via the lumbar lymphatic trunks

✓ The lymphatic vessels accompanying the great saphenous vein end in the vertical group of the superficial inguinal lymph nodes, which parallel the terminal part of the great saphenous vein. This vertical group of nodes receives lymph mainly from the lower limb (both superficial and deep drainage) as far as the toes. There is also the horizontal group of superficial inguinal nodes, which receives lymph from the anterior abdominal wall below the umbilicus, the posterior wall below the iliac crest (hip and buttocks), and the perineum. The deep inguinal lymph nodes connect to the external and common iliac nodes to the lumbar nodes; these drain to the cisterna chili via the lumbar lymphatic trunks

Peripheral cutaneous nerves of the thigh

These nerves are branches of the lumbar and sacral plexuses and reside within the subcutaneous tissue where they (as their name implies) supply innervation to the skin

Clinical notes: There are no medial cutaneous nerves of the thigh (just as there are no anterior cutaneous nerves of the upper limb)

✓ Subcostal nerve (T_{12})—lateral cutaneous branch supplies a small area of skin anterior to the greater trochanter of the femur and the skin over the anterior superior iliac spine

✓ Femoral branch of genitofemoral nerve (L_2-L_3)—supplies skin just inferior to the middle part of the inguinal ligament

✓ Ilioinguinal nerve (L_1)—supplies proximal and medial parts of thigh and the anterior part of the scrotum and labium majus via the anterior scrotal and labial branches, respectively

✓ Lateral femoral cutaneous nerve (L_2-L_3)—direct branch of the lumbar plexus that runs obliquely to the anterior superior iliac spine, closely associated with the inguinal ligament, and has two branches: anterior and posterior

  ◊ Anterior branch—become superficial 10 cm distal to the inguinal ligament and supply lateral and anterior parts of thigh.

  ◊ Posterior branch—supplies skin laterally from greater trochanter to skin located laterally above the knee

✓ Anterior femoral cutaneous nerve (L_2-L_4)—direct branch of the femoral nerve that arises in the femoral triangle, pierces the fascia lata along the length of the sartorius muscle, and supplies skin on the medial and lateral aspects of the thigh.

✓ Posterior cutaneous nerve of the thigh (S_2-S_3)—a branch of the sacral plexus that supplies the posterior aspect of the thigh (note: the S_3 component of the nerve is distributed mostly by its perineal branch, and the medial-most of the inferior cluneal nerves which arise from it)

✓ Cutaneous branch of the obturator nerve (L_2-L_4)—becomes cutaneous after obturator nerve has given rise to all its motor rami and supplies a relatively limited area of skin on the medial aspect of the distal portion of the thigh—just above the knee

✓ Sciatic nerve—arises from sacral plexus, passes through the greater sciatic foramen into the inferior gluteal region, and then into the posterior thigh. At the apex of the popliteal fossa, the sciatic nerve divides into common fibular (peroneal) and tibial nerves; their cutaneous nerves are discussed with the leg

Femoral triangle

Femoral triangle is a triangular fascial space in the superoanterior third of the thigh that appears as a triangular depression inferior to the inguinal ligament when the thigh is flexed, abducted, and laterally rotated

Boundaries

✓ Inguinal ligament (superiorly)—serves as base of the femoral triangle
✓ Sartorius muscle (laterally)—apex of triangle is located where 2 and 3 cross inferiorly
✓ Adductor longus muscle (medially)
✓ Roof: fascia lata, cribiform fascia, subcutaneous tissue, and skin
✓ Floor: formed by iliopsoas mucle (laterally) and pectineus muscle (medially)

Contents (from lateral to medial)

✓ Femoral nerve and its branches (mentioned later in this lecture)
✓ Femoral sheath and its contents (discussed earlier)
✓ Femoral artery (chief artery of lower limb)—passes deep to a point midway between anterior superior iliac spine and pubic tubercle (note: it is a great anatomical location to insert a catheter) just inferior to the inguinal ligament. Lies between the floor musculature in the femoral triangle and bisects the femoral triangle at its apex and enters the adductor canal (deep to the sartorius muscle). Exits the adductor canal by passing through the adductor hiatus and becomes the popliteal artery

 ◊ Continuation of the external iliac artery (changes name under inguinal ligament)

 ◊ Its course marks a "nerve-free" line for incisions—no motor nerves cross it anteriorly within the femoral triangle and only the pectineal branch of the femoral nerve crosses it posteriorly

 ◊ Largest branch—the deep artery of the thigh (profunda femoris artery—the main arterial supply for the thigh) is given off the femoral artery within the femoral triangle. Leaves femoral triangle between the pectineus and adductor longus and descends posterior to the adductor longus muscle circumflex femoral arteries—usually branches of the deep artery of the thigh. They circle the thigh, anastomose with each other and other arteries, and supply the thigh muscles and the proximal end of the femur

  ◆ Medial circumflex femoral artery—supplies most of the blood to the head and neck of the femur. Often torn when femoral neck is fractured or the hip joint is dislocated. Passes deep between the iliopsoas and pectineus muscles

  ◆ Lateral circumflex femoral artery—supplies the head of the femur and muscles on the lateral side of thigh. Passes laterally and deep to the sartorius and rectus femoris muscles

 ◊ Several small branches given off before the origin of the profunda femoris artery: the superficial epigastric artery, the superficial circumflex iliac artery, and the superficial and deep external pudendal arteries

✓ Obturator artery—does not lie within the femoral triangle, but included for completeness. It supplies muscles of the medial compartment (adductors) of the thigh. It arises from the internal iliac artery or as an accessory obturator artery when it arises from the inferior epigastric artery. Passes through the obturator foramen, enters the thigh, and divides into an anterior and posterior branch, the latter of which gives an acetabular branch that supplies the head of the femur

Clinical correlation: The accessory obturator artery is present in approximately 20% of the population. This artery runs close to or across the femoral ring to reach the obturator foramen where it is closely related to the free margin of the lacunar ligament and the neck of the femoral of a femoral hernia. Therefore, this artery can be involved in a strangulated femoral hernia

✓ Femoral vein (and its proximal tributaries, such as the great saphenous and deep femoral veins)

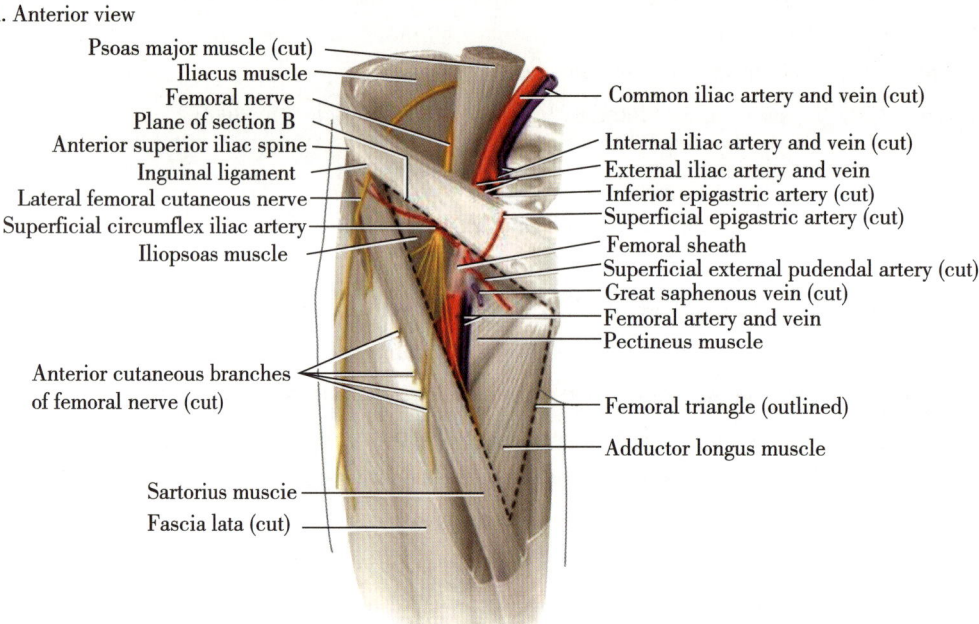

A. Anterior view

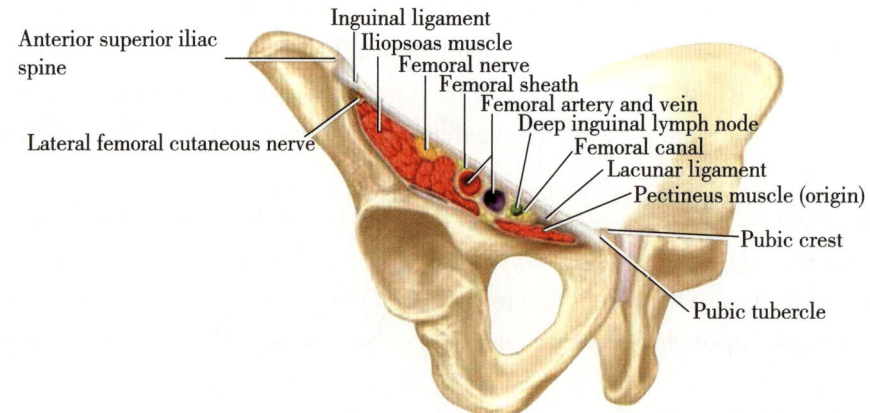

B. Section through the femoral sheath

Adductor canal
Adductor canal is an aponeurotic/musculofibrous canal and/or narrow fascial tunnel beginning at the apex of the femoral triangle and ending in the adductor hiatus, a perforation through the aponeurosis of adductor magnus muscle
Boundaries
✓ Anteromedially: roofed by sartorius muscle (and subsartorius fascia deep to the muscle distally) ✓ Anterolaterally: vastus medialis portion of quadriceps femoris ✓ Posteriorly: aponeurotic tendons of adductors longus and magnus
Contents
✓ Femoral artery—exits adductor canal via adductor hiatus to become popliteal artery in popliteal fossa ✓ Femoral vein—continuation of the popliteal vein from the popliteal fossa ✓ Saphenous nerve—a branch of the femoral nerve and vein; provides cutaneous innervation to medial aspect of knee and leg
Medial compartments of thigh—the femoral artery forms the dividing line between two motor nerve territories
✓ The anterior thigh (quadriceps and sartorius), innervated by the femoral nerve ✓ The medial territory formed by the adductor group and innervated by the obturator nerve (L_2–L_4)
The artery is not crossed by motor branches, but several sensory branches of the femoral nerve pass over it to innervate the skin on the medial side of the thigh
Muscles of the medial compartment—1/2 pectineus, obturator externus, adductors (brevis, longus, and 1/2 magnus), and gracilis
✓ Proximal attachments—all of these muscles attach to the inferior ramus of the pubis, exceptions include the posterior part of the adductor magnus (which is so large that it is innervated posteriorly by the tibial aspect of the sciatic nerve, in addition to its anterior part innervated by the obturator nerve. This posterior part of adductor magnus is included in the posterior compartment with the hamstring muscles, where (like the hamstrings) it arises from the ischial tuberosity. The pectineus muscle is the other exception as it arises from the superior ramus of the pubis, and it is predominately located in the anterior compartment where it will receive its innervation from the femoral nerve; however, it usually does have an obturator nerve component to the muscle that will assist in adduction of the thigh ✓ Distal attachments—all of these muscles attach to the medial aspect of the femur, exceptions include the gracilis muscle (which cross the knee joint to insert of the medial aspect of the tibia) and the obturator externus muscle, which inserts in the trochanteric fossa of the femur in order to stabilize the head of femus in the acetabulum and laterally rotates the thigh ✓ Actions of muscle—the main action of these muscles is to adduct the thigh. The adductors (magnus, longus, and brevis) are used in all movements in which the thighs are adducted (e.g. pressed together when riding a horse). These muscles stabilize other muscles during flexion and extension of the thigh. The exception is the obturator externus (just mentioned), which laterally rotates the thigh and pulls the head of the femur into the acetabulum

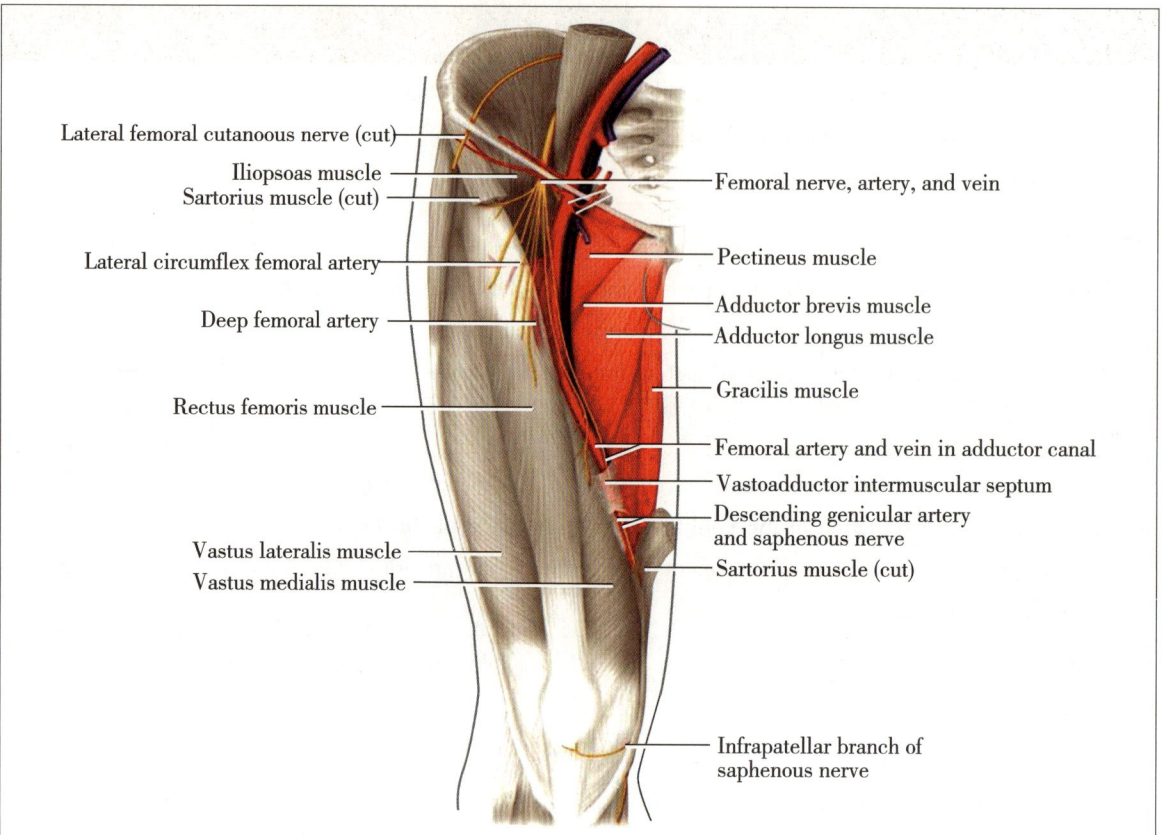

Clinical correlation 1: To test medial compartment muscles—person is lying supine with knee straight and will adduct against resistance. If the adductors are normal, the proximal ends of the gracilis and adductor longus can easily be palpated

Clinical correlation 2: Avulsion fractures of hip bone—these fractures occur when a small part of bone is torn away from the coxal bone by the attachment of a tendon. These fractures occur at apophyses, bony projections that lack secondary ossification center, and where muscles are attached. Most notably, avulsion fractures can be seen at the ischial tuberosity, the hamstring muscles (in the posterior compartment). Avulsion fractures can also occur with the muscles attachments of the medial compartment, where the muscles are torn away from the ischiopubic ramus ("groin" injury). Avulsion fractures can also occur at the anterior superior and inferior iliac spines, where the fracture is called a "hip pointer"

Anterior compartments of thigh—muscles that cause flexion of the hip and extension of the knee that are innervated by the femoral nerve (L_2–L_4)

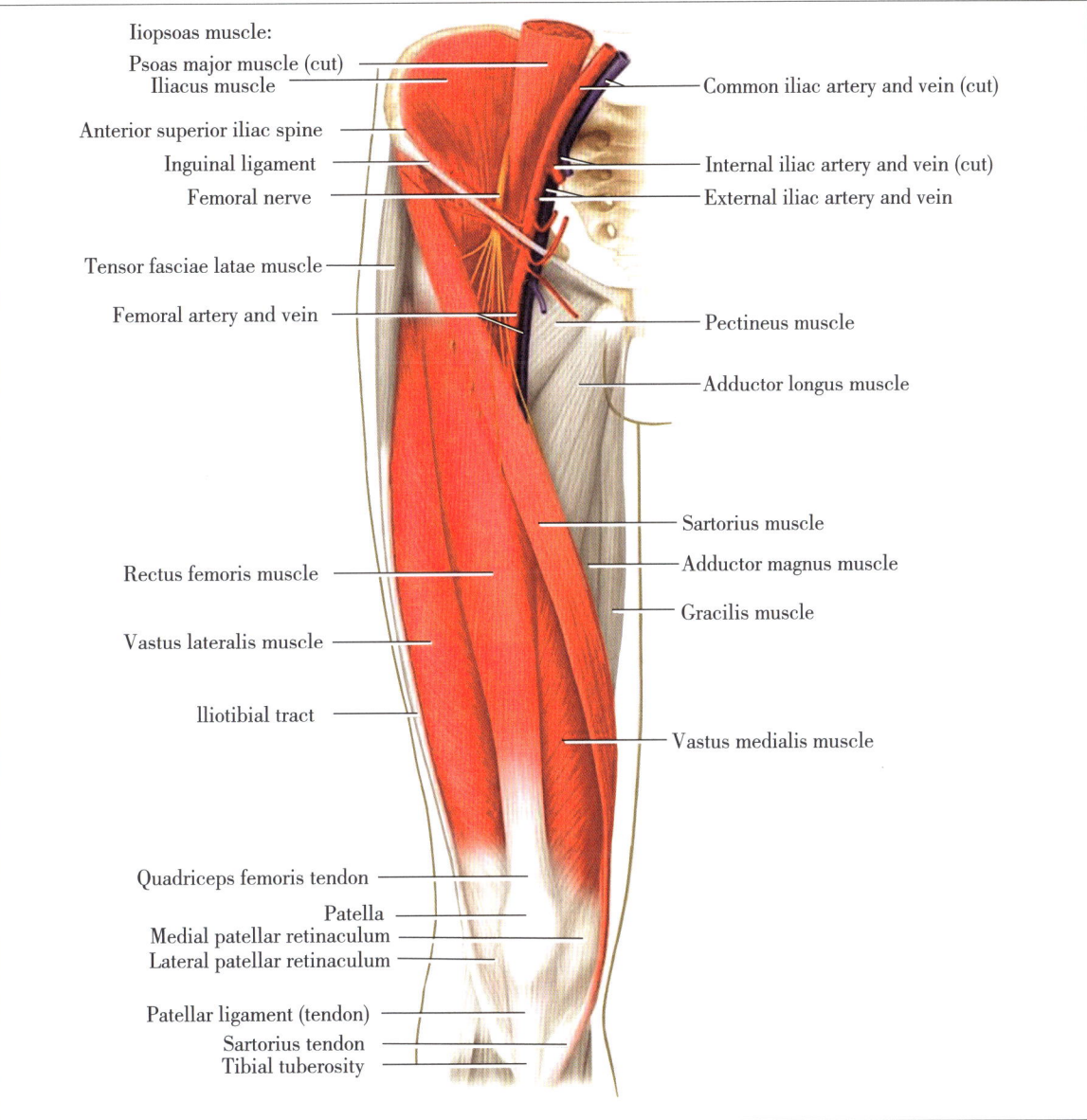

✓ Muscles of the anterior compartment—psoas major and minor, iliacus, articularis genu, rectus femoris, sartorius, vastus (medialis, lateralis, and intermedius) muscles, and 1/3 pectineus muscle. These muscles are innervated by the femoral nerve (L_2–L_4), with exception to the psoas major (L_1–L_3) and psoas minor (L_1 and L_2) muscles, which are innervated by ventral rami before they coalesce to form the femoral nerve. The tensor fascia lata muscle is also considered to be in the anterior compartment, but it is innervated by the superior gluteal nerve (L_4 and L_5)

✓ Proximal and distal attachments—these muscles show much variation in their origin and insertion points. In general, some of these muscles will cross the hip joint and/or the knee in order to cause flexion of the hip and extension of the knee. The iliopsoas muscles flex the thigh at the hip joint and stabilize this joint. The quadriceps femoris (composed of the rectus femoris, vastus lateralis, vastus intermedius, and vastus medialis muscles) attach to the base of the patella and by the patellar ligament to the tibial tuberosity. This distal attachment allows extension of the leg at the knee joint. Since the rectus femoris has a proximal attachment to the inferior iliac spine, this muscle also helps steady the hip joint and helps the iliopsoas to the flex the thigh

Clinical correlation: Psoas abscess—the transversalis fascia in the internal abdominal wall is continuous with the psoas fascia, which forms a fascia covering for the psoas major muscle as the muscle descends into the anterior part of thigh. A retroperitoneal pyogenic (pus-forming) infection in the abdomen may result in a collection of pus (psoas abscess), which passes between the muscle and its fascia into the proximal thigh regions. This should be part of a doctor's differential when edema occurs within the proximal part of the thigh

Muscle	Origin	Insertion	Action	Innervation	Artery	Notes
Adductor brevis	Inferior pubic ramus	Pectineal line and linea aspera (deep to the pectineus and adductor longus, isc)	Adducts, flexes, and medially rotates the femur	Anterior division of the obturator nerve	Obturator artery, deep femoral artery	Anterior and posterior divisions of the obturator nerve lie on the anterior and posterior surfaces of adductor brevis
Adductor longus	Medial portion of the superior pubic ramus	Linea aspera of the femur	Adducts, flexes, and medially rotates the femur	Anterior division of the obturator nerve	Obturator artery, deep femoral artery	The most anterior of the adductor group of muscles
Adductor magnus	Ischiopubic ramus and ischial tuberosity	Linea aspera of the femur; the ischiocondylar part inserts on the adductor tubercle of the femur	Adducts, flexes, and medially rotates the femur; extends the femur (ischiocondylar part)	Posterior division of the obturator nerve; tibial nerve (ischiocondylar part)	Obturator artery, deep femoral artery, medial femoral circumflex artery	The ischiocondylar part of adductor magnus is a hamstring muscle by embryonic origin and action, so it is innervated by the tibial nerve
Articularis genu	Anterior surface of the femur above the patellar surface	Articular capsule of the knee	Elevates the articular capsule of the knee joint	Femoral nerve	Descending genicular artery	Articularis genu is formed by muscle fascicles deep to the vastus intermedius muscle
Gracilis	Pubic symphysis and the inferior pubic ramus	Medial surface of the tibia (via pes anserinus)	Adducts the thigh, flexes and medially rotates the thigh, flexes the leg	Anterior division of the obturator nerve	Obturator artery	The pes anserinus is the common insertion of the gracilis, sartorius, and semitendinosus muscles
Iliacus	Iliac fossa and iliac crest; ala of sacrum	Lesser trochanter of the femur	Flexes the thigh; if the thigh is fixed it flexes the pelvis on the thigh	Femoral nerve	Iliolumbar artery	Inserts in company with the psoas major muscles via the iliopsoas tendon

Iliopsoas	Iliac fossa; bodies and transverse processes of lumbar vertebrae	Lesser trochanter of the femur	Flexes the thigh; flexes and laterally bends the lumbar vertebral column	Branches of the ventral primary rami of spinal nerves $L_2 - L_4$; branches of the femoral nerve	Iliolumbar artery	A combination of the iliacus and psoas major muscles
Obturator externus	The external surface of the obturator membrane and the superior and inferior pubic rami	Trochanteric fossa of the femur	Laterally rotates the thigh	Obturator nerve	Obturator artery	The tendon of the obturator externus muscle passes inferior to the neck of the femur to reach its insertion site
Pectineus	Pecten of the pubis	Pectineal line of the femur	Adducts, flexes, and medially rotates the thigh	Femoral nerve and possibly the anterior division of the obturator nerve	Medial femoral circumflex artery	Pectineus often has a dual innervation
Psoas major	Bodies and transverse processes of lumbar vertebrae	Lesser trochanter of femur (with iliacus) via iliopsoas tendon	Flexes the thigh; flexes and laterally bends the lumbar vertebral column	Branches of the ventral primary rami of spinal nerves L_2-L_4	Subcostal artery, lumbar arteries	The genitofemoral nerve pierces the anterior surface of the psoas major muscle
Psoas minor	Bodies of the T_{12} and L_1 vertebrae	Iliopubic eminence at the line of junction of the ilium and the superior pubic ramus	Flexes and laterally bends the lumbar vertebral column	Branches of the ventral primary rams of spinal nerves L_1-L_2	Lumbar arteries	Absent in 40% of cases
Quadriceps femoris	Anterior surface of the femur and the anterior side of the medial and lateral intermuscular septa	Tibial tuberosity via the patellar ligament	Extends the knee; rectus femoris flexes the thigh	Femoral nerve	Lateral circumflex femoral artery, deep femoral artery	Composed of 4 muscles: rectus femoris, vastus lateralis, vastus intermedius and vastus medialis
Rectus femoris	Straight head: anterior inferior iliac spine; reflected head: above the superior rim of the acetabulum	Patella and tibial tuberosity (via the patellar ligament)	Extends the leg, flexes the thigh	Femoral nerve	Lateral circumflex femoral artery	Rectus femoris is part of the quadriceps femoris muscle

Sartorius	Anterior superior iliac spine	Medial surface of the tibia (pes anserinus)	Flexes, abducts and laterally rotates the thigh; flexes leg	Femoral nerve	Lateral femoral circumflex artery, saphenous artery	Sartorius means "tailor"; its actions put the lower limb in the traditional crosslegged seated position of a tailor
Tensor fasciae latae	Anterior part of the iliac crest, anterior superior iliac spine	Iliotibial tract	Flexes, abducts, and medially rotates the thigh	Superior gluteal nerve	Superior gluteal artery	Tensor fascia latae redirects the rotational forces of the gluteus maximus muscle
Vastus intermedius	Anterior and lateral surface of the femur	Patella	Extends the leg	Femoral nerve	Lateral femoral circumflex artery	Vastus intermedius is part of the quadriceps femoris muscle
Vastus lateralis	Lateral intermuscular septum, lateral lip of the linea aspera and the gluteal tuberosity	Patella and lateral patellar retinaculum	Extends the leg	Femoral nerve	Lateral femoral circumflex artery, perforating branches of the deep femoral artery	Vastus lateralis is part of the quadriceps femoris muscle
Vastus medialis	Medial intermuscular septum, medial lip of the linea aspera	Patella and medial patellar retinaculum	Extends the leg	Femoral nerve	Lateral femoral circumflex artery	Vastus medialis is part of the quadriceps femoris muscle

Clinical correlation 1: Paralysis of the quadriceps femoris—a patient will present with an inability to extend the leg against resistance and usually presses on the distal end of the thigh during walking to prevent inadvertent flexion of the knee joint. Weakness of any of the vastus muscles (due to arthritis or trauma) can result in an abnormal patellar movement and loss of joint stability

Clinical correlation 2: Patellar tendon reflex—a reflex routinely tested during a physical and/or neurological exam to test the L_2 through L_4 nerves. The patient sits with legs dangling of the examination table. The doctor uses a reflex hammer to strike the patellar ligament, which causes the quadriceps femoris muscles to contract (normally). If this reflex is absent or decreased, it will indicate an interruption in the innervation of these muscles (e.g. peripheral nerve disease)

7.6.2 Anterior and lateral compartment of leg, dorsum of foot

Osteology

- ✓ Tibia—leg bone that articulates with the condyles of the femur superiorly and the talus inferiorly.
- ✓ Medially located bone of the leg (pre-axial bone). In embryo, leg rotates 90° medially, placing extensor muscles on its anterior surface and the big toe medially
- ✓ The weight bearing bone of the leg, 2nd largest bone in the body (behind femur)
- ✓ Proximal (upper) end of tibia is flat (the tibial plateau), except for the intercondylar eminence
- ✓ Tibial plateau—consists of medial and lateral tibial condyles (facets)
- ✓ Intercondylar eminence fits into the intercondylar fossa of the femur and consists of the lateral and medial intercondylar tubercles
- ✓ Lateral tibial condyle has a facet inferiorly that articulates with the head of fibula
- ✓ Gerdy's tubercle (lateral)—site of attachment for the iliotibial band
- ✓ Body (shaft) of tibia—triangular in cross-section with medial, lateral, and posterior surfaces (the sides of the triangle) and anterior, medial, and interosseous borders (the points of the triangle)
- ✓ Tibial tuberosity—attachment site of patellar tendon located at crest of anterior border
- ✓ Anterior border of tibia is subcutaneous and the most prominent border ("bumper fractures" occur here). Tibia is most common site of compound fractures
- ✓ Shaft is thinnest at the junction of its middle and distal thirds (its most frequent site of fracture)
- ✓ Interosseous border gives attachment to the interosseous membrane, which unites the two leg bones
- ✓ Distal (lower) end of tibia articulates with the fibula and talus
- ✓ Medial malleolus—inferiorly directed projection from the medial side of tibia
- ✓ Tibialis posterior and flexor digitorum longus tendons run in a groove located posteriorly at the junction of the medial malleolus and distal end of the tibia
- ✓ Fibular notch—articulation site with the fibula
- ✓ Inferior articular facet—the tibial articulation with the talus bone
- ✓ Fibula—slender bone that is important for muscle attachments. It does not bear weight, but its lateral malleolus does help hold the talus in its socket
    - ◊ Head (proximal end) of fibula—articulates with the posterolateral part of the inferior aspect of the lateral condyle of the tibia
    - ◊ Body (shaft) of fibula—is twisted and marked by muscle attachment. Like the tibia, the fibula can have three borders (anterior, posterior, and interosseous) and three surfaces (medial, lateral, and posterior) along its length; however, this bone twists and its shape is not consistent proximally to distally
    - ◊ Lateral malleolus—enlarged, lower end of fibula that is more prominent and more posterior than the medial malleolus of the tibia
    - ◊ This bone along with its nutrient arterial pedicle is frequently removed (since it is non-weight bearing and placed elsewhere (such as in jaw reconstructions after cancer ablation)

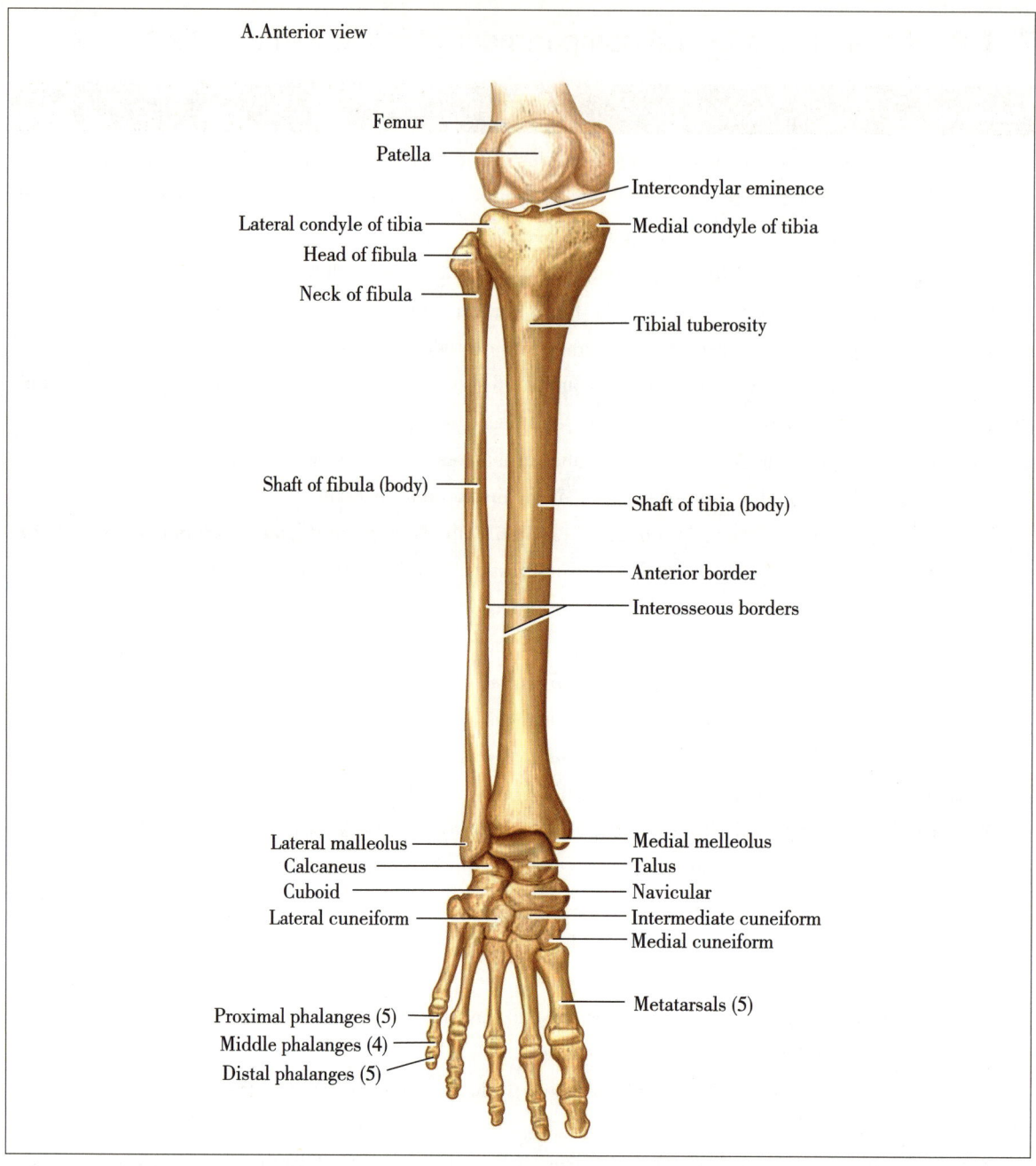

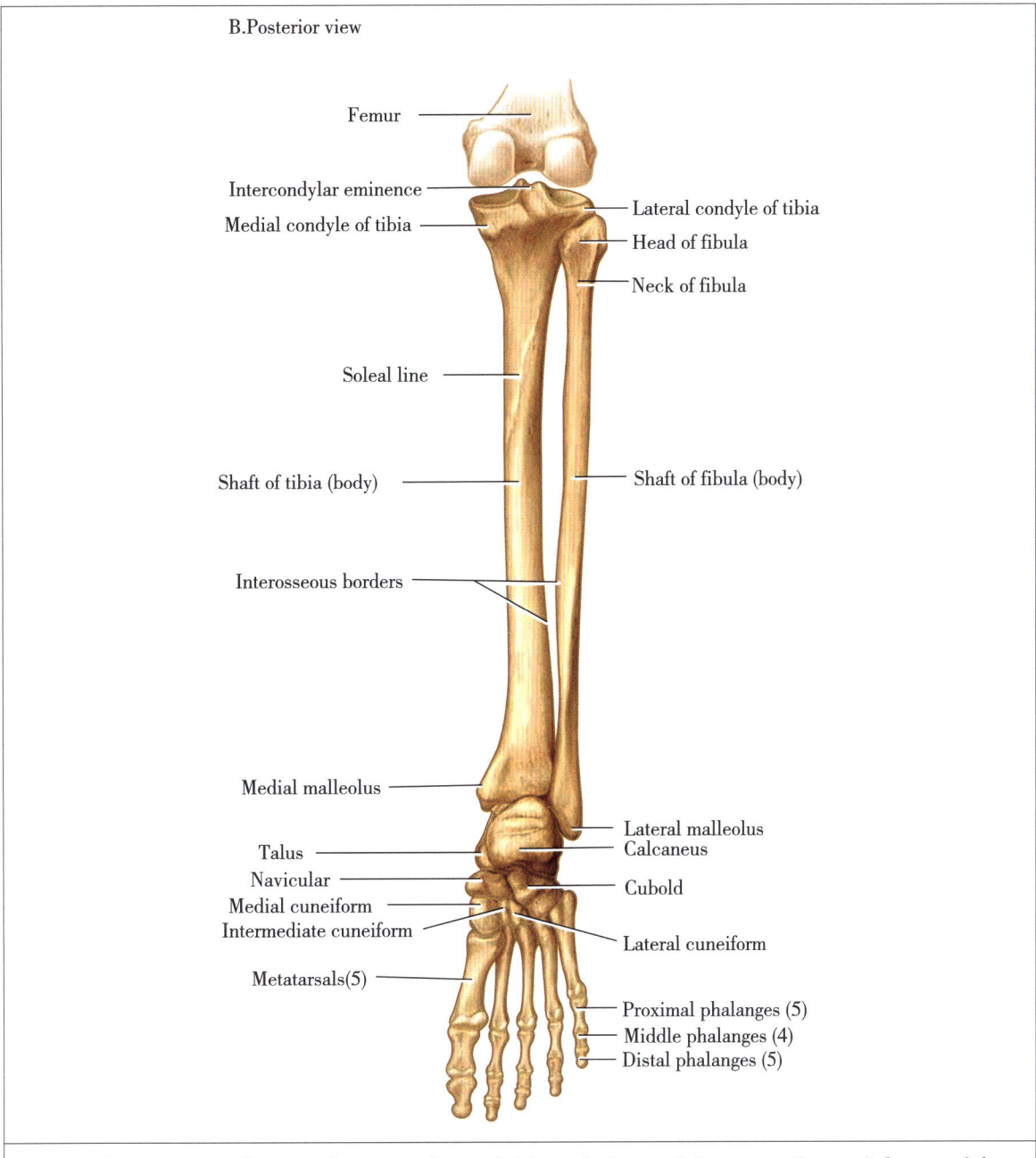

B. Posterior view

✓ Tarsal bones—seven bones: calcaneus, talus, cuboid, navicular, and three cuneiforms. Only one of these bones, the talus, articulates with the leg bones. Talus—bears the weight transmitted by the tibia and spreads the weight to other bones of the foot. Trochlea—proximal surface of bone that helps form, along with fibula and tibia, the talocrural (or tibiotalar) joint
✓ Articulates with calcaneus, navicular, cuboid distally to form the subtalar joint
✓ Only tarsal bone with no muscular or tendinous attachments
✓ Talar head rests on a shelf of bone (sustentaculum tali of the calcaneus bone)
✓ Posterior process with medial and lateral tubercle separated by the groove for the flexor hallucis longus tendon
✓ Calcaneus (heel bone)—largest and strongest bone of the foot, so it transmits most of the weight from the talus to the ground
  ◊ Articulates with the talus superiorly and the cuboid bone anteriorly

◊ Medially located, shelf-like projection, the sustentaculum tali, supports the talar head. The groove for the flexor hallucis longis runs at its base

◊ Calcaneal tuberosity—Achilles' tendon attaches at this posterior tubercle

◊ Fibular trochlea—laterally located tubercle that serves as a pulley for the fibularis (peroneus) longus tendon

✓ Navicular—a flattened, boat-shaped bone that is located between the talus posteriorly and the three cuneiform bones anteriorly

◊ Navicular tuberosity—projects medially and inferiorly to receive the tendon of the tibialis posterior muscle

✓ Cuboid—most lateral bone of the distal row of tarsal bones as it articulates posteriorly with the calcaneus and the 4th-5th metatarsals anteriorly. It contains the groove for the fibularis (peroneus) longus tendon

✓ Three cuneiform bones—lateral, intermediate, medial

◊ Help form the transverse arch of the foot

◊ Articulate with the metatarsals at the tarsometatarsal joint

✓ Metatarsals—5 in number, have a base, a shaft, and a head

✓ Phalanges—14 bones that form the toes. Composed of proximal (1st-5th digit), middle (2nd-5th digit), and distal (1st-5th digit) components. The first toe is the medially located big toe (compare to similar structures in the hand)

Fascial organization/connective tissues

✓ Interosseous membrane—connects the bones of the leg (tibia and fibula) as well as separates anterior and posterior leg compartments

✓ Anterior intermuscular septum—separates anterior and lateral leg compartments

✓ Posterior intermuscular septum—separates lateral and posterior leg compartments

✓ Transverse intermuscular septum—deep fascia that separates the superficial and deep posterior leg compartments

✓ Crural fascia—deep fascia of leg that is a continuation of fascia lata of the thigh

◊ Attaches to the anterior and medial borders of the tibia, where it is continuous with the periosteum

◊ Is connected to tibia and fibular by intermuscular septi

◊ Acts like a compression stocking, preventing muscles from bulging too much during contraction and enables a more efficient pumping of the blood back towards the heart during muscular contractions. Its unyielding nature frequently leads to compartment (compression) syndromes.

◊ Is thickens to form distal extensor retinacula

✓ Superior extensor retinaculum—thickening of deep fascia that prevents tendons of muscles of the anterior compartment from bowstringing anteriorly during dorsiflexion. Connects fibula and tibia proximal to malleoli

✓ Inferior extensor retinaculum—Y-shaped band of deep fascia that attaches laterally to the anterosuperior surface of the calcaneus. It forms a strong loop around the tendons of the extensor digitorum longus and the fibularis tertius muscles

✓ Superior and inferior fibular (peroneal) retinacula—holds down the fibularis longus and brevis tendons between the body of the calcaneus and the lateral malleolus (superior) and the lateral process of the calcaneal tubercle and the fibular trochlea (inferior)

✓ These retinacula prevent bowstringing of the tendons while allowing for gliding movements of the various tendons

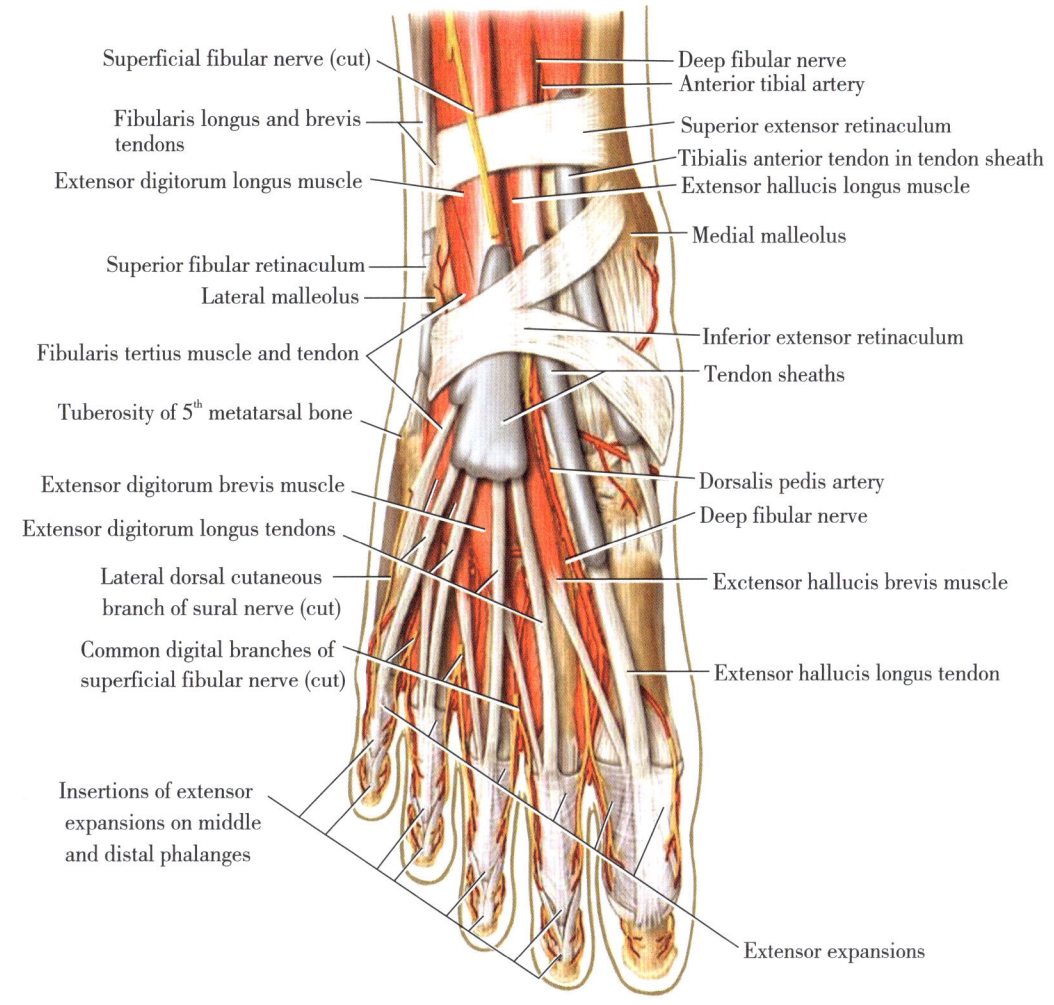

Leg compartments

✓ Anterior leg compartment
  ◊ Muscles—tibialis anterior, extensor digitorum longus, external. hallucis longus
  ◊ Innervation—deep fibular (peroneal) nerve
  ◊ Blood supply—anterior tibial artery and vein
✓ Lateral leg compartment
  ◊ Muscles—fibularis longus, fibularis brevis
  ◊ Innervation—superficial fibular (peroneal) nerve
  ◊ Blood supply—doesn't have its own artery, so the perforating branches of the anterior tibial artery proximally supply it. However, its distal 2/3 are supplied by the perforating branch of the fibular artery (a branch off the posterior tibial artery)
✓ Superficial and deep posterior leg compartments
  ◊ Muscles (7 muscles; 3 superficial and 4 deep muscles)
  ◊ Innervation—tibial nerve
  ◊ Blood supply—posterior tibial artery and vein

Muscles of the anterior leg compartment

Tibialis anterior (TA)

- ✓ Origin—lateral condyle of tibia, upper half/lateral surface of tibia, interosseous membrane
- ✓ Insertion—medial cuneiform, base of 1st metatarsal
- ✓ Nerve—deep fibular (peroneal) (L_4–L_5)
- ✓ Action—ankle dorsiflexion, forefoot inversion

Extensor digitorum longus (EDL)

- ✓ Origin—lateral condyle of tibia, ant surface of fibula, interosseous membrane
- ✓ Insertion—dorsum of base of middle phalanx, dorsum of base of distal phalanx
- ✓ Nerve—deep fibular (peroneal) (L_5–S_1)
- ✓ Action—extension of toes, dorsiflexion of ankle

Fibularis (peroneus) tertius—a lateral slip off the extensor digitorum

- ✓ Origin—distal 1/3 anterior fibula, interosseous membrane
- ✓ Insertion—dorsum shaft of 5th metatarsal
- ✓ Nerve—deep fibular (peroneal) (L_5–S_1)
- ✓ Action—forefoot eversion, weak ankle dorsiflexion

Extensor hallucis longus (EHL) origin—middle 1/2 of anterior fibula

- ✓ Insertion—distal phalanx of the great toe
- ✓ Nerve—deep fibular (peroneal) (L_5–S_1)
- ✓ Action—extend the great toe, dorsiflex ankle

Muscles of the lateral leg compartment

Fibularis (peroneus) longus (FL)

- ✓ Origin—head, upper 2/3 lateral surface of fibula
- ✓ Its tendon courses behind lateral malleolus, underneath the fibular trochlea, and lies in the groove in the cuboid bone before going to its place of insertion
- ✓ Insertion—inferolateral surface of medial cuneiform 1st metatarsal on its inferior surface
- ✓ Nerve—superficial fibular (peroneal) (L_5–S_1)
- ✓ Action—forefoot eversion, ankle plantar flexion

Fibularis (peroneus) brevis (FB)

- ✓ Origin—lower 2/3 lateral fibula
- ✓ Courses behind lateral malleolus and underneath the fibular trochlea
- ✓ Insertion—tuberosity on base of 5th metatarsal
- ✓ Nerve—superficial fibular (peroneal) (L_5–S_1)
- ✓ Action—forefoot eversion, ankle plantar flexion

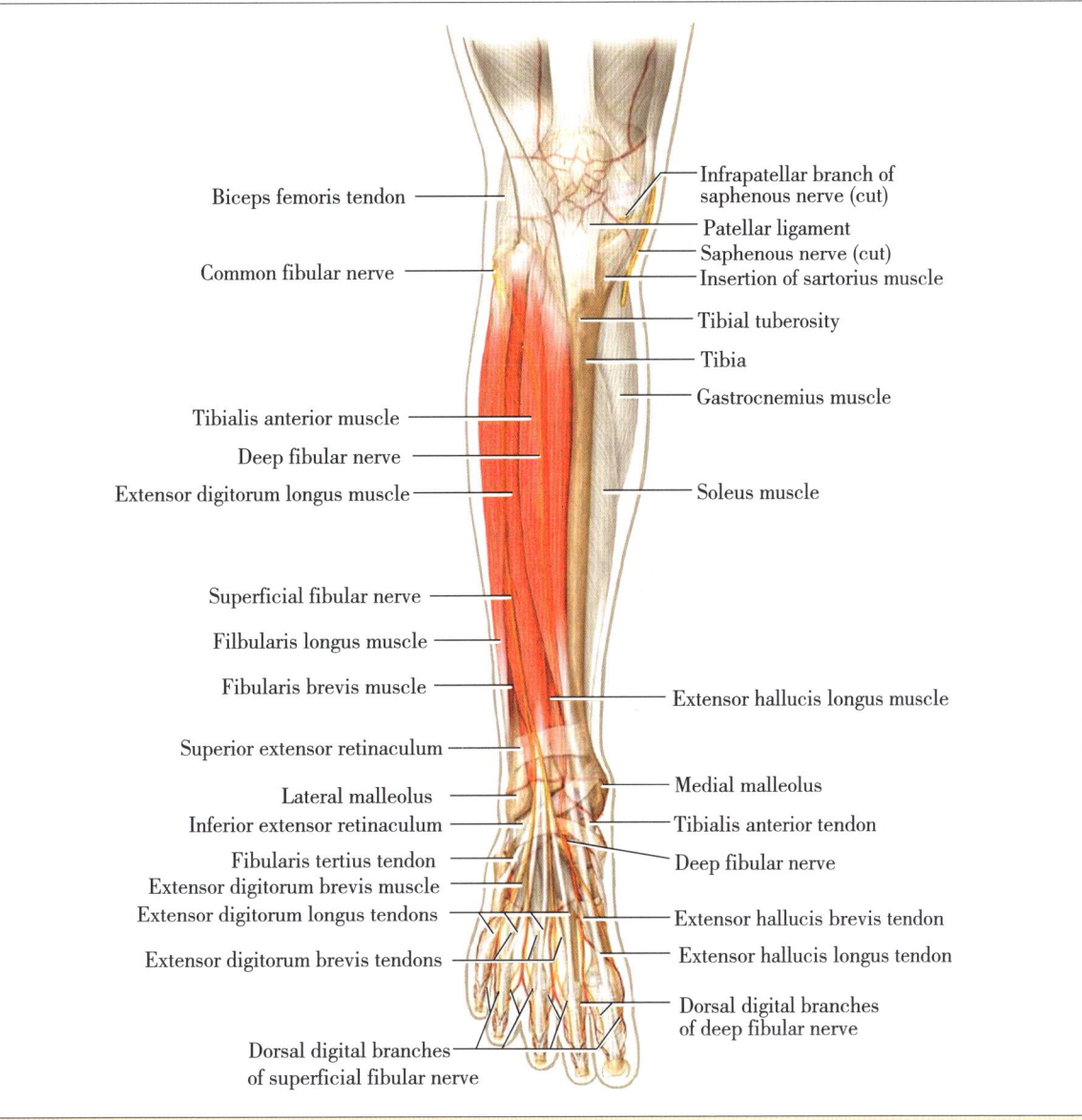

Vascular/neural supply

Superficial (cutaneous) venous drainage great saphenous vein—formed by the union of the dorsal vein of the great toe and the dorsal venous arch of the foot

✓ Passes anterior to medial malleolus
✓ Passes posterior to medial condyle of femur (one hand-width posterior to the medial border of the patella)
✓ Anastomoses freely with the small saphenous vein
✓ Traverses the saphenous opening in the fascia lata
✓ Empties into the femoral vein
✓ Contains 10–12 valves along its length
✓ Accompanied by the saphenous nerve

Small saphenous vein

✓ Formed by the union of the dorsal vein of the small

- ✓ Toe and the dorsal venous arch of the foot
- ✓ Ascends posterior to lateral malleolus
- ✓ Passes along the lateral border of the calcaneal tendon
- ✓ Ascends between the heads of the gastrocnemius and penetrates the deep fascia
- ✓ Empties into the popliteal vein in the popliteal fossa
- ✓ Accompanied by the medial sural nerve distally

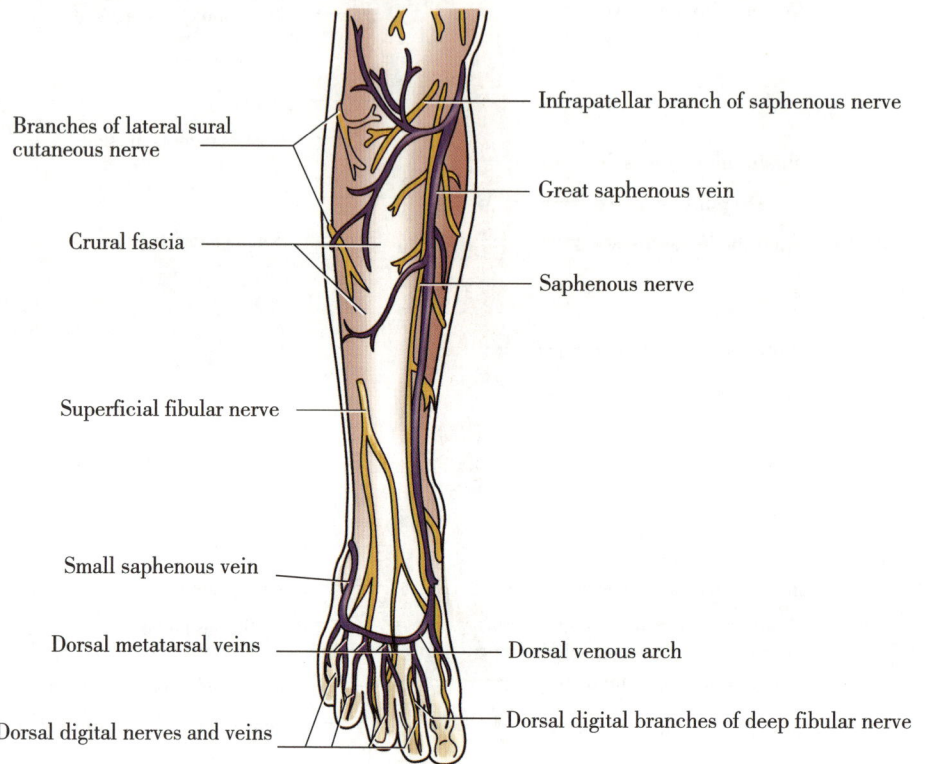

Arterial inflow

✓ Anterior tibial artery—arises from the popliteal artery and passes anteriorly through a gap in the superior part of the interosseous membrane to lie in the anterior compartment of the leg
  ◊ Accompanied along its length by the deep fibular nerve
  ◊ Runs between tibialis anterior and extensor digitorum longus muscle proximally and between TA and extensor hallucis longus tendon distally
  ◊ Midway between the malleoli, it becomes the dorsalis pedis artery
  ◊ Gives off branches at the knee and ankle that participate in collateral circulation
  ◊ Its perforating branches supply the lateral compartment of the leg proximally
✓ Posterior tibial artery—arises from the popliteal artery and provides main blood supply to the foot. This artery has perforating branches that will supply the lateral compartment distally (more information on this artery in upcoming lectures)

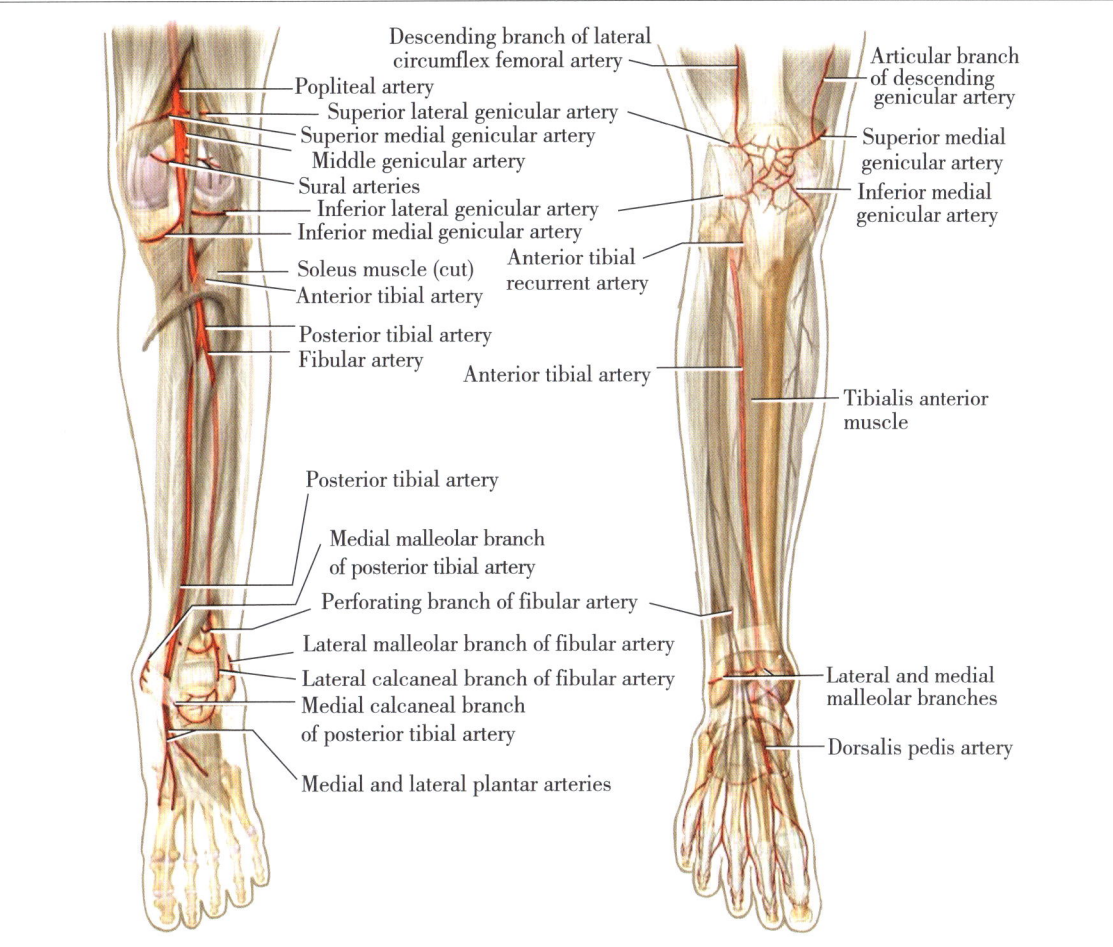

Deep venous drainage

✓ The deep veins have the same names and courses as the major arteries
✓ Thrombi from these deep veins and the sural lakes (DVT) can travel upward and lodge in the pulmonary circuit
✓ Occlusions and poor circulation are very common in the elderly. These patients develop non-healing ulcers from venous insufficiency

Neural supply

✓ Common fibular nerve (peroneal) origin—typically separates from the sciatic nerve along with the tibial nerve at apex of popliteal fossa. These nerves may separate at a higher level
✓ Bifurcates behind neck of fibula into deep and superficial branches
  ◊ Deep fibular nerve—nerve of the anterior compartment
    ◆ Motor to TA, EDL, EHL, FT, extensor digitorum brevis, extensor hallucis longus
    ◆ Sensory—web space between 1st and 2nd toes
  ◊ Superficial fibular nerve—nerve of the lateral compartment
    ◆ Motor—fibularis longus and brevis
    ◆ Sensory—lateral leg, dorsum of foot

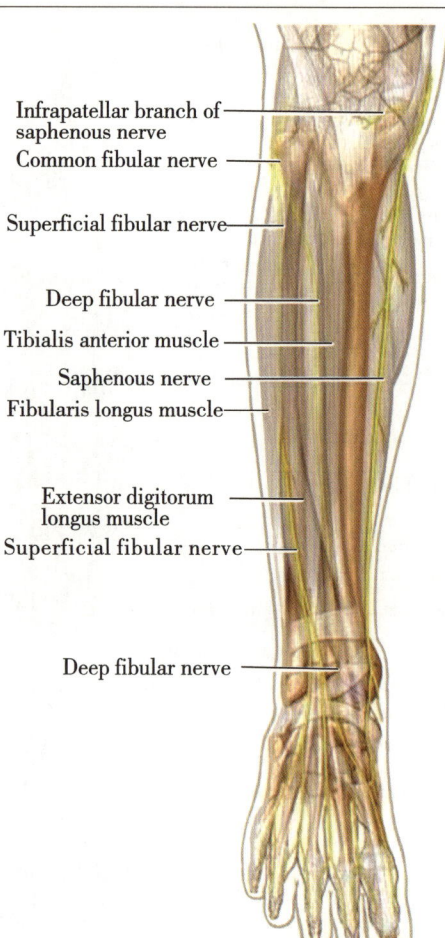

Typical injuries to the common fibular nerve
Compression/injuries
✓ In popliteal space ✓ Near fibular head (superficial location) ✓ In anterior compartment (deep branch) ✓ In lateral compartment (superficial branch)
Anterior compartment syndrome
✓ Mechanism—overuse, trauma ✓ Affects deep fibular nerve, anterior tibial artery ✓ Diagnosed by pressure readings
Diabetes
✓ Diabetic neuropathy results in an insensate foot that cannot detect that the shoes fit improperly or that too much weight is producing ischemia over the weightbearing portions of the foot

Dorsum of foot

Retinacula

✓ Superior extensor retinaculum

✓ Inferior extensor retinaculum
Intrinsic muscles
Extensor digitorum brevis and extensor hallucis brevis
✓ Origin—anterolateral superior surface of calcaneus and inferior extensor retinaculum ✓ Insertion—middle and distal phalanges of toes ✓ Nerve—deep fibular nerve (L_5–S_2) ✓ Action—extend the toes
Neurovasculature on dorsum of foot

✓ Superficial fibular nerve—enters in the superficial fascia and supplies skin except web space between 1st and 2nd toes and sural contribution
✓ Deep fibular nerve—emerges in dorsum between EDL and EHL
   ◊ Innervates EDB and EHB
   ◊ Sensory to skin of web space between 1st and 2nd toes
✓ Arteries on dorsum of foot—dorsalis pedis artery—a continuation of anterior tibial artery that gives off lateral/medial tarsal arteries. Between 1st and 2nd toes, it becomes the arcuate artery which gives off the dorsal metatarsal arteries and dorsal digital arteries. The dorsalis pedis artery may continue onward penetrating the webspace between 1st and 2nd toe and contributing to the deep arterial arch in the foot (note the similarities to the radial artery in the hand)
✓ All the above mentioned arteries can become very small and progressively occluded due to atherosclerosis. This produces a symptom called claudication. This condition produces pain when a patient exerts the muscles in his lower extremities as in minor walking
✓ The above mentioned arteries often become damaged in diabetic patients who are then prone to diabetic foot ulcers and eventual amputations (correlate with what you remember from the emphasis course)

7.6.3 Gluteal region

Overview
✓ Surface anatomy/bony landmarks ✓ Cutaneous innervation ✓ Osteology ✓ Muscles ✓ Nerve and blood supply
Gluteal and hip regions
✓ Parts of the body that link the free lower limb to the trunk ✓ The purpose of the lower limb is locomotion ✓ The bony pelvis consists of the hip bones (ilium, pubis and ischium) and the sacrum ✓ The gluteal region is posterior and includes the buttocks, also called the cluneal and natal regions

Surface anatomy/bony landmarks
Iliac crest
✓ The highest level of the iliac crest is at the L_4 vertebra ✓ The iliac crest serves as a guide to physicians performing spinal punctures ✓ The L_4 vertebral level is also the bifurcation of the abdominal aorta into the common iliac arteries
Posterior superior iliac spine
✓ Deep to the visible venusian dimple above the medial aspect of the buttock ✓ A line joining the diples crosses the 2nd sacral spine, which marks the most inferior extent of the dural and subarachnoid sacs with the contained CSF ✓ This line also crosses the sacro-iliac articulation (SI joint)
Greater trochanter
✓ Palpable bony process on the proximal, lateral femur, especially during passive abduction of the hip. The abductor muscles (hip) and iliotibial band cover the greater trochanter. Therefore, it cannot be palpated while standing on one leg ✓ Constitutes the commonly described "width of the hips"
Intergluteal (natal) cleft
✓ The sulcus between the buttocks
Tip of the coccyx
✓ Palpable bony prominence within the intergluteal (natal) cleft ✓ 3-4 cm posterosuperior to the anus ✓ The 4th sacral spine and sacral cornu define the area of the sacrococcygeal ligament (sacral hiatus)
Ischial tuberosities
✓ Bony prominences covered by the lower border of the gluteus maximus during extension of the hip (in standing), but is uncovered during flexion so that it bears the weight while in a sitting position ✓ To palpate, sit on your fingertips ✓ Serves as the origin (proximal attachment) of the hamstring muscles
Sciatic nerve
✓ L_4-L_5, S_1-S_3 ✓ Passes midway between the ischial tuberosity and greater trochanter.
Gluteal fold and sulcus
✓ Gluteal fold—formed by the inferior margin of the gluteus maximus muscle ✓ Separates gluteal region from the posterior thigh

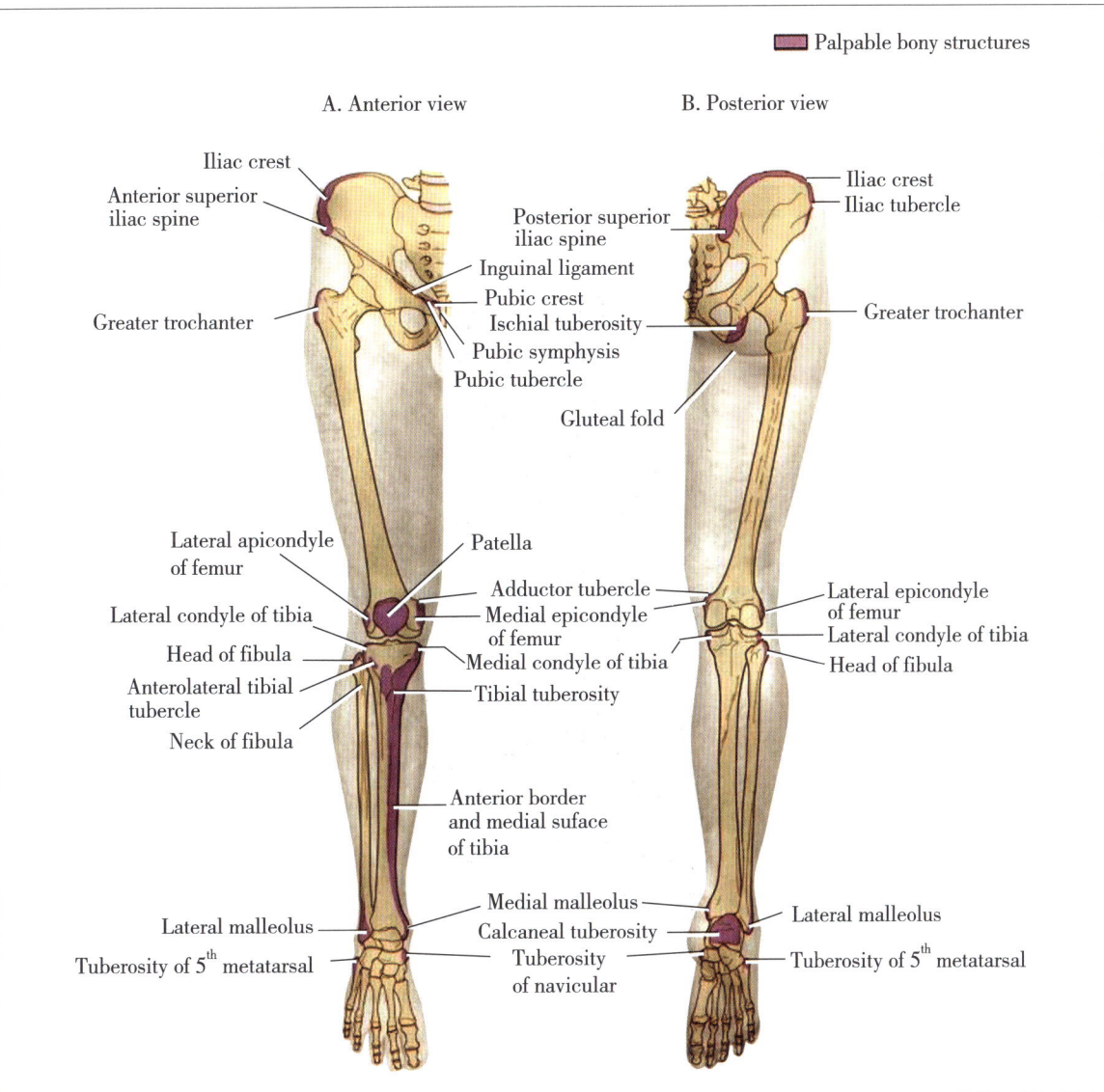

Cutaneous innervation

Gluteal region

✓ Superior cluneal nerves
  ◊ Lateral branches of the upper lumbar posterior rami (L_1–L_3)
  ◊ Supply most of the skin of the buttock

✓ Medial cluneal nerves
  ◊ A series of loops formed between adjacent lateral branches of the lower lumbar posterior rami together with those of the first four sacral nerves
  ◊ Lies immediately posterior to the sacrum and coccyx
  ◊ The medial branches of these posterior rami innervate the erector spinae and transversospinalis muscles
  ◊ These nerves pierce the gluteus maximus muscle and supply the skin of the medial buttock near the intergluteal cleft

- ✓ Inferior cluneal nerves
  - ▷ Arise deep to the gluteus maximus from the posterior cutaneous nerve of the thigh (anterior primary rami, S_1–S_2)
  - ▷ Supply the lower portion of the buttock

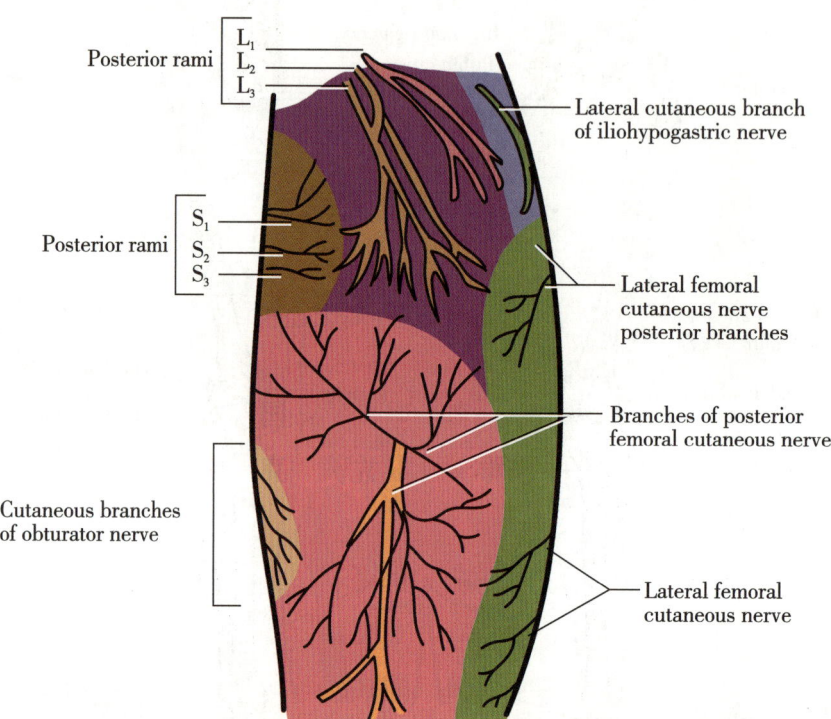

Posterior compartment of the thigh

- ✓ Posterior cutaneous nerve of the thigh (posterior femoral cutaneous nerve)
- ✓ S_1 and S_2 from the anterior primary rami
- ✓ S_3 can also contribute via the perineal branch
- ✓ This nerve runs deep to the fascia lata with branches penetrating the superficial fascia

Superficial lymphatic drainage

- ✓ Skin of buttocks—mainly to horizontal group of superficial inguinal nodes
- ✓ Skin over posterior compartment of the thigh—mainly to the vertical group of superficial inguinal nodes

Bones of the gluteal region

Hip bone (os coxae)

- ✓ Formed from the fusion of the ilium, ischium and pubis
- ✓ 3 separate bones at birth joined by hyaline cartilage
- ✓ At puberty, still separated by triradiate cartilage centered in the acetabulum
- ✓ Fusion begins at 15–17 years; complete by 20–25 years

Ilium—3 parts, each with a special function

- ✓ Ala (wing)—broad area of thin bone for attachment of limb muscles

- ◊ Gluteal muscles laterally
- ◊ Iliacus muscle medially
- ✓ Iliac crest—long curved superior border of ala, running from the anterior superior iliac spine (ASIS) to the posteior superior iliac spine (PSIS)
  - ◊ Internal, intermediate and external lips—for attachment of abdominal muscles
  - ◊ ASIS—sartorius
  - ◊ AIIS—rectus femoris
  - ◊ Auricular facet—articulates with sacrum
  - ◊ Forms a protective wall around the abdominal viscera
  - ◊ Provides attachment for thin, sheet or strap like muscles and for fascia
  - ◊ Tubercle of the iliac crest—upper attachment of the iliotibial tract (thickening of the fascia lata)
- ✓ Body of ilium—thickest, most massive part
  - ◊ Receives weight of upper body via sacroiliac ligaments at iliac tuberosity
  - ◊ Transfers weight of upper body to the head of the femur
  - ◊ Body contributes to the acetabulum

Ischium

- ✓ Body—helps form the acetabulum and the lateral wall of the pelvic cavity
- ✓ Ramus—forms posteroinferior margin of obturator foramen
- ✓ Ischial spine—junction of ramus and body
- ✓ Ischial tuberosity—posteroinferior margin of ramus
- ✓ Greater sciatic notch (foramen)
- ✓ Lesser sciatic notch (foramen)

Pubis

- ✓ Forms the anterior or ventral component of the pelvic girdle
- ✓ Body
  - ◊ Pubic crest
  - ◊ Pubic tubercle
- ✓ Ramus
  - ◊ Superior—fuses with ilium and ischium to form the acetabulum
  - ◊ Inferior—fuses with ramus of ischium

Sacrum

- ✓ 5 fused sacral vertebra
- ✓ Wedged between 2 hip bones to form the pelvis
- ✓ Transmits weight of body to these bones at the SI joint
- ✓ Base articulates with L_5 to form the lumbosacral joint (L_5–S_1)
- ✓ Bony prominences
  - ◊ Base
  - ◊ Sacral promontory–prominent anterior lip
  - ◊ Superior articular facet
  - ◊ Sacral foramina

- ◊ Medial sacral crest
- ◊ Sacral tuberosity
- ◊ Auricular facet (SI joint)
- ◊ PSIS

Femur

Upper end

- ✓ Head—ball like, covered with articular cartilage
- ✓ Fovea capitis—depression in the head, ligament of the head of the femur
- ✓ Greater trochanter—upper margin of neck that joins with the shaft
- ✓ Lesser trochanger—lower margin of neck that joins with the shaft
- ✓ Intertrochanteric crest
- ✓ Intertrochanteric line
- ✓ Gluteal tuberosity

Shaft or body of the femur

- ✓ Linea aspera—longitudinal ridge, posterior surface; medial lip; lateral lip

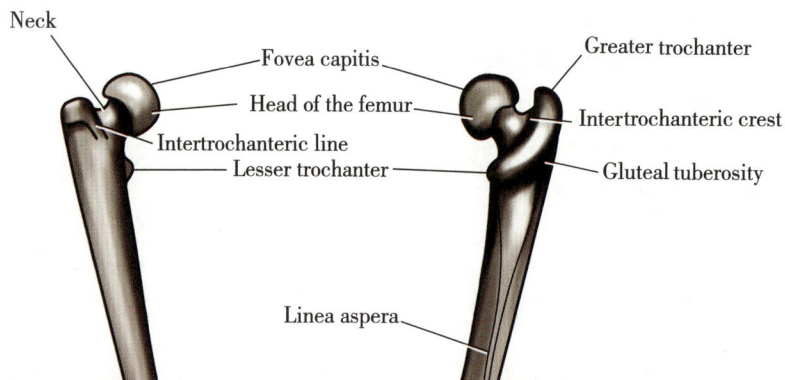

Gluteal ligaments

- ✓ Sacrotuberous ligament—ischial tuberosity to sacrum
- ✓ Sacrospinous ligament—ischial spine to sacrum
- ✓ Ligaments convert notches into greater and lesser sciatic foramen
- ✓ Sciatic hernias—also exit via greater and lesser sciatic foramen
- ✓ These ligaments also support the SI joint

Muscles of the gluteal region

Muscle	Origin	Insertion	Action	Innervation	Artery	Notes
Gemellus, inferior	Ischial tuberosity	Obturator internus tendon	Laterally rotates the femur	Nerve to the quadratus femoris muscle	Inferior gluteal artery	Gemellus is a Latin word that means "little twin"

Muscle	Origin	Insertion	Action	Innervation	Blood supply	Notes
Gemellus, superior	Ischial spine	Obturator internus tendon	Laterally rotates the femur	Nerve to the obturator internus muscle	Inferior gluteal artery	Gemellus is a Latin word that means "little twin"
Gluteus maximus	Posterior gluteal line, posterior surface of sacrum and coccyx, sacrotuberous ligament	Upper fibers: iliotibial tract. Lowermost fibers: gluteal tuberosity of the femur	Extends the thigh; laterally rotates the femur	Inferior gluteal nerve	Superior and inferior gluteal arteries	Gluteus maximus is a site of intramuscular injection
Gluteus medius	External surface of the ilium between the posterior and anterior gluteal lines	Greater trochanter of the femur	Abducts the femur; medially rotates the thigh	Superior gluteal nerve	Superior gluteal artery	The angle at which the gluteus medius tendon approaches the greater trochanter of the femur is anterior to the axis of rotation of the thigh, resulting in medial rotation
Gluteus minimus	External surface of the ilium between the anterior and inferior gluteal lines	Greater trochanter of the femur	Abducts the femur; medially rotates the thigh	Superior gluteal nerve	Superior gluteal artery	The angle at which the gluteus minimus tendon approaches the greater trochanter of the femur is anterior to the axis of rotation of the thigh, resulting in medial rotation
Obturator externus	The external surface of the obturator membrane and the superior and inferior pubic rami	Trochanteric fossa of the femur	Laterally rotates the thigh	Obturator nerve	Obturator artery	The tendon of the obturator externus muscle passes inferior to the neck of the femur to reach its insertion site
Obturator internus	The internal surface of the obturator membrane and margin of the obturator foramen	Greater trochanter on its medial surface above the trochanteric fossa	Laterally rotates and abducts the thigh	Nerve to the obturator internus muscle	Obturator artery	The obturator internus muscle leaves the pelvis by passing through the lesser sciatic foramen; the superior and inferior gemellus muscles Insert on the obturator internus tendon

Piriformis	Anterior surface of sacrum	Upper border of greater trochanter of femur	Laterally rotates and abducts thigh	Ventral rami of S_1–S_2		Piriformis leaves the pelvis by passing through the greater sciatic foramen
Quadratus femoris	Lateral border of the ischial tuberosity	Quadrate line of the femur below the intertrochanteric crest	Laterally rotates the thigh	Nerve to the quadratus femoris muscle	Inferior gluteal artery	The nerve to the quadratus femoris muscle also innervates the inferior gemellus muscle
Tensor fasciae latae	Anterior part of the iliac crest, anterior superior iliac spine	Iliotibial tract	Flexes, abducts, and medially rotates the thigh	Superior gluteal nerve	Superior gluteal artery	Tensor fascia latae redirects the rotational forces of the gluteus maximus muscle
Gemellus, inferior	Ischial tuberosity	Obturator internus tendon	Laterally rotates the femur	Nerve to the quadratus femoris muscle	Inferior gluteal artery	Gemellus is a Latin word that means "little twin"
Gemellus, superior	Ischial spine	Obturator internus tendon	Laterally rotates the femur	Nerve to the obturator internus muscle	Inferior gluteal artery	Gemellus is a Latin word that means "little twin"
Gluteus maximus	Posterior gluteal line, posterior surface of sacrum and coccyx, sacrotuberous ligament	Upper fibers: iliotibial tract. Lowermost fibers: gluteal tuberosity of the femur	Extends the thigh; laterally rotates the femur	Inferior gluteal nerve	Superior and inferior gluteal arteries	Gluteus maximus is a site of intramuscular injection
Gluteus medius	External surface of the ilium between the posterior and anterior gluteal lines	Greater trochanter of the femur	Abducts the femur; medially rotates the thigh	Superior gluteal nerve	Superior gluteal artery	The angle at which the gluteus medius tendon approaches the greater trochanter of the femur is anterior to the axis of rotation of the thigh, resulting in medial rotation

Muscle	Origin	Insertion	Action	Innervation	Blood supply	Notes
Gluteus minimus	External surface of the ilium between the anterior and inferior gluteal lines	Greater trochanter of the femur	Abducts the femur; medially rotates the thigh	Superior gluteal nerve	Superior gluteal artery	The angle at which the gluteus minimus tendon approaches the greater trochanter of the femur is anterior to the axis of rotation of the thigh, resulting in medial rotation
Obturator externus	External surface of the obturator membrane and the superior and inferior pubic rami	Trochanteric fossa of the femur	Laterally rotates the thigh	Obturator nerve	Obturator artery	The tendon of the obturator externus muscle passes inferior to the neck of the femur to reach its insertion site
Obturator internus	The internal surface of the obturator membrane and margin of the obturator foramen	Greater trochanter on its medial surface above the trochanteric fossa	Laterally rotates and abducts the thigh	Nerve to the obturator internus muscle	Obturator artery	The obturator internus muscle leaves the pelvis by passing through the lesser sciatic foramen; the superior and inferior gemellus muscles insert on the obturator internus tendon
Piriformis	Anterior surface of sacrum	Upper border of greater trochanter of femur	Laterally rotates and abducts the thigh	Ventral rami of S_1–S_2		Piriformis leaves the pelvis by passing through the greater sciatic foramen
Quadratus femoris	Lateral border of the ischial tuberosity	Quadrate line of the femur below the intertrochanteric crest	Laterally rotates the thigh	Nerve to the quadratus femoris muscle	Inferior gluteal artery	The nerve to the quadratus femoris muscle also innervates the inferior gemellus muscle
Tensor fasciae latae	Anterior part of the iliac crest, anterior superior iliac spine	Iliotibial tract	Flexes, abducts, and medially rotates the thigh	Superior gluteal nerve	Superior gluteal artery	Tensor fascia latae redirects the rotational forces of the gluteus maximus muscle

Nerve and blood supply of gluteal region

Nerve supply of gluteal region

Nerve	Source	Branches	Motor	Sensory	Notes
Gluteal, inferior	Sacral plexus (ventral primary rami of spinal nerves L_5, S_1–S_2)	No named branches	Gluteus maximus muscle	None	Inferior gluteal nerve passes through the greater sciatic foramen inferior to the piriformis muscle
Gluteal, superior	Sacral plexus (ventral primary rami of spinal nerves L_4–L_5, S_1)	Superior and inferior branches	Gluteus medius muscle, gluteus minimus muscle, tensor fasciae latae muscle	None	Superior gluteal nerve passes through the greater sciatic foramen superior to the piriformis muscle
Sciatic nerve	Sacral plexus (ventral primary rami of spinal nerves L_4–L_5 and S_1–S_3)	Tibial nerve, common fibular (peroneal) nerve	Semitendinosus muscle, semimembranosus muscle, biceps femoris muscle, ischioconylar part of the adductor magnus muscle; its branches supply all muscles of the leg and foot	Its branches supply the skin of the leg and foot (excluding the medial side of leg and foot)	Sciatic nerve is composed of tibial and common fibular divisions; branches to muscles come from one of the two divisions, so that the sciatic nerve is considered to have no direct muscular branches, only 2 terminal branches
To obturator internus muscle	Sacral plexus (ventral primary rami of spinal nerves L_5–S_2)	Nerve to the superior gemellus muscle	Obturator internus muscle, superior gemellus muscle	None	Nerve to obturator internus muscle crosses the ischial spine and enters the ischioanal fossa by passing through the lesser sciatic foramen
To quadratus femoris muscle	Sacral plexus (ventral primary rami of spinal nerves L_4–L_5, S_1)	Nerve to the inferior gemellus muscle	Quadratus femoris muscle, inferior gemellus muscle	None	Nerve to the quadratus femoris muscle passes anterior to the obturator internus tendon

Arteries supplying gluteal region				
Artery	Source	Branches	Supply to	Notes
Femoral	External iliac artery	Superficial epigastric artery, superficial circumflex iliac artery, superficial external pudendal artery, deep external pudendal artery, deep femoral artery, descending genicular artery, popliteal artery	Thigh, leg and foot	Femoral artery is continuous with the popliteal artery, the name change occurs at the adductor hiatus
Femoral, deep	Femoral artery	Medial circumflex femoral artery, lateral circumflex femoral artery, perforating a artery (3 or 4)	Hip joint, proximal thigh, posterior thigh	Deep femoral artery is the primary blood supply to muscles of the posterior compartment of the thigh
Gluteal, inferior	Internal iliac artery, anterior division	Unnamed muscular branches	Gluteus maximus muscle, hip joint	Inferior gluteal artery participates in the formation of the cruciate anastomoses of the hip
Gluteal, superior	Internal iliac, posterior division	Superficial branch, deep branch	Gluteus maximus muscle, gluteus medius muscle, gluteus minimus muscle, hip joint	Superior gluteal artery participates in the formation of the cruciate anastomoses of the hip
Obturator	Internal iliac artery, anterior division	Pubic branch, acetabular branch, anterior branch, posterior branch	Medial thigh and hip	Anterior and posterior branches pass on the anterior and posterior sides of the adductor brevis muscle; aberrant obturator artery arises from the inferior epigastric artery in 30% of cases

7.6.4 Posterior compartment of leg and sole of foot

Overview
✓ Fascia of the leg and foot
✓ Muscles of the posterior compartment of the leg
✓ Tibial nerve and posterior tibial artery
✓ Plantar aspect of the foot (sole)
✓ Arches of the foot
✓ Foot deformities
✓ Laboratory exercise
Fascia of the leg and foot
Crural fascia—continuation of the fascia lata of the thigh, attaches to medial and lateral malleoli

- ✓ Lateral sural cutaneous nerve
- ✓ Small saphenous vein
- ✓ Great saphenous vein
- ✓ Saphenous nerve
- ✓ Sural communicating branch of lateral sural cutaneous nerve

Fascial compartments of the leg

- ✓ Interosseous membrane—connects tibia and fibula; separates anterior and posterior compartments
- ✓ Anterior intermuscular septum—separates anterior and lateral compartments
- ✓ Posterior intermuscular septum—separates lateral and posterior compartments
- ✓ Transverse intermuscular septum—separates superficial and deep posterior compartments

Superficial posterior compartment

- ✓ Medial and lateral gastrocnemius
- ✓ Soleus
- ✓ Plantaris
- ✓ Medial sural cutaneous nerve

Deep posterior compartment

- ✓ Flexor digitorum longus (FDL)
- ✓ Tibialis posterior
- ✓ Flexor hallucis longus (FHL)
- ✓ Popliteus
- ✓ Posterior tibial artery and vein
- ✓ Tibial nerve
- ✓ Fibular (peroneal) artery and vein

Extensor retinaculum

- ✓ Muscles of the posterior compartment of the leg
- ✓ Superficial posterior compartment muscles
- ✓ Gastrocnemius
- ✓ Origin—medial and lateral heads from medial and lateral femoral condyles
- ✓ Insertion—tendocalcaneus, lower part of posterior surface of calcaneus
- ✓ Innervation—tibial nerve (lateral L_5–S_1, medial S_1–S_2)
- ✓ Action—ankle plantar flexion (PF), assist in knee flexion

Soleus

- ✓ Origin—posterior aspect of head of fibula, superior fourth of posterior surface of fibula at soleal line, medial border of tibia
- ✓ Insertion—posterior surface of calcaneus via calcaneal tendon
- ✓ Innervation—tibial nerve (S_1–S_2)
- ✓ Action—PF ankle, steadies leg on foot

Plantaris

- ✓ Origin—inferior end of lateral supracondylar line of femur and oblique popliteal ligament
- ✓ Insertion—posterior surface of calcaneus via calcaneal tendon

- ✓ Innervation—tibial nerve (S_1–S_2)
- ✓ Action—assist gastroc in PF ankle and knee flexion

Popliteus

- ✓ Origin—lateral surface of lateral condyle of femur and lateral meniscus
- ✓ Insertion—posterior surface of tibia superior to soleal line
- ✓ Innervation—tibial (L_4–L_5, S_1)
- ✓ Action—weakly flexes knee, unlocks knee from extension

Deep posterior compartment of the leg muscles

Flexor hallucis longus (FHL)

- ✓ Origin—inferior 2/3 of posterior surface of fibula and inferior part of IM
- ✓ Insertion—base of distal phalanx of great toe (hallux)
- ✓ Innervation—tibial nerve (S_1–S_3)
- ✓ Action—flexes great toe at all joints, weak ankle PF, supports medial longitudinal arch of the foot

Flexor digitorum longus (FDL)

- ✓ Origin—medial part of posterior surface of tibia inferior to soleal line, fibula
- ✓ Insertion—bases of distal phalanges of lateral four digits (2nd–5th)
- ✓ Innervation—tibial nerve (S_1–S_3)
- ✓ Action—flexes lateral four digits (2nd–5th) and PF ankle, supports longitudinal arches of foot

Posterior tibial

- ✓ Origin—IM, posterior surface of tibia inferior to soleal line, posterior surface of fibula
- ✓ Insertion—tuberosity of the navicular, cuneiform, cuboid, and bases of 2nd–4th metatarsals
- ✓ Innervation—tibial nerve (L_4–L_5)
- ✓ Action—PF ankle, inverts foot
- ✓ Orientation as the deep posterior compartment muscles traverse around the medial malleous
  - ◊ Tom—posterior tibial
  - ◊ Dick—FDL
  - ◊ AN—tibial nerve and posterior tibial artery
  - ◊ Harry—FHL

Tibial nerve and posterior tibial artery

Tibial nerve

- ✓ Formed by the anterior divisions of L_4–S_3
- ✓ Medial component of the sciatic nerve in thigh
- ✓ Motor
  - ◊ Thigh—hamstrings (LH biceps, semitendinosus, semimembranosus)
  - ◊ Leg—superficial and deep posterior compartments
- ✓ Sensory
  - ◊ Articular branch to knee joint
  - ◊ Medial sural cutaneous nerve
- ✓ Divides in the posterior tarsal tunnel to form the medial and lateral plantar nerves

Posterior tibial artery

✓ Arises as terminal branch of popliteal artery
 ✓ Runs through deep posterior compartment of the leg with tibial nerve
 ✓ Branches
     ◊ Anterior tibial artery—anterior compartment
     ◊ Fibular (peroneal) artery—deep posterior compartment
     ◊ Blood supply to deep and superficial compartments of leg
     ◊ Branches at the ankle
     ◊ Medial malleolar artery
     ◊ Calcaneal artery
     ◊ Terminates in medial and lateral plantar arteries

Plantar aspect of the foot = sole

✓ Plantar fascia and plantar aponeurosis and four layers of muscles
✓ Plantar fascia and aponeurosis

Superficial fascia

✓ Tough and thick padding over sole of the foot
✓ Skin ligaments—tethers the skin to the plantar aponeurosis

Deep fascia = plantar aponeurosis

✓ Extends forward and divides for digitations of toes
✓ Attaches proximally to calcaneus
✓ Digitations united by transverse fasciculi
✓ Superficial transverse metatarsal ligaments
✓ Deep transverse metatarsal ligaments
✓ Lateral (5th toe) and medial (great toe) plantar fascia

Clinical correlation: plantar fascitis

Superficial (1st layer)—deep to the plantar aponeurosis

Abductor hallucis

✓ Origin—medial tubercle of tuberosity of the calcaneus, flexor retinaculum and plantar aponeurosis
✓ Insertion—medial side of base of proximal phalanx of 1st toe
✓ Innervation—medial plantar nerve (S_2–S_3)
✓ Action—abduct the great toe

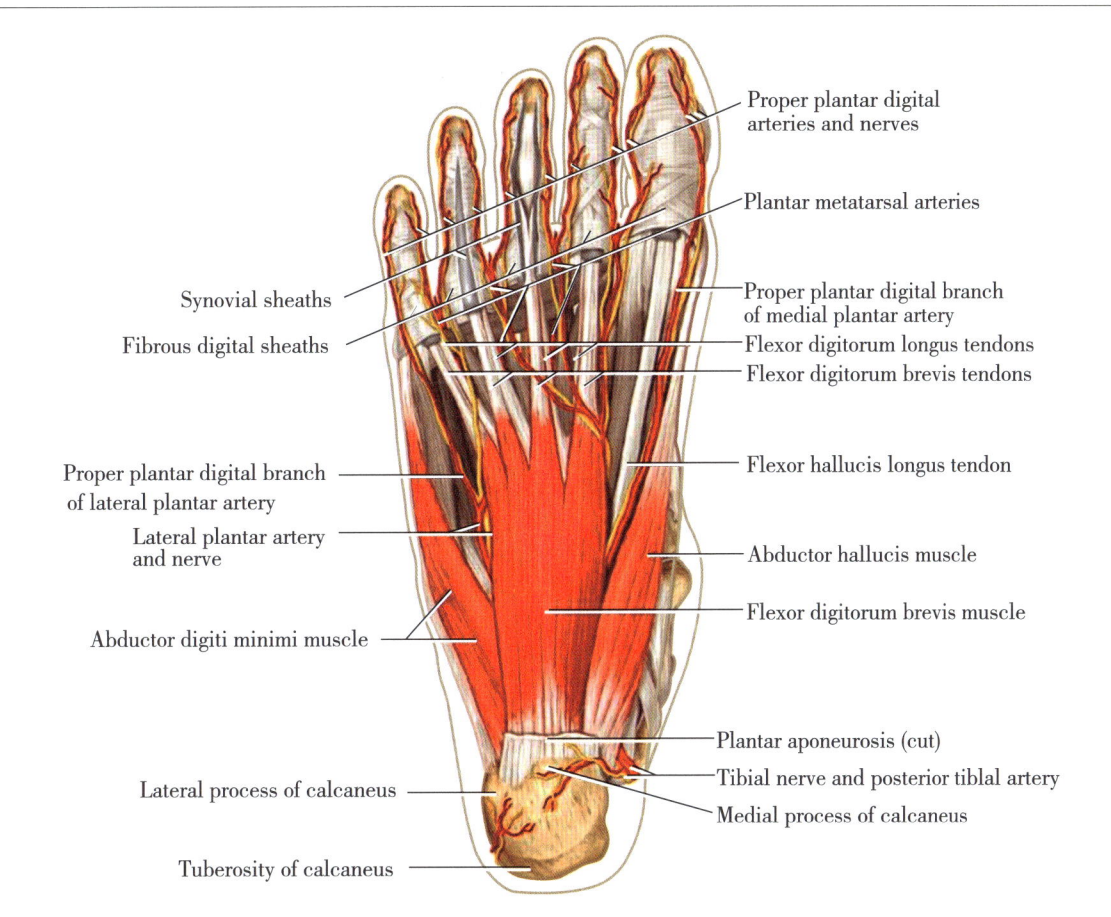

Flexor digitorum brevis (FDB)

✓ Origin—medial tubercle of the tuberosity of the calcaneus, plantar aponeurosis, and intermuscular septa
✓ Insertion—tendons to 2nd–5th toes, inserting on both sides of middle phalanges (forms fibrous sheath that splits to allow FDL tendons to pass through to distal phalanx)
✓ Innervation—medial plantar nerve (S_2–S_3)

Abductor digiti minimi (quinti)

✓ Origin—medial and lateral tubercles of tuberosity of calcaneus, plantar aponeurosis, and intermuscular septa
✓ Insertion—lateral side of base of proximal phalanx of little toe
✓ Innervation—lateral plantar nerve (S_2–S_3)
✓ Action—abduct and flexes the little toe

2nd layer

Tendons of FDL

Quadratus plantae—accessory flexor muscle, no equivalent in hand

✓ Origin—medial surface and lateral margin of plantar surface of calcaneus
✓ Insertion—posterolateral margin of tendon of FDL
✓ Innervation—lateral plantar nerve (S_2–S_3)
✓ Action—assist FDL in flexing lateral four digits; modify the effects of the FDL by pulling the toes medially

478   Regional Anatomy

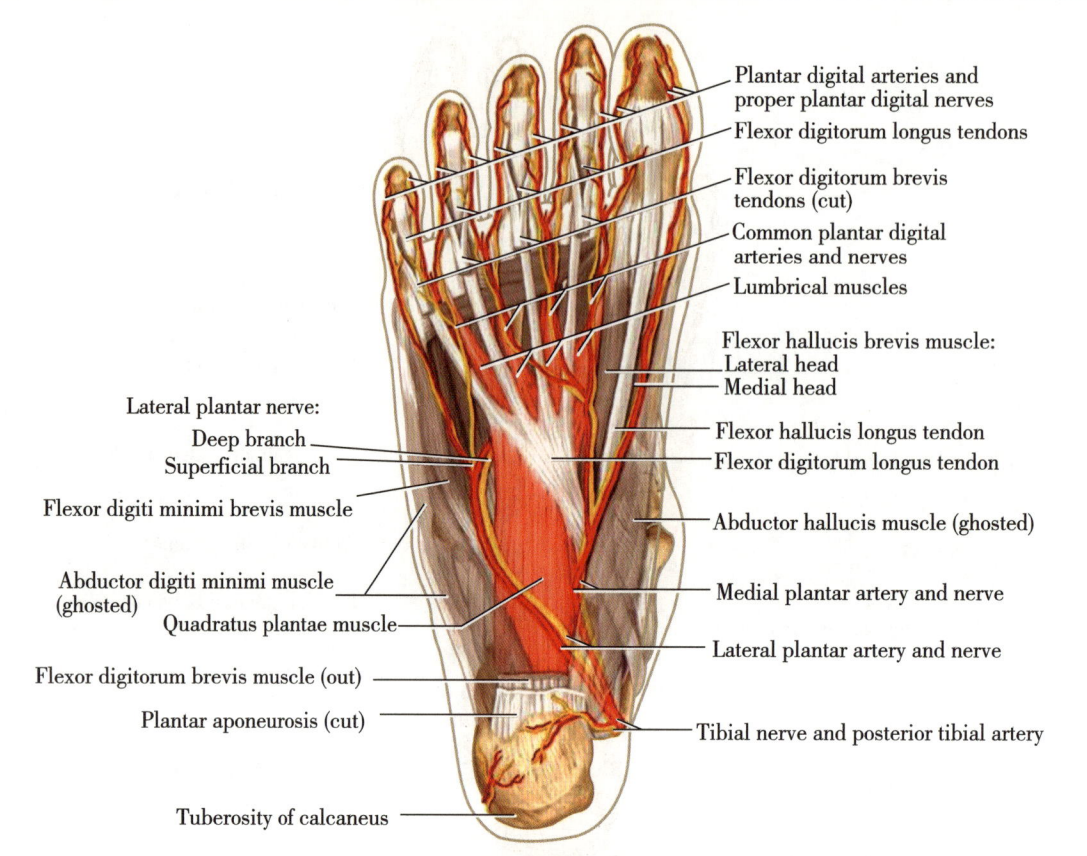

Lumbricales

- ✓ Origin—tendons of the FDL (like FDP in hand)
  - ◊ 1st (medial)—medial side of FDL
  - ◊ $2^{nd}-4^{th}$—between tendons lying each side of muscle
- ✓ Insertion—medial aspect of expansion over lateral four digits
- ✓ Innervation
  - ◊ 1 medial plantar nerve (S_2-S_3)
  - ◊ 2-4 lateral plantar nerve (S_2-S_3)
  - ◊ Based on axis of foot being 2nd toe
- ✓ Action—flex proximal phalanges and extend middle and distal phalanges of lateral four digits

3rd layer

Flexor hallucis brevis

- ✓ Origin—plantar surfaces of cuboid and lateral cuneiform
- ✓ Muscle belly divides into two parts: medial and lateral heads
- ✓ Insertion—both sides of medial side of proximal phalanx of great toe
  - ◊ Medial with abdomen hallucis into medial side of proximal phalanx great toe
  - ◊ Lateral with heads of adductor into lateral side of proximal phalanx great toe
  - ◊ Innervation—medial plantar nerve (S_2-S_3)
  - ◊ Action—flex great toe

Adductor hallucis

- ✓ Origin
  - ◊ Oblique head—base of 2nd–4th metatarsals
  - ◊ Transverse head—no bony origin, plantar and deep transverse plantar ligaments (2nd–5th toes)
- ✓ Insertion—tendons of both heads join with FHB (lateral head) and insert into the base proximal phalanx of great toe
- ✓ Innervation—lateral plantar nerve (S_2–S_3)
- ✓ Action—adduct the great toe, assists in maintaining transverse arch of foot

Flexor digiti minimi brevis

- ✓ Origin—base of 5th metatarsal
- ✓ Insertion—base of proximal phalanx of 5th digit
- ✓ Innervation—lateral plantar nerve (S_2–S_3)
- ✓ Action—flexes proximal phalanx of 5th digit

4th layer

Plantar interossei–3

- ✓ Origin—bases and medial side of 3rd–5th metatarsals
- ✓ Insertion—medial side and bases of proximal phalanges of 3rd–5th toes
- ✓ Innervation—lateral plantar nerve (S_2–S_3)
- ✓ Action—adducts digits 3rd–5th and flexes metatarsalphalangeal joints

Dorsal interossei–4

- ✓ Origin—adjacent sides of 1st–5th metatarsals
- ✓ Insertion
  - ◊ First—medial side of proximal phalanx of 2nd digit
  - ◊ Second to fourth—lateral sides of 2nd–4th digits
- ✓ Innervation—lateral plantar nerve (S_2–S_3)
- ✓ Action—abduct 2nd–4th toes and flex MP joints

Plantar nerves

- ✓ Terminal branches of tibial nerve at the medial malleolus—usually lie between 1st and 2nd layers
- ✓ Medial plantar nerve
  - ◊ Motor—ABD hallucis, FDB, FHB, 1st lumbricale
  - ◊ Sensory—sole of medial foot and 1st–3rd toes
- ✓ Lateral plantar nerve
  - ◊ Motor—ADM, quadratus plantae, 2nd–4th lumbricales, adductor hallucis, FDM, interossei
  - ◊ Sensory—sole of lateral foot and 4th–5th toes
- ✓ Plantar arteries arise from posterior tibial artery (medial malleolus)
- ✓ Medial plantar artery—medial side of foot

- ✓ Lateral plantar artery—lateral side of foot
  - ◊ Forms plantar arch with deep plantar branch of dorsal pedis artery (dorsum of the foot)
  - ◊ Plantar metatarsal arteries
  - ◊ Common plantar digital arteries
  - ◊ Proper plantar digital arteries

Arches of the foot

Transverse arch—across the bases of the metatarsals

- ✓ Medial, intermediate, lateral cuneiforms; cuboid

Medial longitudinal arch—higher arch

- ✓ Medial 3 metatarsals; medial and intermediate cuneiform, navicular (anterior pillar)
- ✓ Calcaneus (posterior pillar)

Lateral longitudinal arch—lower arc

- ✓ Lateral 2 metatarsals; lateral cuneiform, cuboid (anterior pillar)
- ✓ Calcaneus (posterior pillar)

Maintenance of arches

- ✓ Long and short plantar ligaments
- ✓ Spring ligament (calcaneonavicular)
- ✓ Plantar aponeurosis
- ✓ Extrinsic muscles—tibialis posterior, fibularis longus, FDL, FHL
- ✓ Intrinsic muscles

Foot deformities

- ✓ Equinus = foot points downward (PF)
- ✓ Calcaneus = calcaneus down, foot DF
- ✓ Varus—foot deviates toward midline (inversion, adduction, supination)
- ✓ Valgus—foot deviates away from midline (eversion, abduction, pronation)
- ✓ Pes planus = flat feet, arches flattened
- ✓ Pes cavus = arches exaggerated, "high arches"
- ✓ Clubfoot = talipes equinovarus–PF, inversion, adduction, supinated with heel inverted
- ✓ Hallux valgus
  - ◊ Valgus deformity at 1st (great toe) MP joint
  - ◊ Varsudeformity 1st metatarsal
  - ◊ Metatarsal head hypertrophied and rotated medially

Chen Xi, Cui Xiaojun

Chapter 8

The Back and Vertebral Region

8.1 Introduction

8.1.1 Boundaries and divisions

The back, which extends from the skull to the tip of the coccyx, can be defined as the posterior surface of the trunk. Superimposed on the upper part of the posterior surface of the thorax are the scapulae and the muscles that connect the scapulae to the trunk (Figure 8-1).

8.1.2 Surface anatomy

The surface anatomy of this region may be studied on a living subject or on a cadaver. In the cadaver, fixation may make it difficult to distinguish bone from well-preserved soft tissues. Turn the cadaver to the prone position (face down) and attempt to palpate the following structures.
- External occipital protuberance
- Superior border of the trapezius muscle
- Spinous process of the seventh cervical vertebra (vertebra prominens)
- Spine of the scapula (at vertebral level T_3)
- Acromion of the scapula
- Medial (vertebral) border of the scapula
- Inferior angle of the scapula (at vertebral level T_7)
- Spinous processes of thoracic vertebrae
- Erector spinae muscle (most noticeable in the lumbar region)
- Medial furrow
- Lateral border of the latissimus dorsi muscle (posterior axillary fold)
- Iliac crest (at vertebral level L_4)
- Posterior superior iliac spine

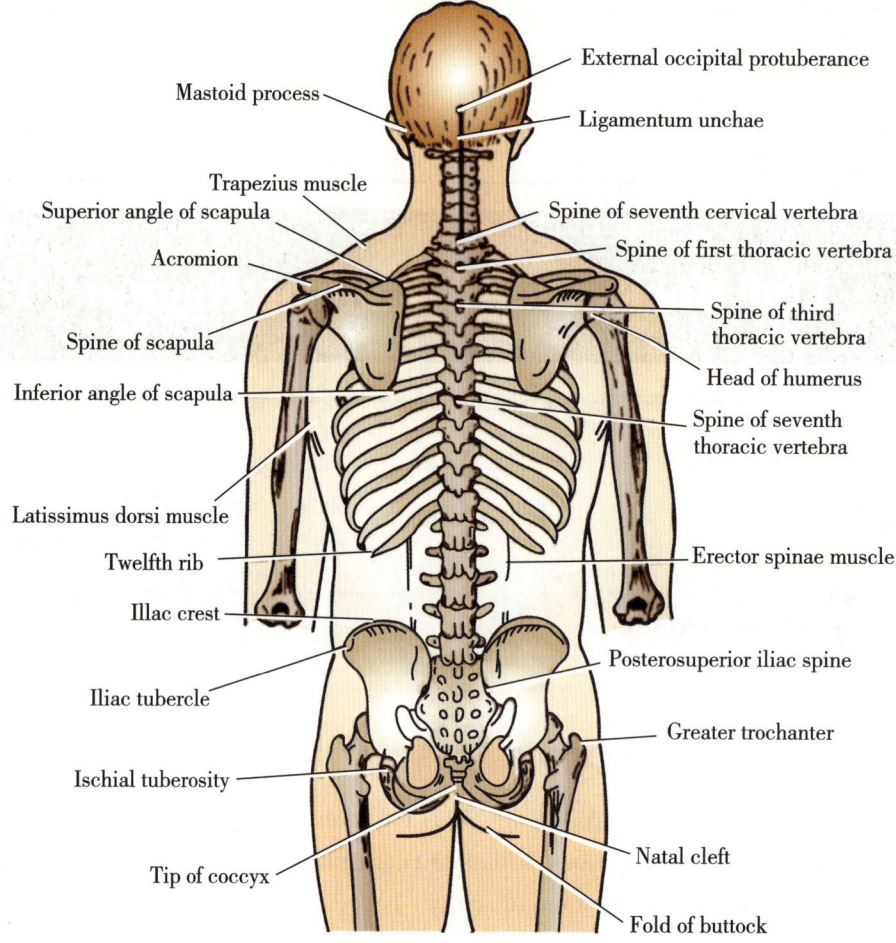

Figure 8-1　Posterior view of the skeleton showing the surface markings on the back

8.2　The layers and structures of the back

8.2.1　The skin

It is thicker, less movable and abundant of hair sac and sebaceous glands.

8.2.2　The superficial fascia

(1) The cutaneous nerves.
(2) The superficial blood vessels.

8.2.3　The deep fascia

(1) The nuchal fascia.
(2) The thoracolumbar fascia (deep fascia of the back). The lumbar part of the deep fascia is situated in the interval between the iliac crest and the 12th rib. It forms a strong aponeurosis and laterally gives origin to the middle fibers of the transversus and the upper fibers of the internal oblique muscles of the abdominal wall. Medially, the lumbar part of the deep fascia splits into three lamellae. The posterior lamella covers the deep muscles of the back and is attached to the lumbar spines. The middle lamella passes medially, to be

attached to the tips of the transverse processes of the lumbar vertebrae; it lies anterior to the deep muscles of the back and posterior to the quadratus lumborum. The anterior lamella passes medially and is attached to the anterior surface of the transverse processes of the lumbar vertebrae; it lies anterior to the quadratus lumborum muscle.

8.2.4 The muscles of the back

Figure 8-2 shows the muscles of the back.

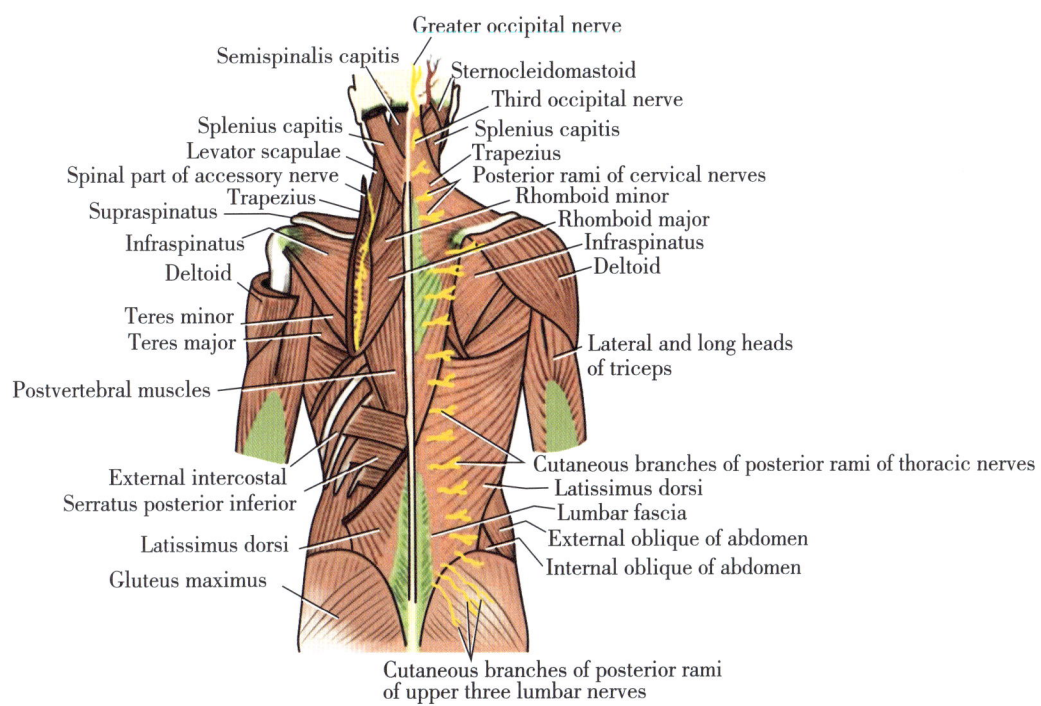

Figure 8-2 Superficial and deep muscles of the back

(1) Trapezius

It is a large, triangular and superficial muscle lying on the back of the neck and thorax. It is responsible for the sloping ridge of the neck. The trapezius arsies from the external occipital protuberance, superior nuchal line, spine of seventh cervical vertebra, ligamentum nuchae, the spinous processes and supraspinal ligaments of all thoracic vertebrae. The trapezius is attached to the lateral one third of the clavicle, the acromion and the spine of scapila.

Actions: steadies, raises, descends, retracts and rotates the scapula and extends the head. Their weakness results in dropping shoulder.

(2) Latissimus dorsi

It is a large, wide, triangular muscle, and superficially placed, except in its uppermost part where it is covered by the trapezius. It arises from the spinous processes of the lower six thoracic vertebrae, the thoracolumbar fascia, by which it is attached to the spinous processes of the lumbar and sacral vertebrae, and the iliac crest. The muscle spirals around the lower edge of the teres major and is inserted into the floor of the intertubercular sulcus.

Actions: extends, adducts and medially rotates humerus at shoulder joint, it plays a considerable role in the downstroke of the arm in swimming, and is also used in rowing, climbing, hammering and supporting the weight of the body on the hand.

(3) Levator scapulae and rhomboideus

The levator scapulae, thin and straplike, arises from the transverse processes of the first four cervical vertebrae. It is inserted into the medial border of the scapula at the level of and above the spine of scapula. The insertions of the levator scapulae and the rhomboideus are usually continuous along the medial border of the scapula. The rhomboideus arises from the spinous processes of the 7th cervical and upper five thoracic vertebrae and the supraspinal ligaments of those regions.

Actions: the levator scapulae elevares the scapula and may act in concert with the trapezius in shrugging the shoulders. However, it may also retract and fix the scapula with the rhomboideus.

(4) Erector spinae (sacrospinalis)

It is a collective name for a group of deep muscles of the back. It lies in the vertebral groove on each side of vertebral spines. The muscle begins at the sacrum, the ilium, and associated ligaments. It becomes thick as it ascenfs alongside the spinous processes of lumbar vertebrae. At about the level of the last rib, it divides into three parts that ascend on the back of the chest, where they are inserted into ribs and vertebrae. From these bones, it runs continuously upward to insert into the mastoid process of the temporal bone.

Actions: when acting on one side, it bends and rotates the spinal column toward the opposite side. When acting on both sides, it extends the spinal column.

(5) Thoracolumbar (lumbar) fascia

It covers the deep muscles of the back of the trunk (Figure 8-3). In the thoracic region, the thoracolumbar fascia is thin fibrous lamina covering the extensor muscles of the vertebral column. It is attached, medialy, to the spinous processes of the thoracic vertebrae, laterally, to the angles of the ribs. In the lumbar region, the thoracolumbar fascia is divided into three layers. The posterior layer is attached to the spinous processes of the lumbar and sacral vertebrae and to the supraspinous ligament; the middle layer is attached, medially, to the tips of the transverse processes of the lumbar vertebrae and intertransverse ligament, below, to the iliac crest, and above, to the lower border of the twelfth rib and the lumbocostal ligament. The anterior layer covers the quadratus lumborum and is attached medially to the anterior surface of the transverse processes of lumbar vertebrae. Below, it is attached to the iliolumbar ligament and the adjoining part of the iliac crest; above, it forms the lateral arcuate ligament. The posterior and middle layers unite at the lateral margin of the erector spinae, and at the lateral border of the quadratus lumborum them are joined by the anterior.

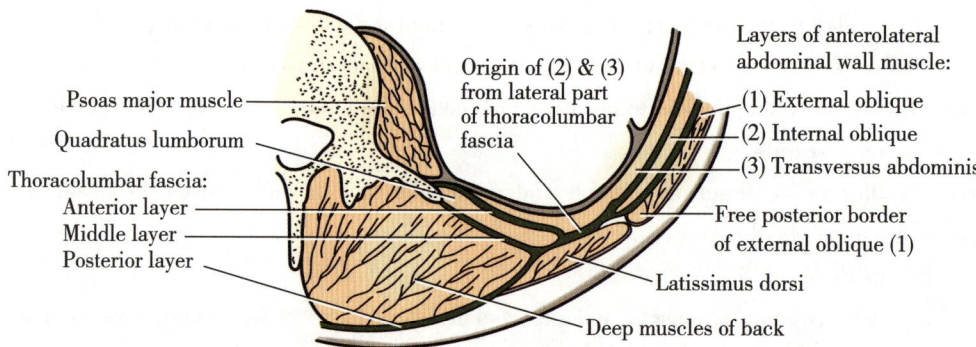

Figure 8-3 Transverse section of the intrinsic back muscles and layers of thoracolumbar fascia

8.2.5 The triangles of the back and nape

(1) Auscultatory triangle

The auscultatory triangle is the site on the back where breath sounds may be most easily heard with a stethoscope. The boundaries are the latissimus dorsi, the trapezius, and the medial border of the scapula.

(2) Lumbar triangle

The lumbar triangle is the site where pus may emerge from the abdominal wall. The boundaries are the latissimus dorsi, the posterior border of the external oblique muscle of the abdomen, and the iliac crest.

8.2.6 Blood supply of the back

8.2.6.1 Arteries

(1) In the cervical region, branches arise from the occipital artery, a branch of the external carotid; from the vertebral artery, a branch of the subclavian; and from the deep cervical artery, a branch of the costocervical trunk.

(2) In the thoracic region, branches arise from the posterior intercostal arteries.

(3) In the lumbar region, branches arise from the subcostal and lumbar arteries.

(4) In the sacral region, branches arise from the iliolumbar and lateral sacral arteries, branches of the internal iliac artery.

8.2.6.2 Veins

The veins draining the structures of the back form plexuses extending along the vertebral column from the skull to the coccyx.

(1) The external vertebral venous plexus lies external and surrounds the vertebral column.

(2) The internal vertebral venous plexus lies within the vertebral canal but outside the dura mater of the spinal cord.

The external and internal vertebral plexuses form a capacious venous network whose walls are thin and whose channels have incompetent valves or are valveless. They communicate through the foramen magnum with the venous sinuses within the skull. Free venous blood flow may therefore take place between the skull, the neck, the thorax, the abdomen, the pelvis, and the vertebral plexuses, with the direction of flow depending on the pressure differences that exist at any given time between the regions. This fact is of considerable clinical significance.

The internal vertebral plexus receives tributaries from the vertebrae by way of the basivertebral veins and from the meninges and spinal cord. The internal plexus is drained by the intervertebral veins, which pass outward with the spinal nerves through the intervertebral foramina.

8.2.7 Lymph drainage of the back

The deep lymph vessels follow the veins and drain into the deep cervical, posterior mediastinal, lateral aortic, and sacral nodes. The lymph vessels from the skin of the neck drain into the cervical nodes, those from the trunk above the iliac crests drain into the axillary nodes, and those from below the level of the iliac crests drain into the superficial inguinal nodes.

8.2.8 Nerve supply of the back

The skin and muscles of the back are supplied in a segmental manner by the posterior rami of the 31 pairs of spinal nerves. The posterior rami of the first, sixth, seventh, and eighth cervical nerves and the fourth and fifth lumbar nerves supply the deep muscles of the back and do not supply the skin. The posterior ramus of the second cervical nerve (the greater occipital nerve) ascends over the back of the head and supplies the skin of the scalp.

The posterior rami run downward and laterally and supply a band of skin at a lower level than the intervertebral foramen from which they emerge. Considerable overlap of skin areas supplied occurs so that section of a single nerve causes diminished, but not total loss of sensation. Each posterior ramus divides into a medial and a lateral branch.

8.2.9 Spinal cord

The spinal cord is a cylindrical, grayish white structure that begins above at the foramen magnum, where it is continuous with the medulla oblongata of the brain. It terminates inferiorly in the adult at the level of the lower border of the first lumbar vertebra. In the young child, it is relatively longer and ends inferiorly at the upper border of the third lumbar vertebra. The spinal cord in the cervical region, where it gives origin to the brachial plexus, and in the lower thoracic and lumbar regions, where it gives origin to the lumbosacral plexus, has fusiform enlargements called cervical and lumbar enlargements.

Inferiorly, the spinal cord tapers off into the conus medullaris, from the apex of which a prolongation of the pia mater, the filum terminale, descends to be attached to the back of the coccyx. The cord possesses in the midline anteriorly a deep longitudinal fissure, the anterior medial fissure, and on the posterior surface a shallow furrow, the posterior medial sulcus (Figure 8-4).

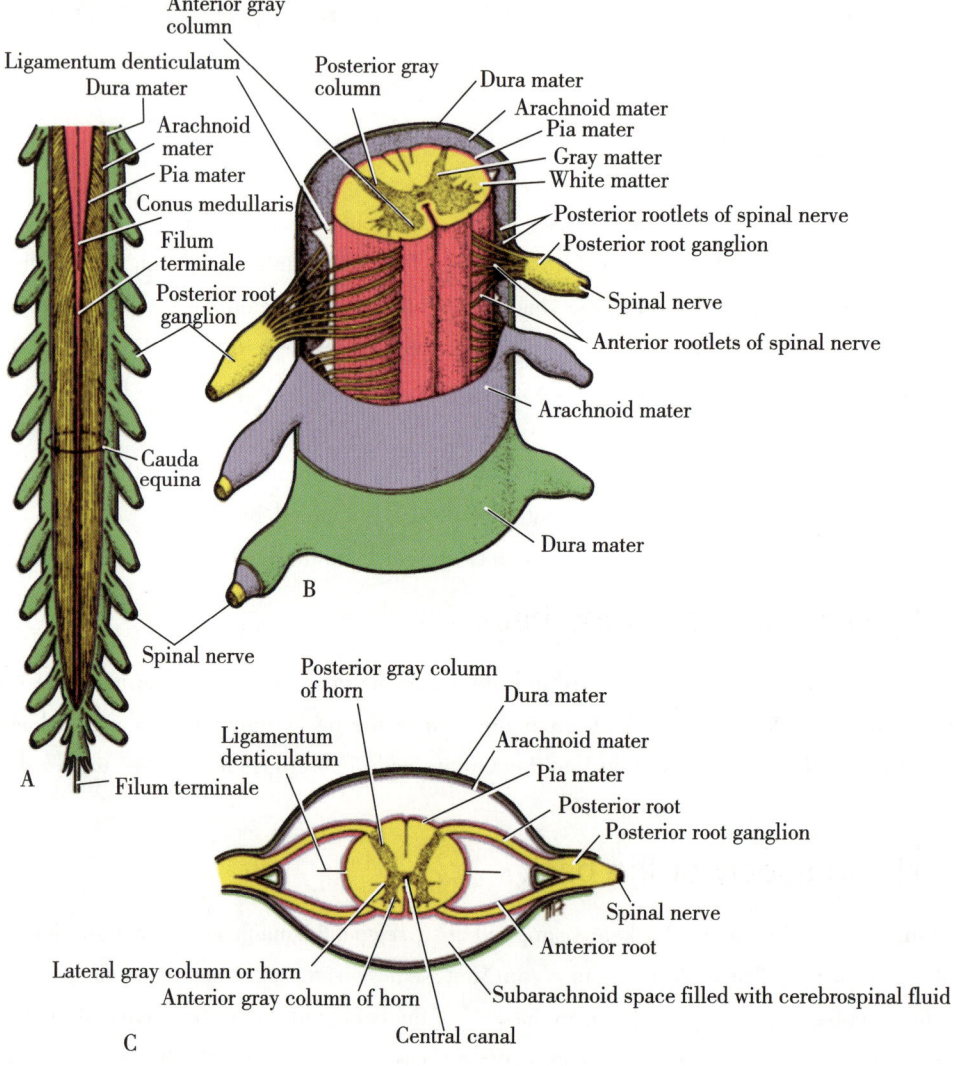

A. Lower end of the spinal cord and the cauda equina; B. Section through the thoracic part of the spinal cord showing the anterior and posterior roots of the spinal nerves and meninges; C. Transverse section through the spinal cord showing the meninges and the position of the cerebrospinal fluid.

Figure 8-4 Spinal cord

8.2.9.1 Roots of the spinal nerves

Along the whole length of the spinal cord are attached 31 pairs of spinal nerves by the anterior, or motor, roots and the posterior, or sensory, roots. Each root is attached to the cord by a series of rootlets, which extend the whole length of the corresponding segment of the cord. Each posterior nerve root possesses a posterior root ganglion, the cells of which give rise to peripheral and central nerve fibers (Figure 8-5).

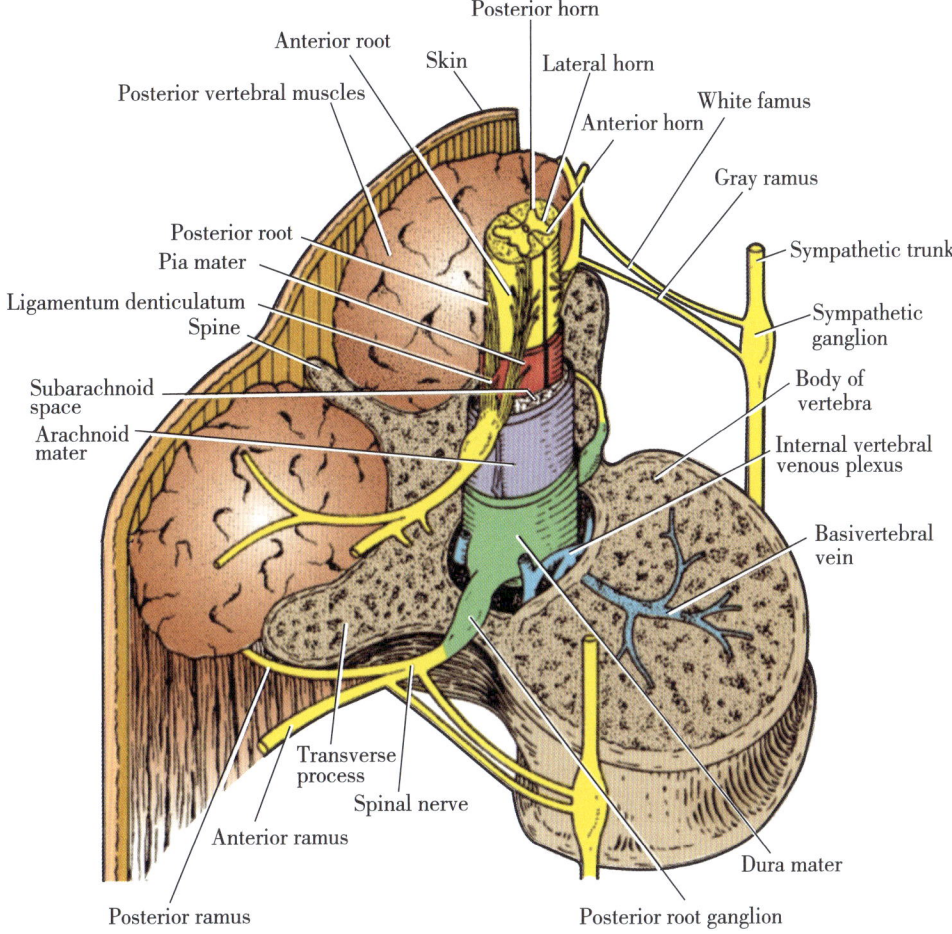

Figure 8-5 Oblique section through the first lumbar vertebra showing the spinal cord and its covering membranes

(Note the relationship between the spinal nerve and sympathetic trunk on each side. Note also the important internal vertebral venous plexus)

The spinal nerve roots pass laterally from each spinal cord segment to the level of their respective intervertebral foramina, where they unite to form a spinal nerve. Here, the motor and sensory fibers become mixed so that a spinal nerve is made up of a mixture of motor and sensory fibers. Because of the disproportionate growth in length of the vertebral column during development compared to that of the spinal cord, the length of the roots increases progressively from above downward. In the upper cervical region, the spinal nerve roots are short and run almost horizontally, but the roots of the lumbar and sacral nerves inferior to the level of the termination of the cord (lower border of the first lumbar vertebra in the adult) form a vertical leash of nerves around the filum terminale. The inferior nerve roots together are called the cauda equina.

After emergence from the intervertebral foramen, each spinal nerve immediately divides into a large anterior ramus and a smaller posterior ramus, which contain both motor and sensory fibers.

8.2.9.2 Blood supply of the spinal cord

The spinal cord receives its arterial supply from three small, longitudinally running arteries: the two posterior spinal arteries and one anterior spinal artery. The posterior spinal arteries, which arise either directly or indirectly from the vertebral arteries, run down the side of the spinal cord, close to the attachments of the posterior spinal nerve roots. The anterior spinal arteries, which arise from the vertebral arteries, unite to form a single artery, which runs down within the anterior medial fissure.

The posterior and anterior spinal arteries are reinforced by radicular arteries, which enter the vertebral canal through the intervertebral foramina.

The veins of the spinal cord drain into the internal vertebral venous plexus.

8.2.9.3 Meninges of the spinal cord

The spinal cord, like the brain, is surrounded by three meninges: the dura mater, the arachnoid mater, and the pia mater.

(1) Dura mater

The dura mater is the most external membrane and is a dense, strong, fibrous sheet that encloses the spinal cord and cauda equina. It is continuous superiorly through the foramen magnum with the meningeal layer of dura covering the brain. Inferiorly, it ends on the filum terminale at the level of the lower border of the second sacral vertebra. The dural sheath lies loosely in the vertebral canal and is separated from the walls of the canal by the extradural space (epidural space). This contains loose areolar tissue and the internal vertebral venous plexus. The dura mater extends along each nerve root and becomes continuous with connective tissue surrounding each spinal nerve (epineurium) at the intervertebral foramen. The inner surface of the dura mater is separated from the arachnoid mater by the potential subdural space.

(2) Arachnoid mater

The arachnoid mater is a delicate impermeable membrane covering the spinal cord and lying between the pia mater internally and the dura mater externally. It is separated from the dura by the subdural space that contains a thin film of tissue fluid. The arachnoid is separated from the pia mater by a wide space, the subarachnoid space, which is filled with cerebrospinal fluid. The arachnoid is continuous above through the foramen magnum with the arachnoid covering the brain. Inferiorly, it ends on the filum terminale at the level of the lower border of the second sacral vertebra.

Between the levels of the conus medullaris and the lower end of the subarachnoid space lie the nerve roots of the cauda equina bathed in cerebrospinal fluid. The arachnoid mater is continued along the spinal nerve roots, forming small lateral extensions of the subarachnoid space.

(3) Pia mater

The pia mater is a vascular membrane that closely covers the spinal cord. It is continuous superiorly through the foramen magnum with the pia covering the brain; inferiorly, it fuses with the filum terminale. The pia mater is thickened on either side between the nerve roots to form the ligamentum denticulatum, which passes laterally to be attached to the dura. It is by this means that the spinal cord is suspended in the middle of the dural sheath. The pia mater extends along each nerve root and becomes continuous with the connective tissue surrounding each spinal nerve.

8.2.9.4 Cerebrospinal fluid

The cerebrospinal fluid is a clear, colorless fluid formed mainly by the choroid plexuses, within the lateral, third, and fourth ventricles of the brain. The fluid circulates through the ventricular system and enters the subarachnoid space through the three foramina in the roof of the fourth ventricle. It circulates both upward over the surface of the cerebral hemispheres and downward around the spinal cord. The spinal part of the subarachnoid space extends down as far as the lower border of the second sacral vertebra, where the arachnoid fuses with the filum terminale. Eventually, the fluid enters the bloodstream by passing through the arachnoid villi into the dural venous sinuses, in particular the superior sagittal venous sinus.

In addition to removing waste products associated with neuronal activity, the cerebrospinal fluid provides a fluid medium that surrounds the spinal cord. This fluid, together with the bony and ligamentous walls of the vertebral canal, effectively protects the spinal cord from trauma.

Xian Dehai, Zhang Yanru

References

[1] MARIEB E N, HOEHN K. Human anatomy & physiology[M]. 9th edition. New York: Person, 2012.

[2] MOORE K L, AGUR A M R, DALLEY A F. Essential clinical anatomy[M]. 2th edition. Baltimore: Lippincott Williams & Wilkins, 2002.

[3] SNELL R S. Clinical anatomy: an illustrated review with questions and explanations[M]. 4th edition. London: Churchill Livingstone, 2004.

[4] SNELL, R S. Clinical anatomy for medical students[M]. 6th edition. Baltimore: Lippincott Williams & Wilkins, 2000.

[5] STANDRING S. Gray's anatomy[M]. 39th edition. London: Churchill Livingstone, 2004.

[6] TANK P W. Grant's dissector[M]. 15th edition. Baltimore: Lippincott Williams & Wilkins, 2012.

[7] 王怀经,刘勇. 局部解剖学:Regional anatomy[M]. 长春:吉林科学技术出版社, 2009.